SUDDEN CARDIAC DEATH
in the
ATHLETE

Edited by

N.A. Mark Estes III, MD
Professor of Medicine
Tufts University School of Medicine
Chief, Division of Cardiovascular Medicine
New England Medical Center
Boston, Massachusetts

Deeb N. Salem, MD
Professor of Medicine
Tufts University School of Medicine
Chief Medical Officer
New England Medical Center
Boston, Massachusetts

Paul J. Wang, MD
Associate Professor of Medicine
Tufts University School of Medicine
Director, Cardiac Arrhythmia Service
New England Medical Center
Boston, Massachusetts

**Futura Publishing
Company, Inc.**
Armonk, NY

Library of Congress Cataloging-in-Publication Data

Sudden cardiac death in the athlete / edited by N. A. Mark Estes III,
   Deeb N. Salem. Paul J. Wang.
          p.   cm.
     Includes bibliographical references and index.
     ISBN 0-87993-691-8 (alk. paper)
     1. Cardiac arrest.   2. Athletes—Diseases.   3. Arrhythmia.
   I. Estes, N. A. Mark (Nathan Anthony Mark), 1949–   .
   II. Salem, Deeb N.   III. Wang, Paul J.
     [DNLM: 1. Death, Sudden, Cardiac—etiology.   2. Heart
   Diseases—complications.   3. Heart Diseases—therapy.
   4. Sports Medicine. WG 205 S941247   1998]
   RC885.C173S7715   1998
   616.1'23025'088796—dc21
   DNLM/DLC
   for Library of Congress   97-52288
                                                              CIP

Copyright © 1998
Futura Publishing Company, Inc.

Published by
Futura Publishing Company
135 Bedford Road
Armonk, New York 10504

LC#: 97-52288
ISBN#: 0-87993-6916

Every effort has been made to ensure that the information in this book
is as up to date and accurate as possible at the time of publication.
However, due to the constant developments in medicine, neither the
author, nor the editors, nor the publisher can accept any legal or any
other responsibility for any errors or omissions that may occur.

Printed in the United States of America on acid-free paper.

Dedication

To my wife Noël, and my children Elise, Chace, and Kathryn,
and the memory of my parents, Nathan and Ione Estes.
N.A.M.E. III

To Patti, Nicole, Deeb, Michael, Mark, and Cam, the joys of my life.
D.N.S.

To my wife Gloria, my children Margaret and Catherine,
my mother Lillian L. Wang,
and the memory of my father, Samuel S.M. Wang.
P.J.W.

Contributors

Cristina Basso, MD Assistant Professor, Cardiovascular Pathology, University of Padua, Padua, Italy

Charles A. Berul, MD Associate in Electrophysiology, Department of Cardiology, Boston Children's Hospital; Assistant Professor of Pediatrics, Harvard Medical School, Boston, MA

Saroja Bharati, MD Director, Maurice Lev Congenital Heart and Conduction System Center, The Heart Institute for Children, Christ Hospital and Medical Center, Oak Lawn, IL; Professor of Pathology, Rush Medical College, Rush University, Rush-Presbyterian-St. Luke's Medical Center; Clinical Professor of Pathology, Finch University of Health Science, Chicago Medical School; Visiting Professor of Pathology, University of Illinois at Chicago, Chicago, IL

David S. Cannom, MD Medical Director of Cardiology, Good Samaritan Hospital; Clinical Professor of Medicine, UCLA School of Medicine, Los Angeles, CA

Agustin Castellanos, MD Professor of Medicine, University of Miami School of Medicine, Miami, FL

Melvin D. Cheitlin, MD Professor of Medicine, University of California, San Francisco; Chief, Cardiology Division, San Francisco General Hospital, San Francisco, CA

Domenico Corrado, MD Associate Director, Cardiac Electrophysiology and Pacing Laboratory, Contract Professor, Cardiovascular Pathology, University of Padua, Padua, Italy

J. Gregory Corrodi, MD Division of Cardiology, Department of Medicine, New England Medical Center; Assistant Professor of Medicine, Tufts University School of Medicine, Boston, MA

Richard O. Cummins, MD, MPH, MSc Professor of Medicine, University of Washington, Seattle, WA

N.A. Mark Estes III, MD Professor of Medicine, Tufts University School of Medicine; Chief, Division of Cardiovascular Medicine, New England Medical Center, Boston, MA

Gerald Fletcher, MD Professor of Medicine, Mayo Medical School, Jacksonville, FL

Caroline B. Foote, MD Co-director, Cardiac Arrhythmia Service, New England Medical Center; Assistant Professor of Medicine, Tufts University School of Medicine, Boston, MA

Paul C. Gillette, MD Medical Director, Cardiology, Cook Children's Heart Center, Fort Worth, TX

Irakli Giorgberidze, MD Arrhythmia and Pacemaker Service, Eastern Heart Institute, Passaic, NJ, and Electrophysiology Research Foundation, Millburn, NJ

Mary Fran Hazinski, RN, MSN Pediatric Critical Care, Department of Surgery and Trauma, Vanderbilt University Medical Center, Nashville, TN

Munther K. Homoud, MD Co-director, Cardiac Electrophysiology and Pacemaker Laboratory, New England Medical Center; Assistant Professor of Medicine, Tufts University School of Medicine, Boston, MA

Alberto Interian, Jr., MD Associate Professor of Medicine, University of Miami School of Medicine, Miami, FL

Michael S. Katcher, MD Clinical Fellow, Section of Pacing and Electrophysiology, New England Medical Center, Boston, MA

Carey D. Kimmelstiel, MD Assistant Professor of Medicine, Tufts University School of Medicine; Associate Director, Cardiac Catheterization Lab, Director Ambulatory Cardiology, New England Medical Center, Boston, MA

George J. Klein, MD, FRCPC, FACC Director, Electrophysiology Laboratory, Division of Cardiology, Department of Medicine, University of Western Ontario, London Ontario, Canada

Robert A. Kloner, MD, PhD Director of Research, The Heart Institute, Professor of Medicine, Section of Cardiology, University of Southern California, Los Angeles, CA

Andrew D. Krahn, MD, FRCPC, FACC Director, Arrhythmia Monitoring Unit, Division of Cardiology, Department of Medicine, University of Western Ontario, London Ontario, Canada

Susan B. Kyle, PhD Project Manager, Sports and Recreation, US Consumer Product Safety Commission, Bethesda, MD

Mark S. Link, MD Director, Cardiovascular Center for the Athlete, Cardiac Arrhythmia Service, New England Medical Center; Assistant Professor of Medicine, Tufts University School of Medicine, Boston, MA

Frank I. Marcus, MD Professor of Medicine, University of Arizona College of Medicine, Tucson, AZ

Barry J. Maron, MD Director, Cardiovascular Research Division, Minneapolis Heart Institute Foundation, Minneapolis, MN

Christopher A. McGrew, MD Associate Professor, Department of Orthopaedics and Rehabilitation, Division of Sports Medicine, and Department of Family and Community Medicine, University of New Mexico Health Sciences Center, Albuquerque, NM

Michael E. Mendelsohn, MD Director, Molecular Cardiology Research Center, New England Medical Center; Associate Professor of Medicine, Tufts University School of Medicine, Boston, MA

Gregory F. Michaud, MD Clinical and Research Fellow in Cardiac Electrophysiology, Cardiac Arrhythmia Service, New England Medical Center; Instructor of Medicine, Tufts University School of Medicine, Boston, MA

Raul Mitrani, MD Associate Professor of Medicine, University of Miami School of Medicine, Miami, FL

Matthew J. Mitten, JD Professor of Law, South Texas College of Law, Houston, TX

Robert J. Myerburg, MD Professor of Medicine and Physiology, Director, Division of Cardiology, American Heart Association Chair in Cardiovascular Research, University of Miami School of Medicine, Miami, FL

Richard D. Patten, MD Division of Cardiology, New England Medical Center; Assistant Professor of Medicine, Tufts University School of Medicine, Boston, MA

David Portugal, MD Fellow in Cardiovascular Diseases, New England Medical Center; Instructor of Medicine, Tufts University School of Medicine, Boston, MA

John C. Richmond, MD Associate Professor, Orthopaedic Surgery, Tufts University School of Medicine, New England Medical Center, Boston, MA

Gregory D. Russell, MD Fellow in Cardiovascular Medicine, New England Medical Center; Instructor of Medicine, Tufts University School of Medicine, Boston, MA

Sanjeev Saksena, MD, FACC Arrhythmia and Pacemaker Service, Eastern Heart Institute, Passaic, NJ, and Electrophysiology Research Foundation, Millburn, NJ

Deeb N. Salem, MD Professor of Medicine, Tufts University School of Medicine; Chief Medical Officer, New England Medical Center, Boston, MA

Steven B. Sloan, MD Clinical and Research Fellow in Cardiac Electrophysiology, Cardiac Arrhythmia Service, New England Medical Center; Instructor of Medicine, Tufts University School of Medicine, Boston, MA

John J. Smith, MD, PhD Director, Adult Cardiac Catheterization Laboratory, Co-director, Heart Failure and Cardiac Transplantation Center, New England Medical Center; Assistant Professor of Medicine, Pharmacology, and Experimental Therapeutics, Tufts University School of Medicine, Boston, MA

Gaetano Thiene, MD Professor, Cardiovascular Pathology, University of Padua, Padua, Italy

Paul D. Thompson, MD Director of Preventive Cardiology, Division of Cardiology, Hartford Hospital, Hartford, CT

Geoffrey H. Toffler, MD Associate Professor of Medicine, Harvard Medical School; Director, Institute for the Prevention of Cardiovascular Disease, Beth Israel Deaconess Medical Center, Boston, MA

James Udelson, MD Director, Nuclear Cardiology Laboratory, Division of Cardiology, Department of Medicine, New England Medical Center; Associate Professor of Medicine, Tufts University School of Medicine, Boston, MA

Paul J. Wang, MD   Associate Professor of Medicine, Tufts University School of Medicine; Director, Cardiac Arrhythmia Service, New England Medical Center, Boston, MA

Richard A. Williams, MD   Clinical Professor of Medicine, UCLA School of Medicine, Los Angeles, CA

Raymond Yee, MD, FRCPC, FACC   Chief, Division of Cardiology, Department of Medicine, University of Western Ontario, London Ontario, Canada

Preface

Sudden death in the athlete has intrigued the medical community and the public since the initial report of the unexpected death of the Greek soldier Pheldippides on completing his historic run from Marathon to Athens to deliver the message of victory over the Persians in 490 B.C. The unexpected death of an athlete during exercise is tragic irony. Exercise should serve as a protective measure against cardiovascular events rather than as a triggering mechanism for them. These deaths seem perplexing, as the athlete epitomizes the most vigorous and healthiest segment of our society. Because sudden death in an athlete is relatively uncommon, the identification of athletes at risk remains a considerable challenge. Recently, the instantaneous deaths of several high-profile athletes from cardiac arrest during sports activities has focused attention on this problem. Although approaches to the prediction and prevention of sudden cardiac death in the athlete have evolved in the last few years, much remains unknown regarding optimal screening strategies, pathophysiologic mechanisms, and prevention.

Many of the underlying cardiovascular diseases responsible for sudden death with exercise are now identified; they include hypertrophic cardiomyopathy, arrhythmogenic right ventricular dysplasia, Wolff-Parkinson-White syndrome, anomalous origin of the coronary arteries, and the inherited long QT syndromes. Guidelines for screening to detect predisposing cardiovascular conditions now exist for high school and college athletes. Appropriately designed epidemiologic studies and a prospective registry are needed to monitor the efficacy and cost of this strategy. In order to prevent fatalities and unnecessary restriction on athletic participation, the best available information has been used to update consensus recommendations regarding the eligibility for competition of athletes with cardiovascular disease.

This book was conceived to fulfill the need for a comprehensive text that would serve as an authoritative reference for the medical and athletic community and the public with an interest in the issues involved in the screening, evaluation, or care of athletes. It is written to provide scholarly yet practical reference for the family practitioner, pediatrician, internist, sports medicine physician, cardiologist, team physician, and athletic trainer. The prediction and prevention of sudden cardiac death in the athlete is viewed from multiple perspectives. The book uses a multidisciplinary approach to incorporate current information on epidemiology, cardiovascular pathophysiology, screening guidelines, recommendations for participation, and the vexing legal and ethical issues.

Recognition is due with appreciation to the expert authors who contributed excellent chapters and thereby made this effort possible. The superb organizational skills of Denise Kirk and the helpful assistance of Jacques Strauss and his staff at Futura merit grateful acknowledgment. A special note of thanks is due to our wives and children for their continued understanding and support of this and other medical and academic efforts. As editors, we have the sincere hope that this book serves to contribute to the growing body of cardiovascular knowledge and stimulates support for the intensification of applied research which ultimately allows effective prevention of sudden cardiac death in the athlete.

Contents

Part II
Strategies for Identification and Response

Part III
Arrhythmias in the Athlete:
Evaluation and Management

Part V
Pathologic Observations and Commotio Cordis

Part VI
Legal, Medical, and Organizational Considerations

Part I

Mechanisms of Sudden Cardiac Death and Identification of the Athlete at Risk

Mechanisms of Sudden Cardiac Death in the Athlete

Michael S. Katcher, MD, Deeb N. Salem, MD, Paul J. Wang, MD, and N.A. Mark Estes III, MD

Introduction

Sudden death in the athlete is always an emotionally disturbing event, especially when it occurs in the young and previously healthy. Trained athletes represent our image of the picture of health and, in the case of professional athletes, are often our heroes. The sudden, unexpected loss of an athlete, while rare, produces not only grief, but fear and anxiety in other athletes and in the community at large, as they are forced to face their own mortality. Usually, underlying cardiovascular disease is present and contributory, but is often not recognized prior to the tragic event. A multitude of underlying conditions have been identified in autopsy series, as well as in sudden death survivors, that have helped further the understanding of this condition. An important distinction in exercise related sudden death must be made on the basis of age.[1,2] There is usually evidence of congenital cardiovascular disease, most often hypertrophic cardiomyopathy (HCM) or anomalous coronary arteries in young athletes who died suddenly. In contrast, in older athletes who died suddenly there is usually evidence of atherosclerotic coronary artery disease.

From Estes NAM, Salem DN, Wang PJ (eds). *Sudden Cardiac Death in the Athlete.* Armonk, NY: Futura Publishing Co., Inc.; ©1998.

Definitions

Sudden cardiac death has been defined as an abrupt unexpected death of cardiovascular etiology in which there is loss of consciousness within 1 hour of onset of symptoms.[3] Others have included in the diagnosis those individuals dying within 6 to 12 hours of loss of consciousness or onset of symptoms.[2,4,5] Although the majority of sudden death in the athlete occurs during or immediately after exercise, sudden death can occur at rest or sleep in this population and therefore a distinction must be made between exercise-related sudden death and sudden death in the athlete. One difficulty with any definition or classification of sudden death is in the confirmation of a cardiac etiology. Often there is not preexisting history or sufficient time from onset of symptoms to perform diagnostic tests prior to death. Autopsy, while quite useful, is not always successful at establishing a diagnosis.[1,2,4–7] Certain conditions are difficult (Wolff-Parkinson-White syndrome) or impossible (long QT syndrome) to diagnose solely postmortem.[8]

The definition of *athlete* is even less specific. Exercise-related deaths have been seen at varying levels of activity and training. Distinction should be made between well-trained competitive athletes who exercise regularly and intensely and the unconditioned individuals who exercise infrequently and when doing so, overexert themselves. Exercise-related mortality would be expected to be different in these two groups, regardless of age. The focus of this chapter is predominantly on the former group, the trained athlete.

Incidence

Fortunately, the incidence of sudden death in the athlete is extremely rare. In the high school male athlete, the risk of sudden death is less than 1 in 100,000 per year, and it is much lower in the female athlete.[9,10] This accounts for approximately 12 deaths per year in the United States, in which approximately 4 million high school students participate in competitive sports each year.[6,11] There are also 25 million children and young adults who participate in competitive sports each year, and approximately one-half million collegiate and professional athletes, also with a very low incidence of sudden death.[12] In comparison, there are approximately 14,700 deaths per year in young people secondary to motor vehicle accidents, 1500 deaths related to drowning, and 500 deaths related to firearms.[13] In most series of unexpected death in young people, less than one third of episodes occurred during exertion and exertional death may represent as little as 5% to 15% of unexpected deaths in young people when a comprehen-

Table 1
Noncardiovascular Causes of Death in High School
and College Athletes

- Hyperthermia
- Rhabdomyolysis (sickle cell trait)
- Asthma
- Gastrointestinal bleed
- Exercise anaphylaxis
- Unknown

sive review of unexpected deaths is performed.[5,14,15] Also, approximately 15% of sudden death in the young athlete may be noncardiac in nature, representing a multitude of conditions including asthma, sickle cell trait, and cerebrovascular events (Table 1).[7] A precise estimate of noncardiac sudden death is impossible since noncardiac etiology has been an exclusion criteria for several retrospective series. The risk of exercise-related sudden death is higher in older athletes, but it is still quite low. Estimates range from 1 in 15,000 joggers to 1 in 50,000 marathoners, representing 1 death per 50,000 to 375,000 man-hours of exercise.[16] There are approximately 10 million regular joggers/runners in the United States. Therefore, although the risk per individual is quite low, the absolute number of jogging-related deaths is not insignificant and reflects an estimated several hundred deaths per year.

Characteristics

Over the last two decades, several studies have reported on series of athletes and physically fit young soldiers who have died suddenly.[2,4,7,17–22] An important limitation to any such study is the potential for referral bias. There is the potential for a higher degree of reporting of events that occur during formal practice sessions or competition relative to informal or recreational exercise. Despite these limitations, there is much information that can be gleaned from these retrospective series.

First, young athletes who die suddenly are predominantly male; females represent only approximately 10%. It is unclear if this represents merely a higher participation in formal athletics by males or a true gender-related predilection for exertional death.[7] Most episodes have been reported in junior high or high school athletes.[4] Episodes most often occur during exercise or immediately following formal exercise and therefore tend to occur between 3 pm and 9 pm, the hours that practice and competitions tend to occur. This is in contrast to sudden death in the nonathlete, which tends to have a higher incidence during the morning hours.[23] Sudden death has been reported with a variety of sports but has most often been reported with basketball and football, which combined, may represent over two thirds of cases.[7] The intensity of exercise may also be a factor in sudden death, as most episodes in young athletes occur at competitions or formal practices rather than at purely recreational activities. This may, in part, reflect reporting biases of these more public high-profile deaths. In the older athlete, exercise-related sudden death tends to occur during non-team athletics such as jogging, which may reflect the exercise preference in this age group. As will be discussed in detail, the vast majority of athletes who die suddenly have underlying structural heart disease. Most concerning is the fact that the majority of young athletes who died suddenly did not have a history of preexistent cardiovascular symptoms; sudden death was their initial presenting symptom.[7] An exception to this is the series by Corrado et al[17] in which 45% of young athletes who died suddenly had preexistent symptoms. Other studies show a history of preexistent symptoms in less than one third of patients.[4,7] It is possible that premonitory symptoms would be under-reported, as an athlete concerned that he or she will be prevented from further participation may hide his or her symptoms or not recognize the importance of these symptoms. Despite these possibilities, since most series report the majority to have been previously asymptomatic, it is likely that at least a significant number of athletes truly manifest initially with sudden death. In contrast, approximately half of athletes over age 35 who die suddenly have a known history of underlying disease (usually coronary artery disease) or prodromal symptoms.[2] Since a disproportionate number of sudden deaths occur during or immediately after exercise, it is presumed that factors associated with exercise must act as a trigger for sudden death, superimposed on an underlying substrate.[16] It is impossible to ascertain whether exercise actually increases mortality in these individuals or only acts to uncover an underlying predisposition for death that would otherwise manifest at some point without exercise as a trigger.

Physiology and Pathology of Exercise

Before discussing specific causes and mechanisms of sudden death in the athlete, it is important to review the physiologic and pathologic changes associated with short- and long-term exercise. Short-term exercise produces significant increase in sympathetic tone and withdrawal of parasympathetic tone with associated increase in heart rate, ventricular contractility, cardiac output, and oxygen consumption.[24] In the setting of structural heart disease (including coronary disease), the autonomic and physiologic demands of exercise may not be well tolerated, producing ischemia, hemodynamic embarrassment, and/or a trigger for arrhythmias. In the vast majority of individuals, however, there are multiple benefits to regular exercise.[24–27] These benefits include improvement in lipid profile, weight loss, insulin resistance, and risk of cardiovascular disease, myocardial infarction, and cardiovascular death, as well as a decreased adrenergic response to exercise. The National Institute of Health has therefore recommended a goal of 30 minutes of moderate activity daily.[26]

In response to the repetitive work of training, the athlete's ventricle develops physiologic hypertrophy. This occurs within several weeks of regular exercise.[28] This should not be confused with HCM, since in physiologic hypertrophy of the athlete there is no myocardial disarray.

There are several risks associated with exercise that can contribute to pathologic states.[29] Exercise can induce coronary vasospasm. The response of normal coronary arteries is to vasodilate during exercise; however, regions of arteries with atherosclerosis (including mild) may paradoxically spasm and precipitate an acute ischemic event or produce plaque rupture. The increased shear forces during increased coronary flow during exercise have also been postulated as a cause for plaque rupture. Platelet aggregation has also been shown to increase with extreme exercise and this has also been postulated as a contributor to exercise-related infarction. Acidosis, hypokalemia, and increased adrenergic states during exercise have all been postulated as contributing to exertional arrhythmias. Exercise therefore can contribute to pathologic states, and acute events, including sudden death, do occur with relation to exercise. However, as will be discussed in more detail later, the benefits of exercise outweigh the risks in the vast majority of individuals.

Acquired Abnormalities in Young Athletes

The vast majority of sudden deaths in young athletes occur in individuals with previously undetected structural heart disease (Table 2). This most often represents congenital cardiovascular disease in these young athletes.[2,4,7,17–19,22] One notable exception to this is sudden death in young soldiers.[20,21] While not strictly athletes, these individuals do participate in regular exertion, and because of preparticipation screening, are all considered healthy prior to death. In series of young people in the military, congenital cardiovascular disease is still common as an underlying cause, but in addition there is a disproportionate representation of myocarditis in comparison to other series (>20%, including a high incidence of rheumatic myocarditis). It is believed that the detailed screening process prior to military service would potentially identify

Table 2
Cardiovascular Causes of Sudden Death

- Hypertrophic cardiomyopathy
- Coronary artery disease
- Arrhythmogenic right ventricular dysplasia
- Anomalous coronary artery
- Left ventricular hypertrophy
- Myocarditis
- Conduction system abnormalities
- Mitral valve prolapse
- Congenital heart disease
- Valvular heart disease
- Aortic dissection
- Cerebral embolus
- Pulmonary embolus
- Arteriovenous malformation
- Berry aneurysm
- Wolff-Parkinson-White syndrome
- Myocardial bridge
- Coronary aneurysm
- Subvalvular aortic stenosis
- Long QT syndrome
- Idiopathic ventricular fibrillation
- Dilated cardiomyopathy

and thus exclude some individuals with congenital disease and thus lower their representation in the mortality statistics. Also, the close living quarters in the military may contribute to an increase in upper respiratory infections and thus increase the potential for myocarditis.[9] Another acquired cardiac disease occasionally seen in young athletes who die suddenly is atherosclerotic coronary artery disease. Severe atherosclerotic coronary disease is quite uncommon in the very young athlete and when present, often represents a manifestation of a familial dyslipidemia syndrome, usually severe heterozygous or homozygous type II hypercholesterolemia.[6]

Hypertrophic Cardiomyopathy

The underlying condition most often associated with sudden death in the young athlete is HCM (Table 2). When death occurs during exercise in young people, in comparison to at rest, HCM is more likely to be the underlying cause.[15] Approximately one half of young athletes who die suddenly have HCM.[2] Unfortunately, they usually have no history of preceding symptoms.[30] HCM is a relatively common congenital disease, affecting approximately 1 in 500 individuals.[31] It is actually a heterogeneous mix of genetically transmitted diseases that affect the myocardial sarcomere.[32] Most genetic abnormalities associated with this disease produce missense mutations in the β-myosin heavy chain gene, although other components of the sarcomere have been shown to be affected in some families. The phenotypic expression of these abnormalities is manifested as ventricular hypertrophy, usually asymmetrical, with decreased compliance. Occasionally there is subvalvular left ventricular outflow obstruction. Histology of these ventricles shows disordered cellular architecture with myocyte disarray. There is also evidence of abnormal intramural arteries with lumenal narrowing. The classic physical exam finding is an ejection murmur increased by maneuvers that decrease preload. Unfortunately, the physical exam is usually not sensitive, as most patients do not develop obstructive physiology and full phenotypic expression of the disease with maximal hypertrophy often does not develop until age 18.[10,33]

The mortality in HCM is approximately 4% to 6% per year in children and adolescents and 1% to 3% per year in adults.[32] The exact mechanism of death in these individuals remains unknown but is presumed to be arrhythmia related. Mortality is not associated with the degree of obstruction.[13] Holter monitors worn at the time of sudden death have shown polymorphic ventricular tachycardia degenerating into ventricular fibrillation.[34] The myocardial disarray and degeneration contribute to inhomogeneity in the ventricle and can act as a substrate for arrhythmias.[30,35] Patients at high risk of death often have inducible sustained ventricular tachycardia at electrophysiologic studies.[36] There is, however, controversy as to whether electrophysiologic studies can reliably predict sudden death.[30] Other risk factors for sudden death may include young age, history of syncope, malignant family history, inducible ischemia, and nonsustained ventricular tachycardia.

The potential trigger mechanisms for sudden death during exercise in this population are multiple. The stiff ventricle seen in this condition can contribute to diastolic dysfunction and increased wall stress, which would be exacerbated by the increased ventricular rates and shorter diastole with exercise. This increased wall stress can contribute to regional subendocardial ischemia and secondary arrhythmias. Exertional ischemia may also play a role. Despite normal epicardial vessels, the increased myocardial mass and abnormal intramuscular arteries can contribute to insufficient perfusion to meet the demands of exercise. Dilsizian et al[37] have shown a very high incidence of inducible ischemia on thallium stress testing in HCM patients who have survived sudden death or have had syncopal episodes.[37] There may also be a direct arrhythmogenic effect of catecholamines in this abnormal myocardium. Animal studies have confirmed β-adrenergic–related delayed afterdepolarizations and triggered activity in HCM.[38] Exercise, especially when upright, can markedly affect hemodynamics, especially in those with obstructive HCM. Increased contractility and decreased preload in upright exercise contributes to functional obstruction, producing twice the pressure gradient seen at rest.[32,39] Even in patients without obstruction at rest, rapid rates can contribute to marked hemodynamic embarrassment.[40] Also the hyperdynamic and underfilled ventricle, when upright, can trigger neurocardiogenic reflexes and syncope. Tilt testing in HCM patients with a history of syncope is often remarkable for sustained or transient hypotension with bradycardia or lack of appropriate tachycardia.[41] Whether neurocardiogenic reflexes ever act as the initial event cascading into total hemodynamic collapse and sudden death remains unclear. Finally, supraventricular arrhythmias, including atrial fibrillation, can contribute to hemodynamic compromise and risk of sudden death.[30]

Idiopathic Left Ventricular Hypertrophy

A condition possibly related to HCM and occasionally seen in sudden death in athletes is idiopathic concentric left ventricular hypertrophy.[1,2] The degree of hypertrophy seen in individuals with this condition is beyond that seen in physiologic hypertrophy of the highly trained athlete. These individuals also lack a history or pathologic evidence of conditions that would predispose to pathologic hypertrophy (eg, hypertension or aortic stenosis). In idiopathic concentric left ventricular hypertrophy, unlike in HCM, the hypertrophy is concentric and symmetrical. Fibromuscular hyperplasia of the arteries that supply the atrioventricular node and sinus nodes, with lumenal narrowing, has been seen in this condition; however, it remains unclear if this contributes to sudden death in these individuals. Unlike HCM, there is no evidence of genetic transmission and at autopsy there is no histologic evidence of myocardial disarray. It has been proposed that this condition may represent a nonfamilial variant of HCM.[2] In the absence of other evident pathologic causes, idiopathic concentric left ventricular hypertrophy is considered a potential underlying cause of sudden death in athletes. In life, making the distinction between physiologic hypertrophy of the athlete's heart, idiopathic hypertrophy, and HCM (especially in young athletes prior to full phenotypic expression or those with only modest hypertrophy) can be difficult; however, history, physical exam, and diagnostic testing often help to make the distinction.[33]

Congenital Coronary Artery Anomalies

Congenital anomaly of a coronary artery or arteries is another common underlying finding in young athletes with sudden death.[2,4,7,17–22]

One frequent anomaly found is origin of the left main coronary artery from the anterior/right sinus of Valsalva. This condition was first described in detail by Cheitlin et al[42] in the 1970s. Cheitlin et al noted that exercise-related death was particularly associated with only those in whom the anomalous left main passes acutely between the aorta and pulmonary artery. The acute angle that this coronary takes produces a slitlike orifice at its origin. With exercise, it has been presumed that expansion of the aorta and pulmonary arteries from increased stroke volume changes the geometry and produces an exaggeration of the take-off angle and a valvular ridge to act as a flap, partially closing the orifice.[12,42,43] Although not originally reported in the series by Cheitlin et al, a mirror image of this anomaly has subsequently been described. In these patients the right coronary artery originates from the left sinus of Valsalva and passes between the aorta and the pulmonary trunk. This condition has also been reported in sudden death in the athlete with a presumed similar mechanism.[2,4,7,43] Even in the absence of a truly anomalous origin of a vessel, coronary arteries with an abnormal acute angle of origin can produce this slitlike orifice with exercise, and have been reported in cases of sudden cardiac death in young people.[43] An alternative hypothesis for the mechanism of sudden death in these individuals is the possibility of compression of the coronary artery as it runs between the expanded aorta and pulmonary trunk during exercise. Compression is thought to be unlikely in most cases because systolic pressure is greater in the coronary artery than in the pulmonary trunk; however, sudden death has been reported in individuals in whom left main coronary arises from the right coronary artery and passes between the aorta and the pulmonary trunk *without* an oblique angle of take off. Therefore, exercise-related compression may play a role in certain anomalies.[12]

Other coronary anomalies seen in exercise-related cardiac death include hypoplasia or absence of a coronary artery, coronary arteries originating from the pulmonary trunk, and coronary intussusception.[1,2] Fibromuscular stenosis of coronary branches including those supplying the conduction system have also been reported.[2,22] Myocardial bridging, in which otherwise normal coronary arteries tunnel through the myocardium, has occasionally been seen in young athletes who have died suddenly. It is unclear what role, if any, such a variant plays in sudden death, as it is a common variant in normals (up to 20%).[1,2] The lumen of the vessel may be compromised by myocardial squeeze during systole; however, during diastole, when most coronary flow occurs, the vessel is not compromised. The presumed mechanism of sudden death in athletes with anomalous coronaries is ischemia contributing to hemodynamic embarrassment and/or malignant arrhythmias. In anomalies affecting vessels that supply the conduction system, acute bradyarrhythmias from such localized ischemia is another potential mechanism. It would seem that individuals who have anomalies that are severe enough to someday contribute to sudden death might be limited by symptoms when attempting to exercise. Surprisingly, many athletes with these conditions are able to engage in strenuous exercise for years with infrequent or no symptoms. A striking example was Pete Maravich, a professional basketball superstar who after retirement died suddenly during recreational play and was found to have severe hypoplasia of his coronary circulation and diffuse fibrosis. Presumably, other factors must also come into play at the time of the fatal event, since the potential trigger (ischemia) can be present every time these athletes exercise.

Atherosclerotic Coronary Artery Disease

In contrast to the young, athletes over age 35 who die suddenly during exercise usually have underlying coronary atherosclerotic disease. The degree of coronary stenosis is usually severe, there is often evidence of multivessel disease, and atherosclerosis in involved vessels tends to be fairly diffuse.[2,19] Left main coronary artery disease, however, is usually not present. This may reflect functional limitation, which could preclude exercise, that left main coronary artery disease often places on individuals. Individuals who die suddenly with coronary atherosclerotic disease often have a history of multiple coronary artery disease risk factors and approximately half have a history of known coronary artery disease or prodromal symptoms.[1,2] Almost half have evidence of healed infarcts.

Several mechanisms can contribute to coronary artery-related deaths during exercise (Table 3). First, as discussed above, exercise can precipitate an acute myocardial infarction. Exercise-related coronary spasm and increased shear forces from increased coronary flow can produce plaque rupture and thrombosis.[1] Evidence of acute infarction is seen in up to three quarters of all sudden death; however, acute infarction may represent a much lower percentage of sudden death occurring

Table 3
Mechanisms of Acute Coronary Events with Exercise

- Plaque rupture and coronary thrombosis
- Contraction of noncompliant atherosclerotic plaque producing rupture
- Alterations of epicardial contour of coronary plaques
- Increased shear force
- Enhanced catecholamine-induced platelet aggregation
- Exercise-induced coronary artery spasm

during exercise.[19,35,44] A rare cause of acute coronary occlusion and sudden death in the absence of significant atherosclerotic disease is acute coronary dissection during exercise.[45] The presumed mechanism for sudden death in acute occlusion of a coronary vessel is a malignant arrhythmia, usually ventricular fibrillation.

Exercise can precipitate cardiac ischemia in the presence of coronary disease by increasing myocardial oxygen demand while fixed coronary stenoses prevent an adequate compensatory increase in blood flow. Ischemia can act as a trigger for malignant arrhythmias, especially in the presence of an appropriate substrate such as a prior infarction. In highly trained athletes who have died suddenly during exercise, even in the absence of a history of known infarction, at autopsy, evidence of prior old (silent) infarction is common.[19] Ischemia need not always be the trigger for sudden death in the setting of old infarction. Ventricular arrhythmias in patients with prior infarction are not infrequently induced with exercise. Formal exercise testing in these patients has shown that electrocardiographic evidence of ischemia is usually absent preceding development of their arrhythmia.[46] The increase in catecholamines and the other physiologic changes of exercise can be significant in the mechanism of sudden death in the absence of inducible ischemia.

Therefore, sudden death during exercise can occur in the presence or the absence of evidence of an acute infarction at the time of death. In individuals with no history of coronary artery disease symptoms, acute infarction is more common. When a history of such symptoms is present, no evidence of acute infarction is usually found at autopsy, however previous infarction may be present.[9]

There is clearly some increased risk of sudden death related to exercise in adult men, of which most is related to coronary artery disease. Even in frequent exercisers, the relative risk of sudden death occurring during exercise as compared to other times may be as high as five- to sevenfold.[9,47,48] In individuals who do not exercise regularly, the relative risk of sudden death occurring during vigorous activity is much higher.[47] While the relative risk of sudden death occurring during exercise is high, the absolute risk is in fact quite low. It has been estimated to be as low as 1 in 50,000 marathon runners or 1 in 7620 joggers per year (1 death per 400,000 man-hours of jogging). In fact, frequent exercise appears to be protective. Active men have less coronary artery disease than their sedentary counterparts.[49] The overall risk of sudden cardiac death in those who exercise regularly appears to be about half that seen in sedentary individuals. This exercise-related difference is especially true in older, hypertensive, and obese males.[50] Although exercise can be a trigger for myocardial infarction and sudden death, frequent exercise appears to reduce the risk of triggering of these events during subsequent exercise.[51]

Aortic Rupture

Another important underlying abnormality reported in young athletes with sudden cardiac death is aortic rupture. Sudden rupture of aneurysms of the ascending aorta usually leads to circulatory collapse from cardiac tamponade as a result of bleeding into the pericardial space. Aortic rupture is often a sequela of Marfan syndrome, in which decrease in elastic tissue in the aortic media (cystic medial necrosis) produces dilatation and weakness with potential for rupture. Marfan syndrome affects connective tissue in a variety of systems.[6,12,13,52] Musculoskeletal abnormalities are most evident with extreme height, arachnodactyly, hyperextensible joints, and abnormalities of the sternum and palate. Cardiac abnormalities include mitral and aortic regurgitation. Ocular abnormalities are also prominent. Aortic rupture can occur in athletes who do not otherwise have signs of Marfan syndrome.[4,7,12] Presumably, the increase in blood pressure and stroke volume with exercise can contribute to rupture occurring preferentially during exercise. Occasionally, individuals with undiagnosed Marfan syndrome have participated in competitive sports for years without symptoms prior to their fatal event. One such example is Flo Hyman, a tall Olympic volleyball player who died of aortic rupture and tamponade during a competition. One proposed explanation for sudden death after years of participation in sports is that progressive aortic dilation may occur with this syndrome and only when a critical point is reached is there a marked increase in risk for rupture.[12]

Arrhythmogenic Right Ventricular Dysplasia

Arrhythmogenic right ventricular dysplasia (ARVD) has been an uncommon underlying condition in young athletes who have died suddenly.[1,2,6,7] However, Corrado et al[17] report a series of sudden deaths in young competitive athletes in the Veneto region of Italy, in which ARVD was the most common underlying condition seen, occurring in 27% of cases. It is unclear whether this represents familial clustering of this condition localized to this region of Italy or a referral bias. While most cases of ARVD are sporadic, familial forms have been reported. The disease represents a right ventricular myopathy in which there is fatty infiltration of the myocardium with potential for thinning, dilatation, and hypokinesia.[53] Right ventricular hypokinesis and dilatation are associated with an increased risk of sudden death in this condition.[54] The mechanism of exercise-related death in this condition is felt to be malignant ventricular arrhythmia. Delayed activation in parts of the right ventricle is occasionally seen on surface electrocardiogram (ECG) (epsilon waves) and signal-averaged ECG in this condition. Abnormal conduction in the diseased right ventricle can represent the substrate for serious arrhythmias. Ventricular tachycardia of a left bundle branch block morphology is often seen in this condition, consistent with a right ventricular site of tachycardia. Right ventricular stretch during exercise, as well as increased catecholamines, are felt to contribute to arrhythmogenicity. Exercise testing in ARVD has been shown to precipitate ventricular tachycardia in about half of cases.[53,55] High-dose isoproterenol induces sustained or nonsustained (usually polymorphic) ventricular tachycardia in most cases.[53,56] In light of the ease of induction of nonfatal arrhythmias with exercise and catecholamines in this condition, it is not surprising that more than half of individuals with ARVD in the series by Corrado et al had a history of previous symptoms, usually palpitations.[17]

Myocarditis

Myocarditis is an infrequent underlying condition in sudden death of the young athlete. The etiology is usually viral (Coxsackie B) or idiopathic and is associated with an inflammatory infiltration with associated myocardial damage and necrosis.[30] Illicit drug use has also occasionally been associated with myocarditis.[33] While regular exercise has been associated with an improved immune system, excessive extreme exercise can impair the immune system and theoretically increase susceptibility to viral upper respiratory infections which can subsequently cause myocarditis.[57,58] A fulminant dilated cardiomyopathy can occasionally result. It is believed that during active myocarditis and during healing, there is an increased risk of malignant arrhythmia from regions of injured myocardium. Therefore, avoidance of vigorous exercise during or immediately following a viral illness is often recommended to avoid potential exercise-related triggers of arrhythmia. However, it is now realized that a fully healed region and its surrounding tissue may contribute to electrical instability and therefore, once myocarditis is recognized, at least 6 months of convalescence should be considered and hemodynamic and arrhythmia evaluation should be considered prior to return to competitive sports.[30]

Valvular Heart Disease

Previously undiagnosed congenital valvular disease is occasionally found in athletes who died suddenly. Congenital aortic stenosis was previously considered a common cause of sudden death in young people; however it has only rarely been identified in young athletes.[12]

This discrepancy may relate to the relative ease of early diagnosis based on the usually loud murmur on physical exam, with subsequent prohibition of strenuous athletics.

Mitral Valve Prolapse

Mitral valve prolapse (MVP) has occasionally been reported in athletes who died suddenly. In light of the high prevalence of MVP in the general population (approximately 5%), a causal relationship of MVP with sudden death is not usually clear. Approximately 12 previously asymptomatic individuals with isolated MVP have been reported to die suddenly during exercise.[30] The presumed mechanism for sudden death in this hemodynamically insignificant valvular abnormality is arrhythmic. Ventricular ectopy has been reported with this condition, however, symptoms and sudden death are uncommon even in these individuals.[6] The proposed means in which this condition could contribute to malignant arrhythmia include abnormal tension on the papillary muscles, redundant chordae tendinae mechanically stimulating the endocardium, and valvular microthrombi embolizing down coronary arteries.[35]

Ventricular Arrhythmias

Arrhythmias are an important cause of sudden death in the athlete. As described earlier, in patients with structurally abnormal hearts malignant arrhythmias are often the presumed mechanism of death. In fact, when life-threatening tachyarrhythmias are detected, an evaluation for structural heart disease is essential. An underlying substrate is almost always found.[59] Low-grade ventricular arrhythmias are often seen in athletes with structurally normal hearts. This may be related in part to exercise and training, since in athletes who stop training, there is a trend to decreased ectopy.[60] However, ventricular ectopy may be no more common in athletes than in age-matched controls.[61] In the absence of structural heart disease, exercise-related modest ventricular ectopy, including slow, very brief, assymptomatic nonsustained ventricular tachycardia, has been associated with no worse prognosis, and occasionally after cardiac evaluation and monitoring, subsequent exercise is not prohibited.[60,62–64]

Exercise-related sustained monomorphic ventricular tachycardia has been seen in patients without structural heart disease. The tachyarrhythmia is often reproduced with isoproterenol, suggesting a catecholamine-related mechanism.[65] Catecholamine-sensitive increased automaticity and triggered activity related to delayed afterdepolarizations are presumed mechanisms of the arrhythmia. A subset of these tachyarrhythmias is suppressible with calcium channel blockers. Most commonly, exertional ventricular tachycardia in the absence of structural heart disease originates in the right ventricle, usually from the right ventricular outflow tract, but occasionally can originate from the left ventricle. Although the prognosis in these conditions is usually benign, sudden death occasionally occurs.[65,66] Patients with symptomatic ventricular tachycardia and no structural heart disease have increased QT dispersion compared with other athletes, and this may contribute to their potential for malignant arrhythmias.[67] Sudden death survivors without structural heart disease are often resuscitated from ventricular fibrillation. While most of these individuals are considered to have idiopathic ventricular fibrillation, a frequent finding in these individuals is tightly coupled premature ventricular depolarizations and nonsustained polymorphic ventricular tachycardia.[68]

Because of the potential risk of exercise-related death, most athletes with ventricular tachycardia should be prohibited from subsequent competitive athletics for at least 6 months without recurrence and should undergo a formal evaluation including exercise testing and electrophysiologic testing prior to consideration of return to competitive sports.[63] A less restrictive recommendation can be considered in athletes with slow brief asymptomatic runs of nonsustained ventricular tachycardia only. However, structural heart disease should still be excluded.

Long QT Syndrome

One rare arrhythmic cause of sudden death in the young athlete is the long QT syndrome. The low reported prevalence of this underlying condition in athletes who die suddenly may in part reflect the fact that pathologic evidence on autopsy is usually lacking. Therefore, without family history or premortem ECG or diagnosis, the postmortem diagnosis is difficult and a portion of sudden deaths of unknown etiology after autopsy may represent this condition. Also, once individual cases are detected, family screening is recommended and therefore prohibition from competitive sports may occur in asymptomatic individuals once detected.

In the majority of cases, inheritance is autosomal dominant in congenital long QT syndrome. Jervell and Lange-Nielsen syndrome is an autosomal recessive form associated with congenital deafness. Sporadic nonfamilial cases occur occasionally as well. Life-threatening arrhythmias including torsade de pointes and ventricular fibrillation are associated with the QT prolongation seen in this condition.[69] Arrhythmia, syncope, and sudden death are often precipitated by sympathetic stimulation, and exercise-related deaths have been seen. Ventricular tachyarrhythmias occurring with exertion or stress are seen in the majority of patients.[14] Therefore, once diagnosed, avoidance of vigorous exercise is recommended.[63] The risk of sudden death in this condition is approximately 1.3% per year with highest risk in patients with female sex, congenital deafness, or history of syncope or malignant arrhythmias.[69]

Bradyarrhythmias

Bradyarrhythmias are also occasionally the presumed mechanism of sudden death in the athlete. Increased vagal tone at baseline is a common finding in the trained athlete. First-, second-, and third-degree AV block have been seen in trained athletes and can be symptomatic. Postexertional- and hyperventilation-related transient asystole greater than 20 seconds and occasionally treated with chest thump has been associated with syncope in athletes.[70,71] The presumed mechanism is an excessive vagal response. A classic neurocardiogenic response to tilt testing is often lacking and electrophysiologic studies, including sinus node function, are usually within normal limits.[70,72] Whether this condition is a mechanism for sudden cardiac death remains unclear.

Conduction System Abnormalities

Intrinsic structural abnormalities of the conduction system are occasionally found in athletes with sudden death, raising the possibility of bradyarrhythmias as a mechanism of sudden death in these individuals.[73,74] These findings are occasionally found in the presence of other structural heart disease, therefore raising the possibility of an alternative to tachyarrhythmia as the mechanism for sudden death in structural heart disease patients. Other times conduction system disease is the only abnormality found in athletes who have died suddenly. These abnormalities can only be detected when a detailed autopsy, with particular attention to the conduction system, is performed. Abormalities include fibrosis and fatty metamorphosis of cells of the conduction system including the AV node and His-Purkinje system and mononuclear cell infiltration to regions of the sinus and AV nodes. Abnormal location of the AV node with limitations to communication to the rest of the conduction system have also been seen.[73] Narrowing of arteries to the sinus and AV nodes has also been seen with necrosis and fibrosis of the associated node.[22] Sudden worsening of conduction or intrinsic pacemaker function is the presumed potential mechanism of bradyarrhythmic-related death in these individuals; however, strict evidence of a causal relationship remains lacking.

Supraventricular Arrhythmias

Supraventricular tachycardia (SVT) is also the presumed mechanism of sudden death in some patients. In the presence of certain forms of structural heart disease such as hypertrophic cardiomyopathy, hemodynamic tolerance of SVT can be dramatically impaired. Cerebral and/or cardiac hypoperfusion and secondary ventricular arrhythmias are potential contributors to SVT-related death.[40] Even in patients without structural heart disease, SVT is occasionally the presumed mechanism of sudden death. Sudden death survivors have been identified in whom SVT has been shown to deteriorate into ventricular fibrillation.[75] AV nodal reciprocating tachycardia has been seen to degenerate into ventricular fibrillation in some of these patients. Atrial fibrillation with accelerated AV nodal conduction (in the absence of Wolff-Parkinson-White syndrome) has been associated with very rapid ventricular response and ventricular fibrillation. Shortest R-R intervals less than 250 milliseconds have been seen in these patients.[75] Given the potential for exercise-related SVT and the altered hemodynamic state during and after exercise, it is possible that SVT occasionally contributes to sudden cardiac death in the athlete.

Wolff-Parkinson-White Syndrome

A special case of supraventricular tachycardia contributing to sudden death is in patients with Wolff-Parkinson-White syndrome (WPW). WPW is usually not familial and it affects up to 0.1% to 0.3% of the population, with twice as many males as females affected.[76] The presence of the atrioventricular bypass tract in this condition contributes to AV reciprocating tachycardia and atrial arrhythmias with rapid ventricular response. WPW is rarely reported as the underlying cause in exercise-related sudden death. This may reflect the difficulty in making a post mortem diagnosis in this condition. While WPW does reflect a form of structural heart disease, the disease is microscopic and very focal. Identification at autopsy requires thousands of histologic sections around the entire mitral and tricuspid annuli. This specialized level of autopsy is not usually performed and therefore, some cases of unexplained sudden death may reflect undiagnosed WPW.

It is estimated that sudden death occurs approximately once per 1000 patient years and is very rare in asymptomatic patients.[8] The presumed mechanism in most instances is atrial fibrillation with rapid ventricular response degenerating into subsequent ventricular fibrillation. Atrial fibrillation can occur spontaneously in WPW, but it is often preceded by AV reciprocating tachycardia. Analysis of patients with aborted sudden death has shown that the shortest R-R interval during atrial fibrillation less than 250 milliseconds, consistent with a bypass tract with particularly short refractory period. In patients with aborted sudden death, cardiac arrest was occasionally their first presentation; however on careful questioning, some patients acknowledge previous minor palpitations.[8] When atrial fibrillation is induced in patients with WPW in the electrophysiology lab, most patients tolerate the arrhythmia well, even when ventricular rates are rapid. Therefore upright posture and neurohumoral factors may play a part in sudden death in this condition, especially in exercise-related cases. Lack of symptoms does not predict a long refractory period of the bypass tract.[77] Approximately 20% of asymptomatic individuals with WPW have "high-risk" characteristics of their bypass tract and short R-R intervals during atrial fibrillation.[8]

Exercise, with its associated change in autonomic tone, improves conduction and shortens refractoriness in bypass tracts (as well as in the AV node), and thus increases the potential for rapid ventricular rates should atrial fibrillation occur.[78] During exercise in sinus tachycardia, the AV node is usually more affected than the bypass tract, producing preferential conduction via the AV node with less preexcitation or loss of manifest preexcitation. Athletic training in patients with WPW has not been shown to negatively affect electrophysiologic effects of a bypass tract at rest.[79] Specifically, after training, there is no increased incidence of inducibility of atrial fibrillation or change in the shortest R-R intervals during atrial fibrillation. Because of the potential for sudden death with exercise and the ability to treat or cure this condition, consideration of an evaluation to assess characteristics of the bypass tract or to consider treatment has been suggested for some competitive assymptomatic athletes.[63,76]

Conclusions

Fortunately, sudden death in the athlete is a rare occurrence. When it does occur, underlying structural heart disease is usually present but usually not detected prior to death. The age at which exercise-related sudden death occurs is the greatest predictor of underlying etiology. In young athletes, hypertrophic cardiomyopathy and anomalous coronary artery anatomy are most commonly found. In older athletes over age 35, coronary artery disease is the most common underlying cause. When no clear underlying etiology is identified, consideration of arrhythmia-related factors not easily identified on autopsy, such as WPW and long QT syndrome, should be considered.

References

1. Burke AP, Farb A, Virmani R. Causes of sudden death in athletes. *Cardiol Clin* 1992;10:303–317.
2. Maron BJ, Epstein SE, Roberts WC. Causes of sudden death in competitive athletes. *J Am Coll Cardiol* 1986;7:204–214.
3. Myerburg RJ, Castellanos A. Cardiac arrest and sudden cardiac death. In Braunwald E (ed): *Heart Disease: A Textbook of Cardiovascular Medicine, 4th Edition.* Philadelphia: W.B. Saunders Co.; 1992:756–789.
4. Maron BJ, Roberts WC, McAllister HA, et al. Sudden death in young athletes. *Circulation* 1980;62:218–229.
5. Topaz O, Edwards JE. Pathologic features of sudden death in children, adolescents, and young adults. *Chest* 1985;87:476–482.
6. McCaffrey FM, Braden DS, Strong WB. Sudden cardiac death in young athletes: A review. *Am J Dis Child* 1991;145:177–183.
7. Maron BJ, Shirani J, Poliac LC, et al. Sudden death in young competitive athletes: Clinical, demographic and pathological profiles. *JAMA* 1996;276:199–204.
8. Munger TM, Packer DL, Hammill SC, et al. A population study of the natural history of Wolff- Parkinson-White syndrome in Olmsted County, Minnesota, 1953–1989. *Circulation* 1993;87:866–873.
9. Thompson PD. The cardiovascular complications of vigorous physical activity. *Arch Intern Med* 1996;156:2297–2302.
10. Epstein SE, Maron BJ. Sudden death and the competitive athlete: Perspectives on preparticipation screening studies. *J Am Coll Cardiol* 1986; 7:220–230.
11. Maron BJ, Thompson PD, Puffer JC, et al. Cardiovascular preparticipation screening of competitive athletes: A statement for health professionals from the sudden death committee (clinical cardiology) and congenital cardiac defects committee (cardiovascular disease in the young), American Heart Association. *Circulation* 1996;94:850–856.
12. Maron BJ, Roberts WC. Causes and implications of sudden cardiac death in athletes. In Akhtar M, Myerburg RJ, Ruskin JN (eds): *Sudden Cardiac Death: Prevalence, Mechanisms, and Approaches to Diagnosis and Management.* Philadelphia: Williams and Wilkins.
13. Rowland TW. Sudden unexpected death in sports. *Pediatr Ann* 1992;21:189,193–195.
14. Liberthson RR. Sudden death from cardiac causes in children and young adults. *N Engl J Med* 1996;334:1039–1044.
15. Burke AP, Farb A, Virmani R, et al. Sports-related and non-sports-related sudden cardiac death in young adults. *Am Heart J* 1991;121:568–575.
16. Willich SN, Maclure M, Mittleman M, et al. Sudden cardiac death: Support for a role of triggering in causation. *Circulation* 1993;87:1442–1450.
17. Corrado D, Thiene G, Nava A, et al. Sudden death in young competitive athletes: Clinicopathologic correlations in 22 cases. *Am J Med* 1990;89: 588–596.
18. Tsung SH, Huang TY, Chang HH. Sudden death in young athletes. *Arch Pathol Lab Med* 1982;106:168–170.
19. Waller BF, Roberts WC. Sudden death while running in conditioned runners aged 40 years or over. *Am J Cardiol* 1980;45:1292–1300.
20. Phillips M, Robinowitz M, Higgins JR, et al. Sudden cardiac death in air force recruits: A 20-year review. *JAMA* 1986;256:2696–2699.
21. Kramer MR, Drori Y, Lev B. Sudden death in young soldiers: High incidence of syncope prior to death. *Chest* 1988;93:345–347.

22. James TN, Froggatt P, Marshall TK. Sudden death in young athletes. *Ann Intern Med* 1967;67:1013–1021.
23. Thakur RK, Hoffmann RG, Olson DW, et al. Circadian variation in sudden cardiac death: Effects of age, sex and initial cardiac rhythm. *Ann Emerg Med* 1996;27:29–34.
24. Wight JN, Salem D. Sudden cardiac death and the 'athlete's heart.' *Arch Intern Med* 1995;155:1473–1480.
25. Fletcher GF, Balady G, Blair SN, et al. Statement on exercise: Benefits and recommendations for physical activity programs for all Americans: A statement for health professionals by the committee on exercise and cardiac rehabilitation of the council on clinical cardiology, American Heart Association. *Circulation* 1996;94:8ɔ1–862.
26. NIH consensus development panel on physical activity and cardiovascular health. Physical activity and cardiovascular health. *JAMA* 1996;276:241–246.
27. Rauramaa R, Leon AS. Physical activity and risk of cardiovascular disease in middle-aged individuals. *Sports Med* 1996;22:65–69.
28. Ehsani A. Loss of cardiovascular adaptations after cessation of training. *Cardiol Clin* 1992;10:257–266.
29. Wolff LJ, Brodsky MA. Arrhythmia in athletes. In Podrid PJ, Kowey PR (eds): *Cardiac Arrhythmia: Mechanisms, Diagnosis and Management.* Boston: Williams and Wilkins; 1995; 1175–1187.
30. Maron BJ, Isner JM, McKenna WJ. Task force 3: Hypertrophic cardiomyopathy, myocarditis and other myopericardial diseases and mitral valve prolapse. *J Am Coll Cardiol* 1994;24:845–899.
31. Maron BJ, Gardin JM, Flack JM, et al. Prevalence of hypertrophic cardiomyopathy in a general population of young adults: Echocardiographic analysis of 4111 subjects in the CARDIA study-Coronary Artery Risk Development in (Young) Adults. *Circulation* 1995;92:785–789.
32. Wigle ED, Rakowski H, Kimball BP, et al. Hypertrophic cardiomyopathy: Clinical spectrum and treatment. *Circulation* 1995;92:1680–1692.
33. Maron BJ, Pelliccia A, Spirito P. Cardiac disease in young trained athletes: Insights into methods for distinguishing athlete's heart from structural heart disease, with particular emphasis on hypertrophic cardiomyopathy. *Circulation* 1995;91:1596–1601.
34. Gardin LL, Nanton MA, Hanna BD. Ambulatory monitoring of the sudden death of an adolescent with hypertrophic cardiomyopathy. *Can J Cardiol* 1994;10:548–550.
35. Furlanello F, Bettini R, Cozzi F, et al. Ventricular arrhythmias and sudden death in athletes. *Ann N Y Acad Sci* 1984;427:253–279.
36. Fananapazir L, Chang AC, Epstein SE, et al. Prognostic determinants in hypertrophic cardiomyopathy: Perspective evaluation of a therapeutic strategy based on clinical, Holter, hemodynamic, and electrophysiologic findings. *Circulation* 1992;86:730–740.
37. Dilsizian V, Bonow RO, Epstein SE, et al. Myocardial ischemia detected by thallium scintigraphy is frequently related to cardiac arrest and syncope in young patients with hypertrophic cardiomyopathy. *J Am Coll Cardiol* 1993;22:796–804.
38. Samson RA, Lee HC. Delayed afterdepolarizations and triggered arrhythmias in hypertrophic cardiomyopathic hearts. *J Lab Clin Med* 1994;124:242–248.
39. Schwammenthal E, Schwartzkopff B, Block M, et al. Doppler echocardiographic assessment of the pressure gradient during bicycle ergometry in hypertrophic cardiomyopathy. *Am J Cardiol* 1992;69:1623–1628.

40. Madariaga I, Carmona JR, Mateas FR, et al. Supraventricular arrhythmia as the cause of sudden death in hypertrophic cardiomyopathy. *Eur Heart J* 1994;15:134–137.
41. Gilligan DM, Nihoyannopoulos P, Chan WL, et al. Investigation of a hemodynamic basis for syncope in hypertrophic cardiomyopathy. *Circulation* 1992;85:2140–2148.
42. Cheitlin MD, De Castro CM, McAllister HA. Sudden death as a complication of anomalous left coronary origin from the anterior sinus of Valsalva: A not-so-minor congenital anomaly. *Circulation* 1974;50:780–787.
43. Steinberger J, Lucas RV, Edwards JE, et al. Causes of sudden unexpected cardiac death in the first two decades of life. *Am J Cardiol* 1996;77: 992–995.
44. Davies MJ. Anatomic features in victims of sudden coronary death: Coronary artery pathology. *Circulation* 1992;85(1 suppl):I19–I24.
45. Sherrid MV, Mieres J, Mogtader A, et al. Onset during exercise of spontaneous coronary artery dissection and sudden death. *Chest* 1995;108: 284–287.
46. O'Hara GE, Brugada P, Rodriguez LM, et al. Incidence, pathophysiology and prognosis of exercise-induced sustained ventricular tachycardia associated with healed myocardial infarction. *Am J Cardiol* 1992;70:875–878.
47. Siscovick DS, Weiss NS, Fletcher RH, et al. The incidence of primary cardiac arrest during vigorous exercise. *N Engl J Med* 1984;311:874–877.
48. Thompson PD, Funk EJ, Carleton RA, et al. Incidence of death during jogging in Rhode Island from 1975 through 1980. *JAMA* 1982;247: 2535–2538.
49. Ciampricotti R, Deckers JW, Taverne R, et al. Characteristics of conditioned and sedentary men with acute coronary syndromes. *Am J Cardiol* 1994;73:219–222.
50. Siscovick DS, Weiss NS, Fletcher RH, et al. Habitual vigorous exercise and primary cardiac arrest: Effect of other risk factors on the relationship. *J Chronic Dis* 1984;37:625–631.
51. Mittleman MA, Siscovick DS. Physical exertion as a trigger of myocardial infarction and sudden cardiac death. *Cardiol Clin* 1996;14:263–270.
52. Johnson RJ. Sudden death during exercise: A cruel turn of events. *Postgrad Med* 1992;92:195–206.
53. Marcus FI, Fontaine G. Arrhythmogenic right ventricular dysplasia/cardiomyopathy: A review. *PACE* 1995;18:1298–1314.
54. Peters S, Reil GH. Risk factors of cardiac arrest in arrhythmogenic right ventricular dysplasia. *Eur Heart J* 1995;16:77–80.
55. Daubert C, Vauthier M, Carre F, et al. Influence of exercise and sport activity on functional symptoms in ventricular arrhythmias in arrhythmogenic right ventricular disease. *J Am Coll Cardiol* 1994;23:34A. Abstract.
56. Haissaguerre M, Le Metayer P, D'Ivernois C, et al. Distinctive response of arrhythmogenic right ventricular disease to high dose isoproterenol. *PACE* 1990;13(part II):2119–2126.
57. Friman G, Wesslen L, Karjalainen J, et al. Infectious and lymphocytic myocarditis: Epidemiology and factors relevant to sports medicine. *Scand J Med Sci Sports* 1995;5:269–278.
58. Shephard RJ, Shek PN. Infectious diseases in athletes: New interest for an old problem. *J Sports Med Phys Fitness* 1994;34:11–22.
59. Furlanello F, Bertoldi A, Bettini R, et al. Life-threatening tachyarrhythmias in athletes. *PACE* 1992;15:1403–1411.
60. Palatini P, Scanavacca G, Bongiovi S, et al. Prognostic significance of ventricular extrasystoles in healthy professional athletes: Results of a 5-year follow-up. *Cardiology* 1993;82:286–293.

61. Zehender M, Meinertz T, Keul J, et al. ECG variants and cardiac arrhythmias in athletes: Clinical relevance and prognostic importance. *Am Heart J* 1990;119:1378–1391.
62. McGovern BA, Liberthson R. Arrhythmias induced by exercise in athletes and others. *Cardiovasc J Southern Afr* 1996;(suppl 2):C78–82.
63. Zipes DP, Garson A Jr. Task force 6: Arrhythmias. *J Am Coll Cardiol* 1994;24:892–899.
64. Committee on Sports Medicine and Fitness. Cardiac dysrhythmias and sports. *Pediatrics* 1995;95:786–788.
65. Sung RJ, Huycke EC, Lai W, et al. Clinical and electrophysiologic mechanisms of exercise-induced ventricular tachyarrhythmias. *PACE* 1988;11: 1347–1357.
66. Wesley RC Jr, Taylor R, Nadamanee K. Catecholamine-sensitive right ventricular tachycardia in the absence of structural heart disease: A mechanism of exercise-induced cardiac arrest. *Cardiology* 1991;79:237–243.
67. Jordaens L, Missault L, Pelleman G, et al. Comparison of athletes with life-threatening ventricular arrhythmias with two groups of healthy athletes and a group of normal control subjects. *Am J Cardiol* 1994;74: 1124–1128.
68. Wellens HJ, Lemery R, Smeets JL, et al. Sudden arrhythmic death without overt heart disease. *Circulation* 1992;85(1 suppl):I92–97.
69. Moss AJ, Schwartz PJ, Crampton RS, et al. The long QT syndrome: A prospective international study. *Circulation* 1985;71:17–21.
70. Buja G, Folino AF, Bittante M, et al. Asystole with syncope secondary to hyperventilation in three young athletes. *PACE* 1989;12:406–412.
71. Huycke EC, Card HG, Sobol SM, et al. Postexertional cardiac asystole in a young man without organic heart disease. *Ann Intern Med* 1987;106: 844–845.
72. Hirata T, Yano K, Okui T, et al. Asystole with syncope following strenuous exercise in a man without organic heart disease. *J Electrocardiol* 1987;20: 280–283.
73. Bharati S, Lev M. The conduction system findings in sudden cardiac death. *J Cardiovasc Electrophysiol* 1994;5:356–366.
74. Thiene G, Pennelli N, Rossi AL. Cardiac conduction system abnormalities as a possible cause of sudden death in young athletes. *Hum Pathol* 1983;14:704–709.
75. Wang Y, Scheinman MM, Chien WW, et al. Patients with supraventricular tachycardia presenting with aborted sudden death: Incidence, mechanism and long-term follow-up. *J Am Coll Cardiol* 1991;18:1711–1719.
76. Zardini M, Yee R, Thakur RK, et al. Risk of sudden arrhythmic death in Wolff-Parkinson-White syndrome: Current perspectives. *PACE* 1994;17: 966–975.
77. Brembilla-Perrot B, Ghawi R. Electrophysiological characteristics of asymptomatic Wolff-Parkinson-White syndrome. *Eur Heart J* 1993;14:511–515.
78. Crick JCP, Davies DW, Holt P, et al. Effect of exercise on ventricular response to atrial fibrillation in Wolff-Parkinson-White syndrome. *Br Heart J* 1985;54:80–85.
79. Mezzani A, Giovannini T, Michelucci A, et al. Effects of training on the electrophysiologic properties of atrium and accessory pathway in athletes with Wolff-Parkinson-White syndrome. *Cardiology* 1990;77:295–302.

2

Identification of Risk of Cardiac Arrest and Sudden Cardiac Death in Athletes

**Robert J. Myerburg, MD, Raul Mitrani, MD,
Alberto Interian, Jr., MD,
and Agustin Castellanos, MD**

Approaches to the problem of sudden cardiac death (SCD) have broadened in recent years.[1] As it is one of the dominant manifestations of coronary heart disease, epidemiologic considerations of SCD initially began as a derivation from population studies on risk of development, and of clinical manifestations, of coronary atherosclerosis.[2,3] The model expanded with the addition of risk markers such as cardiac arrhythmias after myocardial infarction,[4-6] but epidemiologic concepts specific to SCD as an entity did not develop until recently.[1,7-11] During the past 10 years, attention has expanded beyond studies of population characteristics to include: (1) time relationships between index cardiovascular events and sudden or total cardiovascular mortality; (2) conditioning risk factors for SCD, or the structural basis of risk; (3) transient risk factors, or the identification of triggering events; and (4) response risk, or predetermination of individuals at risk of responding adversely to triggering events (Figure 1).[10] These expanded concepts are relevant

Dr. Myerburg is supported in part by the American Heart Association Chair in Cardiovascular Research at the University of Miami.

From Estes NAM, Salem DN, Wang PJ (eds). *Sudden Cardiac Death in the Athlete.* Armonk, NY: Futura Publishing Co., Inc.;©1998.

EPIDEMIOLOGY OF CARDIAC ARRHYTHMIAS

◎ POPULATION DYNAMICS

    * Classic epidemiology; control of risk factors

◎ TIME-DEPENDENT INFLUENCES

    * Temporal nonuniformity of deaths after index
      cardiovascular events

◎ CONDITIONING RISK FACTORS

    * Risks related to identifiable structural disorders

◎ TRANSIENT RISK FACTORS

    * Dynamic functional changes: Inciting events

◎ RESPONSE RISK

    * Individual clinical susceptibility:
      Random events vs genetic predetermination

Figure 1. Epidemiology of sudden cardiac death. Epidemiologic perspectives range from classic population-based epidemiology to individual susceptibility based on pathophysiologic response characteristics that may be genetically determined. Each of these levels of epidemiologic analysis may contribute to risk profiling. The conditioning and transient risk factors are very closely related to clinical factors. Response risk is an evolving approach based on progress in the genetics of cardiovascular diseases and physiology. Reproduced from Reference 10, with permission from Futura Publishing Co., Inc., Armonk, NY.

for the population generally, as well as for adolescents and young adults—including athletes. In this chapter, current concepts of the epidemiology of SCD among the general population are summarized and application of these principles to younger age groups[12] and to athletes is provided where information is available.

Definition and Magnitude of the Problem

General Population

SCD is defined as unexpected death that occurs instantaneously or up to a maximum of 1 hour (24 hours if not witnessed) after the onset of an abrupt change in clinical status.[8] It accounts for approximately 50% of all cardiac deaths.[2,3,7,8] This represents 300,000 SCD events in the United States each year.[8,9] An order-of-magnitude incidence figure for the adult population 35 years and older, based upon these numbers, is in the range of 0.1% to 0.2% per year (Figure 2).

Despite the significant reduction in cardiovascular mortality during the past 20 to 30 years,[2,7,8] due, at least in part, to public and professional education and attention to control of risk factors for atherosclerosis and coronary artery disease, cardiovascular disease remains the single largest categorical cause of natural death in the Western hemisphere. Moreover, the proportion of deaths which are sudden appears to have remained constant at 50%. The majority of SCDs are caused by acute fatal arrhythmias—ventricular tachycardia/ventricular fibrillation (VT/VF)[8]—and thus, in order to achieve an alteration in cardiovascular death rates attributable to a specific reduction in SCD, the interactions between preventive epidemiology and the pathophysiology of ventricular tachyarrhythmias and fibrillation must be devel-

SUDDEN DEATHS - INCIDENCE AND TOTAL EVENTS

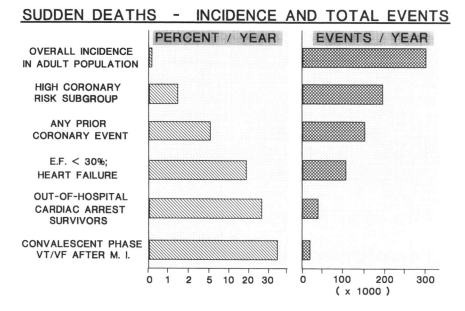

Figure 2. Sudden cardiac deaths among population subgroups. Estimates of incidence (percent per year) and total number of sudden cardiac deaths per year are shown for the overall adult population in the United States and for higher risk subgroups. The overall estimated incidence is 0.1% to 0.2% per year, totaling more than 300,000 deaths per year. Within subgroups identified by increasingly powerful risk factors, the increasing incidence is accompanied by progressively decreasing total numbers. Practical interventions for the larger subgroups will require identification of higher risk clusters within the groups. EF = ejection fraction; MI = myocardial infarction; VT/VF = ventricular tachycardia/ventricular fibrillation. The horizontal axis for the incidence figures is nonlinear. See text for details. Reproduced from Reference 9, with permission from the American Heart Association.

oped as a specific scientific and clinical discipline.[10] However, among the segment of the population who die suddenly with far-advanced heart diseases, the fraction of SCDs caused by mechanisms other than acute tachyarrhythmias (eg, bradyarrhythmias/asystole or pulseless electrical activity) is proportionately higher,[13] representing a different clinical and epidemiologic entity.

Adolescents, Young Adults, and Athletes

Far less epidemiologic data are available for the younger population and athletes than for the general adult population, but it is certain that the sudden *cardiac* death risk is considerably lower—likely in the range of 5 to 10 deaths per 1,000,000 at risk per year (Figure 3). Unfortunately, many of the reports do not distinguish between sudden natural death and sudden unnatural death,[14] and between SCD and sudden natural

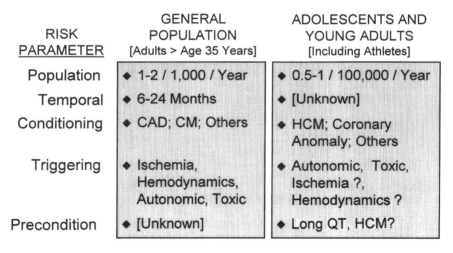

RISK PARAMETER	GENERAL POPULATION [Adults > Age 35 Years]	ADOLESCENTS AND YOUNG ADULTS [Including Athletes]
Population	◆ 1-2 / 1,000 / Year	◆ 0.5-1 / 100,000 / Year
Temporal	◆ 6-24 Months	◆ [Unknown]
Conditioning	◆ CAD; CM; Others	◆ HCM; Coronary Anomaly; Others
Triggering	◆ Ischemia, Hemodynamics, Autonomic, Toxic	◆ Autonomic, Toxic, Ischemia ?, Hemodynamics ?
Precondition	◆ [Unknown]	◆ Long QT, HCM?

Figure 3. Risk profile for sudden cardiac death. The risk parameters outlined in Figure 1 are used to compare the general population of adults >35 years to adolescents and young adults, including athletes, in these younger age groups. Although data are limited, estimates of sudden cardiac death risk in adolescents and young adults are of an order of magnitude less than 1% of the risk attributable to the older age group. No data are available on temporal patterns of cardiac arrest in adolescents and young adults comparable to those in the older groups because of the infrequency of nonfatal index events and the lack of sharply defined onset of disease. The conditioning and triggering parameters appear to differ, although the data for the triggering events are less clear cut than for underlying disease in adults (see text). Preconditioning response risk based on genetically determined susceptibility is well defined in some syndromes in adolescents and young adults, but remains uncertain among the general population. CAD = coronary artery disease; CM = cardiomyopathy; HCM = hypertrophic cardiomyopathy.

death due to noncardiac causes.[15–18] One report approximates the annual incidence of sudden deaths among younger populations in the range of 100 deaths per 1,000,000 population at risk, an estimate that includes traumatic and noncardiac deaths.[14] SCDs were a minority of the events reported. In a study of nontraumatic deaths among athletes, a risk of 7.5 sudden deaths per 1,000,000 male athletes per year and 1.3 per 1,000,000 per year among females was reported.[17] This contrasts with the SCD risk cited for the general adult population $\geq$35 years of age of 1000 to 2000 per 1,000,000 population annually (Figure 3). In addition, the probability that a sudden natural death in adolescents and young adults will be of cardiac origin is smaller than that in older adults. In one study, 19% of sudden natural deaths in children aged 1 to 13 years were due to cardiac causes, while the corresponding figure among the 14- to 21-year age group was 30%.[19] However, the probability that a cardio vascular death will be sudden is proportionally higher when measured as a fraction of total cardiovascular mortality. The distribution of diseases responsible for SCD also differs among different age groups, especially among those under the age of 30 years (see below).

Population Dynamics and the Risk of Life–Threatening Arrhythmias

General Population

Among 5209 men and women in the Framingham, Massachusetts population who were 30 to 59 years of age and free of identified heart disease at baseline observation, a 26-year follow-up demonstrated that SCD accounted for 46% of the coronary heart disease deaths among men and 34% among women.[20] The *incidence* of SCD increased with age, but the *proportion* of coronary heart disease deaths that were sudden and unexpected was greater in the younger age groups. Pooled data from Albany, New York and Framingham, Massachusetts (4120 men) identified SCD as the initial and terminal manifestation of coronary heart disease in more than one half of all sudden death victims.[21] In the Tecumseh, Michigan study of 8641 subjects, 46% of all coronary heart disease deaths occurred within 1 hour of onset of acute symptoms[22]; and in the Yugoslavian cardiovascular disease study involving 6614 men aged 35 to 62 and free of coronary disease at entry, 75% of all coronary deaths occurred suddenly. Two of every three victims had had no documented coronary events prior to death.[11]

Much of the clinical information available on risk of SCD is derived from the highest risk subgroups such as patients with low ejection fractions, a history of heart failure, and survivors of out-of-hospital cardiac arrests. However, when SCD is analyzed in terms of the absolute number of events annually within both the general population and defined subpopulations, it is clear that the majority of SCDs do not come from the highest risk subgroups.[9] Thus, subgroups with the highest case fatality rates have the lowest population attributable risk. In contrast, the larger population subgroups, with much lower relative fatality rates, generate the largest absolute numbers of SCD events because of the size of the population pools from which the events emerge. The magnitude of risk, expressed as incidence, is compared to the total number of events annually under six different conditions as shown in Figure 2. These estimates are based on published epidemiologic and clinical data.[8,9] When the 300,000 SCDs that occur annually among an unselected adult population in the United States is expressed as a fraction of the total adult population, the overall incidence is 0.1% to 0.2% per year. However, after the more easily identified high-risk subgroups are removed from this total population base, the calculated incidence for the remaining population decreases and the identification of specific individuals at risk becomes more difficult. Based on these estimates, a preventive intervention designed for the general adult population would have to be applied to the 999 of 1000 people who will not have an event during the course of a year in order to reach and potentially influence the unidentified 1 of 1000 who will. A model of such limited efficiency prohibits the application of many active interventions[1] and highlights the need for more sensitive and specific markers of risk, which can be applied to large segments of the general population.

The public health relevance of this point lies within the relationship between the size of the denominator in any population pool and the number of events occurring within that subgroup. For example, with escalation from high coronary risk subgroups without prior clinical events (risk = 1% to 2% per year, see Figure 2) to groups with prior coronary events, low ejection fraction and heart failure, or survival after out-of-hospital cardiac arrest, the probability of identifying individuals at higher risk becomes progressively greater, but the absolute number of individuals who can be identified for interventions decreases with each escalation. The relevance for clinical therapeutics embodies a distinction between therapeutic efficacy (relative risk reduction) and efficiency (absolute risk reduction), a distinction which influences interpretation of population impact of clinical intervention trials.[1] Thus, the major challenge resides not simply in the need to focus on the highest risk clinical subgroups, but rather to develop methods which will identify high-risk clusters within subgroups that have lesser degrees of excess risk. Such strategies will provide better resolution of SCD risk, and greater efficiency for preventive and therapeutic interventions. To approach this problem, it is necessary to know the total number of SCDs within a specified population, the fraction of deaths that are sudden, and total mortality. Diagnostic or screening procedures that are easily applied to larger populations and have specific implications for risk of VT/VF or SCD are needed to resolve these population-based limitations.

Adolescents, Young Adults, and Athletes

Limited data are available on the general risk of SCD among this population subgroup. It is appreciated that the absolute numbers are very small relative to the older adult population,[23] and that the probability of a sudden natural death being of cardiac origin increases in adolescence and young adulthood, compared to younger children.[19] Compared to adults ≥35 years of age, who have a cumulative annual risk of 1000 to 2000 per 1,000,000 population, the younger groups have a reported risk of approximately 100 per 1,000,000 at risk. This figure includes traumatic deaths and noncardiac deaths. The rate of cardiac sudden deaths in adolescents and young adults is considerably smaller, likely in the range of 5 to 10 per 1,000,000. Among athletes who died suddenly, the apparent risk was found to be 7.5 per 1,000,000 at risk in males and 1.3 per 1,000,000 among females.[17] The rate was higher among college athletes than among high school athletes. However, noncardiac causes of natural sudden deaths were included, reducing the risk of SCD in male athletes to approximately 5.6 per 1,000,000 at risk, and in female athletes to approximately 0.9 per 1,000,000 at risk. Structural heart disease is usually present in SCD, either identified before the event or characterized during postmortem examination.[15–19]

Time Dependence of Risk

General Population

The risk of SCD after survival of a major change in cardiovascular status is usually nonlinear over time.[1,9] Survival estimates for both SCD and total cardiac mortality demonstrate that the highest secondary death rates occur during the first 6 to 18 months after an index event. By 18 to 24 months, the configurations of survival curves begin to approach the slopes of survival curves that describe a similar population that has remained free of interposed cardiovascular events (Figure 4). The curves may also be influenced by the magnitude of increased risk after an index event. The data from CAST[26,27] demonstrate linear survival curves for the placebo population during long-term follow-up, while data from the multicenter postinfarction program[24,28] demonstrate that subgrouping postmyocardial infarction patients according to increasing risk, based on interaction between premature ventricular contraction (PVC) frequency and ejection fractions, resulted in progressively higher risk as the number and power of risk factors increased. The added mortality in the

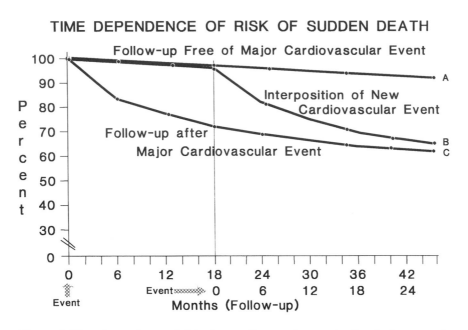

Figure 4. Time dependence of risk after cardiovascular events. Survival curve patterns for patients with known cardiovascular disease free of a major index event (curve A) and for patients surviving major cardiovascular events (curve C). Attrition is accelerated during the initial 6 to 24 months after the event. Curve B shows the dynamics of risk over time in low-risk patients with an interposed major event that is normalized to a time point (for example, 18 months). The subsequent attrition is accelerated for 6 to 24 months. Reproduced from Reference 9, with permission from the American Heart Association.

higher risk subgroups was expressed early. Thus, among the higher risk subgroups, time-dependent risk provides the greatest opportunity for effective intervention strategies in the early period after conditioning cardiovascular events. Mortality patterns having these characteristics have been observed among survivors of out-of-hospital cardiac arrest,[25] among patients with recent onset of heart failure, and among those who have high-risk markers after myocardial infarction.[29] In contrast, data from one of the angiotensin converting enzyme inhibitor trials (SAVE) suggest that mortality benefit, as a result of limiting the delayed onset of cardiac enlargement, is expressed late after the index event.[30] Similarly, a lipid-lowering trial in postmyocardial infarction patients (CARE)[31] also demonstrated late benefit, presumably because of influence on developing structural disease, rather than shorter-term influences.

Time as a dimension for estimating risk must be integrated into strategies designed for population interventions. Ignoring this characteristic of the clinical epidemiology of VT/VF and SCD may preselect study groups that are composed of lower risk components. When merged into a population defined by high-risk characteristics, the predicted risk of the population is diluted by the time dynamics. For instance, studies that permit (or favor) the enrollment of patients more than 12 to 18 months after an index event will be characterized by lower than predicted event rates if late entrants are heavily represented in the study population. The greater the increase in early mortality related to the index event, the greater is the potential for distortion of event rates caused by late entrants.

Adolescents, Young Adults, and Athletes

Although the data are much more limited for these population groups, young survivors of cardiac arrest appear to have similar time relationships for recurrent events.[32] However, the events to which risk is indexed differ in the younger groups. Rather than recent myocardial infarction, onset of heart failure, or unstable angina pectoris, the more common index events are syncope (Figure 5) (see below), onset of new ventricular arrhythmias, acute heart diseases such as myocarditis,

---

SYNCOPE or NEAR SYNCOPE IN ADOLESCENTS AND YOUNG ADULTS

◆ **Neurocardiogenic syncope**

    * Primary vasodepressor

    * Mixed vasodepressor and cardioinhibitory

◆ **Tachycardias without defined heart diseases; benign**

◆ **Life-threatening syndromes**

Figure 5. Causes of syncope in adolescents and young adults. Syncope is a common cardiovascular symptom in adolescents and young adults. The majority of syncopal events are benign and the most common cause is neurocardiogenic syncope. A less common category is the benign tachycardias such as paroxysmal supraventricular tachycardia in patients without defined structural heart disease. The least common category is syncope due to life-threatening syndromes (see text). Electrocardiography and echocardiography can often suggest the presence of specific abnormalities, but the yield from general screening is very low (see text). In this category, the first episode of loss of consciousness may be a fatal arrhythmic event or it may forewarn of a forthcoming event.

and progression of chronic diseases such as hypertrophic cardiomyopathy or right ventricular dysplasia.

Conditioning Risk Factors: The Structural Basis of Sudden Death

In recent years, a distinction has emerged between preconditions for VT/VF (Figure 6) and acute functional events responsible for the initiation of potentially fatal arrhythmias (Figure 7).[1,33] It is now generally agreed that: (1) established structural diseases provide the cardiac substrate for the genesis of VT/VF and SCD in the overwhelming majority of events; and (2) virtually all structural cardiac abnormalities, and likely some functional ones as well, can serve this function. Moreover, new knowledge of the genetic control of ion channel function in cardiac myocytes among patients with congenital long QT interval

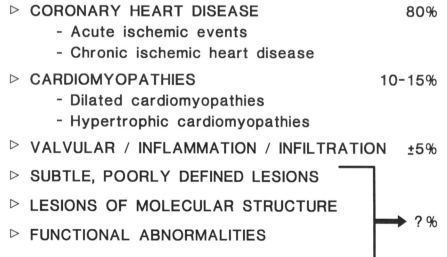

ETIOLOGIC BASIS OF SUDDEN CARDIAC DEATH

▷ CORONARY HEART DISEASE   80%
    - Acute ischemic events
    - Chronic ischemic heart disease

▷ CARDIOMYOPATHIES   10-15%
    - Dilated cardiomyopathies
    - Hypertrophic cardiomyopathies

▷ VALVULAR / INFLAMMATION / INFILTRATION   ±5%

▷ SUBTLE, POORLY DEFINED LESIONS

▷ LESIONS OF MOLECULAR STRUCTURE

▷ FUNCTIONAL ABNORMALITIES   ? %

▷ "NORMAL" HEARTS - IDIOPATHIC VF

Figure 6. Etiologic basis for potentially fatal arrhythmias. Structural heart disease establishes the long-term basis of risk of potentially fatal arrhythmias. It is the conditioning substrate that allows functional abnormalities to initiate a potentially fatal arrhythmia under specific conditions. Collectively, coronary artery disease and the myopathies account for 90% to 95% of the structural causes of sudden cardiac death in the United States. All of the remaining causes listed account for the remainder. Genetically determined abnormalities of structure at a molecular level is a recent addition to the list of identifiable specific causes (eg, long QT interval syndrome). VF = ventricular fibrillation.

TRANSIENT RISK FACTORS

• Ischemia and Reperfusion
> Ischemic Ventricular Tachycardia/Fibrillation
> Initiation of Monomorphic VT by Ischemia
> Reperfusion Arrhythmias

• Systemic Inciting Factors
> Hemodynamic Dysfunction
> Hypoxemia, Acidosis
> Electrolyte Imbalance

• Neurophysiologic Interactions
> Central and Systemic Factors
> Local Cardiac Factors - Transmitters/Receptors

• Toxic Cardiac Effects
> Idiosyncratic Proarrhythmia
> Dose-dependent Proarrhythmia
> Transient Proarrhythmic Risk

Figure 7. Triggering events for cardiac arrest. The four general categories listed include most of the functional factors responsible for initiating cardiac arrest. These factors are responsible for initiating electrophysiologic disturbances which interact with structural preconditions for cardiac arrest. They may also contribute to maintenance of life-threatening arrhythmias after their initiation. VT = ventricular tachycardia.

syndromes[34] now defines structural abnormalities at a molecular level. The principle of a structural basis applies to both general (older) populations and to the younger groups, including athletes. However, the specific structural entities differ greatly.

General Population

Coronary atherosclerosis and its major structural consequences—acute and healed myocardial infarction—constitute the most common structural bases of SCD in the general adult population. Accounting for approximately 80% of SCD events, it was the first category of disease to receive attention, and initially was almost exclusively equated with cause of SCD. More recently, insights have been emerging into other structural abnormalities such as left ventricular hypertrophy and the cardiomyopathies. The role of left ventricular hypertrophy as a risk factor for SCD has been recognized in epidemiologic studies,[35,36] and clinical associations have been described.[37,38] New information on alteration of membrane channel function and arrhythmogenic electrophysiologic changes in hypertrophied myocardium is emerging,[39,40] providing insight into mechanisms by which this structural abnormality may contribute to the genesis of potentially fatal arrhythmias. The fact that regional hypertrophy is common after healing of myocardial infarction[41,42] carries further implications for the role of hypertrophy-related electrical disturbances in the generation of life-threatening arrhythmias.

The proportion of SCDs caused by the various etiologies approximates the prevalence estimates of various cardiac diseases. Thus, 80% of SCDs are associated with coronary artery disease, 10% to 15% with the various cardiomyopathies, and only small fractions by the less common disorders (see Figure 6). However, the small numbers of less

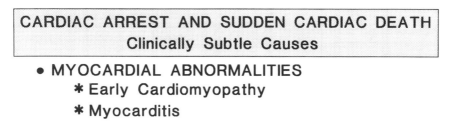

CARDIAC ARREST AND SUDDEN CARDIAC DEATH
Clinically Subtle Causes

- MYOCARDIAL ABNORMALITIES
  - * Early Cardiomyopathy
  - * Myocarditis
  - * Left Ventricular Hypertrophy

- VENTRICULAR DYSPLASTIC SYNDROMES

- MYOCARDIAL ISCHEMIA/REPERFUSION
  - * Coronary Artery Spasm
  - * Anomalous Origin of Coronary Arteries

- VASCULAR ABNORMALITIES (eg, Marfan syndrome)

- MITRAL VALVE PROLAPSE (?)

- UNRECOGNIZED ACCESSORY PATHWAYS

Figure 8. Clinically subtle causes of cardiac arrest. Among the group of cardiac arrest and sudden cardiac death victims without coronary artery disease or defined cardiomyopathies, a small subgroup has clinically subtle causes which may be difficult to define clinically or even pathologically. Among these are early cardiomyopathies and myocarditis. Left ventricular hypertrophy (without a defined hypertrophic cardiomyopathy) may be a contributing factor, but the risk distinction between left ventricular hypertrophy and hypertrophic cardiomyopathy has not yet been clearly defined. Among the other causes are ventricular dysplasias, myocardial ischemia due to coronary artery spasm or anomalous origin of coronary arteries, and perhaps mitral valve prolapse. Undiagnosed accessory pathways may also be a cause.

common diseases (Figure 8) often provide excellent models for understanding pathophysiology, and commonly affect younger individuals without a variety of comorbid states. Their recognition clinically is important beyond their numbers because the affected individuals can often survive long-term if the conditions are recognized and therapy is initiated before an unexpected fatal event.

Most of the major studies of risk factors for SCD have focused upon this etiologic category because coronary heart disease accounts for approximately 80% of SCDs in Western societies.[8] Data from multiple studies have demonstrated a concordance between risk factors for coronary atherosclerosis, total cardiovascular mortality, and SCD.[2,3,12,43,44] In most studies, approximately 50% of all deaths related to coronary heart disease are sudden and unexpected, although proportions of sudden deaths to nonsudden deaths may vary as a function of the severity of left ventricular dysfunction and functional impairment.[45] Among patients who have cardiomyopathies, those with better preserved functional capacity (Functional Classes I and II) have lower total death rates, but the fraction of all deaths that are sudden and unexpected is higher. Among class IV patients, total death rates are higher, but the fraction that are sudden is lower. There is a *competing risk* between sudden and nonsudden deaths, which implies that the extent to which SCD mortality improvement will influence total mortality may be inherently limited by other mechanisms of death.[1,10,46]

For patients with coronary heart disease, the evolution of the structural abnormalities that condition risk are the physical expression of conventional coronary risk factors. The magnitude of risk relates well to the number of risk factors present. In the Framingham study,[8] there was a 14-fold increase in risk from the lowest risk decile to the highest risk decile; and in the Yugoslavian cardiovascular disease study, the probability of SCD was 11 times higher in the top quintile than in the bottom quintile of multivariate risk distribution.[20] Thus, risk factors such as age, family history, gender, cigarette smoking, the hypertension/hypertrophy complex, hyperlipidemias, and the other conventional coronary risk factors provide easily identifiable markers for risk of SCD. These markers may be viewed as static because of their potential to be continuously present over time. Their limitation is that they primarily identify the risk of developing the underlying disease responsible for SCD, rather than for the pathophysiologic event responsible for its expression. The ability of conventional risk factors to identify high-risk subgroups in epidemiologic terms is unquestioned; and it is likely that for some of these risk factors, active preventive interventions will influence risk and significantly alter the number of events occurring among the population. However, pathophysiologic susceptibility does not necessarily equate with risk of developing structural heart disease risk (see below), and thus the ability of these long-term risk factors to identify specific individuals who will manifest VT/VF or SCD is limited. Therefore, while conventional risk factors relate well to the anatomic basis for VT/VF and SCD and provide important preventive opportunities, they lack the specific focus required for efficient preventive strategies in large subgroups and in individual patients.

A higher power of risk is provided by the presence of established structural abnormalities. When present, they constitute the substrate upon which triggering events (Figure 7) can initiate unstable cardiac electrophysiologic disturbances. The clinical recognition of structural disease defines individual risk much more specifically than do the conventional risk factors for coronary artery disease. At a different level of resolution, specific myocardial pathways that form the myocardial structural support for VT or VF (ie, potential reentrant circuits) have been well studied.[47] These might provide a much more specific anatomic description of risk but lack direct clinical or epidemiologic accessibility short of extensive and costly testing techniques.

Adolescents, Young Adults, and Athletes

The structural conditioning risk basis for SCD in younger populations differ markedly from the general population and older groups. In people under the age of 30 years, coronary atherosclerosis is a minor contributor among the causes of SCD. It is replaced by the cardiomyopathies, especially the hypertrophic forms, as the most common cause among athletes, with a wide array of other entities included on the list (Figure 8).[48] For unselected children and younger adolescents, the relative proportion of the hypertrophic cardiomyopathies is smaller, and myocarditis, coronary artery anomalies, dysplastic syndromes, and long QT interval syndromes are relatively more common (Figure 9).[15–18] Since many of these entities are familial, degenerative, and progressive (but often clinically subtle), case findings and preventive measures are important but often difficult. Even among patients who present with ventricular tachyarrhythmias

---

Figure 9. Age-frequency distribution of various etiologies of sudden cardiac death. The vertical order of the listed causes of sudden cardiac death reflects the relative frequency of each, with atherosclerosis far ahead of all others. The horizontal bars

A. Adolescents and Young Adults

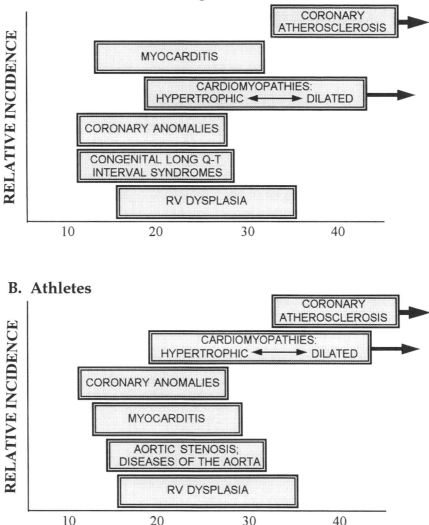

B. Athletes

indicate the age range of preponderance of each of these causes. **A.** Unselected adolescents and young adults. Myocarditis and the cardiomyopathies are the most commonly reported causes. Hypertrophic cardiomyopathy is more common in the younger age range, and dilated, in the older. Coronary artery anomalies follow, except in the very young (ages 10 to 15 years), where it is a more common cause. **B.** Athletes. Coronary artery disease dominates from the early- to mid-30s, and prior to that, hypertrophic cardiomyopathy is the most common cause after the early teenage years, where coronary artery anomalies appear to be more frequent. RV = right ventricular.

and apparently normal hearts, identification of subtle abnormalities is likely, if sought carefully.[49] Recent progress in genetic characterization is providing new approaches, and promises further insights for the future.[34] Warning symptoms for the causes of SCD in these groups are different than those in older groups. The onset of syncopal events, particularly exercise related, is of particular concern. As demonstrated in Figure 5, the causes of most syncopal events in younger individuals are benign, but the subgroup of concern, although small, are those who have causes predictive of (or caused by) life-threatening arrhythmias. This includes a sizeable list of infrequent disorders (Figure 10), for most of which, a screening electrocardiogram (ECG), although imperfect, may provide clues to the presence of the disease.

SYNCOPE AND NEAR SYNCOPE IN ADOLESCENTS AND YOUNG ADULTS: Life-Threatening syndromes

Long QT interval syndromes

Right ventricular dysplasia/cardiomyopathy

Wolff-Parkinson-White syndrome

Cardiomyopathies, hypertrophic or dilated

Coronary vascular anomalies

Inflammatory and infiltrative diseases

Other polymorphic tachycardias,
     including drug-induced

Idiopathic ventricular fibrillation

Figure 10. Life-threatening causes of syncope in adolescents, young adults, and athletes. A broad variety of cardiac disorders may cause warning syncopal events in patients subject to potentially fatal arrhythmias. Collectively, the listed syndromes contribute only a small number to total population of young adults and athletes who have syncopal events, but their life-threatening nature should be actively sought in unexplained or uncertain cases.

Transient Risk Factors

When used in reference to the triggering of VT/VF or SCD, transient risk indicates a time-limited and unpredictable event or state that has the potential to initiate, or allow the initiation of, an unstable electrophysiologic condition (Figure 7). The term *unstable* is used to indicate an increased probability of transition from a normal or benign cardiac rhythm to a potentially fatal VT or VF. Historically, the relationship between PVCs and the initiation of VT/VF was the first use of the concept. The PVC hypothesis evolved as an expression of the premise that PVCs serve a primary triggering function for the initiation of VT/VF, and presumed that PVC suppression would protect against SCD by eliminating the electrophysiologic triggers. Despite consistent data supporting chronic PVCs as a risk factor for SCD in patients with underlying heart disease,[4–6,28] special circumstances are required to demonstrate the initiation of life-threatening arrhythmias by PVCs. Ambulatory recordings of the spontaneous onset of cardiac arrest show a tendency to increases in sinus rate *and* PVC frequency prior to VF,[50–52] likely reflecting a change in sympathetic tone or hemodynamic status functioning as an intermediary in the PVC-VT/VF relationship. This supports the concept of a role for active transient influences in establishing the pathophysiologic conditions for potentially fatal arrhythmias, as opposed to simple fortuitous relationships between chronic PVCs and steady-state structural abnormalities. Transient pathophysiologic changes are proposed as the factor(s) that convert ventricular myocardium from a stable to unstable state at a specific point in time, permitting the genesis of potentially fatal arrhythmias by a definable relationship between acute pathophysiologic changes and chronic abnormalities (Figures 6 and 7). After recognizing that the PVC-VT/VF relationship generally required structural conditioning factors, clinical investigators and physiologists began to study the factors that are directly responsible for the initiation of fatal arrhythmias at a specific point in time. The transient nature of these events makes their prospective elucidation a difficult clinical and epidemiologic chore. Although the general principle of triggering events applies to both the general population and to the younger subgroups, including athletes, the specific triggers differ.

General Population

The most common triggering mechanism among the adult population appears to be myocardial ischemia. The development of a base of experimental information on the role of myocardial ischemia in creating an electrophysiologic risk of VT/VF first led to the concept of an initiating or transitional event, in which the role of PVCs in the initiation of VT/VF could be defined by a predictable set of circumstances.[47] Subsequently, other functional perturbations received attention. Intense functional changes alone may destabilize this system in the absence of structural abnormalities; but the vast majority of cardiac arrests occur in hearts with preceding structural abnormalities. As shown in Figure 7, the major functional influences or categories of transient risk factors may be separated into four groups: (1) ischemia and reperfusion; (2) systemic abnormalities; (3) autonomic factors; and (4) cardiotoxic factors, including the general problem of proarrhythmia. While each of these categories can be viewed as a clinical event or pathophysiologic influence, they are now starting to be modeled and applied as measurable epidemiologic risk factors.[53,54]

Transient Ischemia and Reperfusion

Ischemia occurring at the onset and during the early phase of acute myocardial infarction has a clearly established clinical and experimental association with potentially fatal arrhythmias. However, the majority of SCD victims and survivors of out-of-hospital cardiac arrest do not have acute transmural myocardial infarctions.[55] Approximately 80% of SCDs due to coronary heart disease are *not* associated with acute myocardial infarction,[56] and it is assumed that transient acute ischemia is one of the major triggering factors. However, its transient nature has precluded systematic clinical and epidemiologic studies. Unstable angina pectoris and silent myocardial ischemia also appear to have the capability to initiate potentially fatal arrhythmias,[57–60] although there is only limited clinical documentation of such mechanisms.[61] Both are associated with a statistical increase in the risk of SCD when they accompany preexisting coronary artery disease.

Clinical and epidemiologic data indicating associations between ischemia and potentially fatal arrhythmia are paralleled by experimental data that demonstrate adverse effects of ischemia, especially in the presence of a prior myocardial infarction. For example, a study in dogs with healed myocardial infarction was designed to determine the arrhythmogenic effects of graded reductions in blood flow through a non-infarct–related artery. The study demonstrated that lesser decreases in blood flow resulted in inducible VT or spontaneous VF in the presence of a prior myocardial infarction compared to controls without a prior infarction.[62] These and other[47] experimental data are providing insight into mechanisms responsible for ischemia-mediated arrhythmias. Techniques range from intact in situ hearts to specific membrane channel characteristics studied in isolated myocytes, and serve both as explanations for the deranged electrophysiology and as targets for treatment. In addition, the epidemiologic impact of left ventricular hypertrophy, especially in the presence of coronary artery disease and prior myocardial infarction, is paralleled by observations of specific channel abnormalities in hypertrophied myocytes, some of which become manifest primarily during ischemia. These observations include differences in ATP-sensitive K^+ channels during ischemia in the hypertrophied myocardium compared to normal, and between endocardium and epicardium in normal hearts,[63] as well as changes in Ca^{++} and K^+ currents under conditions of metabolic inhibition as a surrogate for ischemia.[64] Thus, some of the epidemiologic factors that increase risk of SCD are paralleled by abnormalities at the level of membrane channels, which could serve as an explanation for increased risk. While the interaction between epidemiology and membrane physiology is only in its infancy, these relationships warrant further exploration.

Transient ischemia enhances susceptibility to sustained ventricular arrhythmias; and in addition, the role of subsequent or concomitant reperfusion of ischemic muscle is beginning to be clarified. Reperfusion appears to induce electrical instability by several different mechanisms, both reentrant[64] and triggered activity.[40] The former is characterized by rapid electrical activity, which may be due to abrupt changes in refractoriness,[65] while the latter is due to generation of afterdepolarizations, which are experimentally sensitive to Ca^{++} blockade.[66] Hypertrophied myocytes appear to be more prone to generate reperfusion-induced early afterdepolarizations and triggered activity than are normal myocytes, apparently due to depressed delayed rectifier current (I_k) in the hypertrophied myocyte.[40] In situ studies of the frequency of VF during ischemia and reperfusion in previously hypertrophied hearts support the potential clinical relevance of such data.[67]

Systemic Mechanisms of Transient Risk

Acute or subacute systemic abnormalities modulate chronic structural cardiac abnormalities, influencing electrophysiologic stability and susceptibility to VT/VF and SCD.[68] Among the larger studies of survivors of out-of-hospital cardiac arrest, small subgroups have had recognizable reversible systemic abnormalities which contributed to the life-threatening arrhythmias. When transient systemic factors can be identified *and* predictably controlled, no other preventive interventions against recurrences are required.[56] Hypoxemia, acidosis, and electrolyte imbalances may all contribute to destabilization[69–72]; these factors are commonly clinically recognized and reversible with appropriate therapy. Clues regarding the mechanisms by which these forms of transient risk may influence electrophysiology are beginning to evolve. For instance, in myocytes from globally hypertrophied hearts, conductance through ATP-sensitive K^+ channels may be increased by a reduction in pH.[72] When a hypertrophied heart becomes regionally ischemic and acidotic, this characteristic may cause dispersion of electrophysiologic properties, thereby predisposing to reentrant ventricular arrhythmias. Chronic electrolyte disturbances, most prominently hypokalemia associated with long-term use of diuretics, are associated with an increased risk of cardiovascular mortality.[70] Hypokalemia as a cause or contributor to the initiation of polymorphic VT and torsade de pointes is well recognized,[71,73] most commonly in patients with chronically abnormal hearts and in the presence of class I antiarrhythmic drugs and other proarrhythmic substances.

Transient hemodynamic dysfunction in patients with abnormal hearts is likely among the most common of the systemic inciting factors. However, this mechanism is difficult to study clinically in a controlled manner. Severe acute or subacute hemodynamic deterioration may cause a secondary cardiac arrest, which has long been known to carry a very high short-term mortality rate.[69,74] However, the less well-defined relationship between chronically impaired left ventricular function, acute modulations in hemodynamic status, and predisposition to VT/VF is an important focus for the future. It has been shown experimentally that volume loading of isolated perfused canine left ventricles shortens refractory periods,[75,76] and regional disparity in hearts with prior myocardial infarction has been demonstrated.[76] Stretch-induced modulation of membrane channels may play a role in such changes. Clinical studies to define such mechanisms have been limited to date.

Autonomic Fluctuations and Transient Risk

Systemic, central nervous system, and local cardiac neurophysiologic factors are receiving increasing attention as markers for identifying high-risk subgroups and for elucidating mechanisms of fatal arrhythmias.[77] At a local myocardial level, an increasing body of experimental information[78–84] and limited clinical data[85–92] suggest that prior myocardial infarction and other cardiac abnormalities predisposing to SCD are accompanied by changes in cardiac autonomic function. Several patterns of altered regional responses to sympathetic stimulation have been reported in different myocardial infarction models.[78,79,81] Regionally altered β-adrenoceptor numbers and changes in coupling proteins and in adenylate cyclase activity have been observed in hearts with healed myocardial infarction.[83] Experimental and clinical imaging studies have also shown disruption of myocardial sympathetic innervation after acute myocardial infarction, with apparent reinnervation after convalescence.[78,80,81,84] Clinically, isoproterenol-dependent induction of sustained VT among cardiac arrest survivors, and its prevention by β-adrenoceptor blocking drugs,[90] suggest a role for autonomic stimuli in the genesis of potentially fatal arrhythmias.

At a systemic level, qualitative and quantitative estimates of neurophysiologic alterations that may modulate cardiac activity have been proposed as a means of identifying subgroups at increased risk for SCD. Changes in heart rate variability or baroreceptor sensitivity have been studied in selected subgroups. Among myocardial infarction survivors[85–89] and survivors of out-of-hospital cardiac arrest, altered heart rate variability has been suggested as a marker for SCD risk. Power spectrum analysis of heart rate variability in the frequency domain has suggested specific patterns that identify high-risk subgroups,[88] and short-term frequency domain patterns differ before the onset of sustained VT compared to nonsustained VT.[89] A blunted baroreceptor response to phenylephrine infusion has also been suggested as a marker to identify subgroups at risk for SCD and VT after myocardial infarction.[86] An association between sinus node rate immediately following the onset of sustained VT, and the electrophysiologic and hemodynamic stability of the VT, has been reported.[92] In patients with stable VT, sinus node rate during V-A dissociation increases progressively during the first 30 seconds of VT. When VT is unstable, sinus node rate increases more rapidly during the initial 5 seconds of VT, and then decreases abruptly. A role for autonomic dysfunction, either as a cause of or a consequence of the arrhythmia pattern, has been suggested. Finally, autonomic mechanisms have been proposed as explanation for some patterns of nonischemic arrhythmias[93] and deaths during intense environmental stresses.[94] These diverse observations provide strong arguments for abnormal patterns of autonomic function as a controlling factor in risk of VT/VF and SCD.

Effects of Exogenous Substances on the Heart

The risk of VF during chloroform anesthesia was the first recognized relationship between a clinically used substance and potentially fatal arrhythmias.[95,96] Subsequently, relationships between antiarrhythmic drugs and proarrhythmic events, initially described in terms of the risk of torsade de pointes and VF during quinidine therapy,[97] identified a specific clinical circumstance in the ambulatory setting. It is now recognized that classic proarrhythmic responses of this type may occur with any of the class IA antiarrhythmic drugs as well as the class III drugs. More subtle but possibly quite important is the emerging number of clinically used substances other than antiarrhythmic drugs that are recognized to have induced similar proarrhythmic responses. These include such diverse categories of medications as erythromycin, pentamidine, a number of the psychotropic drugs, and ter-fenadine.[98] In addition, limited clinical data suggest an effect on QT interval and the risk of torsade de pointes in the susceptible individual for such diverse other substances as organic phosphate insecticides, cocaine,[99] probucol,[100] and haloperidol.[101] For many of these substances, limited data at this time suggest that the offending substances prolong QT intervals by an effect on repolarizing currents, such as the delayed rectifier current I_K (I_{kR}).[98,99] The combination of an inherent ability of a substance to prolong action potential duration and specific patterns of individual susceptibility to this effect may explain the sporadic occurrence of these responses. It follows that identification of an offending channel effect coupled with an ability to identify individual susceptibility might provide a method to identify risk prospectively. Unfortunately, since such events are more common in patients with underlying heart disease, the distinction between a proarrhythmic response and a confounding clinical arrhythmia caused by the underlying disease is difficult at the present time.

Adolescents, Young Adults, and Athletes

In athletes, and likely among adolescents and young adults generally, functional triggering events appear to relate to the effects of autonomic activity. Exercise-induced shifts in sympathetic and parasympathetic activity occurring at the onset of physical stress, at peak exercise spurts, and after abrupt cessation of activity may initiate electrophysiologic changes in the individual who is susceptible because of an existing conditional basis. The fact that SCD is most common in sports characterized by high-intensity surges of activity[48] supports this concept. However, a study of sudden death risk during marathon runs in unscreened populations has demonstrated that the risk associated with this form of intense exertion is small (1 in 50,000).[102] This supports the concept that a structural substrate is generally required for risk to be expressed, and possibly that the *form* of stress (ie, surges) may also be important, as discussed earlier.

Transient ischemia in SCD in this age group is far less common but nonetheless occurs, particularly among those with some patterns of myocardial bridging[103,104] and congenital coronary artery abnormalities,[104,105] coronary artery spasm,[61] and perhaps the hypertrophic cardiomyopathies. In some forms of the congenital long QT interval syndrome and some degenerative diseases such as right ventricular dysplasia, acute exertion may have a role in the initiation of cardiac arrest. Finally, exogenous substances, particularly cocaine, which can produce a quinidine-like proarrhythmia, may cause sudden death in the young.[99]

Response Variables: Identification
of the Susceptible Individual

The concept of response risk is an attempt to introduce principles of epidemiology to the disciplines of cardiac electrophysiology and myocardial cell membrane function. It refers to the mechanisms by which a *specific individual,* among a subgroup with an established conditioning risk factor (eg, coronary heart disease, left ventricular hypertrophy, congenital long QT interval syndrome), generates arrhythmias when exposed to transient functional risk influences. Based on the premises that the conditioning factors create a persistent substrate for arrhythmic risk and the transient functional factors serve an initiating role (see Figure 7), the epidemiologic question focuses on the identification of those subjects whose inherent physiologic characteristics make the initiation of electrophysiologic instability more likely when these conditions are met. It requires clinically identifiable, genetically based, or acquired individual differences in the responses of membrane channels or receptors in the susceptible individual. In "idiosyncratic" proarrhythmic responses to class IA antiarrhythmic drugs, excessive prolongation of repolarization and generation of torsade de pointes occurs in 1% to 3% of the exposed population. This subgroup, which appears to have a specific susceptibility, may have exaggerated depression of I_{kR}, creating individual susceptibility.[106] The ability to identify abnormal response characteristics of specific channels or receptors under a variety of pathophysiologic conditions holds the promise of identifying individuals at risk for potentially fatal arrhythmias under conditions of specific substance exposures. This extends beyond proarrhythmic effects of antiarrhythmic drugs to include factors such as the response of specific channels to ischemia and reperfusion[39,106,107] and the response of previously conditioned hearts to other stimuli in the environment (eg, cocaine) that can influence specific ion channel function.[99] Therefore, the ability to identify specific individuals who are at risk of responding abnormally to a specific transient stimulus offers the hope of providing increased power for epidemiologic resolution of risk within large population groups.

Conclusions

Classic epidemiology has provided a great deal of useful information regarding the risk of life-threatening ventricular arrhythmias, SCD, and possible approaches to their prevention. The additional emphasis on specific subgroup characteristics, the relationship between absolute numbers and relative risk, and the temporal modulation of risk add power to available epidemiologic information. Continued resolution of the problems of VT/VF and SCD, and their control, will require an interaction with other disciplines, both clinical and basic. Among adolescents and young adults, and athletes in particular, the low prevalence of disease makes efficient screening programs difficult. Even among those with identifiable structural abnormalities, the low incidence of life-threatening arrhythmic events adds to the difficulty of identification of individuals at risk.[108] In addition, the apparent absence of structural abnormalities in the adolescent, young adult, or athlete with symptoms such as palpitations, near syncope, or syncope may mandate an aggressive search for evidence of diverse conditions.[109,110] Even so, risk of idiopathic VF[111,112] may fail to be identified prospectively (Figure 11). The development of innovative screening tools to find susceptible individuals is particularly pressing for this seg-

SUDDEN CARDIAC DEATH IN THE APPARENT ABSENCE OF STRUCTURAL HEART DISEASE

▷ TRANSIENT TRIGGERING EVENTS

  • Toxic, Metabolic, Electrolye Imbalance

  • Autonomic, Neurophysiologic

  • Ischemia/Reperfusion; Hemodynamic

▷ HIGH-RISK REPOLARIZATION ABNORMALITIES

  • Congenital Long QT Interval Syndromes

  • Acquired Long QT Interval Syndromes
    Proarrhythmic drugs; drug interactions

▷ CLINICALLY SUBTLE HEART DISEASE

  • Unrecognized

  • Unrecognizable

▷ IDIOPATHIC VENTRICULAR FIBRILLATION

Figure 11. Sudden cardiac death in the apparent absence of structural heart disease. The adolescent, young adult, or athlete with symptomatic palpitations, near syncope, or syncope in the apparent absence of structural abnormalities, may have a variety of conditions known to confer risk of SCD. Idiopathic ventricular fibrillation is included among those individuals in whom no apparent cause has been identified after survival of a cardiac arrest.

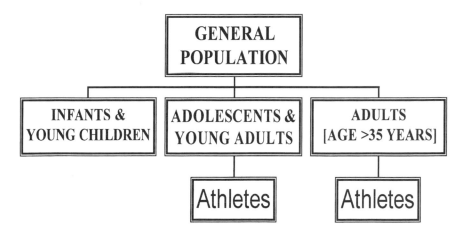

Figure 12. Risk of sudden death among specific population subgroups. Risk of SCD is usually expressed in terms of the general population and the sudden infant death risk subgroup. However, the epidemiology differs across the three subgroups shown, and the risk factors, causes, and characteristics for adolescent and young adult athletes differ from older athletes (see text).

ment of the population, which must be treated as a specific epidemiologic subgroup distinct from the general population of adults ≥35 years of age (Figure 12).

References

1. Myerburg RJ, Kessler KM, Castellanos A. Sudden cardiac death: Epidemiology, transient risk, and intervention assessment. *Ann Intern Med* 1993;119:1187–1197.
2. *Report of the Working Group on Arteriosclerosis of the National Heart, Lung, and Blood Institute (Volume 2): Patient Oriented Research—Fundamental and Applied, Sudden Cardiac Death.* DHEW. NIH Publication No. 83–2035. Washington, DC: US Government Printing Office; 1981;114–122.
3. Epstein FH, Pisa Z. International comparisons in ischemic heart disease mortality. *Proc Conf on the Decline in Coronary Heart Disease Mortality.* DHEW. NIH Publication No. 79–1610. Washington, DC: US Government Printing Office; 1979;58–88.
4. Vismara LA, Amsterdam BA, Mason DT. Relation of ventricular arrhythmias in the late-hospital phase of acute myocardial infarction to sudden death after hospital discharge. *Am J Med* 1975;59:6–12.
5. Ruberman W, Weinblatt M, Goldberg JD, et al. Ventricular premature complexes and sudden death after myocardial infarction. *Circulation* 1981;64:297–305.
6. Schulze RA, Strauss HW, Pitt B. Sudden death in the year following myocardial infarction: Relationship of ventricular premature contractions in the late hospital phase and left ventricular ejection fraction. *Am J Med* 1977;62:192–199.

7. Gillum RF. Sudden coronary deaths in the United States, 1980–1985. *Circulation* 1989;79:756–765.
8. Myerburg RJ, Castellanos A. Cardiac arrest and sudden cardiac death. In Braunwald E (ed): *Heart Disease: A Textbook of Cardiovascular Medicine, 4th Edition.* New York: W.B. Saunders Co.; 1997:742–779.
9. Myerburg RJ, Kessler KM, Castellanos A. Sudden cardiac death: Structure, function, and time-dependence of risk. *Circulation* 1992;85(suppl I):I2–I10.
10. Myerburg RJ, Kessler KM, Castellanos A. Epidemiology of sudden cardiac death: Population characteristics, conditioning risk factors, and dynamic risk factors. In Spooner PM, Brown AM, Catterall WA, et al. (eds): *Ion Channels in the Cardiovascular System.* Armonk, NY: Futura Publishing Co.; 1994:15–33.
11. Demirovic J. *Risk Factors in the Incidence of Sudden Cardiac Death and Possibilities for its Prevention.* Belgrade, YU: University of Belgrade; University of Belgrade Press; 1985. Thesis.
12. Liberthson RR. Sudden death from cardiac causes in children and young adults. *N Engl J Med* 1996;334:1039–1044.
13. Luu M, Stevenson WG, Stevenson LW, et al. Diverse mechanisms of unexpected cardiac arrest in advanced heart failure. *Circulation* 1991;80:1675–1680.
14. Kuisma M, Suominen P, Korpela R. Paediatric out-of-hospital cardiac arrests: Epidemiology and outcome. *Resuscitation* 1995;30:141–150.
15. Anderson RE, Hill RB, Broudy DW, et al. A population-based autopsy study of sudden, unexpected deaths from natural causes among persons 5 to 39 years old during a 12-year period. *Hum Pathol* 1994;25:1332–1340.
16. Whittington RM, Banerjee A. Sport-related sudden natural death in the city of Birmingham. *J Royal Soc Med* 1994;87:18–21.
17. Van Camp SP, Bloor CM, Mueller FO, et al. Nontraumatic sports death in high school and college athletes. *Med Sci Sports Exerc* 1995;27(5):641–647.
18. Steinberger J, Lucas RV Jr, Edwards JE, Titus JL. Causes of sudden unexpected cardiac death in the first two decades of life. *Am J Cardiol* 1996;77:992–995.
19. Neuspiel DR, Kuller LH. Sudden and unexpected natural death in childhood and adolescence. *JAMA* 1985;254:1321–1325.
20. Kannel WB, Thomas HE. Sudden coronary death: The Framingham study. *Ann N Y Acad Sci* 1982;382:3–21.
21. Doyle JT, Kannel WB, McNamara RM, et al. Factors related to suddenness of death from coronary heart disease: Combined Albany-Framingham Studies. *Am J Cardiol* 1976;37:1073–1078.
22. Chiang B, Perlman HV, Fulton M, et al. Predisposing factor in sudden cardiac death in Tecumseh, Michigan: A prospective study. *Circulation* 1970;41:31–37.
23. Klitzer TS. Sudden cardiac death in children. *Circulation* 1990;82:629–632.
24. Bigger JT. Antiarrhythmic therapy: An overview after myocardial infarction. *Am J Cardiol* 1984;53:8B–16B.
25. Furukawa T, Rozanski JJ, Nogami A, et al. Time-dependent risk of and predictors for cardiac arrest recurrence in survivors of out-of-hospital cardiac arrest with chronic coronary artery disease. *Circulation* 1989;80:599–608.
26. The Cardiac Arrhythmia Suppression Trial (CAST) Investigators. Preliminary Report: Effect of encainide and flecainide on mortality in a random-

ized trial of arrhythmia suppression after myocardial infarction. *N Engl J Med* 1989;331:406–412.

27. Echt DS, Liebson PR, Mitchell B, et al, and the CAST Investigators. Mortality and morbidity in patients receiving encainide, flecainide, or placebo. The Cardiac Arrhythmias Suppression Trial. *N Engl J Med* 1991;324: 781–788.

28. Bigger JT, Fleiss JL, Kleiger R, et al, and the Multicenter Post-Infarction Research Group. The relationships among ventricular arrhythmias, left ventricular dysfunction, and mortality in the 2 years after myocardial infarction. *Circulation* 1984;69:250–258.

29. Schechtman KB, Bipone RJ, Kleiger RE, et al, and the Diltiazem Reinfarction Study Research Group. Risk stratification of patients with non-Q wave myocardial infarction. *Circulation* 1989;80:1148–1158.

30. Pfeffer MA, Braunwald E, Moye LA, et al, and the SAVE Investigators. The effect of captopril on mortality and morbidity in patients with left ventricular dysfunction after myocardial infarction: Results of the survival and ventricular enlargement trial. *N Engl J Med* 1992;327:669–677.

31. Sacks FM, Pfeffer MA, Moye LA, et al, for the Cholesterol and Recurrent Events Trial Investigators. The effect of pravastatin on coronary events after myocardial infarction in patients with average cholesterol levels. *N Engl J Med* 1996;335:1001–1009.

32. Silka MJ, Kron J, Walance CG, et al. Assessment and follow-up of pediatric survivors of sudden cardiac death. *Circulation* 1990;82:341–349.

33. Myerburg RJ, Kessler KM, Bassett AL, Castellanos A. A biological approach to sudden cardiac death: Structure, function and cause. *Am J Cardiol* 1989;63:1512–1516.

34. Roden DM, George AL, Bennett PB. Recent advances in understanding the molecular mechanisms of the long Q-T syndrome. *J Cardiol Electrophysiol* 1995;6:1023–1031.

35. Kannel WB, Thomas HE. Sudden coronary death: The Framingham Study. *Ann N Y Acad Sci* 1982;38:3–21.

36. Cupples LA, Gagnon DR, Kannel WB. Long- and short-term risk of sudden coronary death. *Circulation* 1992;85(suppl I):I11–I18.

37. Anderson KP. Sudden death, hypertension, and hypertrophy. *J Cardiovasc Pharmacol* 1984;6(suppl III):S498–S503.

38. Messerli FH, Ventura HO, Elizardi DJ, et al. Hypertension and sudden increased ventricular ectopic activity in left ventricular hypertrophy. *Am J Med* 1984;77:18–22.

39. Furukawa T, Myerburg RJ, Furukawa N, et al. Ionic mechanism of increased susceptibility of hypertrophied feline myocytes to metabolic inhibition. *Circulation* 1990;82(suppl III):III522. Abstract.

40. Furukawa T, Bassett AL, Kimura S, et al. The ionic mechanism of reperfusion-induced early afterdepolarizations in feline left ventricular hypertrophy. *J Clin Invest* 1993;91:1521–1531.

41. Ginzton LE, Conant R, Rodrigues DM, Laks MM. Functional significance of hypertrophy of the non-infarcted myocardium after myocardial infarction in humans. *Circulation* 1989;80:816–822.

42. Cox MM, Berman I, Myerburg RJ, et al. Morphometric mapping of regional myocyte diameters after healing of myocardial infarction in cats. *J Mol Cell Cardiol* 1991;23:127–135.

43. Kannel WB, Doyle JT, McNamara PM, et al. Precursors of sudden coronary death: Factors related to the incidence of sudden death. *Circulation* 1979;51:606–613.

44. Kuller LH. Sudden death: Definition and epidemiologic considerations. *Prog Cardiovasc Dis* 1980;23:1–12.
45. Kjekshus J. Arrhythmias and mortality in congestive heart failure. *Am J Cardiol* 1990;65:42I–48I.
46. Myerburg RJ, Kessler KM, Kimura S, Castellanos A. Sudden cardiac death: Future approaches based on identification and control of transient risk factors. *J Cardiovasc Electrophysiol* 1992;3:626–640.
47. Rosen MR, Janse MJ, Myerburg RJ. Arrhythmias induced by coronary artery occlusion: What are the electrophysiologic mechanisms? In Hearse D, Manning A, Janse M (eds): *Life-Threatening Arrhythmias During Ischemia and Infarction*. New York: Raven Press; 1987:11–47.
48. Maron BJ, Shirani J, Poliac LC, et al. Sudden death in young competitive athletes. *JAMA* 1996;276:199–204.
49. Deal BJ, Miller SM, Scagliotti SG, et al. Ventricular tachycardia in a young population without overt heart disease. *Circulation* 1986;73: 1111–1118.
50. Nikolic G, Bishop RL, Singh JB. Sudden death recorded during Holter monitoring. *Circulation* 1984;66:218–225.
51. Myerburg RJ, Kessler KM, Luceri RM, et al. Classification of ventricular arrhythmias based on parallel hierarchies of frequency and form. *Am J Cardiol* 1984;54:1355–1358.
52. Leclercq JF, Coumel PH, Maisonblanche P, et al. Mise en evidence des mecanismes udetenninants de la morte subite: Enquete cooperative portant sur 69 cas enregistres par la methode de Holter. *Arch Mal Coeur* 1986;79:1024–1036.
53. Muller JE, Tofler GH, Stone PH. Circadian variation and triggers of onset of acute cardiovascular disease. *Circulation* 1989;79:733–743.
54. Maclure M. The case-crossover design: A method for studying transient effects on the risk of acute events. *Am J Epidemiol* 1991;133:144–153.
55. Baum RS, Alvarez H, Cobb LA. Survival after resuscitation from out-of-hospital ventricular fibrillation. *Circulation* 1974;50:1231–1235.
56. Myerburg RJ, Kessler KM, Zaman L, et al. Survivors of prehospital cardiac arrest. *JAMA* 1982;247:1485–1490.
57. Gottlieb SO, Weisfeldt MI, Ouyang P, et al. Silent ischemia as a marker for early unfavorable outcomes in patients with unstable angina. *N Engl J Med* 1986;314:1214.
58. Weintraub RM, Aroesty JM, Paulin S. Medically refractory unstable angina pectoris. 1. Long-term follow-up of patients undergoing intra-aortic balloon counterpulsation and operation. *Am J Cardiol* 1979;43:877.
59. Mulcahy R, Awadhi AHA, deBuitieor M, et al. Natural history and prognosis of unstable angina. *Am Heart J* 1985;109:753.
60. Nademanee K, Intarachot V, Josephson MA, et al. Prognostic significance of silent myocardial ischemia in patients with unstable angina. *J Am Coll Cardiol* 1987;1:1–9.
61. Myerburg RJ, Kessler KM, Mallon SM, et al. Potentially fatal arrhythmias in patients with silent myocardial ischemia due to coronary artery spasm. *N Engl J Med* 1992;326:1451–1455.
62. Furukawa T, Moroe K, Mayrovitz HN, et al. Arrhythmogenic effects of graded coronary blood flow reduction superimposed upon prior myocardial infarction in dogs. *Circulation* 1991;84:368–377.
63. Furukawa T, Kimura S, Furukawa N, et al. Role of cardiac ATP-regulated potassium channels in differential responses of endocardial and epicardial cells to ischemia. *Circ Res* 1991;68:1693–1702.

64. Coronel R, Wilms-Schopman FJG, Opthof T, et al. Reperfusion arrhythmias in isolated perfused pig hearts: Inhomogeneities in extracellular potassium, ST and TO potentials and transmembrane action potentials. *Circ Res* 1992;71:1131–1142.
65. Ideker RE, Klein GJ, Harrison L, et al. The transition to ventricular fibrillation induced by reperfusion after ischemia in the dog: A period of organized epicardial activation. *Circulation* 1981;63:1371–1379.
66. Priori SG, Mantica M, Napolitano C, Schwartz PJ. Early afterdepolarization induced in vivo by reperfusion of ischemic myocardium. *Circulation* 1990;81:1911–1920.
67. Koyha T, Kimura S, Myerburg RJ, Bassett AL. Susceptibility of hypertrophied rat hearts to ventricular fibrillation during acute ischemia. *J Mol Cell Cardiol* 1988;20:159–168.
68. Myerburg RJ, Kessler KM, Castellanos A. Pathophysiology of sudden cardiac death. *PACE* 1991;14(part II):935–943.
69. Packer M. Sudden unexpected death in patients with congestive heart failure: A second frontier. *Circulation* 1985;72:681–685.
70. Multiple Risk Factor Intervention Trial Research Group. Multiple-risk factor intervention, trial: Risk factor changes in mortality results. *JAMA* 1982;248:1465–1477.
71. Gettes LS. Electrolyte abnormalities underlying lethal ventricular arrhythmias. *Circulation* 1992;85(suppl I):I70–I76.
72. Kimura S, Bassett AL, Xi H, et al. Characteristics of ATP-sensitive K+ channels in hypertrophied cells: Effects of pH. *Circulation* 1992;86(suppl I):I-92. Abstract.
73. Jackman WM, Friday KJ, Anderson JL, et al. The long Q-T syndrome: A critical review, new clinical observations, and a unifying hypothesis. *Prog Cardiovasc Dis* 1988;32(2):115–172.
74. Robinson JS, Sloman G, Mathew TH, Goble AJ. Survival after resuscitation from cardiac arrest in acute myocardial infarction. *Am Heart J* 1965;69:740–747.
75. Lab MJ. Contraction-excitation feedback in myocardium: Physiologic basis and clinical relevance. *Circ Res* 1982;50:757–766.
76. Calkins H, Maughan WL, Weissman HF, et al. Effect of acute volume load on refractoriness and arrhythmia development in isolated chronically infarcted canine hearts. *Circulation* 1989;79:687–697.
77. Schwartz PJ, La Rovere T, Vanoli E. Autonomic nervous system and sudden cardiac death: Experimental basis and clinical observations for post-myocardial infarction risk stratification. *Circulation* 1992;85(suppl I):I77–I91.
78. Barber MJ, Mueller TM, Henry DF, et al. Transmural myocardial infarction in the dog produces sympathectomy in non-infarcted myocardium. *Circulation* 1982;67:787–796.
79. Gaide MS, Myerburg RJ, Kozlovskis PL, Bassett AL. Elevated sympathetic response of epicardium proximal to healed myocardial infarction. *Am J Physiol* 1983;14:646–652.
80. Schwartz PJ, Billman GE, Stone HL. Autonomic mechanisms in ventricular fibrillation induced by myocardial ischemia during exercise in dogs with a healed myocardial infarction: An experimental preparation for sudden cardiac death. *Circulation* 1984;69:780–790.
81. Kammerling JJ, Green FJ, Watanabe AM, et al. Denervation supersensitivity of refractoriness in non-infarcted areas apical to transmural myocardial infarction. *Circulation* 1987;76:383–393.

82. Schwartz PJ, Vanoli E, Stramba-Badiale M, et al. Autonomic mechanisms and sudden death: New insights from analysis of baroreceptor reflexes in conscious dogs with and without a myocardial infarction. *Circulation* 1988;78:969–979.
83. Kozlovskis PL, Smets MJD, Duncan RC, et al. Regional beta-adrenergic receptors and adenylate cyclase activity after healing of myocardial infarction in cats. *J Mol Cell Cardiol* 1990;22:311–322.
84. Tull M, Minardo J, Mock BH, et al. SPECT with high purity ^{123}I-MIBG after transmural myocardial infarction (TMI), demonstrating sympathetic denervation followed by reinnervation in a dog model. *J Nucl Med* 1987;28:669.
85. Kleiger RE, Miller JP, Bigger JT, Moss, and the Multicenter Post-Infarction Research Group. Decreased heart rate variability and its association with increased mortality after acute myocardial infarction. *Am J Cardiol* 1987;59:256–262.
86. Le Rovere MT, Specchia G, Mortara A, Schwartz PJ. Baroreflex sensitivity, clinical correlates and cardiovascular mortality among patients with first myocardial infarction: A prospective study. *Circulation* 1988;78:816–824.
87. Huikuri HV, Linnaluoto MK, Seppanen T, et al. Heart rate variability and its circadian rhythm in survivors of cardiac arrest. *Am J Cardiol* 1992;70:610–615.
88. Bigger JT, Fleiss JL, Steinman RC, et al. Frequency domain measures of heart period variability and mortality after myocardial infarction. *Circulation* 1992;85:164–171.
89. Huikuri HV, Valkama JO, Airaksinen KEJ, et al. Frequency domain measures of heart rate variability before the onset of nonsustained and sustained ventricular tachycardia in patients with coronary artery disease. *Circulation* 1993;87:1220–1228.
90. Interian A, Fernandez P, Robinson E, et al. Long-term effect of propranolol in ventricular tachycardia/fibrillation patients with isoproterenol-dependent inducibility. *Circulation* 1990;82(suppl III):435.
91. Huikuri HV, Cox M, Interian A Jr, et al. Efficacy of intravenous propranolol for suppression of inducibility of ventricular tachyarrhythmias with different electrophysiologic characteristics in coronary artery disease. *Am J Cardiol* 1989;64:1305–1309.
92. Huikuri HV, Zaman L, Castellanos A, et al. Changes in spontaneous sinus node rate as an estimate of cardiac autonomic tone during stable and unstable ventricular tachycardia. *J Am Coll Cardiol* 1989;13:646–652.
93. Coumel P, Rosengarten MD, Leclerq JF, Attuel P. Role of sympathetic nervous system in non-ischemic ventricular arrhythmias. *Br Heart J* 1982;47:137–147.
94. Leor J, Poole WK, Kloner RA. Sudden cardiac death triggered by an earthquake. *N Engl J Med* 1996;334:413–419.
95. Hill IGW. Human heart in anaesthesia: Electrocardiographic study. *Edinburgh Med J* 1932;39:533–553.
96. Hill IGW. Cardiac irregularities during chloroform anaesthesia. *Lancet* 1932;1:1139–1142.
97. Selzer A, Wray HW. Quinidine syncope: Paroxysmal ventricular fibrillation occurring during treatment of chronic atrial arrhythmias. *Circulation* 1964;30:17.
98. Woosley RL, Chen Y, Freiman JP, Gillie RA. Mechanism of cardiotoxic actions of terfenadine. *JAMA* 1993;269:1532–1536.

99. Kimura S, Bassett AL, Xi H, Myerburg RJ. Early afterdepolarizations and triggered activity induced by cocaine: A possible mechanism of cocaine arrhythmogenesis. *Circulation* 1992;85:2227–2235.

100. Gohn DC, Simmons TW. Polymorphic ventricular tachycardia (torsade de pointes) associated with the use of probucol. *N Engl J Med* 1992;326: 1435–1436.

101. Wilt JL, Minnema AM, Johnson RF, Rosenblum AM. Torsade de pointes associated with the use of intravenous haloperidol. *Ann Intern Med* 1993;119:391–394.

102. Maron BJ, Poliac LC, Roberts WO. Risk for sudden cardiac death associated with marathon running. *J Am Coll Cardiol* 1996;28:428–431.

103. Morales AR, Romanelli R, Boucek RJ. The mural left anterior descending coronary artery, strenuous exercise, and sudden death. *Circulation* 1980;62:230–237.

104. Corrado D, Thiene G, Cocco P, Frescura C. Non-atherosclerotic coronary arterial disease and sudden death in the young. *Br Heart J* 1992;68: 601–607.

105. Roberts WC. Major anomalies of coronary arterial origin seen in adulthood. *Am Heart J* 1986;111:943–963.

106. Roden DK, Bennett PB, Snyders DJ, et al. Quinidine delays I_k activation in guinea pig ventricular myocytes. *Circ Res* 1988;62:1055–1058.

107. January CR, Riddle JM. Early afterdepolarizations: Mechanisms of induction and block: A role for L-type Ca^{++} current. *Circ Res* 1989;64: 977–990.

108. Maron B, Bodison SA, Wesley YE, et al. Results for screening a large group of intercollegiate competitive athletes for cardiovascular disease. *J Am Coll Cardiol* 1987;10:1214–1221.

109. Brugada P, Brugada J. Right bundle branch block, persistent ST segment elevation, and sudden cardiac death: A distinct clinical and electrocardiographic syndrome—a multicenter report. *J Am Coll Cardiol* 1992;20: 1391–1396.

110. Leenhardt L, Glaser E, Burguera M, et al. Short-coupled variant of torsade de pointes: A new electrocardiographic entity in the spectrum of idiopathic ventricular tachyarrhythmias. *Circulation* 1994;89:206–215.

111. Meissner MD, Lehmann MH, Steinman RT, et al. Ventricular fibrillation in patients without structural heart disease: A multicenter experience with implantable cardioverter-defibrillator therapy. *J Am Coll Cardiol* 1993;21:1406–1412.

112. Consensus Statement of the Joint Steering Committees of the Unexplained Cardiac Arrest Registry of Europe and of the Idiopathic Ventricular Fibrillation Registry of the United States. Survivors of out-of-hospital cardiac arrest with apparently normal heart: Need for definition and standardized clinical evaluation. *Circulation* 1997;95:265–272.

3

Risk Profiling and Screening Strategies

Michael S. Katcher, MD, Barry J. Maron, MD, and Munther K. Homoud, MD

Risk Profiling and Screening Strategies

Introduction

The sudden death of an athlete is a great tragedy, especially when it occurs in the young and previously apparently healthy. Fortunately, it is a rare event, but there is little solace in this knowledge at the time when such devastating events occur. Such deaths incite a strong desire in society and the medical community to prevent future occurrences. Therefore, it is reasonable to attempt to discern when sudden death in the athlete is preventable and to evaluate measures that aim to enact this prevention. The vast majority of athletes who have died suddenly were found to have underlying structural heart disease that is thought to have been contributory to their deaths.[1-6] In individuals under age 35, the most common finding is hypertrophic cardiomyopathy (HCM).[1] Other findings include congenital coronary artery anomalies, aortic rupture related to Marfan syndrome, myocarditis, premature atherosclerotic coronary disease, arrhythmogenic right ventricular dysplasia, and valvular heart disease. The majority of these young athletes, however, lacked preexisting cardiovascular symptoms. Instead, unfortunately,

From Estes NAM, Salem DN, Wang PJ (eds). *Sudden Cardiac Death in the Athlete.* Armonk, NY: Futura Publishing Co., Inc.; ©1998.

sudden death was their initial presentation.[1] Also, most episodes of sudden death in athletes occur during or immediately following exercise.[7]

Goals to prevent or limit sudden death in the athlete must be aimed at identification of asymptomatic athletes who unknowingly are at increased risk. There are two arms to the prevention of sudden cardiac death in the athlete: first, widescale screening of athletes to identify occult structural heart disease, and second, risk assessment and subsequent institution of treatment or prohibition of competitive athletics to modify these risks.

Goals and Feasibility of Screening

In general, the goal of a screening program for any condition is to detect that condition in an asymptomatic or premorbid state. To determine the appropriateness of screening, several conditions should be met.[8]

First, the disease(s) being screened should have significant morbidity or mortality associated if not detected. Sudden death is clearly one such significant outcome. The disease(s) screened should also have available treatment that can affect its outcome, since screening is usually aimed at affecting negative outcomes and not merely prematurely identifying the inevitable.[8] Several underlying causes of sudden cardiac death in athletes meet this condition. One such example is in the case of aortic aneurysm in Marfan syndrome, which can be surgically corrected if detected prior to rupture.

An extrapolation of the idea of "treatment" in athletes is behavior modification. Since most episodes of sudden death in the athlete are exercise related, it is assumed that exercise prohibition or limitation may prevent some sudden cardiac death. By definition, avoidance of all exercise prevents sudden death *during* exercise. What remains to be answered is if such behavior modification reliably affects mortality in general. There is not yet sufficient evidence that prohibition of exercise improves overall survival.[9] Many of the underlying conditions seen in sudden death in athletes are also associated with sudden death occurring outside of activity. It is possible that exercise-related sudden death occurs in those individuals who would otherwise have died suddenly at rest if they were not athletes. Despite the lack of proven efficacy, until evidence to the contrary, the current strategy of prohibition of exercise in those identified with "high-risk" underlying conditions appears to be prudent and reasonable and should be continued.

Another important element in appropriate screening is that the early treatment afforded by early detection produces superior results to the treatment of early symptomatic individuals.[8] This is particularly relevant in screening of athletes. If all athletes who die suddenly had nonfatal symptoms on occasions prior to their fatal event, then screening would be unnecessary. In such a case, it would be prudent to wait for early symptoms and intervene aggressively at that time. Unfortunately, this is not the case in sudden death in young athletes. The initial presenting symptom for many of these underlying conditions is sudden death itself.[1] Therefore, waiting for the "early symptomatic" state can be catastrophic.

Another factor important in screening is a sufficiently high prevalence in the population of the condition to merit screening.[8] Determining just how prevalent a condition needs to be is a decision fraught with multiple emotional, ethical, and practical considerations. Age and state of health of the population at risk, severity of outcome if not detected early, and degree that outcome can be affected are all at least as important as the absolute prevalence of the condition. Approximately 0.2% of young athletes have underlying conditions that *could* predispose to exertional sudden death.[10] Although this prevalence is not insignificant, it must be remembered that only a small minority of these individuals will actually die during exercise. The risk of sudden death in the high school athlete is less than 1 in 100,000.[10,11] Approximately 15 to 25 high school athletes suffer sudden cardiac death during exercise each year in the United States.[9,12] This must be compared to the more than 4 million high school athletes who participate each year in the United States.[7] An additional 25 million children and young adults and one-half million college and professional athletes participate in competitive athletics and they also have a low incidence of sudden death.[13] Epstein and Maron[10] estimate that 200,000 athletes under age 30 would need to be screened to identify 1000 individuals with underlying congenital heart disease. Of these, 10 athletes would have a condition that *could* cause sudden death and 1 of these would actually die of sudden death. Therefore, if screening were 100% sensitive, for every 200,000 individuals screened, 1 life would be saved and 1000 individuals might require additional testing and/or prohibition of competitive athletics.

In older athletes, exercise-related sudden death is also uncommon; however, it is more common than in younger athletes; 6 in 100,000 middle-aged men will die during exertion.[11] Sudden death occurs in approximately 1 in 15,000 joggers and 1 in 50,000 marathoners.[14] In exercise-related death in athletes over age 35, the most common underlying cause is atherosclerotic coronary artery disease and is usually multi-vessel disease.[2,6] Approximately 50% of these individuals have a history of known coronary artery disease or have symptoms consistent with coronary disease.[2,15] Therefore, these 50% of individuals should theoretically not benefit from screening, as they should already be identified. In reality, many of these individuals do not seek medical attention and therefore they would most benefit from preparticipation screening, in which their history could be elucidated.

Truly asymptomatic coronary disease occurs in approximately 3% of men 35 to 55 years old and in a higher percentage of those with multiple coronary artery disease risk factors.[10] Epstein and Maron[10] estimate that if exercise and risk factor screening is performed, for every 10,000 men over 35 years old screened, 100 would be identified for increased risk of sudden death, of which 1 would actually die suddenly each year.

Costs of Screening

Once a condition is felt appropriate for screening, the available tests required must be evaluated.[8] Such tests must be available to be used for the entire population at risk. Therefore, they must be affordable on a mass scale and not be overwhelmingly labor intensive to be practical. Available screening tests for conditions that predispose to exercise-related sudden death are discussed individually below. A multitude of tests are available for the detection of cardiac disease. The cost of large-volume community screening to prevent exercise-related sudden death is dependent on the number of tests incorporated. When more tests are used, the potential for identification of conditions rises but the costs rise markedly as well. For example, in 1986 screening with use of only a detailed history and auscultation was estimated to cost $25 per individual.[10] Unfortunately, with the exception of aortic stenosis, this strategy would fail to identify a majority of individuals with predisposing conditions for sudden death. In contrast, a more elaborate screening regimen including history, auscultation, chest x-ray, electrocardiogram (ECG), exercise test, and M-mode echocardiogram was estimated to cost approximately $250 per individual.[10] Despite this increased effort and cost, most individuals with coronary disease (atherosclerotic and congenital anomalous) as well as some patients with HCM would not be diagnosed. Two-dimensional echocardiography and nuclear stress myocardial perfusion imaging would further increase detection, however, at a marked increase in cost.

In addition to the primary costs of the tests involved, widescale screening is associated with multiple secondary costs that must be taken into consideration. Even when a relatively modest screening program is used (such as assessment of personal and family history and performance of a directed physical exam), further, more expensive tests are required when abnormalities are found on screening. These subsequent tests are required for confirmation as well as risk stratification to determine if prohibition of athletics or treatment is necessary. The vast majority of these confirmatory tests show normal or benign conditions (false-positive results of screening). The costs of these tests must be measured not only in dollars but in resources as well, since they require a significant use of time from health care professionals, and equipment. Once a condition is identified, the prohibition of competitive athletics has financial repercussions as well, especially in professional or collegiate athletes whose livelihoods may be compromised.

In light of the primary and secondary costs and the large number of young athletes participating in competitive sports, mass screening by use of a full battery of tests would be prohibitively expensive for most health care or athletic institutions. An important exception to this belief is the experience in Italy.[16] In Italy comprehensive preparticipation screening is widely practiced. It is provided for by law and financed in part from a national lottery. For 30 years, Italy has supported a preventative medical evaluation for those participating in official organized sports. This screening is rather comprehensive, using annual physical examinations, ECGs, and submaximal exercise tolerance tests under the supervision of physicians specifically trained in sports medicine. Elite athletes also undergo echocardiography and chest x-ray. Approximately 2.5% of athletes are disqualified from participation as a result of this screening. About half of these disqualifications are for cardiovascular conditions, although these have included disqualifications for hypertension and mitral valve prolapse (MVP), conditions which may not significantly increase the risk of exercise-related sudden death.

Despite these great efforts and expenses, sudden death in the athlete has not been eliminated in Italy.[4] First, as would be expected of a program of such massive scale, participation has not been absolute. Less than 50% of the 6 million Italians participating in competitive athletics have undergone preparticipation screening.[16] The extent to which sudden death has been changed in Italy by these massive efforts is difficult to assess. Of interest, HCM is an infrequent underlying cause found in athletes who have died suddenly.[4] In contrast, HCM is commonly found in Americans who have died suddenly during exercise.[1–3] It is not clear if these differences reflect geographic variation or are secondary to screening efforts. The extensive preparticipation evaluation in Italy would be expected to identify a large percent of individuals with silent HCM and therefore, theoretically prevent exercise-related death by prohibiting exercise. In Italy, instead, arrhythmogenic right ventricular dysplasia is the most frequently identified underlying cause in athletes who have died suddenly.[4] There are geographic factors that likely partially contribute to this, as right ventricular dysplasia has an unusually high incidence in the Veneto region of Italy. However, this condition is not unusually common in other regions of Italy. Therefore, it is possible that the high incidence of right ventricular dysplasia in athletes dying suddenly is, in part, related to a decrease in other causes that can be readily identified with screening. In contrast, the premorbid identification of arrhythmogenic right ventricular dysplasia can be quite difficult and therefore may be expected to escape identification with screening, and thus continue to contribute to sudden death in athletes.

History

A wide variety of tests are available for screening to prevent sudden death in athletes. The simplest of these tests is the detailed history. There are two crucial elements to such a history: identification of a personal history of potentially cardiovascular-related symptoms in the athlete, and a family history of inheritable life-threatening conditions or premature and/or sudden death.

A history of symptoms consistent with possible cardiovascular disease are identified retrospectively in a minority of athletes who die suddenly, representing approximately one fifth to one third of such individuals.[1,2,17,18] Accepting this limitation, it appears reasonable to try to identify symptomatic individuals prior to death. Formal preparticipation questionnaires have been developed to identify symptomatic patients by asking appropriate questions. Such questionnaires have been recommended by a variety of organizations including a joint recommendation from the American Academy of Pediatrics, the American Academy of Family Physicians, the American Medical Society for Sports Medicine, the American Orthopaedic Society for Sports Medicine, and the American Osteopathic Academy of Sports Medicine.[12,17] When both a preparticipation history and physical exam are used to screen young athletes, abnormalities in personal history are more frequent than those identified on physical exam.[19] Ideally, all symptomatic athletes would seek medical attention independent of screening; however, it is common for young individuals to minimize such symptoms in their minds, especially in light of the fear of testing or exclusion from sports that might ensue should they come forward. Education of athletes on the importance of honest and complete answers is therefore a prerequisite for the utility of history as a screening test. To help ensure this, history should be obtained from parents or guardians of all athletes who are minors, as well as from the athletes themselves. In older athletes, a history of symptoms as well as a history of coronary artery disease risk factors can be helpful.[3] Even when middle-aged individuals present to a health care professional requesting to start new exercise or requesting a stress test, they may in fact have had symptoms that they are withholding.[10,20]

Dyspnea, lightheadedness, chest discomfort, palpitations, and early fatigue (out of proportion to peers or past performance), can be suggestive of underlying structural heart disease and risk for sudden death and may prompt further evaluation. A history of syncope may also warrant further evaluation to exclude structural heart disease. Syncope is not uncommon in young people, the vast majority of whom suffer from vasodepressor syncope, a relatively benign condition usually not associated with exercise-related sudden death. When young people die suddenly, a previous history of syncope is occasionally seen.[4,21] Although exercise-related syncope may be benign, it may also be suggestive of underlying conditions that are predictive of sudden death, and thus exercise-related syncope should always merit further evaluation.[21]

Unfortunately, the vast majority of athletes who have died suddenly did not have previous symptoms that they declared.[1,17,18] For example, the majority of patients with HCM who die suddenly have no functional limitation prior to death.[2] In fact, even when a screening preparticipation history had been used, there was no preexisting suspicion of cardiovascular disease in almost all athletes who later died suddenly.[1] Therefore, obtaining a personal history of possible cardiovascular symptoms is a relatively insensitive screening test; however, the relative ease to which it can be performed on a widescale adds to its practicality.

A family history of certain conditions or premature or sudden death can also be useful in identifying athletes at risk for sudden death. Several life-threatening conditions associated with exertional death are inheritable. HCM, Marfan syndrome, long QT syndrome, and familial hyperlipidemias and premature coronary artery disease all have familial predilection. Unfortunately, in athletes who die suddenly with these conditions, a known familial history or history of familial sudden death is usually lacking. Most patients with HCM do not have a family history of sudden or premature death.[7,22]

Physical Examination

The role of the physical examination in identification of specific potentially life-threatening conditions in athletes is discussed in detail in chapter 4 this volume. Ideally, the preparticipation physical examination should be performed as part of the patient's regular medical care by someone familiar with the athlete and his or her history.[20] The examination should be performed in a quiet and private environment to best detect subtle findings.[12,20] In contrast, locker room mass physical examinations are less than ideal. Cardiac auscultation in an upright posture with and without Valsalva maneuvers to maximize the murmur of hypertrophic obstructive cardiomyopathy and examination for the stigmata of Marfan syndrome (especially in very tall athletes) should be included in screening physical examinations.[11,20]

The physical examination can identify most individuals with aortic stenosis as well as some individuals with HCM and Marfan syndrome.[17] The loud murmur of aortic stenosis is readily identifiable on physical examination; however, aortic stenosis is rarely seen as the cause of sudden death in athletes. This may reflect early diagnosis in childhood and prohibition from competitive sports prior to any screening.[10] The classic physical examination findings of HCM are very specific for this condition.[10] Unfortunately, the vast majority of patients with this condition lack such findings.[7] These findings, when present, reflect relative obstruction to left ventricular outflow. Most individuals with HCM do not develop obstruction and there may be incomplete phenotypic expression in young athletes prior to adulthood.[10,23]

One limitation of the physical examination for screening is the frequency of findings in normal athletes. Normal athletes frequently have soft murmurs secondary to increased pulmonic flow as well as occasional third or fourth heart sounds.[24] Up to 50% of athletes will have a systolic ejection murmur.[17] Such findings can prompt further expensive testing (such as echocardiography) in a large number of individuals when widescale screening is implemented.

Electrocardiography

Electrocardiography is occasionally used in the screening of athletes. Several factors contribute to its potential role. ECGs are relatively inexpensive. In 1986, Epstein and Maron[10] estimated that routine electrocardiography would add approximately $25 per athlete screened. ECGs can also be performed quickly with only a modest degree of equipment and technical support, and can be performed at the time of the history and physical. A variety of abnormalities can be evaluated using electrocardiography, including evidence of conduction abnormalities, arrhythmias, hypertrophy, infarction, and ischemia.

Conditions whose diagnoses are usually based on ECG criteria, such as Wolff-Parkinson-White syndrome (WPW) and long QT syndrome, can be detected in ECG screening efforts. The diagnosis of WPW on resting ECG can sometimes be difficult, especially when pre-excitation is submaximal at rest. Normal QT measurements, especially at rest, are also seen even in symptomatic patients with known family histories of long QT syndrome. Therefore, even in these conditions, ECG screening is not perfect.

ECGs are often abnormal in several conditions that can predispose to sudden death. Up to 90% of individuals with known arrhythmogenic right ventricular dysplasia have ECG abnormalities.[25] These abnormalities may be subtle and nonspecific. Over 90% of individuals with HCM and 90% of those who die suddenly have an abnormal ECG.[7,10,13] Certain abnormalities including unusual or bizarre ECGs with markedly increased voltage, deep Q waves, or deeply inverted T waves, especially with superior axis, anterior displacement of forces, and loss of septal Q waves, are most suggestive of HCM.[23]

The ECG abnormalities seen in HCM, although sensitive, are not very specific and there is a wide overlap with "abnormalities" seen in the normal athlete.[10] Also, not all patients with HCM have ECG abnormalities and this is especially true in those with the nonobstructive form of the condition.[3,26]

One important factor that limits the utility of electrocardiography in screening is the variety of abnormalities seen on ECG in normal athletes. These abnormalities arise from increased vagal tone and physiologic hypertrophy seen in athletes.[18,24] Resting bradycardia and abnormalities in atrioventricular (AV) conduction can be seen. This includes third-degree AV block, which occurs with a 100-fold increase in frequency over nonathletes, although it is still quite rare and thus structural heart disease must still be excluded in athletes with this condition.[8,24] The increase in ventricular muscle mass seen in athletes frequently contributes to an incomplete right bundle branch block in highly trained athletes.[8,24] ECG criteria for left ventricular hypertrophy are seen in 10% to 80% of athletes.[8,24] ST segment elevation and T wave inversion, the latter, believed in part related to heterogeneity in the action potential due to vagal influence, are also frequently seen in athletes.[8,24] ECG abnormalities are frequent in both athletes with underlying structural heart disease and normal athletes. Therefore, the low specificity of this test significantly limits its utility for widescale screening. In a study by Maron et al[27] evaluating ECG screening (in conjunction with history and physical examination) in 501 college athletes, abnormalities in history, physical examination, and/or ECG were detected in approximately 20% of individuals. Of those that allowed further evaluation, 84% with an abnormal screening test were found to have no definite evidence of cardiovascular disease after more comprehensive testing including echocardiography was performed. No individual in this study was found to have clear evidence of conditions that would predispose to significant risk of exercise-related sudden death, although several subjects were found to have increased ventricular wall thickness, and HCM could not be excluded.

Echocardiography

Echocardiography is another potential screening tool. The visualization of the heart afforded by this technique can identify a multitude of structural abnormalities. Aortic stenosis can be readily diagnosed with two-dimensional echocardiography; however, this condition is usually easily identifiable by physical examination. Coronary artery anomalies can occasionally be identified with careful echocardiographic imaging of their take-off sites. Limited echocardiography, which has been used in some screening studies, is insufficient for identification of anomalous coronary arteries.[9] Echocardiographic screening for asymptomatic coronary artery anomalies has been attempted in elite athletes in Italy.[16] Echocardiography would also be expected to identify most individuals with aortic dilatation secondary to cystic medial necrosis of Marfan syndrome.[10] Echocardiography is a useful test when arrhythmogenic right ventricular dysplasia is suspected; however, the pathology can be quite focal and echocardiographic identification can require imaging in multiple planes with careful attention to regional right ventricular motion. Routine echocardiography may lack sensitivity for this diagnosis.[28] Therefore, the role of echocardiography in screening for this condition may be limited.

Echocardiography is particularly sensitive for detecting HCM.[23] In the absence of other diseases associated with hypertrophy (such as systemic hypertension and aortic stenosis), the echocardiographic appearance is also very specific for HCM.[10] Findings most suggestive of HCM include asymmetric and extreme ventricular hypertrophy and dramatic systolic anterior motion of the mitral valve. Abnormalities in diastolic filling pattern and characteristic ventricular tissue appearance are also helpful in identifying this condition.[24] Septal hypertrophy and systolic anterior motion of the mitral valve can usually be identified on M-mode echocardiography or on parasternal two-dimensional imaging. Therefore, limited echocardiography, without full two-dimensional imaging, has been proposed as a potential screening tool, since it may be performed more rapidly and less costly than more detailed echocardiography.[29,30] Unfortunately, the majority of patients with HCM lack systolic anterior mitral motion.[10] Also, the anterior septum is not always disproportionately hypertrophied and is occasionally of normal thickness (with hypertrophy limited to other regions). M-mode echocardiography can fail to identify these individuals.[10] Finally, adolescents with HCM who have not yet manifested full phenotypic expression may have ventricles whose thickness does not yet exceed upper limits of normal.[7] Therefore, repeat serial studies might be required until adulthood for echocardiography to gain maximal sensitivity as a screening tool, although at great expense.

One important limitation to the use of echocardiography in the screening of athletes is the frequency of findings in normal athletes. The physiologic adaptive changes to frequent exercise include increase in end-diastolic volume and wall thickness.[24] This physiologic hypertrophy is usually not extreme and most athletes' hearts remain within the upper limit of normal thickness. Rarely does wall thickness exceed 15 mm in normal athletes.[10] Unfortunately, there is still some overlap in wall thickness between normal physiologic hypertrophy of the athlete and pathologic HCM. As a result, in some athletes with borderline echocardiographic appearance, HCM cannot be diagnosed, but it cannot be excluded either.[27,31] Echocardiography of nonathletic first-degree relatives or repeat echocardiography after discontinuation of regular exercise can sometimes be helpful in resolving the diagnosis in these individuals.[10]

Several studies have evaluated the utility of primary echocardiography in screening of athletes.[29–32] Weidenbener et al[30] used a limited echocardiogram (single view parasternal long and parasternal short axis) in 2997 athletes. Cardiovascular abnormalities were detected in 64 studies. The majority of these abnormalities were MVP and bicuspid aortic valve, abnormalities without a clear strong association with exercise-related sudden death. Four patients were identified to have a dilated aortic root and one patient was noted to have septal hypertrophy (without a diagnosis of definitive HCM), and none had abnormalities that excluded them from athletic participation. Feinstein et al[32] evaluated 1570 high school athletes by use of two-dimensional echocardiography and identified only one significant abnormality (dextrocardia). Murry et al[29] used limited echocardiography to evaluate 125 college athletes, and identified 11 with MVP and 2 with bicuspid aortic valve. Lewis et al[31] evaluated 265 (predominantly African American) college athletes by using two-dimensional and M-mode echocardiography. No individual had diagnostic evidence of HCM or other cardiovascular conditions that are seen frequently in athletes who die suddenly. Eleven percent of these athletes had ventricular septal thickness of at least 13 mm, making it difficult to distinguish between normal athlete's heart and HCM in some. It is interesting to note that in these four studies, in almost 5000 athletes, no definitive cases of HCM or other diseases that have a strong association with sudden death in the athlete were made, despite significant costs and efforts.

An important limitation to the utility of echocardiography for screening in athletes is cost. In the studies by Weidenbener et al[30] and Murry et al,[29] the estimated cost of portable limited echocardiography was thought to be less than $20 per study. These studies, however, were somewhat dependent on volunteered time and equipment and may not be generalizable. Mass screening using full echocardiography has been estimated to cost an average of $600 per athlete.[7] Therefore, in the United States screening could cost over $250,000 for each new case of HCM identified and over $100 million for each life saved, while using over 50,000 hours of technician time to perform these studies.[7,9] Enactment of echocardiographic screening is therefore prohibitively expensive and labor intensive to recommend on a mass scale.

Exercise Electrocardiography

The principal utility of exercise electrocardiography in athlete screening is the identification of occult atherosclerotic coronary artery disease. Congenital coronary anomalies may be identified as well, but the sensitivity in this population remains unknown.[10] Also, initiation of arrhythmias with exercise can be seen in patients with a variety of cardiac diseases. For example, exercise tests exacerbate ventricular arrhythmias in approximately half of cases of arrhythmogenic right ventricular dysplasia.[28] Significant ectopy during screening exercise testing merits further evaluation.

In young asymptomatic athletes, the likelihood of significant coronary artery disease is extremely low, limiting the usefulness of exercise testing in this population. One possible exception is those individuals with very strong family histories of premature coronary artery disease or known familial dyslipidemias.

In the athletes over age 35 who have died suddenly, the most frequently detected underlying condition has been coronary artery disease.[2,15] As stated previously, half of these individuals have had a history of known coronary disease or symptoms consistent with coronary disease.[2,15] Screening that uses exercise electrocardiography would be directed at identifying the remaining asymptomatic 50% prior to death. Evidence of acute myocardial infarction is often found at autopsy in previously asymptomatic individuals who died during exercise.[11] Not infrequently, plaques responsible for myocardial infarctions are subcritical prior to rupture and secondary thrombosis at the site.[11,33,34] Therefore, identifying such plaques prior to rupture may be difficult, as they may not significantly impede flow enough to induce ischemia on exercise electrocardiography and therefore may escape detection on screening. In addition, exercise electrocardiographic testing has a significant false-positive rate, as high as 10%, especially in young asymptomatic athletes, and therefore further limits its utility in large-scale screening.[20,35] In general, stress electrocardiography has a low predictive value in asymptomatic individuals, especially in those with a low pretest probability of having occult coronary disease, such as younger athletes.[10]

Several studies have evaluated the utility of exercise electrocardiographic testing in screening of athletes over age 35. The Seattle Heart Watch Study evaluated over 2000 men, with coronary artery disease risk factor analysis and exercise testing.[10,36] The investigators identified a subgroup, representing approximately 1% of the individuals, who were at an 18-fold increase in risk of developing symptomatic coronary artery disease or death. The overall sudden death rate was low (0.05%). Therefore, because of the low incidence, efforts to lower the risk further could only have modest absolute benefit. Epstein and Maron[10] estimated that for every 10,000 individuals screened with exercise testing, 100 individuals at increased risk would be identified, of whom only 1 would be expected to die suddenly. An additional 4 individuals per 10,000 screened would be expected to die suddenly, and these four would not be identified with stress electrocardiographic screening. In addition, it must be remembered that not all sudden death would occur during exercise in such a population. It remains unclear the extent to which sudden death in this population would be preventable by treatment or by exercise restriction. To an extent, this would be dependent on more detailed assessment of coronary anatomy. The risk of sudden death is lower in individuals who exercise regularly.[37] Restricting exercise in all asymptomatic individuals who are found to be at increased risk on screening could theoretically increase their risk further, especially if their absolute risk was relatively low.

McHenry et al[38] used exercise testing to prospectively evaluate 916 state troopers, with a follow-up of over 12 years on average.[11,38] Although a positive exercise test was predictive of subsequent angina, most subsequent myocardial infarctions and episodes of sudden death actually occurred in those with a negative initial exercise test.[11,20,38]

Even when the use of exercise electrocardiographic testing for screening is limited to a higher risk population, results remain imperfect. Siscovick et al[39] evaluated over 3600 individuals with an elevated lipid profile who had undergone exercise testing. These individuals underwent repeat exercise testing annually as part of the Lipid Research Clinics Primary Prevention Trial. In follow-up, 62 individuals had an exercise-related myocardial infarction or sudden death and less than 20% of these had a prior positive exercise test.[11,39] Therefore, even in a higher risk population, exercise testing would fail to identify the majority of individuals who will have exercise-related cardiac events.

Recommendations for Preparticipation Screening

The limitations to preparticipation screening in athletes have been discussed in detail. Sudden death in the athlete is an infrequent event and tests available are by no means perfectly sensitive, specific, or inexpensive. However, the loss of a young and previously healthy athlete to sudden death can be devastating. Therefore, respecting the limitations, it is a reasonable goal to attempt to identify those at risk and try to prevent exercise-related sudden death. The means to perform this, however, remain in question with ethical, practical, and economic considerations that must all be weighed into the equation. In Italy, one tact has been chosen. Elaborate preparticipation screening with frequent follow-up evaluation has been accepted as the standard.[16] The large costs and demands on resources have been chosen by the Italian community in an effort to minimize risk to their athletes. No such formal screening system exists in the United States. Screening efforts instead are coordinated at the state, educational, and athletic institution levels.[7] Screening in the United States, to date, has been based on voluntary participation by these agencies and by participating individuals.

The American Heart Association (AHA) recommends *that some form of preparticipation cardiovascular screening for high school and collegiate athletes is justifiable and compelling based on ethical, legal and medical grounds.*[7] The AHA as well as pediatric, family practice, and sports medicine agencies have recommended obtaining a personal history and a family history and performing a physical examination.[7,11,12,17,20] Acknowledging the limitations, it has been felt to be the most practical and cost-effective screening approach for young athletes as well as for older athletes, and the AHA has recommended that such efforts be mandatory for all athletes and that a national standard be developed.[7] The AHA recommends that in high school and collegiate athletes, repeat screening be performed every 2 years and history obtained every year. It must be remembered that even this modest screening approach would not be inexpensive in light of the large number of American athletes.

Additional available tests including electrocardiography, echocardiography, and exercise testing have not been recommended for mass screening of athletes by the AHA. Cost and practical considerations have contributed to this recommendation. An exception to the recommendation regarding additional testing exists for a subset of older athletes. In male athletes over age 40 and female athletes over age 50 with significant coronary artery disease risk factors in whom a physician suspects asymptomatic coronary disease, it has been felt "prudent" to "selectively" perform exercise testing prior to participation in vigorous athletics.[7]

These recommendations were formalized in an official statement by the AHA in 1996 and endorsed by the board of trustees of the American College of Cardiology and the American Academy of Pediatrics Section on Cardiology.[7]

Risk Stratification of Causes of Sudden Cardiac Death

Introduction

Attempts at screening for causes of sudden cardiac death in athletes have been met with limited success.[27,29,31,32] The population of patients engaged in competitive athletics is large and the number of athletes at risk is small.[7] Compared to the population of patients with ischemic heart disease who are at risk for sudden cardiac death, athletes with cardiac disorders that carry the potential for sudden cardiac death are often asymptomatic and may not be aware of their underlying cardiac disease. Hence, any adopted screening policy should be easy to conduct, safe to perform, and inexpensive.

In addition, trained athletes often develop structural changes that help enhance their performance.[24] These changes often lead to the misinterpretation of conventional noninvasive diagnostic tools such as the ECG and the echocardiogram.[23] This raises concern about the risk of labeling a healthy individual as one with a potentially fatal disease with the ensuing emotional, financial, and occupational ramifications.

The diseases that contribute to the bulk of sudden cardiac death in athletes are heterogeneous.[1] Although most cases of sudden cardiac death are arrhythmic in etiology, this final pathway is the culmination of the interplay of a variety of factors. Structural heart disease, the state of neurohumoral milieu at the time of initiation of the arrhythmic event, and other variables such as ischemia and electrolyte imbalance all contrive to precipitate the arrhythmic event.

The risk of sudden cardiac death varies from one individual to another and the identification of these high-risk features should potentially allow the selection of individuals at higher risk for sudden cardiac death and their exclusion from competitive athletics. This concept underlies the recommendations of the 26th Bethesda Conference identifying high-risk features of patients with cardiovascular diseases, and allows guidance in offering patients necessary recommendations.[40]

Hypertrophic Cardiomyopathy

By far, the most common cause of sudden cardiac death in athletes is HCM.[1] The majority of cases are familial, and genetic mutations involving the β-myosin heavy chain, troponin T, α-tropomyosin, and myosin-binding protein C genes have been identified. HCM is described in 2 of 1000 young adults, with the nonobstructive form more prevalent than the obstructive form.[41] The heterogeneous echocardiographic features of HCM suggest that it may be more prevalent than currently appreciated.[41] Although HCM is the leading cause of sudden cardiac death in athletes, it is important to appreciate that the majority of patients with HCM remain asymptomatic and have normal survival.[1,22] The wide distribution, diverse clinical manifestations, and potential for sudden cardiac death characteristic of this disorder prompt the identification of risk factors that may identify potential candidates for prophylactic therapy. Regardless of these risk factors, it is not recommended that patients with HCM engage in athletic activities.[22]

The identification of risk factors for sudden cardiac death in HCM has been influenced by the population studied.[41a] Most studies have been conducted in referral centers where most high-risk cases concentrate, and the low prevalence of the disorder precludes conducting any meaningful long-term natural history study.[42] Most sudden death in HCM occurs in the young and in individuals not known to carry the disease.[42] The incidence of sudden cardiac death varies from 2% to 3%, although numbers as high as 6% have been described; the majority of deaths occur during rest or with minimal physical exertion.[43,44]

The number of cases of sudden cardiac death that occur in individuals while they are being monitored is too small to make possible definitive conclusions as to the mechanism of sudden cardiac death. Proposed mechanisms include ventricular tachyarrhythmias, supraventricular tachyarrhythmias including paroxysmal atrial fibrillation with or without accessory AV conduction, and various bradyarrhythmias.[22,42] The hemodynamic consequences of such arrhythmias are compounded by underlying diastolic dysfunction, outflow tract obstruction, and reduced coronary vascular reserve.

As in other patients with structural heart disease, survival from an arrhythmic sudden cardiac death portends a worse prognosis.[45] Other high-risk features include sustained ventricular tachycardia and a strong family history defined as two or more sudden deaths in young members of the family.[22] Certain families have been described with unusually high sudden death rates in young members.[46] Genetic studies have uncovered certain mutations, such as the Arg403Gln and the cardiac troponin T mutations, that are associated with an adverse prognosis.[47,48] Although the prognostic significance of syncope in the young patient with HCM remains unclear,[22] young age itself has long been defined as an adverse prognostic feature.[49,50]

Holter monitoring of patients with HCM often reveals the presence of nonsustained runs of ventricular tachycardia. Studies conducted in the early 1980s suggest that this finding portends a worse prognosis.[51,52] Recently, Spirito et al[53] prospectively evaluated 151 patients clinically identified as low risk for sudden cardiac death. Patients with nonsustained ventricular tachycardia had a 1.4% annual risk for sudden cardiac death compared to 0.6% for those individuals with no nonsustained ventricular tachycardia. In a group of 230 patients with HCM, less than 45% with history of syncope or sudden cardiac death were found to have ventricular tachycardia on Holter monitor.[54] A history of cardiac arrest and a history of syncope, on the other hand, were the only clinical variables associated with future cardiac events when these patients were followed for a mean of 28 ± 19 months.[54]

The role of primary electrophysiologic study in the identification of high-risk patients with HCM is controversial. In the group followed by Fananapazir et al,[54] there were 17 cardiac events: 8 sudden deaths, 1 cardiac arrest, and 8 episodes of syncope associated with defibrillator discharge. Fourteen out of the 17 patients had inducible arrhythmias on electrophysiologic study, 12 polymorphic, and 2 monomorphic, requiring 3 premature extrastimuli in 10 patients and 2 in 4 patients.[54] The concern raised about the validity of electrophysiologic study lies in the specificity of the test. Polymorphic ventricular tachycardia is not considered a specific response and the use of more aggressive stimulation protocols invariably results in the induction of such nonspecific arrhythmias. Recently, the degree of fractionation of intracardiac right ventricular electrograms in response to prematurely delivered extrastimuli was found to distinguish patients at high risk and those at low risk for future adverse events.[55]

The relation between the extent of left ventricular hypertrophy and the prognosis is unclear. Some studies show an increase prevalence of ventricular tachyarrhythmias and sudden cardiac death with significant left ventricular hypertrophy.[56,57] The heterogeneous morphological manifestations of this disorder[58] and the changes in wall thickening associated with aging[59] preclude the meaningful use of echocardiography to assist in establishing prognosis. Exercise-induced perfusion defects are well described in patients with HCM and, in young patients, portend a poor prognosis.[60] Patients can drop their blood pressure during exercise, due to a reduction in peripheral vascular resistance. In the young individual with a family history of sudden cardiac death, this finding may predispose the individual to sudden cardiac death.[61]

In summary, survivors of cardiac arrest, young patients with a strong family history of sudden cardiac death, and carriers of certain high-risk genes are all at high risk for future adverse cardiac events. Whereas ambient nonsustained ventricular tachycardia, exercise-induced ischemia and hypotension, marked left ventricular hypertrophy, and significant outflow tract gradient suggest a higher risk, their value stems from their negative prognostic value.[22] The absence of these risk factors in an asymptomatic or mildly symptomatic individual should prompt reassurance.[22] Although few restrictions are recommended, strenuous, competitive training or athletics should be proscribed due to the increased risk of sudden cardiac death.

Mitral Valve Prolapse

MVP is the most common cardiac structural disease, affecting up to 6% of the general population with women affected more than men.[62] Pathologically, it is characterized by the myxomatous degeneration of the valve's collagenous layer. The degree of involvement and extension of this process into the chordae and mitral valve annulus is one of the determinants of the diverse clinical presentations of this disorder.[63] MVP is often seen in conjunction with other heritable disorders that affect the connective tissues. A familial form with autosomal dominant transmission appears to exist and is more common in women.[64]

Although MVP is currently the most common cause of mitral valve regurgitation requiring surgical treatment, it is fortunate that most patients with this disorder are asymptomatic.[65,66] Although rare, potential complications of MVP include mitral regurgitation, infective endocarditis, and cerebrovascular accidents. These complications are seen more commonly in older, male patients with this disorder.[67]

Of the varied clinical manifestations of this disease, palpitations are reported commonly. The etiology varies from benign atrial and ventricular premature complexes to the more disabling supraventricular tachycardias. Due to the wide prevalence of MVP and of benign arrhythmias such as atrial or ventricular premature beats in the normal population, it remains unclear whether an increased incidence actually exists in the MVP population. Once mitral regurgitation complicates MVP, on the other hand, the incidence of atrial and ventricular arrhythmia rises.[68]

The increased prevalence of accessory bypass tracts in patients with MVP has been debatable.[69,70] Ware et al[70] detected a higher incidence of dual AV nodal pathways in patients with MVP; AV nodal reentrant tachycardia was the most common inducible arrhythmia in patients with symptomatic supraventricular tachycardia. As in other patients with accessory bypass tracts, tracts with short antegrade refractory periods may conduct atrial fibrillation to the ventricles at rates that may precipitate fatal ventricular arrhythmias. Patients with a history of syncope and manifest bypass tracts on their resting 12-lead ECG should undergo diagnostic electrophysiologic evaluation to establish the refractory period of the bypass tract. Under controlled circumstances in the electrophysiology lab, the induction of atrial fibrillation allows the evaluation of the bypass tract's potential to precipitate life-threatening ventricular arrhythmias.

Sudden cardiac death has been reported in patients with MVP and is believed to be due to ventricular arrhythmias.[71] The annual incidence varies from 0.2% to as high as 0.5%,[63,72] relying heavily on the population of patients selected. Whereas many cases of sudden cardiac death have been reported in patients with mitral regurgitation, the role of mitral regurgitation in patients with prolapse who had suffered sudden cardiac death has been questioned.[73,74] In a study by Nishimura et al,[63] redundancy of the mitral valve leaflet was found to be the only determinant of sudden death in six patients with MVP.

The high prevalence of ventricular arrhythmias in patients with MVP who have mitral regurgitation and the poor prognosis of patients with MVP with reduced left ventricular function indicate that patients with mitral regurgitation are at increased risk for sudden cardiac death.[75] Although mitral regurgitation and complex ventricular arrhythmias are more frequent in patients at risk for sudden cardiac death, the predictive value of ventricular arrhythmias in MVP is poor.[63]

Although an increased incidence of prolonged corrected QT interval has been reported in patients with MVP, this has not been consistently shown and its role in precipitating sudden cardiac death is unclear.[73,76,77] Multiple incidence of sudden death in families with MVP has been reported.[78]

In summary, MVP is a common disorder with a benign prognosis. Survivors of sudden cardiac death and people with a family history of sudden death, especially with familial MVP, should be at a higher risk for future sudden death. Although sudden death has been reported with uncomplicated MVP, redundant leaflets and mitral regurgitation have been associated with a worse prognosis. The role of ambient ventricular arrhythmias remains unknown.

Congenital Long QT Syndrome

Congenital long QT syndrome is a predominantly hereditary disorder. It is most commonly transmitted in an autosomal dominant manner—the Romano Ward syndrome.[79,80] In a smaller number of affected individuals, transmission is autosomal recessive and is associated with congenital sensorineural deafness, the Jervell and Lange-Nielsen syndrome.[81] One third of affected individuals have no clear hereditary pattern and are thought to have a sporadic form of the disorder. Females appear to be affected more often than males.[79]

The incidence of this disorder is unclear, 2 to 3 per 1000 congenitally deaf people carry this disorder.[82] The form associated with congenital deafness constitutes 6% to 10% of the congenital long QT population.[79] The incidence among males and females is equal until the age of 15, when the ratio of females to males rises sharply.[83]

Keating et al[84] classified patients with the long QT into three groups. Those clearly affected either had a QTc >470 ms in asymptomatic individuals or QTc >450 ms in symptomatic individuals. Individuals with QTc <420 ms were classified as unaffected. Distinct genetic markers have been found linking the long QT syndrome to those genetic abnormalities.[85,86]

Syncope is the most common manifestation of the disorder and is caused by torsade de pointes. One of the hallmarks of this disorder is the precipitation of syncope by fright, intense emotional circumstances, or the sudden awakening by a loud sound. Certain physical activities, such as swimming, have become recognized precipitants.[87] Although sudden increases in adrenergic stimulation have been classically recognized as precipitants of syncope, it is becoming increasingly recognized that some forms of syncope occur during sleep or at rest.[88] The mean age at the time of first episode of syncope is lower in males compared to females (11 years versus 16 years).[83]

The mortality in high-risk, untreated symptomatic patients is as high as 5% per year.[82] Recommendations for the management of asymptomatic individuals with this syndrome are not available. Whereas sudden death is usually preceded by a history of recurrent syncope, this syndrome may rarely manifest itself with sudden death as the first sign. Survivors of sudden death, siblings of individuals who have died suddenly, and infants with this syndrome are all considered at high risk.[87] Markers of poor prognosis in the International Prospective Study[79] were congenital deafness, female gender, documented malignant arrhythmias, and history of syncope. Marked prolongation of the QTc interval (>600 ms) and notching of the T wave are also added risk factors.[89,90] Individuals with the congenital long QT syndrome are not advised to engage in any competitive athletics.[40]

Marfan Syndrome

Marfan syndrome is an inherited autosomal dominant disorder that affects the connective tissues.[91] The disease has been found to occur as a result of a mutation in the gene-encoding fibrillin-1 on chromosome 15.[92] The organs involved are the musculoskeletal organs, the eyes, the heart, and the aorta. Cardiovascular involvement results in MVP/mitral valve regurgitation, aortic incompetence, and dissection of the aorta.[93] Six to nine percent of all aortic dissections occur in patients with Marfan syndrome.[94] Death occurs from rupture of the dissected aorta into a hemithorax or into the pericardium. As in MVP, mitral regurgitation may engender ventricular tachyarrhythmias, a less well-defined cause of morbidity and mortality in this disorder.

Life expectancy in Marfan syndrome has improved significantly over the last decade.[95] This has been partially attributed to increased frequency of diagnosis and to cardiovascular surgery.[95] Surgery to replace the ascending arch of the aorta when its diameter reaches 55 mm, and aortic valve replacement when left ventricular dysfunction begins secondary to aortic regurgitation have led to an improvement in the survival of patients with Marfan syndrome.[96] Initiation of β-blocker therapy has led to attenuation of the rate of aortic dilation and a modest improvement in outcome.[97]

Early diagnosis of this condition is paramount, since prognosis is dependent on the prophylactic initiation of therapy and on timely surgical intervention. The clinical variability of its features often makes this relatively common disorder difficult to diagnose. The earlier commencement of therapy with antiadrenergic agents appears to bestow a more favorable prognosis compared with its later initiation.[98] Patients with Marfan syndrome are advised not to participate in activities that may expose them to body collision. These patients should have echocardiography to measure their aortic root diameter every 6 months.[40] Their activities should be limited to low-intensity sports such as golf, billiards, and bowling.[40]

Congenital Coronary Artery Abnormalities

Congenital coronary artery abnormalities represent the second most common cause of sudden death in athletes—death that invariably occurs during exertion.[1] The most common anomaly is the origin of the left coronary artery from the right sinus of Valsalva.[1] Compression of the coronary vessel between the exercise-induced dilated ascending aorta and pulmonary trunk results in myocardial ischemia. Another mechanism for coronary insufficiency is the slitlike opening of the ostium that is further narrowed during exercise.[3,99]

Mortality from this disorder is high, which may be a reflection of the difficulty encountered in screening for it.[15] Exercise-induced chest pain, syncope, or shortness of breath out of proportion to the amount of exertion should lead to its consideration.[15]

Idiopathic Dilated Cardiomyopathy

By definition, this is a form of cardiomyopathy that occurs in the absence of an established cause of left ventricular dysfunction such as coronary artery disease, hypertension, or valvular heart disease. Twenty percent of idiopathic dilated cardiomyopathy is familial.[100] The incidence of idiopathic dilated cardiomyopathy is about 6 per 100,000.[101] Survival figures are difficult to establish due to the biased nature of the reported patients, but figures are generally poor.[102]

Both subjective indices of left ventricular dysfunction such as New York Heart Association class, and objectitive values such as reduced left ventricular ejection fraction portend a poor prognosis.[103,104] The incidence of sudden cardiac death is also increased in patients with a history of syncope.[105]

Although the overwhelming majority of patients with idiopathic dilated cardiomyopathy have baseline ventricular arrhythmias, bradyarrhythmias and electromechanical dissociation are reported terminal events in a large number of individuals with this disorder.[106] The presence of complex ventricular arrhythmias predicts a higher mortality although it does not predict whether death will be arrhythmic or secondary to pump failure.[107,108] The role of electrophysiologic study is not as clear in idiopathic dilated cardiomyopathy as it is in ischemic cardiomyopathy. Monomorphic ventricular tachycardia is seldom induced, and only in those presenting with it, and serial drug testing is not reliable in predicting freedom from arrhythmic events.[109]

Arrhythmogenic Right Ventricular Dysplasia

Arrhythmogenic right ventricular dysplasia is a disease of unclear etiology characterized by recurrent ventricular tachycardia with a left bundle block morphology secondary to fatty degeneration of the right ventricular free wall. In areas where this disorder is endemic, it accounts for approximately 20% of sudden cardiac death in individuals under the age of 35 years, many occurring during physical exertion.[110] Resting 12-lead ECG may reveal widening of the QRS complex in V_1, incomplete or complete right bundle branch block, and occasionally a late wave (epsilon wave) representing delayed depolarization of the right ventricular free wall.[111] T wave inversion in the right precordial leads has been suggested to represent right ventricular cavity dilatation.[112] Magnetic resonance imaging has a distinct role in uncovering fatty infiltration of the right ventricular free wall, a hallmark of arrhythmogenic right ventricular dysplasia.[113] A history of syncope and involvement of the left ventricle appear to portend a poor prognosis.[114,115]

Conclusions

The death of an athlete is often unpredictable. Available screening strategies are far from having attained a status that would allow for universal applicability. Organizations that support competitive athletics should practice some form of screening to identify potential victims of sudden cardiac death. Once a potential victim is identified, risk stratification would allow for appropriate counseling and direction. Until better recommendations for screening become available, venues for competitive athletic events should always have individuals and equipment to provide prompt advanced cardiac life support. The efforts to teach advanced cardiac life support to the public is a step in the right direction to curb the incidence of sudden cardiac death in athletes.

References

1. Maron BJ, Shirani J, Poliac LC, et al. Sudden death in young competitive athletes: Clinical, demographic and pathological profiles. *JAMA* 1996;276:199–204.
2. Maron BJ, Epstein SE, Roberts WC. Causes of sudden death in competitive athletes. *J Am Coll Cardiol* 1986;7:204–214.
3. Maron BJ, Roberts WC, McAllister HA, et al. Sudden death in young athletes. *Circulation* 1980;62:218–229.
4. Corrado D, Thiene G, Nava A, et al. Sudden death in young competitive athletes: Clinicopathologic correlation in 22 cases. *Am J Med* 1990;89: 588–596.
5. Tsung SH, Huang TY, Chang HH. Sudden death in young athletes. *Arch Pathol Lab Med* 1982;106:168–170.
6. Waller BF, Roberts WC. Sudden death while running in conditioned runners aged 40 years or over. *Am J Cardiol* 1980;45:1292–1300.
7. Maron BJ, Thompson PD, Puffer JC, et al. Cardiovascular preparticiption screening of competitive athletes. A statement for health professionals from the sudden death committee (clinical cardiology) and congenital cardiac defects committee (cardiovascular disease in the young), American Heart Association. *Circulation* 1996;94:850–856.
8. Lynn LA. Screening tests for the healthy adult: Guidelines from the American College of Physicians. *Hospital Physician* 1993;50:29–43.
9. Rowland TW. Sudden unexpected death in sports. *Pediatr Ann* 1992; 21:193–195.
10. Epstein SE, Maron BJ. Sudden death and the competitive athlete: Perspectives on preparticipation screening studies. *J Am Coll Cardiol* 1986;7:220–230.
11. Thompson PD. The cardiovascular complications of vigorous physical activity. *Arch Intern Med* 1996;156:2297–2302.
12. McCaffrey FM, Braden DS, Strong WB. Sudden cardiac death in young athletes: A review. *Am J Dis Child* 1991;145:177–183.
13. Maron BJ, Roberts WC. Causes and implications of sudden cardiac death in athletes. In Akhtar M, Myerburg RJ, Ruskin JN (eds): *Sudden Cardiac Death: Prevalence, Mechanisms, and Approaches to Diagnosis and Management.* Philadelphia: Williams and Willkins; 1994.
14. Burke AP, Farb A, Virmani R, et al. Sports-related and non sports-related sudden cardiac death in young adults. *Am Heart J* 1991;121:568–575.
15. Burke AP, Farb A, Virmani R. Causes of sudden death in athletes. *Cardiol Clin* 1992;10:303–317.
16. Pelliccia A, Maron BJ. Preparticipation cardiovascular evaluation of the competitive athlete: Perspectives from the 30 year Italian experience. *Am J Cardiol* 1995;75:827–829.
17. Rich BSE. Sudden death screening. *Med Clin North Am* 1994;78(2): 267–288.
18. Zehender M, Meinertz T, Keul J, Just H. ECG variants and clinical arrhythmias in athletes: Clinical relevance and prognostic importance. *Am Heart J* 1990;119:1378–1391.
19. Rifat SF, Ruffin MT 4th, Gorenflo DW. Disqualifying criteria in a preparticipation sports evaluation. *J Fam Pract* 1995;41:42–50.
20. Fahrenbach MC, Thompson PD. The preparticipation sports examination. Cardiovascular considerations for screening. *Cardiol Clin* 1992; 10(2): 319–328.

21. Driscoll DJ, Edwards WD. Sudden unexpected death in children and adolescents. *J Am Coll Cardiol* 1985;5(6 suppl):118B–121B.
22. Spirito P, Seidman CE, McKenna WJ, Maron BJ. The management of hypertrophic cardiomyopathy. *N Engl J Med* 1997;336(11):775–785.
23. Maron BJ, Pelliccia A, Spirito P. Cardiac disease in young trained athletes. Insights for distinguishing athlete's heart from structural heart disease, with particular emphasis on hypertrophic cardiomyopathy. *Circulation* 1995;91(5):1596–1601.
24. Wight JN Jr, Salem D. Sudden cardiac death and the 'athlete's heart'. *Arch Intern Med* 1995;155:1473–1480.
25. Metzger JT, de Chillou C, Cheriex E, et al. Value of the 12-lead electrocardiogram in arrhythmogenic right ventricular dysplasia, and the absence of correlation with echocardiographic changes. *Am J Cardiol* 1993;72:964–967.
26. Wigle ED, Rakowski H, Kimball BP, Williams WG. Hypertrophic cardiomyopathy: Clinical spectrum and treatment. *Circulation* 1995;92: 1680–1692.
27. Maron BJ, Bodison SA, Wesley YE, et al. Results of screening a large group of intercollegiate athletes for cardiovascular disease. *J Am Coll Cardiol* 1987;10:1214–1221.
28. Marcus FI, Fontaine G. Arrhythmogenic right ventricular dysplasia/cardiomyopathy: A review. *PACE* 1995;18:1298–1314.
29. Murry PM, Cantwell JD, Heath DL, Shoop J. The role of limited echocardiography in screening athletes. *Am J Cardiol* 1995;76:849–850.
30. Weidenbener EJ, Krauss MD, Waller BF, Taliercio CP. Incorporation of screening echocardiography in the preparticipation screening exam. *Clin J Sports Med* 1995;5:86–89.
31. Lewis JF, Maron BJ, Diggs JA, et al. Preparticipation echocardiographic screening for cardiovascular disease in a large predominantly black population of collegiate athletes. *Am J Cardiol* 1989;64:1029–1033.
32. Feinstein RA, Colvin E, Oh KM. Echocardiographic screening as part of a preparticipation examination. *Clin J Sports Med* 1993;3:149–152.
33. Little WC, Constantinescu M, Applegate RJ, et al. Can coronary angiography predict the site of a subsequent myocardial infarction in patients with mild-to-moderate coronary artery disease? *Circulation* 1988;78: 1157–1166.
34. Ambrose JA, Tannenbaum MA, Alexopoulos D, et al. Angiographic progression of coronary artery disease and the development of myocardial infarction. *J Am Coll Cardiol* 1988;12:56–62.
35. Spirito P, Maron BJ, Bonow RO, et al. Prevalence and significance of an abnormal ST-T segment response to exercise in a young athletic population. *Am J Cardiol* 1983;51:1663–1666.
36. Bruce RA, DeRouen TA, Hossack KF. Value of maximal exercise tests in risk assesment of primary coronary heart disease events in healthy men. Five years' experience of the Seattle heart watch study. *Am J Cardiol* 1980;46:371–378.
37. Siscovick DS, Weiss NS, Fletcher RH, et al. Habitual vigorous exercise and primary cardiac arrest: Effect of other risk factors on the relationship. *J Chron Dis* 1984;37:625–631.
38. McHenry PL, O'Donell J, Morris SN, Jordan JJ. The abnormal exercise electrocardiogram in apparantly healthy men: A predictor of angina pectoris as an initial coronary event during long-term follow up. *Circulation* 1984;70:547–551.

39. Siscovick DS, Ekelund LG, Johnson JL, et al. Sensitivity of exercise electrocardiography for acute cardiac events during moderate and strenuous physical activity. The Lipid Research Clinics Coronary Primary Prevention Trial. *Arch Intern Med* 1991;151:325–330.

40. Zipes DP, Garson A Jr. Task Force 6: Arrhythmias. In Maron BJ, Mitchell JH (eds): 26th Bethesda Conference: Recommendations for determining eligibility for competition in athletes with cardiovascular abnormalities. *J Am Coll Cardiol* 1994;24:845–899.

41. Maron BJ, Gardin JM, Flack JM, et al. Prevalence of hypertrophic cardiomyopathy in a general population of young adults. Echocardiographic analysis of 4111 subjects in the CARDIA Study. *Circulation* 1995; 2:785–789.

41a. Maron BJ, Spirito P. Impact of patient selection biases on the perception of hypertrophic cardiomyopathy and its natural history. *Am J Cardiol* 1993;72:970–972.

42. Maron BJ, Cecchi F, McKenna WJ. Risk factors and stratification for sudden cardiac death in patients with hypertrophic cardiomyopathy. *Br Heart J* 1994;72(6 suppl):S13–S18.

43. Maron BJ, Fananapazir L. Sudden cardiac death in hypertrophic cardiomyopathy. *Circulation* 1992;85(suppl I):I57–I63.

44. Kofflard MJ, Waldstein DJ, Vos J, ten Cate FJ. Prognosis in hypertrophic cardiomyopathy observed in a large clinic population. *Am J Cardiol* 1993;72:939–943.

45. De Rose JJ Jr, Banas JS Jr, Winters SL. Current perspectives on sudden cardiac death in hypertrophic cardiomyopathy. *Prog Cardiovasc Dis* 1994;36:475–484.

46. Maron BJ, Lipson LC, Savage DD, Epstein SE. "Malignant" hypertrophic cardiomyopathy: Identification of a subgroup of families with unusually frequent premature deaths. *Am J Cardiol* 1978;41:1133–1140.

47. Watkins H, Rosenzweig A, Hwang D-S, et al. Characteristics and prognostic implications of myosin missense mutations in familial hypertrophic cardiomyopathy. *N Engl J Med* 1992;326:1108–1114.

48. Watkins H, McKenna WJ, Thierfelder L, et al. Mutations in the genes for cardiac troponin T and alpha tropomyosin in hypertrophic cardiomyopathy. *N Engl J Med* 1995;332:1058–1064.

49. McKenna WJ, Deanfield JE, Faruqui A, et al. Prognosis in hypertrophic cardiomyopathy: Role of age and clinical, electrocardiographic and hemodynamic features. *Am J Cardiol* 1981;47:532–538.

50. McKenna WJ, Deanfield JE. Hypertrophic cardiomyopathy: An important cause of sudden death. *Arch Dis Child* 1984;59:971–975.

51. Maron BJ, Savage DD, Wolfson JK, Epstein SE. Prognostic significance of 24 hour ambulatory monitoring in patients with hypertrophic cardiomyopathy: A prospective study. *Am J Cardiol* 1981;48:252–257.

52. McKenna WJ, Harris L, Percy G. Arrhythmias in hypertrophic cardiomyopathy: Comparison of amiodarone and verapamil in treatment. *Br Heart J* 1981;46:173–178.

53. Spirito P, Rapezzi C, Autore C, et al. Prognosis of asymptomatic patients with hypertrophic cardiomyopathy and non sustained ventricular tachycardia. *Circulation* 1994;90:2743–2747.

54. Fananapazir L, Chang AC, Epstein AC, McAreavey D. Prognostic determinants in hypertrophic cardiomyopathy: Prospective evaluation of a therapeutic strategy based on clinical, Holter, hemodynamic, and electrophysiologic findings. *Circulation* 1992;86:730–740.

55. Saumarez RC, Slade AKB, Grace AA, et al. The significance of paced electrogram fractionation in hypertrophic cardiomyopathy. A prospective study. *Circulation* 1995;91:2762–2768.
56. Spirito P, Maron BJ. Relation between extent of left ventricular hypertrophy and occurrence of sudden cardiac death in hypertrophic cardiomyopathy. *J Am Coll Cardiol* 1990;15:1521–1526.
57. Spirito P, Watson RM, Maron BJ. Relation between extent of left ventricular hypertrophy and occurrence of ventricular tachycardia in hypertrophic cardiomyopathy. *Am J Cardiol* 1987;60:1521–1526.
58. Maron BJ, Gottdiener JS, Epstein SE. Patterns and significance of distribution of left ventricular hypertrophy in hypertrophic cardiomyopathy. A wide-angle, two-dimensional echocardiographic study of 125 patients. *Am J Cardiol* 1981;48:418–428.
59. Spirito P, Maron BJ, Bonow RO, Epstein SE. Occurrence and significance of left ventricular wall thinning and relative cavity dilatation in hypertrophic cardiomyopathy. *Am J Cardiol* 1987;60:123–129.
60. Dilsizian D, Bonow RO, Epstein SE, Fananapazir L. Myocardial ischemia is a frequent cause of cardiac arrest and syncope in young patients with hypertrophic cardiomyopathy. *Circulation* 1990;82:35A.
61. Frenneaux MP, Counihan PJ, Caforio ALP, Chikamori T, McKenna WJ. Abnormal blood pressure response during exercise in hypertrophic cardiomyopathy. *Circulation* 1991;82:1995–2002.
62. Procacci PM, Savran SV, Screiter SL, Bryson AL. Prevalence of clinical mitral valve prolapse in 1,169 young women. *N Engl J Med* 1976;294:1086.
63. Nishimura RA, McGoon MD, Shub C, et al. Echocardiographically documented mitral valve prolapse. *N Engl J Med* 1985;313:1305–1309.
64. Devereaux RB, Brown WT, Kramer-Fox R, Sachs I. Inheritance of mitral valve prolapse. Effect of age and sex on gene expression. *Ann Intern Med* 1982;97:826–832.
65. Zuppiroli A, Rinaldi M, Kramer-Fox R, et al. Natural history of mitral valve prolapse. *Am J Cardiol* 1995;75:1028–1032.
66. Cohn LH, Couper GS, Aranki SF, et al. Long-term results of mitral valve reconstruction for the regurgitating myxomatous mitral valve. *J Thorac Cardiovasc Surg* 1994;107:143–150.
67. McMahon SW, Roberts JK, Kramer-Fox R, et al. Mitral valve prolapse and infective endocarditis. *Am Heart J* 1987;113:1291–1298.
68. Klingfield P, Hochreiter C, Kramer H, et al. Complex arrhythmias in mitral regurgitation with and without mitral valve prolapse: Contrast to arrhythmias in mitral valve prolapse without mitral regurgitation. *Am J Cardiol* 1985;55:1545–1549.
69. Josephson ME, Horowitz LN, Kastor JA. Paroxysmal supraventricular tachycardia in patients with mitral valve prolapse. *Circulation* 1977;57:111–115.
70. Ware JA, Magro SA, Luck JC, et al. Conduction system abnormalities in symptomatic mitral valve prolapse: An electrophysiologic analysis of 60 patients. *Am J Cardiol* 1984;53:1075–1078.
71. Klingfield P, Levy D, Devereaux RB, Savage DD. Arrhythmias and sudden death in mitral valve prolapse. *Am Heart J* 1987;113:1298–1307.
72. Duren DR, Becker AE, Dunning AJ. Long-term follow-up of idiopathic mitral valve prolapse in 300 patients; a prospective study. *J Am Coll Cardiol* 1988;11:42–47.
73. Boudoulas H, Schaal SF, Stang JM, et al. Mitral valve prolapse: Cardiac arrest with long term survival. *Int J Cardiol* 1990;26:37–44.

74. Dollar AL, Roberts WC. Morphologic comparison of patients with mitral valve prolapse who died suddenly with patients who died from severe valvular dysfunction or other conditions. *J Am Coll Cardiol* 1991; 17:921–931.

75. Klingfield P, Hochreiter C, Niles N, et al. Relation of sudden death in pure mitral regurgitation, with and without mitral valve prolapse, to repetitive ventricular arrhythmias and right and left ventricular ejection fractions. *Am J Cardiol* 1987;60:397–399.

76. DeMaria AN, Amsterdam EA, Vismara LA, et al. Arrhythmias in the mitral valve prolapse syndrome. Prevalence, nature and frequency. *Ann Intern Med* 1976;84:656–660.

77. Puddu PE, Pasternac A, Tubau JF, et al. QT interval prolongation and increased plasma catecholamine levels in patients with mitral valve prolapse. *Am Heart J* 1983;105:422–428.

78. Shappell SD, Marshall CE, Brown RE, Bruce TA. Sudden death and the familial occurrence of mid-systolic click, late-systolic murmur syndrome. *Circulation* 1973;48(5):1128–1134.

79. Moss AJ, Schwartz PJ, Crampton RS, et al. The long QT syndrome: A prospective international study. *Circulation* 1985;71:17–21.

80. Vincent GM, Timothy K, Leppert M, Keating M. The spectrum of symptoms and QT interval in carriers of the gene for the long QT syndrome. *N Engl J Med* 1992;327:846–852.

81. Jervell A, Lange-Nielsen F. Congenital deaf-mutism, functional heart disease with prolongation of the Q-T interval and sudden death. *Am Heart J* 1957;54:59.

82. Schwartz PJ, Periti M, Malliani A. The long Q-T syndrome. *Am Heart J* 1975;89:378–390.

83. Locati EH, Moss AJ, Schwartz PJ, et al. Age and gender differences in congenital long QT syndrome. A study in 328 LQTS families. *J Am Coll Cardiol* 1992;19:367A.

84. Keating M, Atkinson D, Dunn C, et al. Linkage of a cardiac arrhythmia, the long QT syndrome, and the Harvey *ras*-1 gene. *Science* 1991;252:704–706.

85. Roden DM, George JL Jr, Bennett PB. Recent advances in understanding the molecular mechanisms of the long QT syndrome. *J Cardiovasc Electrophysiol* 1995;6:1023–1031.

86. Russell MW, Dick M 2nd. The molecular genetics of the congenital long QT syndromes. *Curr Opin Cardiol* 1996;11:45–51.

87. Schwartz PJ, Locati EH, Napolitano C, Priori SG. The long QT syndrome. In Zipes DP, Jalife J (eds): *Cardiac Electrophysiology: From Cell to Bedside, 2nd Edition.* Philadelphia, PA: W.B. Saunders Co.; 1995:788–811.

88. Viersma JW, May JF, de Jongste MJL, et al. Long QT syndrome and sudden death during sleep in one family. *Eur Heart J* 1988;9(suppl 1):45–49.

89. Moss AJ, Schwartz PJ, Crampton RS, et al. The long QT syndrome: Prospective longitudinal study of 328 families. *Circulation* 1991;84: 1136–1144.

90. Malfatto G, Beria G, Sala S, et al. Quantitative analysis of T wave abnormalities and their prognostic implications in the idiopathic long QT syndrome. *J Am Coll Cardiol* 1994;23:296–301.

91. Pyeritz RE, McKusick VA. The Marfan syndrome: Diagnosis and management. *N Engl J Med* 1979;300:772–777.

92. Kainulainen K, Pulkkinen L, Savolainen A, et al. The gene defect causing Marfan syndrome is located on chromosome 15. *N Engl J Med* 1990; 323:935–939.

93. Child JS, Perloff JK, Kaplan S. The heart of the matter: Cardiovascular involvement in Marfan's syndrome. *J Am Coll Cardiol* 1989;14:429.
94. Spittell PC, Spittell JA Jr, Joyce JW, et al. Clinical features and differential diagnosis of aortic dissection. Experience with 236 cases (1980 through 1990). *Mayo Clin Proc* 1993;68;642–651.
95. Silverman DI, Burton KJ, Gray J, et al. Life expectancy in the Marfan syndrome. *Am J Cardiol* 1995;75:157–160.
96. Gott VL, Pyeritz RE, Cameron DE, Greene PS, McKusick VA. Composite graft repair of Marfan aneurysm of the ascending aorta: Results in 100 patients. *Ann Thorac Surg* 1991;52:38–44.
97. Shores J, Berger KR, Murphy EA, Pyeritz RE. Progression of aortic dilation and the benefit of long-term beta-adrenergic blockade in Marfan's syndrome. *N Engl J Med* 1994;330:1335–1341.
98. Beighton P, de Paepe A, Danks D, et al. International nosology of heritable disorders of connective tissue, Berlin 1986. *Am J Med Genet* 1988;29: 581–594.
99. Cheitlin MD, De Castro CM, McAllister HA. Sudden death as a complication of anomalous left coronary origin from the anterior sinus of Valsalva: A not so minor congenital anomaly. *Circulation* 1974;50:780–787.
100. Michels VV. Progress in defining the cause of idiopathic dilated cardiomyopathy. Editorial. *N Engl J Med* 1993;329:960–961.
101. Codd MB, Sugrue DD, Gersh BJ, Melton LJ. Epidemiology of idiopathic dilated and hypertrophic cardiomyopathy: A population based study in Olmsted County, Minnesota, 1975–1984. *Circulation* 1989;80:564–572.
102. Manolio TA, Baughman KL, Rodheffer R, et al. Prevalence and etiology of idiopathic dilated cardiomyopathy (summary of a National Heart, Lung, and Blood Institute workshop). *Am J Cardiol* 1992;69:1458–1466.
103. Keogh AM, Baron DW, Hickie JB. Prognostic guides in patients with idiopathic or ischemic dilated cardiomyopathy assessed for cardiac transplantation. *Am J Cardiol* 1990;65:903–908.
104. Hofmann T, Meinertz T, Kasper W, et al. Mode of death in idiopathic dilated cardiomyopathy: A multivariate analysis of prognostic determinants. *Am Heart J* 1988;116:1455–1463.
105. Brembilla-Perrot B, Donetti J, de la Chaise AT, et al. Diagnostic value of ventricular stimulation in patients with idiopathic dilated cardiomyopathy. *Am Heart J* 1991;121:1124–1131.
106. Luu M, Stevenson WG, Stevenson LW, et al. Diverse mechanisms of sudden cardiac arrest in advanced heart failure. *Circulation* 1989;80: 1675–1680.
107. Holmes J, Kubo SH, Cody RJ, Kligfield P. Arrhythmias in ischemic and non ischemic dilated cardiomyopathy: Prediction of mortality by ambulatory electrocardiography. *Am J Cardiol* 1985;55:146–151.
108. Gonska BD, Bethge KP, Figulla HR, Kreuzer H. Occurrence and clinical significance of endocardial late potentials and fractionations in idiopathic dilated cardiomyopathy. *Br Heart J* 1988;59:39–46.
109. Tamburro P, Wiber D. Sudden death in idiopathic dilated cardiomyopathy. *Am Heart J* 1992;124:1035–1045.
110. Thiene G, Nava A, Corrado D, et al. Right ventricular cardiomyopathy and sudden death in young people. *N Engl J Med* 1988;318:129–133.
111. Fontaine G, Guiraudon G, Frank R, et al. Stimulation studies and epicardial mapping in ventricular tachycardia: Study in mechanisms and relation for surgery. In Kulbertus HE (ed): *Reentrant Arrhythmias.* Lancaster: MTP Publishers; 1977:334–350.

112. Nava A, Canciani D, Buja G, et al. Electrocardiographic study of negative t-waves on precordial leads and arrhythmogenic right ventricular dysplasia: Relationship with right ventricular volume. *J Electrocardiol* 1988;21:239–245.
113. Casolo GC, Poggcsi L, Boddi M, et al. ECG-gated magnetic resonance imaging and right ventricular dysplasia. *Am Heart J* 1989;113: 1245–1248.
114. Marcus FI, Fontaine G, Frank R, et al. Long term follow-up in patients with arrhythmogenic right ventricular disease. *Eur Heart J* 1989;10 (suppl D):68–73.
115. Fontaine G, Brestescher C, Fontaliran F, et al. Outcome of arrhythmogenic right ventricular dysplasia. Apropos of 4 cases (French). *Arch Mal Coeur Vaiss* 1995;88:973–979.

4

The Role of History and Physical Examination in Screening for Causes of Sudden Cardiac Death in Athletes

Munther K. Homoud, MD
and Deeb N. Salem, MD

The demise of an athlete is a tragedy and is received with great anguish. The trauma of such an unexpected occurrence is compounded by the age of the individual and his or her presumed good health. There are over 4 million competitive athletes in the United States, the majority of whom are in high school.[1] The estimated death rate among high school and college athletes is 0.75 and 0.13 per 100,000 men and women, respectively, with a slightly higher incidence among college athletes and a disproportionately higher incidence among males.[2] Traumatic death remains the preeminent cause of death in the adolescent population, athletics-related sudden cardiac death being one of the least common causes.[3] Heat-related deaths, rhabdomyolysis in patients with sickle cell trait, asthma, and gastrointestinal hemorrhage constitute the noncardiac causes of nontraumatic deaths among athletes.[3]

From Estes NAM, Salem DN, Wang PJ (eds). *Sudden Cardiac Death in the Athlete.* Armonk, NY: Futura Publishing Co., Inc.; ©1998.

Table 1
Causes of Sudden Cardiac Death in Athletes

Age <35 years

    Hypertrophic cardiomyopathy
    Congenital coronary artery anomalies
    Arrhythmogenic right ventricular dysplasia
    Marfan syndrome
    Mitral valve prolapse
    Congenital long QT syndrome
    Dilated cardiomyopathy
    Myocarditis

Age >35 years

    Coronary artery disease

Etiology of Sudden Cardiac Death in Athletes

Several congenital and acquired diseases either manifest exclusively or include as one of their clinical manifestations with exertion-related sudden cardiac death. Although due to the acute unexpected nature of its presentation in individuals not suspected of having cardiovascular abnormalities, documentation is difficult; it is believed that arrhythmias constitute a common final pathway in the genesis of this entity. In Marfan syndrome, on the other hand, the etiology is acute rupture of the ascending aorta with hemopericardium and acute cardiac tamponade.

The cardiac etiologies of sudden cardiac death can be divided by age (Table 1). The most common abnormality found in patients younger than 35 is hypertrophic cardiomyopathy.[4] Other causes include anomalous origin of the left coronary artery from the right sinus of Valsalva, ruptured aorta (Marfan syndrome), myocarditis, dilated cardiomyopathy, arrhythmogenic right ventricular dysplasia, mitral valve prolapse, and coronary artery disease.[1,4] Among patients older than 35, coronary artery disease predominates as the cause of sudden cardiac death.[1]

Cardiovascular Adaptation to Exercise

Athletes' hearts undergo morphological changes that account for changes in their baseline physical examination, electrocardiographic, and echocardiographic features.[5] These changes are highly dependent upon the predominant type of exercise they participate in. Athletes whose predominant activity is isotonic exercises (such as long distance runners) undergo hypertrophic changes. These changes are characterized by an increase in left ventricular cavity size, manifest by an increase in end-diastolic volume and diameter.[6] Such changes are most marked in cyclists.[7] There is concomitant increase in left ventricular wall thickness, especially of the posterior wall and septum. This results in an increase in left ventricular mass and a normal mass-to-volume ratio.[6] Although a gray area exists between values consistent with endurance training and those consistent with hypertrophic cardiomyopathy, the values for trained athletes usually falls in the normal zone.[8]

Isometric exercises such as weight lifting result in a pressure load on the heart, raising both systolic and diastolic blood pressure. Hypertrophy is concentric; maximal oxygen consumption is not increased since energy is provided by anaerobic metabolism.[9] Left ventricular cavity is not increased and the ratio of mass to volume is increased.[9] Compared to patients with structural heart disease, the morphological changes seen in trained athletes regress with time once exercise is halted.[10]

The cardiovascular examination of trained athletes often uncovers findings that would be considered abnormal in nonathletes. Resting heart rates are low and occasionally a pulmonic flow murmur can be heard if the examination is conducted while the patient is in the supine position.[5] While controversy exists as to the presence of an S_4 in highly trained athletes, S_3 can often be heard.[5] The enhanced baseline resting parasympathetic tone often can manifest as sinus bradycardia, wandering pacemaker rhythm, Wenckebach atrioventricular block and, rarely, higher degrees of atrioventricular block.[11] Some of these findings can be detected by neck vein examination.

The History and Physical Examination in Preparticipation Screening

The History

The history should be directed toward uncovering significant cardiovascular abnormalities with particular emphasis at causes of exercise-related death (Table 2). A history of exertion-related chest pain may suggest hypertrophic cardiomyopathy or, in an older individual, ischemic heart disease. The occurrence of syncope, presyncope, or lightheadedness during or shortly after exertion may suggest exercise-related arrhythmias, obstructive cardiomyopathy, aortic stenosis, or congenital long QT syndrome. Shortness of breath or sudden fatigue out of proportion to the degree of physical activity should also raise suspicion of an acute rise in left ventricular filling pressure or a sudden

Table 2
Proposed Outline for the Use of History and Physical
Examination in Preparticipation Screening

History:
- Race and gender
- Type of anticipated sport participation
- History of syncope, especially if during or immediately after exertion
- History of exertional chest pain or shortness of breath out of proportion to amount of exertion
- History of palpitations with or without lightheadedness
- Family history of premature sudden cardiac death
- Family history of premature coronary artery disease
- Family history of Marfan, hypertrophic cardiomyopathy, long QT syndrome/congenital deafness

drop in cardiac output. This may occur secondary to structural heart disease or to an acute exercise-related arrhythmia. It is important to consider that these symptoms are commonly seen in athletes and may be extracardiac in origin.[12] The history should include an attempt at elucidating the possible use of illicit drugs or anabolic steroids.

Certain sports, such as football and basketball, carry an inherently higher risk of sudden cardiac death than others.[4] The risk of sudden cardiac death, by contrast, is low enough in marathon runners to question the necessity of routine preparticipation screening.[13] Some sports tend to attract individuals with physical features seen advantageous to a particular sport shared by some of the causes of athlete-related sudden cardiac death. One such example is basketball or volleyball and individuals with Marfan syndrome.[3] Some individuals, particularly in the older age group, are prompted to start engaging in physical activity shortly after the inception of symptoms of cardiac disease.[14]

A family history should be obtained and, in high school athletes, the parents should be involved in the interview process for a thorough history. A family history of syncope may suggest long QT syndrome. Marfan syndrome, hypertrophic cardiomyopathy, and long QT syndrome are familial. In older individuals, a family history of premature coronary artery disease or sudden cardiac death should raise the possibility of coronary artery disease.

The Physical Examination

The examination should be performed in a quiet, comfortable environment (Table 3). Blood pressure should be measured in both arms. The general habitus should be inspected for stigmata of Marfan syndrome.

Table 3
Proposed Outline for the Use of History and Physical
Examination in Preparticipation Screening

Physical examination:
* In a quiet, warm room
* Body height, arm span/total body height, lower/upper body height
* Xanthomas, xanthelesmas
* Eye exam for myopia, ectopia lentis
* Thoracic bony abnormalities, abnormal joint laxity
* Cardiac examination in the sitting-up or standing position
* Employ dynamic maneuvers such as Valsalva, squatting
* Midsystoloc clicks, apical systolic murmurs, early decrescendo diastolic murmurs
* Inguinal hernias

These include an arm span greater than total body height and an increased lower body (pubis to foot) to upper body (pubis to head) ratio. Patients with hypercholesterolemia may have eyelid xanthomas and xanthelesmas. Ectopia lentis, a manifestation of Marfan syndrome, results in myopia and the need for corrective lenses. The presence of contact lenses, masking myopia, should be excluded.[14] The jugular venous wave should be inspected in the 45° recumbent position, while looking for abnormal elevation seen in right heart failure or a prominent a wave in hypertrophic cardiomyopathy. A brisk upstroke carotid pulse helps differentiates hypertrophic cardiomyopathy from the delayed weak upstroke seen in aortic stenosis. The chest wall should be inspected for deformities such as pectus excavatum or pectus carinatum.

Cardiac examination should be conducted with the patient sitting up or standing to reduce the incidence of benign venous murmurs and enhance the murmur of hypertrophic cardiomyopathy.[3,14] Precordial palpation in hypertrophic cardiomyopathy may reveal a sustained precordial heave and, less commonly, a palpable presystolic bulge coinciding with the rapid filling of the stiff left ventricle during late diastole.

The obstructive form of hypertrophic cardiomyopathy is characterized by a systolic ejection murmur that is best heard between the apex and left sternal border and does not radiate to the neck. Maneuvers that reduce left ventricular volume, such as standing and performing the Valsalva maneuver, enhance the murmur, whereas squatting and isometric handgrip exercises reduce the murmur by increasing afterload. The auscultatory findings of mitral valve prolapse vary from one examination to another. The systolic click is best heard with the diaphragm in the left lateral position at the apex. Interventions that reduce left ventricular size, such as standing or performing the Valsalva maneuver, move the click closer to S_1 and lengthen the systolic murmur. On the other hand, squatting, lying down from the standing position, or raising the legs, by enhancing venous return and afterload, all increase left ventricular size, shifting the click and murmur toward mid- or late systole. To differentiate the systolic murmur of obstructive hypertrophic cardiomyopathy from mitral valve prolapse, one must note that whereas after the Valsalva maneuver, the systolic murmur becomes louder in the former, it becomes longer in the latter disorder and not necessarily louder. The Valsalva maneuver is best performed with the operator placing his hand against the patient's abdomen. The patient is instructed to push against the operators hand, and the murmur can be enhanced by performing this maneuver with the patient standing up.

During diastole, auscultation must be carefully performed while looking for extra sounds and/or murmurs. An S_3 or S_4 can normally be heard in a young, athletic population.[5] A loud S_4, especially in a patient with the nonobstructive form of hypertrophic cardiomyopathy, may be the only auscultatory finding. Diastolic murmurs are never innocent and, if decrescendo, blowing, and best heard in the right second intercostal space, should suggest aortic incompetence. In a young individual this would most probably occur in the context of Marfan syndrome.

Hypertrophic Cardiomyopathy

Hypertrophic cardiomyopathy is the leading cause of sudden cardiac death in athletes, accounting for one third of all cases in athletes younger than 35 years of age.[4] The prevalence of this disorder is estimated at 1 in 500 people.[15] Fifty percent of cases of hypertrophic cardiomyopathy are inherited in the autosomal dominant form.[16]

The significance of diagnosing this condition rests on the increased risk of sudden cardiac death. Most patients are asymptomatic and are often diagnosed in the course of screening family members of an individual with this disorder (Table 4). Dyspnea is the most common symptom and is a consequence of the elevated left ventricular pressure secondary to diastolic dysfunction. Angina is another common symptom and can occur in the absence of epicardiac coronary disease. Increased myocardial mass and elevated end-diastolic pressure are some of the causes of this symptom.

Syncope carries a worse prognosis for the occurrence of sudden death in children, compared to adults.[17,18] The mechanisms of sudden death are not uniform and include ventricular tachyarrhythmias, severe hypotension during atrial tachycardia, bradycardia, and myocardial ischemia resulting in hypotension.[19] Despite the difficulty of predicting the incidence of sudden death in patients with hypertrophic

Table 4
Hypertrophic Cardiomyopathy

History	Exertional dyspnea (most common symptom)
	Exertional chest pain
	History of syncope*
	Premature sudden cardiac death in the family*
	Family history of hypertrophic cardiomyopathy
Physical exam.	Elevated jugular venous pressure, prominent a wave
	Brisk upstroke carotid pulse
	Spike and dome contour of carotid pulse
	Bi- or triphasic apical beat
	Harsh systolic murmur between the apex and left sternal border
	Murmur increased by standing, Valsalva maneuver decreased by squatting, elevation of lower limbs
	Loud S_4

*along with young age at presentation, these features are considered to portend an adverse prognosis.

cardiomyopathy, certain risk factors have been identified.[18,19] These factors include a family history of sudden cardiac death occurring in at least two first-degree relatives under 55 years old, young age at presentation, nonsustained ventricular tachycardia on Holter monitor, especially if associated with symptoms of impaired consciousness, and a history of cardiac arrest or syncope. Recent evidence suggests that inducible ischemia on exercise perfusion imaging is a risk factor in children with hypertrophic cardiomyopathy.[19]

Physical examination reflects the essential hemodynamic features of hypertrophic cardiomyopathy: midsystolic obstruction to cardiac output, diastolic dysfunction, and increased myocardial mass. The carotid pulse has a characteristic rapid upstroke followed by an abrupt decline coinciding with maximal outflow obstruction, followed by a second wave resulting from completion of systole "spike and dome." The jugular venous wave may show a prominent a wave due to increased right ventricular late diastolic filling pressure. A left precordial heave can be felt, along with a palpable fourth heart sound due to increased ventricular stiffness.

The systolic murmur heard in obstructive hypertrophic cardiomyopathy is harsh, best heard between the apex and left heart border, and S_1 can be distinctly heard. Maneuvers that increase preload, such as squatting and elevation of the lower limbs while lying down, attenuate the murmur. The Valsalva maneuver, standing up, and amyl nitrate, enhance the murmur. A holosystolic murmur can be heard over the apex if the patient has concomitant mitral regurgitation. A loud S_4 can also be heard over the apex. It is important to note that the nonobstructive form of hypertrophic cardiomyopathy is the more prevalent form in the 24- to 35-year population.[15]

Congenital Coronary Artery Abnormalities

Congenital coronary artery abnormalities are the second most common cause of sudden death in athletes younger than 30 years.[20] The incidence of sudden death is high, with a 46% incidence of sudden death when the left main coronary artery arises from the right sinus of Valsalva. Eighty-six percent of deaths in this disorder occur during exercise.[20] Since physical examination is unrevealing in this disorder (Table 5), suspicion must be raised when a child or athlete loses consciousness during activity, shows signs of ischemia on exercise, or develops acute, exercise-related shortness of breath out of proportion to the exercise he or she is engaged in.[20]

Arrhythmogenic Right Ventricular Dysplasia

Arrhythmogenic right ventricular dysplasia is a disorder of unclear etiology characterized by heterogeneous infiltration of the right ventricular free wall with adipose and fibrous tissue.[21] This disorder usually presents in young people with palpitations, presyncope, and syncope. The mechanism of these symptoms is ventricular tachyarrhythmia. There are no distinct physical findings (Table 5), and the diagnosis is usually established by magnetic resonance scanning.[22]

Table 5
Congenital Coronary Anomalies and
Arrhythmogenic Right Ventricular Dysplasia

Congenital Coronary Artery Anomalies	
History	Syncope and/or chest pain on exertion Dyspnea disproportional to amount of exertion
Physical exam.	Noncontributory

Arrhythmogenic Right Ventricular Dysplasia	
History	Palpitations, presyncope, syncope
Physical exam.	Noncontributory

Marfan Syndrome

This entity is important to recognize not only for the potential incidence of sudden cardiac death due to aortic rupture, but because certain sports such as volleyball and basketball attract players with features common to this disorder.[3] There is a failure to diagnose this disorder outside of families known to carry this disorder because it is a familial disorder with marked clinical variability.[23] Thirty percent of cases represent new mutations. The cardiovascular features of Marfan syndrome include mitral valve prolapse, resulting in mitral regurgitation and dilatation of the sinuses of Valsalva.[24] The latter results in aortic regurgitation and dissection of the aorta in nonhypertensive individuals.

The history and physical examination should provide a strong clue to the existence of Marfan syndrome (Table 6). Affected individuals are tall and thin, have long arms with the arm span exceeding their height, and have a pubis-to-foot length greater than the length from crown to pubis. Arachnodactyly is manifest by the overlap between thumb and fifth finger when the wrist is encircled. Ocular manifestations include myopia and ectopia lentis. Joint hypermobility, pectus excavatum, scoliosis, and reduced thoracic kyphosis are some of the other skeletal deformities associated with Marfan syndrome.

Variability exists in the cardiovascular findings of mitral valve prolapse associated with Marfan syndrome, the two main features being a mid- to late-systolic click and/or systolic murmur of mitral regurgitation. The click can best be heard by the diaphragm of the stethoscope with the patient in the left lateral position. The click results from the tensing of the redundant chordae and valve leaflets. Any decrease in left ventricular cavity size such as by reduction in venous return or

Table 6
Marfan Syndrome

History	Familial incidence (aut. dominant)
Physical exam.	Disproportionate lower body/upper body height
	Retinal detachment
	Ectopia lentis, myopia, elongated globe
	Scoliosis, pectus excavatum/carinatum
	Reduced thoracic kyphosis
	Mitral valve prolapse
	Mitral regurgitation
	Aortic regurgitation
	Inguinal, incisional hernias
	Striae atrophicae

increased contractility, moves the systolic click earlier into systole, also lengthening the duration of the systolic regurgitant murmur. The Valsalva maneuver, standing upright, and the inhalation of amyl nitrite will advance the click and murmur, whereas squatting, isometric exercise, and leg raising will delay the click and murmur.

Mitral Valve Prolapse

Prevalent in approximately 5% of the population, mitral valve prolapse is probably the most common valvular heart disease.[25] While most patients remain asymptomatic throughout their lives, the most common complication is mitral regurgitation.[26] Patients may complain of a variety of symptoms such as palpitations, dyspnea, and atypical chest pain. The hallmark of this disorder is the midsystolic click (Table 7). If accompanied by mitral regurgitation, a late systolic murmur may be heard. The click is best heard in the apex and can be moved earlier by reducing the size of the left ventricle. Whereas the Valsalva maneuver and standing up will shift the click earlier, squatting, elevation of lower limbs, and isometric arm exercised will delay it. Sudden cardiac death during exercise has been reported in individuals with mitral valve prolapse.[27] Although it is distinctly rare, Kligfield and Devereux[28] have identified certain risk factors for sudden death in patients with mitral valve prolapse.

Table 7
Mitral Valve Prolapse and Congenital Long QT Syndrome

Mitral Valve Prolapse	
History	Palpitations, dyspnea, atypical chest pain
Physical exam.	Thoracic bony abnormalities, hypomastia, Apical mid-to-late systolic click, late SEM, Click advanced by standing, Valsalva delayed by squatting, elevating lower limbs
Congenital Long QT Syndrome	
History	Deafness, family history of sudden cardiac death, Syncope in response to fright, exertion, or emotional stress
Physical exam.	Noncontributory

SEM = systolic ejection murmur.

Other Disorders

Patients with the congenital long QT syndrome have a history of recurrent loss of consciousness. These attacks are characteristically precipitated by fright, emotional stress, and sudden, loud noises (Table 7). Exertion, notably swimming, may be a precipitant.[29] There is often a familial history of recurrent syncope and/or of sudden cardiac death. The long QT syndrome is usually transmitted in an autosomal dominant or, rarely, autosomal recessive form. The latter is associated with sensorineural deafness. Patients with myocarditis or dilated cardiomyopathy may be asymptomatic (Table 8). Patients with significant myocardial decompensation may complain of chest discomfort, shortness of breath, or palpitations. Physical examination may reveal inappropriate sinus tachycardia, premature ventricular beats, or narrow pulse pressure. Auscultation may be unremarkable or show an S_4 or an S_3 beat over the apex.

Summary

Sudden cardiac death during or shortly after engaging in competitive sports is, fortunately, a rare occurrence. The cause is usually an as yet undiscovered cardiac disease. The nature of the constellation of

Table 8
Myocarditis and Dilated Cardiomyopathy

Myocarditis	
History	Asymptomatic Chest discomfort Palpitations Dyspnea
Physical exam.	Tachycardia out of proportion to fever Ventricular arrhythmias Pericardial friction rub Protodiastolic gallop
Dilated Cardiomyopathy	
History	Fatigue, dyspnea
Physical exam.	Tachycardia, narrow pulse pressure Jugular venous distension Displaced apex, apical heave S_4, S_3, mitral/tricuspid valve murmur(s) Hepatomegaly, ascites, lower-limb edema

diseases leading to this entity does not readily lend itself to early detection. The alterations in cardiac structure that result from the consistent engagement in competitive athletics result in physical and electrocardiographic changes, blurring the margin that separates what is considered normal from what is not. Screening studies on small populations have not proved beneficial. Until larger studies are conducted to evaluate the efficacy of screening studies, these authors recommend, and in keeping with the recommendations of the American Heart Association/American College of Cardiology, urging a policy of screening using history and physical examination. The authors believe that a history directed at uncovering potentially lethal diseases will allow for the identification of individuals who would further benefit from cardiovascular work-up.

References

1. Maron BJ, Thompson PD, Puffer JC, et al. Cardiovascular preparticipation screening of competitive athletes. A statement for health professionals from the sudden death committee (clinical cardiology) and congenital cardiac defects committee (cardiovascular disease in the young), American Heart Association. *Circulation* 1996;94:850–856.
2. van Camp SP, Bloor CM, Mueller FO, et al. Non traumatic sports death in high school and college athletes. *Med Sci Sports Exerc* 1995;27:641–647.
3. Thompson PD. The cardiovascular complications of vigorous physical activity. *Arch Intern Med* 1996;156:2297–2302.
4. Maron BJ, Shirani J, Poliac LC, et al. Sudden death in young competitive athletes: Clinical, demographic and pathological profiles. *JAMA* 1996; 276:199–204.
5. Wight JN Jr, Salem D. Sudden cardiac death and the 'athlete's heart.' *Arch Intern Med* 1995;155:1473–1480.
6. Shapiro LM. Morphologic consequences of systematic training. *Cardiol Clin* 1992;10(2):219–226.
7. Fagard R, Aubert A, Staessen J, et al. Cardiac structure and function in runners. Comparative echocardiographic study. *Br Heart J* 1984;52(2): 124–129.
8. Maron BJ, Pelliccia A, Spirito P. Cardiac disease in young trained athletes. Insights for distinguishing athlete's heart from structural heart disease, with particular emphasis on hypertrophic cardimyopathy. *Circulation* 1995;91(5):1596–1601.
9. Longhurst JC, Stebbins CL. The isometric athlete. *Cardiol Clin* 1992; 10(2):281–293.
10. Ehsani AA, Hagberg JM, Hickson RC. Rapid changes in left ventricular dimensions and mass in response to physical conditioning and deconditioning. *Am J Cardiol* 1978;42(1):52–56.
11. Oakley CM. The electrocardiogram in the highly trained athlete. *Cardiol Clin* 1992;10(2):295–302.
12. Rich BSE. Sudden death screening. *Med Clin North Am* 1994;78(2): 267–288.
13. Maron BJ, Poliac LC, Roberts WO. Risk for sudden cardiac death associated with marathon running. *J Am Coll Cardiol* 1996;28:428–431.

14. Fahrenbach MC, Thompson PD. The preparticipation sports examination. Cardiovascular considerations for screening. *Cardiol Clin* 1992;10(2): 319–328.
15. Maron BJ, Gardin JM, Flack JM, et al. Prevalence of hypertrophic cardiomyopathy in a general population of young adults. Echocardiographic analysis of 4111 subjects in the CARDIA Study. *Circulation* 1995;2: 785–789.
16. Davies MJ, McKenna WJ. Hypertrophic cardiomyopathy: An introduction to pathology and pathogenesis. *Br Heart J* 1994;72(6 suppl):S2–S3.
17. Nienaber CA, Hiller S, Spielmann RP, et al. Syncope in hypertrophic cardiomyopathy: Multivariate analysis of prognostic determinants. *J Am Coll Cardiol* 1990;15(5):948–955.
18. Maron BJ, Cecchi F, McKenna WJ. Risk factors and stratification for sudden death in patients with hypertrophic cardiomyopathy. *Br Heart J* 1994;72(6 suppl):S13–S18.
19. Fananapazir L, McAreavey D, Epstein ND. Hypertrophic cardiomyopathy. In Zipes DP, Jalife J (eds): *Cardiac Electrophysiology: From Cell to Bedside, 2nd Edition.* Philadelphia, PA: W.B. Saunders Co.; 1995:769–779.
20. Burke AP, Farb A, Virmani R. Causes of sudden death in athletes. *Cardiol Clin* 1992;10(2):303–317.
21. McKenna WJ, Thiene G, Nava A, et al. Diagnosis of arrhythmogenic right ventricular dysplasia/cardiomyopathy. Task force of the Working Group Myocardial and Pericardial Disease of the European Society of Cardiology and of the Scientific Council on Cardiomyopathies of the International Society and Federation of Cardiology. *Br Heart J* 1994;71(3):215–218.
22. Blake LM, Scheinman MM, Higgins CB. MR features of arrhythmogenic right ventricular dysplasia. *AJR* 1994;162(4):809–812.
23. Pereira L, Levran O, Ramirez F, et al. A molecular approach to the stratification of cardiovascular risk in families with Marfan's syndrome. *N Engl J Med* 1994;331(3):148–153.
24. McKusick VA. The cardiovascular aspects of Marfan's syndrome: A heritable disorder of connective tissues. *Circulation* 1955;11:321.
25. Levy D, Savage DD. Prevalence and clinical features of mitral valve prolapse. *Am Heart J* 1987;113(5):1281–1290.
26. Devereux RB. Recent developments in the diagnosis and management of mitral valve prolapse. *Curr Opin Cardiol* 1995;10(2):107–116.
27. Maron BJ, Mitchell JH. 26th Bethesda Conference: Recommendations for determining eligibility for competition in athletes with cardiovascular abnormalities. *J Am Coll Cardiol* 1994;24:845–899.
28. Kligfield P, Devereux RB. Arrhythmia in mitral valve prolapse. In Podrid PR, Kowey PR (eds): *Cardiac Arrhythmia: Mechanisms, Diagnosis and Management.* Baltimore: Williams and Wilkins Co.; 1995.
29. Schwartz PJ, Locati EH, Napolitano C, Priori SG. The long QT syndrome. In Zipes DP, Jalife J (eds): *Cardiac Electrophysiology: From Cell to Bedside, 2nd Edition.* Philadelphia, PA: W.B. Saunders Co.; 1995:788–811.

5

The Athlete's Electrocardiogram:

Distinguishing Normal from Abnormal

Caroline B. Foote, MD and
Gregory F. Michaud, MD

Current recommendations for preparticipation screening of competitive athletes as put forth in a consensus statement for health care professionals by the American Heart Association include a careful history and physical examination.[1] In athletes with a personal history, family history, or physical examination suggestive of organic heart disease, further diagnostic evaluation including resting 12-lead electrocardiogram (ECG) is indicated. In athletes older than 35 years of age, the International Federation of Sports Medicine recommends a resting 12-lead ECG (International Federation of Sports Medicine Web Site). Some authors suggest a resting 12-lead ECG as a standard preparticipation screening measure.[2,3] This presupposes that the interpreting physician has full knowledge of the normal athlete's ECG.

In athletes under 35 years of age, the organic cardiovascular cause most frequently associated with sudden death is hypertrophic cardiomyopathy (HCM).[4–6] Less commonly reported are anomalous coronary arteries, Marfan syndrome, myocarditis, and dilated cardiomyopathy.[7] In one series, arrhythmogenic right ventricular dysplasia (ARVD) had a high incidence.[8] Valvular heart disease, conduction abnormalities,

From Estes NAM, Salem DN, Wang PJ (eds). *Sudden Cardiac Death in the Athlete.* Armonk, NY: Futura Publishing Co., Inc.; ©1998.

and sarcoid are rarely associated with sudden cardiac death in the young athlete.[6] Long QT syndrome and the Wolff-Parkinson-White syndrome are associated with an increased risk of sudden death, but may be under-reported in athletes because autopsy findings are absent or easily overlooked. In athletes over 35 years of age, coronary artery atherosclerosis is the predominant cause of sudden death.[9]

The athlete's ECG frequently shows abnormalities that mimic organic heart disease. The importance of distinguishing ECG abnormalities due to organic heart disease from the normal athletic heart has profound implications. Athletes may be unnecessarily removed from competition or may undergo expensive diagnostic work-ups for abnormalities that fall within the normal range for athletes. Alternatively, clues to important organic heart disease may be misinterpreted as normal variants of an athlete's ECG. Certainly, the ECG must be interpreted in light of an athlete's medical history, physical examination, family history of cardiovascular disease and sudden death, and review of symptoms. Even with full knowledge of the common abnormalities encountered in the athlete's ECG, it may be impossible to distinguish organic heart disease from normal cardiac adaptation to chronic strenuous physical exertion without further diagnostic evaluation.

Athletic conditioning leads to a predictable cardiac adaptive response. An increase in left ventricular (LV) mass is accomplished by increasing LV wall thickness or diastolic cavity dimension or both.[10] These changes are of small magnitude, but are statistically significant when athletes and nonathletic controls are compared. In most competitive athletes, LV wall thickness is ≤12 mm.[11] In some sports, such as distance running, swimming, cycling, and rowing, LV wall thickness may reach 16 mm. Patients with HCM usually have LV wall thicknesses in excess of 20 mm,[12] but a minority have wall thicknesses within the upper range of athletic hearts. LV end-diastolic cavity dimension is usually within 53 to 58 mm in athletes, but may occasionally be larger.[11] Absence of systolic dysfunction in the athlete distinguishes a normal adaptive response from dilated cardiomyopathy in athletes with a dilated LV cavity. A decrease in resting heart rate (HR) and exercise HR mediated by an increase in vagal tone and a reduction in sympathetic tone is seen in all athletes. The chronic physiologic response to exercise may underlie many of the common ECG abnormalities in athletes, as outlined below.

Sinus Bradycardia/Arrhythmia

Sinus bradycardia, as defined by a HR less than 60 bpm, is common in athletes. Depending on the sport sampled and the level of competition, 50% to 91% of athletes will have a resting sinus brady-cardia.[13-21] Athletes' resting HRs are generally lower in endurance sports such as long distance running, and inversely correlate with the level of fitness of the individual athlete. Mean resting HRs are usually in the 50s. In one electrocardiographic analysis of 20 elite distance run-ners, the mean HR was 47 bpm.[19] The lowest reported HR was 25 bpm in an asymptomatic distance runner.[22] Asymptomatic sinus pauses greater than 2 seconds are common in athletes.[23] Sinus bradycardia is easily overcome by exercise.

Although sinus bradycardia is largely a result of increased resting vagal tone and decreased sympathetic tone, it is interesting to note that chemically denervated hearts in athletes have significantly lower intrinsic HRs than those of sedentary controls.[24] This suggests that si-nus pacemaker cells are influenced by athletic conditioning indepen-dent of neural input.

Sinus arrhythmia is reported with widely varying frequency, from 13% to 69%.[13,14,25] With long-term monitoring, the incidence may be as high as 91%.[23] Such a wide spectrum of frequency can probably be ex-plained by the individual athlete's autonomic state and level of fitness, as well as the definition of sinus arrhythmia used by the various au-thors when the resting ECG was obtained. Sinus arrhythmia is gener-ally believed to represent high vagal tone.

Atrioventricular Block

First-degree atrioventricular (AV) block is seen in 10% to 33% of athletes,[14,26,27] and normalizes with exercise.[15,19,20,27] On a random resting ECG, 2% to 10% of endurance runners will exhibit Mobitz type I second-degree AV block.[27,28] On ambulatory monitoring, up to 40% of such athletes will demonstrate Mobitz type I block and up to 8% will also demonstrate Mobitz type II block.[23] Complete heart block is rare in athletes (approximately 0.02%),[29] but is 100-fold higher than in the healthy general population.[30] As with sinus bradycardia, AV block is overcome with exercise or atropine, suggesting that high vagal tone causes block at the level of the AV node.[31]

Intraventricular Conduction Delay/Incomplete Right Bundle Branch Block

The mean QRS duration in most series of normal athletes is 0.09 milliseconds to 0.10 milliseconds.[16,17] Complete left bundle branch block and right bundle branch block are rare, as are intraventricular conduction delays with QRS duration ≥0.12 milliseconds. Incomplete right bundle branch block (IRBBB) is prevalent in athletes, as it is in young healthy controls, and it has been reported to occur in up to 35% to 51% of athletes[14,27] as compared to 10% of young, healthy controls.[30] In a report comparing female athletes to male athletes, a striking difference in the incidence of IRBBB was reported: 17% in males, and only 2% in females.[32] Males and females were not matched according to type of sport or level of training, and these nongender factors may have played a role in the observed difference. It has been proposed that the right ventricular conduction delay is not within the His-Purkinje system, but is due to hypertrophy of the right ventricular apex.[33]

P Wave

P wave amplitude has been demonstrated in multiple studies to be greater in athletes than in control subjects.[14,16,19] One study[19] reports 4 of 20 elite distance runners with a P wave voltage between 2.5 mm and 3 mm, with marked orthostatic and respiratory variation. Notched P waves in the inferior limb leads are common. In another study,[27] 18 out of a group of 25 elite distance runners showed notched P waves with the interpeak distance >1 mm. Forty-one of 651 Finnish athletes showed notching of the P waves.[34]

Ventricular Hypertrophy

The incidence of precordial lead voltage satisfying criteria for right ventricular hypertrophy (RVH) in athletes not well studied. In one study, Sokolow-Lyon voltage criteria for RVH (R-V_1+S-V_5>10.5 mm)[35] was seen in 9 of 46 Olympic endurance athletes.[36] Four athletes had an R/S ratio greater than 1.0 in lead V_1. Of 3000 healthy athletes studied in Israel[13] and in an early series of 165 athletes, 20% and 18%, respectively, met criteria for RVH.[37]

Voltage criteria for left ventricular hypertrophy (LVH) have been studied more extensively and have been compared to echocardiographic findings. Studies report a 10% to 80% incidence of LVH[14,15,17,18,25,27,38] if the criteria of Sokolow and Lyon are used (S wave in V_1+R wave in V_5>35 mm).[39] In a study of 44 triathletes, there was echocardiographic evidence of LVH in 17 of 29 (59%) male triathletes and 8 of 15 (53%) female triathletes as compared with 0 of 20 male controls. Overall, 25 of 44 (57%) of athletes met Sokolow-Lyon criteria (S-V_1+R-V_5) for LVH; 17 of these athletes had concurrent echocardiographic evidence. Sokolow-Lyon criteria showed only a 65% sensitivity and 61% specificity in diagnosing echocardiographically confirmed LVH in athletes. The Cornell voltage (R-aVL+S-V_3>2.8 mV in men and >2.0 mV in women)[40] showed very low sensitivity (8%) but relatively high specificity (95%). Left axis deviation, a "strain" pattern of repolarization, and delayed intrinsicoid deflection were not seen in any athlete in this series. The Romhilt-Estes score (≥4),[41] since it incorporates such nonvoltage criteria, also showed a low sensitivity (16%) and higher specificity (84%).

When endurance athletes are compared to sprinters, who are mainly power trained, a significantly higher incidence of LVH by Sokolow-Lyon criteria is found in the endurance group (44% versus 32%).[18] Both groups have similar LV cavity dilatation, but the endurance group has greater wall thickness. It is unclear whether the thinner chest wall or the greater myocardial wall thickness seen in endurance athletes accounts for the increased precordial voltage. Similarly, in a series of football players studied while at training camp, the incidence of voltage satisfying Sokolow-Lyon criteria for LVH (35% overall) varied inversely with body mass.[17]

Despite the increase in LV mass seen in athletes, the QRS axis in athletes is more vertical than that seen in control subjects; but it is still within the normal range.[14,25] In controlled studies where the difference did not reach statistical significance, the right axis trend was still apparent.[15,16]

QT Interval

In controlled studies, the QT interval is longer in athletes than in nonathletic controls.[13,15–17,42] The difference lies mainly in the lower resting HRs, but the QTc (corrected by the Bazett formula) shows a smaller but significant difference in some series. In all surveys, the mean QTc of the athletic group is within normal limits, but is usually toward the upper limit of 0.42 seconds. Some athletes may have corrected QT intervals up to 0.47 seconds. In comparing athletes with ventricular arrhythmias to normal athletes, QT and QTc do not differ significantly. Measurements of dispersion of the QT interval on the surface ECG, however, are statistically significant when the two groups of athletes are compared.[42]

ST Segment and T Wave Abnormalities

Patterns of early repolarization or J-point elevation are described well and reported frequently in ECGs of athletes. In one study of 20 elite distance runners, 14 showed an early repolarization pattern,[19] compared to ECGs from over 49,000 healthy pilots in whom the incidence of ST segment elevation was 2.4%.[43] In a study of 289 professional American football players, only 5% had no J-point elevation on ECG.[17] The majority of J-point elevation was 1 mm to 3 mm, but it reached as high as 5 mm in some tracings. In one study,[27] 25 endurance athletes in the Japanese Army (80%) showed J-point elevation, compared to 32% of controls. These repolarization changes normalize with exercise. Tall or peaked T waves accompanied the J-point elevation in many athletes in these series.

Resting ST segment depressions are rarely reported in athletes. In one series of cyclists, 3% showed up to 0.1 mm J-point depressions.[26] In many series, ST segment depression is lumped together with T wave abnormalities,[17,27,44] making the true incidence unknown.

T wave inversions are reported to occur commonly in the limb or precordial leads or both[14,17,19,27,44–46] in up to 30% of endurance athletes. Of the previously mentioned 289 professional American football players, 39 players (13%) also had ST segment and T wave abnormalities that mimicked ischemia.[17] Twenty-three of these players were African American (24% of that subpopulation) and the remaining 16 players were white (9%). A persistent juvenile pattern was seen in 9 players, isolated T wave inversions in the inferior limb leads in 22 players, and an anterior "ischemia" pattern with deep precordial T wave inversions in 8 players. Most studies do not attempt to further characterize the T wave abnormalities, although they often appear in conjunction with ST segment elevation and, less commonly, with ST depression.

Exercise nearly uniformly abolishes the resting T wave abnormalities. In a survey of Israeli athletes, seven were found to have striking T wave inversions.[45] Four of seven had normalization of T waves with exercise testing. The remaining three may not have been stressed adequately with conventional exercise protocols. None of the athletes had evidence of heart disease with 3-years follow-up. Eight top-ranking healthy Italian athletes referred for repolarization abnormalities underwent echocardiographic evaluation and stress testing. Some athletes received isoproterenol infusion and atropine bolus.[46] One asymptomatic athlete had mitral valve prolapse and the remaining seven had structurally normal hearts. All of the athletes showed normalization of T wave inversions with exercise or isoproterenol infusion, but none did with the administration of atropine, suggesting that an imbalance of sympathetic tone is responsible for the T wave abnormalities and that a low sympathetic input is necessary for the persistence of these abnormalities. All 39 of the aforementioned professional American football players showed normalization of the T wave abnormalities with exercise.[17]

Distinguishing Normal from Abnormal

Striking abnormalities may be seen as variants of normal in the ECGs of healthy athletes (Figure 1), and it may not be possible to exclude heart disease without further diagnostic evaluation such as stress testing, perfusion imaging, and echocardiography. The common abnormalities associated with a competitive athlete's ECG are summarized in Table 1. Cardiac diseases associated with sudden death are often in the differential diagnosis of an asymptomatic athlete with ST segment and T wave abnormalities. These include, but are not limited to, HCM and ARVD.

In 55% of patients with ARVD, the ECG shows a QRS duration greater than 110 milliseconds and a complete or IRBBB pattern.[47] Athletes rarely have QRS durations >100 milliseconds, although incomplete right bundle branch patterns are common. In the original series of patients with ARVD, 30% were reported to have a small, discrete potential seen just after the QRS in the right precordial leads, most often V_1. The so-called epsilon wave is thought to represent delayed activation of a portion of the right ventricle.[48] This finding is absent in athletes. Up to 50% of patients have inverted T waves in the right precor-

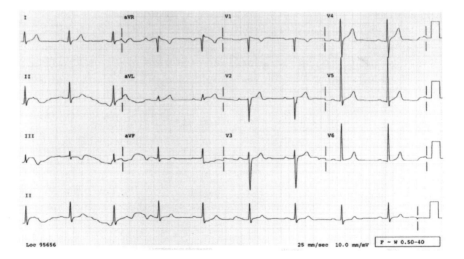

Figure 1. This electrocardiogram of a 45-year-old African American male competitive cyclist shows abnormalities often seen in highly trained athletes, including sinus bradycardia, first-degree atrioventricular block, high voltage, and J-point elevation.

Table 1
Common Electrocardiographic Abnormalities Found in Athletes

Sinus bradycardia
Sinus arrhythmia
First-degree AV block
Second-degree AV block types I and II
Incomplete right bundle branch block
Notched p waves
Voltage criteria for left and right ventricular hypertrophy
ST segment elevation and depression
Corrected QT interval at upper limit of normal
Tall, peaked, and inverted T waves

AV = atrioventricular.

dial leads (Figure 2). T wave inversions are common in healthy athletes as well; further testing is warranted if ARVD is suspected. Exercise almost uniformly abolishes the ST segment and T wave abnormalities seen in normal athletes. Exercise is associated with ventricular arrhythmias in patients with ARVD.

HCM is the leading cause of sudden death in competitive, apparently healthy athletes under 35 years of age. Unfortunately, there are no diagnostic ECG features for HCM, although most people with the disease will have an abnormal ECG. The 12-lead ECG is, normal, however, in up to 25% of asymptomatic individuals with HCM.[49,50] Most individuals with HCM exhibit an intraventricular conduction delay and voltage criteria for LVH associated with ST segment depressions and T wave inversions (Figure 3). Few will have complete left or right bundle branch block. Twenty percent will exhibit left axis deviation and abnormal Q waves in the inferior limb leads or anterior precordial leads.[50] These abnormalities overlap significantly with electrocardiographic findings in healthy athletes. Therefore, it may be impossible to exclude HCM when confronted with an athlete's ECG showing repolarization abnormalities and voltage criteria for LVH. A careful physical examination demonstrating absence of an obstructive murmur, echocardiogram showing LV wall thickness < 13 mm, and stress test that shows normalization of ST segment and T wave abnormalities with exercise should be sufficient to diagnose HCM in an athlete.

Likewise, athletes with other organic heart disease such as myocarditis, dilated cardiomyopathy, and coronary artery atherosclerosis will show nonspecific electrocardiographic abnormalities that overlap significantly with the common abnormalities seen in a healthy athlete. Although rarely the cause of sudden death in apparently healthy athletes under the age of 35 years, these diseases usually cause symptoms that mandate further evaluation.

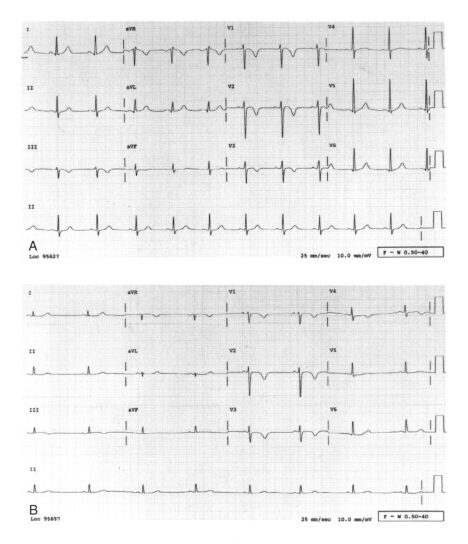

Figure 2. Both electrocardiograms (ECGs) are taken from individuals with arrhythmogenic right ventricular dysplasia (ARVD). The first tracing (**A**) is an ECG of a 31-year-old Caucasian male who presented with palpitations and syncope while playing basketball. Note the moderately prolonged QRS duration of 110 milliseconds as well as the T wave inversions in the right precordial leads. The second tracing (**B**) is an ECG from a 36-year-old Caucasian female who presented with exercise-induced palpitations and presyncope. She was treated with an implantable cardioverter defibrillator and antiarrhythmic therapy, but she continued to have infrequent episodes of exercise-related ventricular tachycardia documented and treated by the device. While the QRS duration is normal in this tracing, right precordial leads show T wave inversions typical of ARVD. The sinus bradycardia is secondary to sotalol therapy superimposed on a preexisting resting bradycardia attributed to her aerobic conditioning.

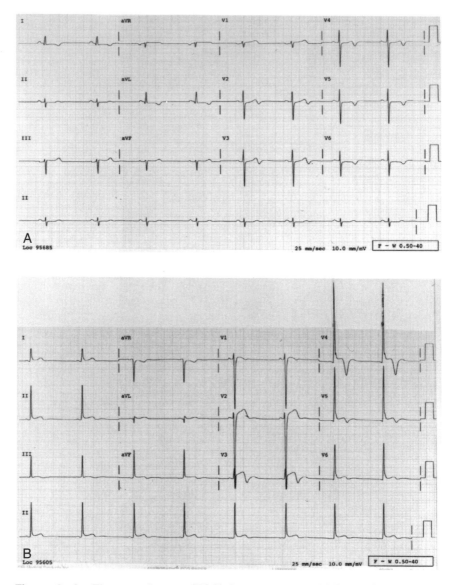

Figure 3. A., Electrocardiogram (ECG) from a 42-year-old Caucasian male with echocardiogram-documented hypertrophic cardiomyopathy who developed presyncope associated with documented nonsustained ventricular tachycardia. Note the leftward axis secondary to left anterior fascicular block and the anterolateral T wave inversions, the latter being an abnormality also seen in highly trained athletes. **B.,** ECG from a 17-year-old African American male competitive basketball player who experienced syncope while warming up prior to a game. Note the extremely high QRS voltage and associated ST and T wave abnormalities suggestive of left ventricular hypertrophy. Evaluation demonstrated hypertrophied myocardium that regressed with deconditioning, making hypertrophic cardiomyopathy an unlikely diagnosis. Increased left ventricular mass due to physical conditioning combined with young age and thin body habitus are therefore more likely responsible for these ECG abnormalities.

Summary

In summary, healthy athletes commonly exhibit abnormalities on a resting 12-lead ECG. These abnormailities include sinus bradycardia, sinus arrhythmia, first- and second-degree AV block, ST segment elevation or depression, T wave peaking and inversion, IRBBB, corrected QT interval at the upper limit of normal, and voltage criteria for left and RVH. As such, the ECG is a poor screening tool for organic heart disease in competitive athletes and should be used as part of a diagnostic evaluation in individuals with a personal history, family history, or physical examination suggestive of organic heart disease.

References

1. Maron B, Thompson P, Puffer J, et al. Cardiovascular preparticipation screening of competitive athletes. A statement for health professional from the Sudden Death Committee (clinical cardiology) and Congenital Cardiac Defects Committee (cardiovascular diseases in the young), American Heart Association. *Circulation* 1996;94:850–856.
2. Rich BSE. Sudden death screening. *Med Clin North Am* 1994;78:267–288.
3. Epstein SE, Maron BJ. Sudden death and the competitive athlete: Perspectives on preparticipation screening studies. *J Am Coll Cardiol* 1986; 7:220–230.
4. Maron B, Roberts W, McAllister H, et al. Sudden death in young athletes. *Circulation* 1980;62:218–229.
5. Maron J, Epstein S, Roberts WC. Causes of sudden death in competitive athletes. *J Am Coll Cardiol* 1986;7:204–214.
6. Maron BJ, Pelliccia A, Spirito P. Cardiac disease in young trained athletes: Insights into methods for distinguishing athlete's heart from structural heart disease, with particular emphasis on hypertrophic cardiomyopathy. *Circulation* 1995;91:1596–1601.
7. Corrado D, Thiene G, Nava A. Sudden death in young competitive athletes: Clinicopathologic correlation in 22 cases. *Am J Med* 1990;89:588–596.
8. Thiene G, Nava A, Corrado D, et al. Right ventricular cardiomyopathy and sudden death in young people. *N Engl J Med* 1988;318:129–133.
9. Burke AP, Farb A, Virmani R. Causes of sudden death in athletes. *Cardiol Clin* 1992;10:303–317.
10. Maron B. Structural features of the athlete's heart as defned by echocardiography. *J Am Coll Cardiol* 1986;7:190–203.
11. Pelliccia A, Maron BJ, Spataro A, et al. The upper limit of physiological hypertrophy in highly trained elite athletes. *N Engl J Med* 1991;324: 295–301.
12. Maron B, Gottdiener J, Epstein S. Patterns and significance of the distribution of left ventricular hypertrophy in hypertrophic cardiomyopathy: A wide-angle, two-dimensional study of 125 patients. *Am J Cardiol* 1981; 48:418–428.
13. Hanne-Paparo N, Drory Y, Schoenfeld Y, YS, Kellerman J. Common ECG changes in athletes. *Cardiology* 1976;61:267–278.
14. Venerando A, Rulli V. Frequency morphology and meaning of the electrocardiographic anomalies found in Olympic marathon runners and walkers. *J Sports Med Phys Fitness* 1964;4:135–141.

15. Van Ganse W, Versee L, Eylenbosch W, Vuylsteek K. The electrocardiogram of athletes: Comparison with untrained subjects. *Br Heart J* 1970;32:160–164.

16. Northcote R, Canning GP, Ballantyne D. Electrocardiographic findings in male veteran endurance athletes. *Br Heart J* 1989;61:155–160.

17. Balady GJ, Cadigan JB, Ryan TJ. Electrocardiogram of the athlete: An analysis of 289 professional football players. *Am J Cardiol* 1984;53: 1339–1343.

18. Ikaheimo M, Palatsi I, Takkunen J. Noninvasive evaluation of the athletic heart: Sprinters versus endurance runners. *Am J Cardiol* 1979;44: 24–30.

19. Gibbons L, Cooper K, Martin R, Pollock M. Medical examination and electrocardiographic analysis of elite distance runners. *Ann N Y Acad Sci* 1977;301:283–296.

20. Bjornstad H, Storstein L, Dyre Meen H, Hals O. Electrocardiographic findings of heart rate and conduction times in athletic students and sedentary control subjects. *Cardiology* 1993;83:258–267.

21. Bjornstad H, Smith G, Storstein L, et al. Electrocardiographic and echocardiographic findings in top athletes, athletic students and sedentary controls. *Cardiology* 1993;82:66–74.

22. Chapman J. Profound sinus bradycardia in the athletic heart syndrome. *J Sports Med Phys Fitness* 1982;22:45–48.

23. Hanne-Paparo N, Kellerman J. Long-term Holter ECG rnonitoring of athletes. *Med Sci Sports Exerc* 1981;13:294–298.

24. Smith M, Hudson D, Graitzer H, Raven P. Exercise training bradycardia: The role of autonomic balance. *Med Sci Sports Exerc* 1989;21:40–44.

25. Parker B, Londeree B, Cupp G, Dubiel JP. The noninvasive cardiac evaluation of long-distance runners. *Chest* 1978;73:376–381.

26. Huston T, Puffer J, Rodney WM. The athletic heart syndrome. *N Engl J Med* 1985;313:24–32.

27. Nakamoto K. Electrocardiograms of 25 marathon runners before and after 100 meter dash. *Jpn Circ J* 1969;33:105–126.

28. Myetes I, Kaplinsky E, Yahini J, et al. Wenckenbach AV block: A frequent feature following heavy physical training. *Am Heart J* 1975;990:426–430.

29. Zehender M, Meinertz T, Keul J, Just H. ECG variants and cardiac arrhythmias in athletes: Clinical relevance and prognostic importance. *Am Heart J* 1990;119:1378–1391.

30. Hiss R, Lamb L. Electrocardiographic findings 122,043 indiduals. *Circulation* 1962;25:947–961.

31. Zeppilli P, Fenici R, Sassasra M, et al.Wenckenbach second degree AV block in top-ranking athletes: An old problem revisited. *Am Heart J* 1980; 100:281–294.

32. Storstein L, Bjornstad H, Hals O, Dyre Meen H. Electrocardgraphic findings according to sex in athletes and controls. *Cardiology* 1991;79: 227–236.

33. Moore EN, Boineau JP, Patterson DF. Incomplete right bundle branch block: An electrocardiographic enigma and possible misnomer. *Circulation* 1971;44:678–687.

34. Klemola E. Electrocardiographic observations on 650 Finnish athletes. *Ann Med Finn* 1951;40:121–132.

35. Sokolow M, Lyon T. The ventricular complex in right ventricular hypertrophy as obtained by unipolar precordial and limb leads. *Am Heart J* 1949;38:273.

36. Arstila M, Koivikko A. Electrocardiographic and vectorcardiographic signs of left and right ventricular hypertrophy in endurance athletes. *J Sport Med Phys Fitness* 1964;4:166–175.
37. Beckner G, Winsor T. Cardiovascular adaptations to prolonged physical effort. *Circulation* 1954;9:835–846.
38. Douglas PS, O'Toole ML, Hiller DB, et al. Electrocardiogaphic diagnosis of exercise-induced left ventrular hypertrophy. *Am Heart J* 1988;116: 784–790.
39. Sokolow M, Lyon T. The ventricular complex in left ventricular hypertrophy as obtained by unipolar precordial and limb leads. *Am Heart J* 1949; 37:161.
40. Casale P, Devereux R, Kligfield P, et al. Electrocardgraphic detection of left ventricular hypertrophy: Development and prospective validation of improved criteria. *J Am Coll Cardiol* 1985;6:572.
41. Romhilt D, Bove KE, Norris R, et al. A critical appraisal of the electrocardiographic criteria for the diagnosis of left ventricular hypertrophy. *Circulation* 1969;40:185.
42. Jordaens L, Missault L, Pelleman G, et al. Comparison of athletes with life-threatening arrhythmias with two groups of healthy athletes and a group of normal control subjects. *Am J Cardiol* 1994;74:1124–1128.
43. Parisi A, Beckmann C, Lancaaster M. The spectrum of ST segment elevation in the electrocardiograms of healthy adult men. *J Electrocardiol* 1971;4:137–144.
44. Oakley DG, Oakley CM. Significance of abnormal electrograms in highly trained athletes. *Am J Cardiol* 1982;50:985–989.
45. Hanne-Paparo N, Wendkos MH, Brunner D. T wave abnormalities in the electrocardiogram of top-ranking athletes without demonstrable organic heart disease. *Am Heart J* 1971;81:743–747.
46. Zeppilli P, Pirrami MM, Sassara M, Fenici R. T wave abnormalities in top ranking athletes: Effects of isoproterenol, atropine, and physical exercise. *Am Heart J* 1980;100:213–222.
47. Marcus FI, Gontaine G. Arrhythmogenic right ventricular dysplasia. In Podrid PJ, Kowey PR (eds): *Cardiac Arrhythmia: Mechanisms, Diagnosis, and Management. Volume 1.* Boston, Philadelphia: Williams and Wilkins; 1995:1121–1130.
48. Fontaine G, Guiraudon G, Frank R, et al. Stimulation studies and epicardial mapping in ventricular tachycardia: Study of mechanisms and selection for surgery. In Kulbertus H (ed): *Reentrant Arrhythmias.* Lancaster: MTP Publishers; 1977:334–350.
49. Saumarez RC, Slade AK, McKenna WJ. Arrhythmias in hypertrophic cardiomyopathy. In Podrid PJ, Kowey PR (eds): *Cardiac Arrhythmia: Mechanisms, Diagnosis, and Management, Volume 1.* Boston, Philadelphia: Williams and Wilkins; 1995;1095–1109.
50. Savage D, Seides S, Clark C, et al. Electrocardiographic findings in patients with obstructive and nonobstructive hypertrophic cardiomyopathy. *Circulation* 1978;58:402–408.

6

Ambulatory Monitoring in the Athlete

Gerald F. Fletcher, MD

History of Ambulatory ECG Monitoring

The use of Holter recording dates back many years and has been clinically revealing with regard to cardiac arrhythmias, conduction disturbances seen in athletes, and evaluation of the etiology of sudden cardiac death (SCD).[1] Norman Holter was one of the important contributors to electrocardiography, along with Einthoven, Lewis, and Wilson. Holter was a physicist from Helena, Montana. In his basic observations he noted that there was a universal need for a method of recording the electrocardiogram (ECG) in "real life activity"; this should be done without "cumbersome" leads and with a mechanism to store such data for subsequent analysis and medical interpretation for the patient. Since Holter's time, many sophisticated systems of ambulatory ECG recording have evolved that are widely used in patient care. The most complete systems record blood pressure and heart rate variability, as well as provide analysis of heart rate and rhythm and ST segment change, to near perfection.

In the current era of interest in the summer Olympics, which were held in America on 1996, there are continued concerns about arrhythmias[2] in professional athletes, and about the definition of "normal range" versus those conditions that might predispose to critical events or SCD.

From Estes NAM, Salem DN, Wang PJ (eds). *Sudden Cardiac Death in the Athlete.* Armonk, NY: Futura Publishing Co., Inc.; ©1998.

Normal Findings in Ambulatory Electrocardiogram Monitoring in Athletes

A number of cardiac rhythm alterations are detected in normal athletes.[3] These include sinus bradycardia of 30 to 45 beats per minute (bpm), sinus arrhythmia, atrial ectopy, and atrial couplets, as well as ventricular ectopy and ventricular couplets. The heart rate may vary from the 30 to 45 bpm at rest to rates of 140 to 160 bpm with exercise. However, as athletes become more highly "trained" the exercise heart rates are often in the range of 110 to 130 bpm. Brief periods of supraventricular rhythm and idioventricular rhythm may also occur. Conduction disturbances also occur in normal athletes.[3] First-degree atrioventricular block has been described, as have atrioventricular junctional rhythm and atrioventricular Wenckebach conduction.

Examples of the aforementioned conditions are seen on ECG in Figure 1, a 38-year old runner (40 miles/wk) with documented sinus bradycardia and sinus arrhythmia, Figure 2, a 23-year-old male athlete with bradycardia and a low atrial rhythm, Figure 3, a 52-year-old "athlete" (runner of 25 miles/wk) with "dropped beats" and atrioventricular Wenckebach conduction, and Figure 4, a high school football player, age 17, with syncope, diagnosed with primary myocardial disease. In the latter patient, Holter recording revealed a short PR interval with ectopic atrial and ventricular beats.

Several studies have been done in normal runners.[4-6] In one study, Talan et al[4] obtained 24-hour continuous ECG recordings in 20 young (19- to 28-year-old) male long-distance runners (50 miles/wk) during activities other than running. All 20 runners had premature atrial complexes, but only one had >100 per 24 hours. Fourteen (70%) had premature ventricular complexes, but only two (10%) had >50 in 24 hours and none had ventricular couplets or tachycardia.

In a study[6] by Pantano and Oriel,[5] 60 high-level runners (24 to 177 km/wk, median 48.5 km) had Holter recordings only during the period of exercise. Sixty percent had ventricular arrhythmias during the recorded run: bigeminy in 10%, couplets in 10%, and multiform premature ventricular contractions in 5%. Forty percent of the group had atrial arrhythmias during the recorded run. Occasional to frequent premature atrial complexes were the most common; however, seven subjects had atrial couplets or paroxysmal atrial tachycardia. This study is limited in scope, however, because of the brief time of Holter recording.

In a larger study by Pilcher et al,[6] 80 healthy runners were studied with continuous ECG recording during both exercise and free activity. In this study, group 1 consisted of 20 runners (0 to <5 miles/wk); group 2, 19 (>5 to ≤15 miles/wk); group 3, 21 (>15 to≤30 miles/wk);

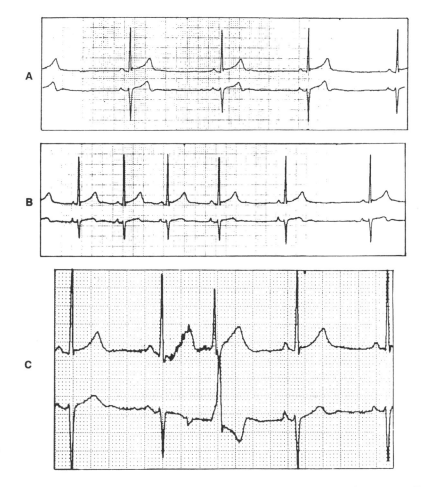

Figure 1. Recordings taken from a 38-year-old high-level runner (20 to 60 miles/ week) with no symptoms. They reveal **A** sinus bradycardia of 30 bpm at 4:30 am, **B** periods of sinus arrhythmia, and **C** infrequent single, ventricular ectopic beats.

and group 4, 20 (>30 miles/wk). The continuous electrocardiography during both running and other activity, revealed no significant differences in the occurrence of rhythm and conduction disturbances in the different groups. The most common abnormalities were ventricular ectopic complexes, seen in 40 subjects, less than 50 per minute in 34 and greater than 50 per minute in 6. The high-grade ventricular ectopic activity—five-beat run of ventricular tachycardia (immediately after exercise) and two instances of ventricular couplets during exercise—were of concern and subjects were referred for further medical evaluation. However, no data are available on the follow-up medical evaluation.

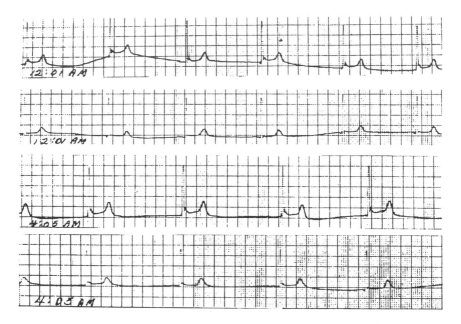

Figure 2. A 23-year-old, well-trained male athlete with no clinical evidence of cardiac disease was evaluated because of "slow heart beat." Extreme bradycardia (34 to 42 bpm), either sinus or low atrial, was recorded during sleep. No treatment was administered and the subject has remained healthy. From Fletcher GF, with permission.

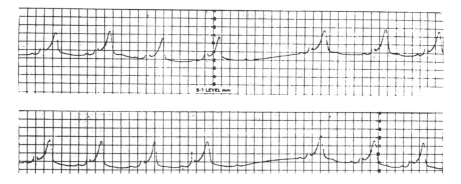

Figure 3. A 52-year-old subject who regularly ran 25 to 30 miles/week presented with "dropped beats." Holter recording revealed sinus bradycardia of 50 bpm with periods of atrioventricular block, probably Wenckebach (type 1). No therapy was initiated and the subject continues to run regularly without any difficulty.

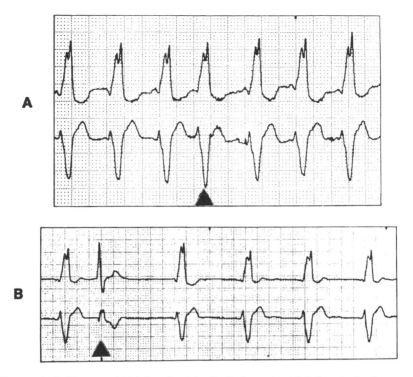

Figure 4. A 17-year-old high school football player had brief periods of syncope. Clinical evaluation revealed a resting ECG consistent with preexcitation. **A.** A two-channel Holter recording of the preexcitation pattern (extremely short PR interval) with rare supraventricular ectopic contractions (▲). **B.** A rare ventricular ectopic beat (▲). Variable supraventricular tachycardias were documented by electrocardiography and electrophysiologic studies. Further evaluation by echocardiography revealed global hypokinesis with a dilated left ventricle and paradoxical septal motion consistent with the preexcitation. Arrhythmias were treated with 1000 mg procainamide (long-acting) three times daily and physical activity was decreased. The patient was believed to have a cardiomyopathy, but has done well clinically with no recurrence of high-grade arrhythmias.

Indications for Ambulatory Electrocardiogram Monitoring

There are certain indications for Holter recording that include but are not limited to the following:

History

1. Syncope and dizziness
2. Subjective palpitations
3. Concerns about heart disease in the family

Physical examination

1. Irregular pulse
2. Certain cardiac murmurs
3. Evidence of cardiomegaly (with a significant history)

The indications for Holter recording in athletes should be placed in proper perspective. A detailed history should be taken at the outset with appropriate physical examination emphasizing certain findings, specifically, irregular pulse, heart murmurs, and heart enlargement. A standard 12-lead ECG then may be indicated. If arrhythmias are documented, further analysis may be in order with use of the Holter recording. This may be done during the time of the athletic activity such as running or hurdling. At this time, however, electrode lead systems are not effective in recording during water sports.

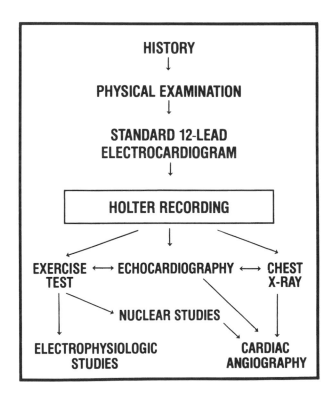

Figure 5. Step-by-step guide to the cardiovascular evaluation of athletes. The arrows depict rational alternatives in evaluation based on variables of the clinical setting and the initial data base. Evaluation may be completed at any point or level, at which time treatment is prescribed or disposition is made.

In certain clinical situations, event monitoring over a longer period may be more effective, especially when symptoms that suggest arrhythmias are less frequent. This is done by having the subject "self initiate" an ECG recording with a portable system that has the technical capabilities of "storing" the rhythm data for subsequent analysis.

Regardless of the athletic setting, whether running, gymnastics, or other "land sports," the technique of lead application must include proper skin preparation (usually including shaving of hair) and support of the lead system with wrapping of the lead wires and cable securely around the body. In recording of women athletes, the support and stability of the breasts adjacent to the lead system are mandatory; this is usually accomplished with tight-fitting undergarments.

Other studies such as echocardiography, electrophysiologic studies, and even coronary and left ventricular angiography, may be ultimately considered based on the results of the initial evaluation. Figure 5 displays a proposed format for use of the Holter recording in the evaluation of arrhythmia and conduction disturbances in an athlete.

It must be repeatedly emphasized that disturbances of heart rate and rhythm are very common and normal in our population of athletes. Such disturbances are often related to changes and alterations in parasympathetic and sympathetic tone that develop in athletes with the training effect. Therefore, the proper medical evaluation by health professionals prior to instigation of costly studies should be done as described. This will put the Holter recording in the proper perspective in the medical evaluation of athletes.

References

1. Fletcher GF. *Dynamic Electrocardiographic Recording.* Mount Kisco, NY: Futura Publishing Co.; 1979.
2. Josephson ME, Schibgilla VH. Athletes and arrhythmias: Clinical considerations and perspectives. *Eur Heart J* 1996;17:498–509.
3. Fletcher GF. Holter recording in athletes: Purposes and applications. In Waller BF, Harvey WP (eds): *Cardiovascular Evaluation of Athletes.* Newton NJ: Laennec Publishing; 1993:87–94.
4. Talan DA, Bauernfeind RA, Ashley WW, et al. Twenty-four-hour continuous ECG recordings in long-distance runners. *Chest* 1982;82:19–24.
5. Pantano JA, Oriel FJ. Prevalence and nature of cardiac arrhythmias in apparently normal well-trained runners. *Am Heart J* 1982;104:762–768.
6. Pilcher GF, Cook AJ, Johnston BL, Fletcher GF. Twenty-four-hour continuous electrocardiography during exercise and free activity in 80 apparently healthy runners. *Am J Cardiol* 1983;52:859–861.

7

The Role of Exercise Testing in the Evaluation of the Athlete

Stephen B. Sloan, MD and Paul J. Wang, MD

Exercise testing may play an important role in the evaluation of both the competitive and the noncompetitive athlete. The technique may be particularly valuable because of its ability to evaluate the hemodynamic and electrocardiographic changes that occur with exertion. Furthermore, a symptom-limited protocol of exercise testing may simulate athletic activity over a range of increasing workloads and durations. The noninvasive nature of exercise testing makes this technique particularly suitable for evaluation of the athlete with a known cardiovascular disorder or to uncover disease in the asymptomatic athlete who nonetheless has risk factors for developing cardiovascular disease.

This chapter reviews the potential role of exercise testing in athletes with a variety of documented cardiovascular disorders. Also reviewed in this chapter is the literature on exercise-induced hemodynamic, electrocardiographic, and arrhythmic abnormalities in each of these disorders, and the relative effectiveness of exercise testing in uncovering these findings. In addition, this chapter discusses the potential role and limitations of screening for conditions that have a low prevalence in asymptomatic individuals who do not have risk factors for developing cardiovascular disease. To complement this discussion of the literature and of clinical experience with each of these individ-

From Estes NAM, Salem DN, Wang PJ (eds). *Sudden Cardiac Death in the Athlete.* Armonk, NY: Futura Publishing Co., Inc.; ©1998.

ual disorders, two recent documents on the evaluation of athletes are referred to: *The 26th Bethesda Conference Recommendations for Determining Eligibility for Competition in Athletes with Cardiovascular Abnormalities*[1] and the American Heart Association's document entitled *Cardiovascular Preparticipation Screening of Competitive Athletes.*[2] These documents provide an important framework for defining a practical role for exercise testing and other forms of evaluation of the athlete.

Normal and Abnormal Responses to Exercise

Physiologic Changes that Occur During Exercise Testing

Exercise testing can produce numerous physiologic changes that may have important consequences related to underlying cardiovascular disease. Most of these changes arise from the increased metabolic demands that occur during exercise. The primary response to these increased demands is an increase in both the cardiac output and the blood flow to exercising muscles. As a result of vasodilatation of the blood vessels in the exercising skeletal muscles, there is a marked reduction in systemic vascular resistance. These changes may be mediated not only by local metabolic stimuli, but also by increased parasympathetic stimulation of the arterioles that supply the exercising muscle. Although arterioles vasodilate in the extremities during exercise, other vascular beds, such as the splanchnic bed, will vasoconstrict. As a result, there is an overall increase in systemic arterial pressure. The marked increase in cardiac output also contributes to the increase in systemic arterial pressure.[3,4] Contraction of exercising skeletal muscle and sympathetic regulation of venous capacitance vessels may contribute to increased venous return.[5]

During exercise, cardiac output may increase to 25 L/min.[6] During maximal exertion in the upright position, stroke volume increases to twice the level at rest.[7,8] Indices such as ventricular ejection fraction, left ventricular end-diastolic volume, and cardiac output all increase with maximal exercise in normal subjects, while end-systolic volume decreases. In addition, the heart rate increases markedly during exercise, an additional factor that contributes to the increased cardiac output. The increase in stroke volume results, in part, from increased contractility due to activation of the sympathetic nervous system. Myocardial oxygen consumption also increases markedly during exercise.[9] The increased heart rate, contractility, and wall tension that are observed in exercise contribute to the increased myocardial oxygen demands. In order to meet the increased myocardial oxygen demand associated with exercise, coronary blood flow increases approximately fivefold. This increase is predominantly due to decreases in the resistance of the intramural "resistance" vessels. Because of the magnitude of the coronary flow reserve during gradually increasing exercise, myocardial ischemia is not observed in normal individuals.

Abnormalities in Physiologic Response to Exercise

Failure to increase systemic arterial pressure during exercise most commonly results from an impaired ability to increase cardiac output in the presence of vasodilatation. In fact, a fall in systemic pressure may indicate severe left ventricular dysfunction. Myocardial ischemia is the most common cause of such an abnormal response to exercise. Such falls in systemic pressure frequently reflect a large region of myocardial ischemia such as in left main coronary artery disease, three-vessel coronary artery disease, or their equivalents. Prognostically, such declines in blood pressure have been associated with increased mortality following myocardial infarction.[10] In the presence of a severe coronary artery stenosis, the intramural vessels' inability to adequately reduce their resistance in order to allow increased coronary blood flow leads to myocardial ischemia. A failure to increase the systolic blood pressure may also reflect conditions associated with a limited ability to increase cardiac output. In severe aortic stenosis there may be an impaired ability of the left ventricle to augment the stroke volume against the aortic valve pressure gradient during exercise. There may also be a limitation in the ability to increase cardiac output in severe dilated cardiomyopathy.

Maximal work capacity is a measure of functional capacity that may have prognostic value. Numerous factors such as exercise training and physical conditioning influence this index. In large part, the measurement reflects the ability of the heart to increase cardiac output adequately without resultant myocardial ischemia. Patients with myocardial ischemia at 3 minutes or less (approximately 5 metabolic equivalents [METS]) have a fourfold increase in cardiovascular progression or death.[11] Assessment of the maximal work capacity of the athlete may be useful for the development of training programs and the evaluation of the effects of the programs.

In the healthy state there is no significant impairment of diastolic properties of the ventricles during exercise. Decreases in ventricular compliance during exercise that produce elevations in left ventricular end-diastolic pressure, and as a result, pulmonary congestion, may reflect one of several disorders: severe myocardial ischemia; ischemia in the presence of prior infarction; or severe left ventricular dysfunction.

Exercised-induced elevations of left ventricular end-diastolic pressure may be reflected in the exercise-induced lung uptake of thallium during radionuclide scintigraphy. While the conditioned athlete may have left ventricular hypertrophy, elevations of left ventricular diastolic pressure leading to pulmonary congestion are not observed. Restrictive cardiomyopathies may also exhibit elevations in left ventricular diastolic pressure due to abnormalities in compliance.

The failure of the heart rate to increase as expected during exercise may reflect intrinsic sinus node dysfunction or impaired sympathetic stimulation; the phenomenon is termed *chronotropic incompetence*. An impairment of heart rate response may lead to decreases in exercise tolerance and maximal work capacity since increased heart rate is an important contributor to increased cardiac output during exercise. Poorly conditioned individuals or those unable to exercise may also exhibit an impaired heart rate response to exercise testing.

The maximal predicted heart rate declines with age. A commonly used approximation of maximal predicted heart rate is provided by the formula:

$$\text{maximal predicted heart rate} = 220\text{-age (in years)}$$

Gender may be considered when calculating maximal predicted heart rate.[12] The standard deviation provided by the commonly used formulas are large enough so that some authors feel that judging the level of exertion as a percentage of maximally predicted heart rate may be misleading in some subjects.

Exercise-Induced Arrhythmias

Arrhythmias may occur during exercise and frequently reflect the altered electrophysiologic properties of myocardial tissue that result from myocardial ischemia, hemodynamic effects, or changes in autonomic tone produced by exercise. These changes may increase automaticity, lead to triggered activity, or create conditions favoring reentry. Exercise-induced arrhythmias are discussed individually later in this chapter.

Exercise Test Procedures

Exercise testing most frequently uses either a treadmill or bicycle protocol. A motor-driven treadmill permits the controlled and timed increase in grade and speed. Continuous electrocardiographic monitoring is used and blood pressure response is usually monitored at each stage of exercise. The Bruce and the Naughton protocols are two of the more commonly used treadmill protocols. Published guidelines for clinical exercise testing that can serve as a reference are available.[13] Numerous books that provide a more thorough discussion of exercise testing procedures and protocols are available.[11,14] A joint statement regarding physician competence in exercise testing was issued by the American College of Physicians, the American College of Cardiology, and the American Heart Association.[15]

Patient Selection: Contraindications

Prior to initiation of an exercise test, a history and physical examination should be performed. Information regarding the patient's medications should be obtained. The history and physical examination may provide information about the presence of relative or absolute contraindication to exercise testing. A consensus statement issued in 1990 by the American Heart Association lists the following absolute contraindications: acute myocardial infarction, recent change in electrocardiogram, acute unstable angina, serious cardiac arrhythmias, acute pericarditis, endocarditis, severe aortic stenosis, severe left ventricular dysfunction, acute pulmonary embolism or infarction, acute or serious noncardiac disorder, and severe physical handicap or disability. Relative contraindications include: less serious noncardiac disorders, significant systemic or pulmonary hypertension, tachyarrhythmias, bradyarrhythmias, moderate valvular or myocardial heart disease, left main coronary obstruction or its equivalent, hypertrophic cardiomyopathy, and psychiatric disease.[16] While many of these contraindications continue to apply, exercise testing of patients with left ventricular dysfunction, hypertrophic cardiomyopathy, and cardiac arrhythmias may be performed safely if considerable caution is used.

Exercise Testing in Known Cardiovascular Disorders or for Screening of these Disorders

Coronary Artery Disease

Exercise testing has been more extensively employed in the evaluation of patients with known or suspected coronary artery disease than in any other condition. Indeed, for decades exercise testing has been part of the routine evaluation of such patients. It is useful for making the diagnosis of coronary artery disease, as well predicting the occurrence of future cardiac events. It may also be used to guide therapy in coronary artery disease and to monitor cardiac rehabilitation following myocardial infarction. Because coronary artery disease is the predominant cause of sudden death in athletes over the age of 35 years,[17–22] there is interest in the use of the exercise test to screen athletes for the prevention of sudden death.

Several parameters of exercise testing provide important prognostic and diagnostic information. These parameters include: electrocardiographic changes, heart rate response, blood pressure response, and exercise capacity. These parameters are frequently combined with clinical information to provide more accurate probability of the presence and severity of coronary artery disease. Emphasis has been placed on the electrocardiographic changes. Criteria have been developed to maximize the sensitivity and specificity of exercise testing. The criterion of a flat ST segment depression of 0.10 mV (1 mm) that persists for 1 or more minutes after exercise is felt to provide the best balance between sensitivity and specificity. By contrast, upsloping ST segment depression may be observed in normal individuals as well as in patients with ischemia.

Unfortunately, numerous abnormalities confound the interpretation of electrocardiographic changes during exercise. The presence of pressure overload of the left ventricle, most commonly due to systemic hypertension (or less commonly, left ventricular outflow obstruction), may cause ST segment depression. In addition, metabolic abnormalities, such as hypokalemia, may produce ST segment changes during exercise.[23] Digitalis is also known to produce exertional ST segment depression—even when the baseline ECG is normal; however, digitalis is not felt to produce false-negative test results.[24] Conditions that are associated with repolarization abnormalities, such as left bundle branch block and Wolff-Parkinson-White syndrome, can result in false-positive ST segment shifts during exercise.

Screening for Coronary Artery Disease and Sudden Cardiac Death

Because of its ability to detect coronary artery disease, exercise testing of the athlete may be considered for several purposes: (1) to identify the presence of coronary artery disease at the time of the exercise test; (2) to predict the risk of future cardiac events; and (3) to determine the safety of exercise. While exercise testing may have a high sensitivity and specificity for detecting coronary artery disease,[25–31] its ability to predict future cardiac events such as myocardial infarction and sudden death is more limited. Due to the low prevalence of coronary artery disease in the asymptomatic athletic population, exercise tests will identify far more false-positive test results than true-positive test results. For example, assuming a 90% sensitivity and specificity and a prevalence of 0.5%, if 10,000 individuals are tested, 45 out of 1040 positive tests will be true positives (giving a positive predictive value of only 4.3%) even though the sensitivity is high and 45 out of 50 individuals with coronary artery disease might be detected. Exercise testing may have a much lower sensitivity for the detection of individuals at risk for sudden death. Epstein and Maron's analysis of the Seattle Heart Watch Study[32,33] population highlights this limitation. With combination of risk factor analysis and exercise test results, a subgroup of 100 patients (out of 10,000 tested) could be identified as having an 18-fold increased risk for sudden death. With an annual incidence of sudden cardiac death of 0.05%, only one patient with sudden death would be identified in the high-risk group, while four deaths would occur in the low-risk group. The ability to identify patients at risk for sudden death is more limited than is the identification of patients with coronary artery disease for several reasons. First, patients may not have flow-limiting stenosis at the time of exercise testing but may acutely develop coronary occlusion, leading to myocardial infarction or sudden death in the future. Second, patients with coronary artery disease may have other mechanisms of sudden death that may not be detected by exercise testing. Third, coronary artery disease is a progressive disorder.

Studies, such as that involving Indiana state police performed by McHenry et al,[34] demonstrate the value of exercise tests for predicting future cardiac events. During 5 years of follow-up, of the 61 (6.6%) individuals with a positive exercise test, 18 (29.5%) developed angina, 1 (1.6%) had a myocardial infarction, and 1 (1.6%) died suddenly. Of the 833 individuals with a normal exercise test, 12 (1.4%) developed angina, 25 (3.0%) had a myocardial infarction, and 7 (0.8%) died suddenly.[34] Thus, it is possible to use exercise testing to stratify patients who are at increased risk for developing cardiac events. Cardiac events that occur in patients with normal exercise tests may reflect the imperfect sensitivity of the technique or the progression of coronary artery disease. It is possible that repeated exercise testing might be useful in identifying the progression of coronary artery disease.

Exercise Testing in Patients with Known Coronary Artery Disease

Exercise testing has a particularly important role in guiding individuals with documented coronary artery disease. Patients with inducible ischemia at a low workload, impaired exercise tolerance, impaired blood pressure response to exercise, or pulmonary congestion with exercise have been shown to have an increased risk of future cardiac events. Although there is an increased risk of myocardial infarction, cardiac arrest, and sudden cardiac death during physical exertion,[35–40] it is difficult to identify the individual who may experience sudden death. While exercise testing may assess the severity of ischemia and provoke serious arrhythmias, it is neither sensitive nor specific in identifying the risk for sudden death. As a result there are only limited data demonstrating the relationship between the risk of athletic participation and the severity of coronary artery disease. Nevertheless, the ability of exercise testing both to identify inducible ischemia and to predict future cardiac events, including myocardial infarction and total cardiac mortality, justifies its use in all athletes with documented coronary artery disease.

It is believed that all patients with established coronary artery disease are at increased risk for future cardiovascular events. The 26th Bethesda Conference divides these patients into two categories or groups: those judged to be at only mildly increased risk, and those at substantially increased risk. Three findings at exercise testing are required for the classification of mildly increased risk: (1) normal age-adjusted exercise tolerance; (2) absence of exercise-induced ischemia; and (3) absence of exercised-induced complex ventricular arrhythmias (Table 1). In addition to findings at exercise testing, the results of studies of left ventricular systolic function and coronary angiography are used in the classification of the athlete.

Coronary Artery Vasospasm

Left main coronary artery spasm has been described in a single case report as a cause of postexertional syncope.[41] In this study, exercise testing was abnormal with both ischemic ST segment depression and an abnormal blood pressure response to exercise. Coronary angiography demonstrated 25% distal left main coronary artery stenosis. Ergonovine challenge resulted in a 90% left main coronary artery stenosis associated with hypotension and presyncope. Treatment with nitrates and a calcium channel blocker led to normalization of this patient's exercise test. Unfortunately, there are limited data regarding the ability of exercise testing to detect coronary vasospasm or to predict syncope or cardiac arrest.

Patients with angiographically normal coronaries and coronary vasospasm (documented either at rest or with exercise) should be restricted to low intensity-sports, according to the 26th Bethesda Conference. Coronary vasospasm most often occurs in patients with concomitant coronary artery disease. Athletes with both coronary artery

Table 1
Acquired Valvular Disease*

Disorder	Role of Exercise Test
Mitral stenosis	Indicated if atrial fibrillation with mild mitral stenosis or moderate mitral stenosis to assess peak pulmonary artery systolic pressure; if <50 mm Hg, can participate in low and moderate static and low and moderate dynamic sports. Indicated to assess pulmonary artery pressure with exercise; if PA sys >80 mm Hg, no competitive sports are permitted
Mitral regurgitation	Indicated if atrial fibrillation is present to assess control of ventricular rate
Aortic stenosis	Indicated in mild and moderate AS to assess for ST segment depression, blood pressure response, and arrhythmias Not indicated in severe AS
Aortic regurgitation	Indicated in athletes with nonspecific symptoms to evaluate functional capacity
Tricuspid regurgitation	Not indicated
Tricuspid stenosis	Indicated at least to level anticipated of sport
Postoperative prosthetic or bioprosthetic cardiac valve	Not indicated
Postoperative with valvuloplasty	Indicated at least to level of anticipated activity to assess exercise tolerance
Mitral valve prolapse	Possible role to assess for increase in arrhythmias with exercise

Coronary Artery Disease*

Role of Exercise Test	Recommendations
Routinely performed	If exercise-induced ischemia, exercise-induced ventricular arrhythmias, EF <40%, or coronary stenosis >50%, athletes are restricted to low dynamic and low/moderate static competitive sports. If severe abnormalities, no competitive sports.

*Adapted from Reference 1. PA = pulmonary artery; AS = aortic stenosis, EF = ejection fraction.

disease and coronary vasospasm should be managed with the same guidelines as those with obstructive coronary artery disease.

Coronary Artery Disease in Cardiac Transplant Recipients

As discussed in the task force report of the 26th Bethesda Conference, maximal exercising testing is used in transplant patients to judge exercise tolerance and to help determine eligibility for competitive sports. It appears that the exercise test can also be used to evaluate patients for inducible ischemia.

Coronary Artery Disease in Kawasaki Disease

Kawasaki disease is a systemic vasculitis that can result in coronary artery aneurysms in up to 25% of untreated patients.[42] In a recent review of the long-term sequelae of Kawasaki disease, 18 of 74 patients died during follow-up. Exercise-related sudden death occurred in 13 of these cases.[43]

To detect inducible ischemia in patients with Kawasaki's disease, exercise testing with nuclear perfusion imaging is preferred over standard ECG exercise testing. Currently, the 26th Bethesda Conference does not recommend exercise testing for athletes with coronary artery disease related to Kawasaki disease, but evidence of inducible ischemia may warrant the suggestion that the athlete refrain from participation in all competitive sports.

Intramyocardial Coronary Arteries

Intramyocardial coronary arteries, sometimes referred to as *myocardial bridging* are commonly observed as an incidental finding at autopsy.[44,45] This condition has only rarely been reported as a cause of sudden cardiac death[44,46] or as a cause of ventricular arrhythmias. Feld et al[47] described a 41-year-old man with atypical chest pain who developed ventricular tachycardia during stage 5 of a Bruce protocol. Ischemic ECG changes occurred before the ventricular tachycardia developed. At coronary angiography, the patient had midsystolic compression of his left anterior descending coronary artery. During electrophysiologic studies, ventricular tachycardia was induced during isoproterenol infusion.

Exercise testing may be used to detect inducible ischemia if intramyocardial coronary arteries are seen angiographically. Patients without inducible ischemia are permitted to participate in all competitive sports, according to the suggestions of the 26th Bethesda Conference.

Hypertrophic Cardiomyopathy

Exercise-related sudden death accounts for a substantial portion of death in patients with hypertrophic cardiomyopathy. In several studies of sudden death of athletes younger than 35, hypertrophic cardiomyopathy is usually the most common cardiac structural abnormality detected.[18–20,22] Hemodynamic changes, ischemia, and catecholamines may all contribute to ventricular arrhythmias, which are probably the cause of exercise-induced sudden death in this condition.

Exercise-induced ischemia, as detected by thallium scintigraphy, may be predictive of sudden cardiac death, ventricular arrhythmias, and syncope in selected patients with hypertrophic cardiomyopathy.[48–51]

The 26th Bethesda Conference suggests the exclusion of all athletes with definite hypertrophic obstructive cardiomyopathy from participation in all but the least strenuous competitive sports. Individual judgment is permitted for the athlete over the age of 30 who is free of risk factors for sudden cardiac death. Included in the risk factors, by the 26th Bethesda Conference, is the absence of an exercise-induced myocardial perfusion abnormality (Table 2).

Mitral Valve Prolapse

Mitral valve prolapse has not been definitively associated with increased risk of sudden death. In the presence of syncope documented

Table 2
Hypertrophic Cardiomyopathy, Myocarditis, Other Myopericardial Diseases*

Disorder	Role of Exercise Test
Hypertrophic cardiomyopathy	Possibly indicated to assess myocardial perfusion (with radionuclide imaging)
Myocarditis	Indicated for assessment of ventricular function with exercise (with radionuclide imaging)
Pericarditis	Indicated

System Hypertension*

Role of Exercise Test
Not required

*Adapted from Reference 1.

to be arrhythmogenic, a family history of sudden death associated with mitral valve prolapse, repetitive supraventricular or ventricular arrhythmias (particularly if exaggerated by exercise), moderate to severe mitral regurgitation, or prior embolic event, athletes should be restricted to low-intensity sports, according to the suggestions of the 26th Bethesda Conference. The role of exercise testing in such patients is largely limited to assessing if arrhythmias are aggravated by exertion. Exercise may result in worsening or provocation of mitral regurgitation which, in turn, has been associated with an increased incidence of syncope.[52,53]

Systemic Hypertension

While hypertension is a risk factor for the development of coronary artery disease and sudden death, there are no data to suggest that it is a primary cause of sudden death in athletes. Therefore, exercise testing is not routinely required for assessment of eligibility for sports participation of hypertensive patients. Exercise testing may be useful in assessing the blood pressure response during exertion in athletes with known or suspected hypertension. A hypertensive blood pressure response during exercise testing (variously defined as a systolic blood pressure >240 mm Hg; or >210 mm Hg in men and >190 mm Hg in women) may be predictive of the development of hypertension in a normotensive population.[54,55] Similarly, severe hypertension during stress testing may indicate the need for increased pharmacological control of hypertension (Table 2).

Arrhythmias

Exercise frequently facilitates or precipitates arrhythmias—even in individuals without underlying structural heart disease. The mechanisms underlying exercise-induced arrhythmias are complex. They involve changes in autonomic tone that result from stimulation of both α- and β-adrenergic receptors and from decreases in parasympathetic tone. Induction of ischemia may also play a role. These factors can result in increased automaticity, provoke triggered activity, or favor reentry.[56–58]

The 26th Bethesda Conference and the Council on Child and Adolescent Health both recommend exercise testing for most athletes with documented arrhythmias (Table 3).[59] Exercise testing helps to evaluate the effects of exercise on the arrhythmia as well as on the hemodynamic status of the athlete during the arrhythmia. Often the exercise test should be modified to simulate more accurately the sport that is being contemplated. In this respect, ambulatory monitoring during

Table 3
Arrhythmias*

Disorder	Role of Exercise Test	Interpretation/Recommendation
Sinus pauses >3.0 sec, sinoatrial exit block	Indicated	Assess appropriate increase of the heart rate; if present, athlete can participate in all sports
Atrial flutter	Indicated if no structural heart disease	Assess adequate rate control; if present, low-intensity sports May participate if no atrial flutter 3–6 months
Atrial fibrillation (without WPW)	Indicated	Assess adequate rate control; if present, may participate in all sports (if anticoagulated, no bodily collision)
Atrial tachycardia	Indicated	Assess adequate rate control; if present, may participate in all sports
Supraventricular tachycardia	Indicated	Assess rate during exercise and control by therapy; if asymptomatic and controlled by therapy; can participate in all sports
Ventricular preexcitation (WPW)	Indicated	To exclude associated abnormalities
Ventricular tachycardia	Indicated	For most, adjunctive to EP study For asymptomatic athlete with <8–10 beats nonsustained VT, rates <150 bpm, and no structural heart disease, evidence of suppression of VT, may participate in all sports

Table 3 (continued)

Disorder	Role of Exercise Test	Interpretation/Recommendation
First-degree AV block	Indicated	In absence of symptoms or structural heart disease, no evidence of worsening of AV block with exercise, may participate in all sports
Type I second-degree AV block	Indicated	If no structural heart disease and no worsening of AV block with exercise, may participate in all sports
Type II second-degree AV block	Not indicated	
Congenital complete AV block	Indicated	If structurally normal heart, normal cardiac function, no history of syncope, narrow QRS complex, ventricular rates >40–50 bpm that increase with exertion, without ventricular ectopy, may participate in all sports
Acquired complete AV block	Not indicated	
Right bundle branch block	Indicated	If no ventricular arrhythmias, no symptoms and no AV block with exercise, may participate in all sports
Left bundle branch block	Indicated	If no ventricular arrhythmias, no symptoms, and no AV block with exercise, may participate in all sports; younger athletes should also have EP study
Congenital long QT interval syndrome	Not indicated	

*Adapted from Reference 1. WPW = Wolff-Parkinson-White; AV = atrioventricular; EP = electrophysiologic; VT = ventricular tachycardia.

sports participation, if it can be safely performed, has advantages over formal exercise testing.

Syncope

Syncope is an important cardiovascular symptom and should prompt a thorough cardiovascular evaluation. Syncope is frequently reported before sudden death in young athletes.[18] Of athletes or soldiers who die suddenly, 9% to 25%[20,60,61] have a history of syncope.

Syncope in the athlete is a particularly challenging diagnostic problem because it may occur in up to 15% of the young population,[62,63] however, syncope that occurs during or immediately after exercise suggests an arrhythmic etiology, and should prompt an evaluation for structural heart disease.[1,61] In an epidemiologic study of syncope in children and adolescents, six cases of exertional syncope occurred out of a total of 194 episodes of syncope. Of those 6, 1 died suddenly and 1 was found to have the long QT syndrome.[64] The occurrence of syncope in athletes who have evidence of significant structural heart disease is associated with a high incidence of potentially life-threatening ventricular arrhythmias. In such patients, electrophysiologic testing should be strongly considered. In patients with exertional syncope, exercise testing is routinely performed, although the value of the test is not well defined.

There are many etiologies for syncope that occurs during exertion. In the presence of structural heart disease, syncope may be due to arrhythmias. In the absence of structural heart disease, a neurocardiogenic mechanism has been implicated. In neurocardiogenic syncope[65] a stimulus, such as prolonged standing, leads to venous pooling. The decreased blood return to the heart results in sympathetic nervous system stimulation. The increase in catecholamines leads to increased inotropy. The increased inotropy results in increased stimulation of unmyelinated mechanoreceptors (C-fibers) located in the heart. These C-fibers are believed to be the afferent neural input for the initiation of the neurocardiogenic reflex.[63,66] The neural output from this reflex results in inappropriate withdrawal of sympathetic tone and enhanced vagal tone. The change in autonomic tone causes vasodilatation, hypotension, bradycardia, and finally syncope.

Neurocardiogenic syncope occurs in three forms: cardioinhibitory (predominant bradycardia), vasodepressor (predominant hypotension), and mixed. Exertion-related neurocardiogenic syncope that occurs after exertion may more frequently be of the cardioinhibitory type and may occur as long as 1 to 10 minutes after exertion. Vagal reactions have been reported to occur in 0.2% of exercise tests, but profound bradycardia resulting in syncope has been infrequently reported.[67] Neurocardiogenic syncope that occurs during exertion may be of the

Table 4
Use of the Exercise Test in Exercise-Induced
Neurocardiogenic Syncope

Author	Year	Number of Patients	Type of Syncope	Number w/ ETT	Num. ETT w/ Syncope
Rassmussen[118]	1978	4	—	4	0
Fleg[119]	1983	1	CI	1	1
Yerg[120]	1985	1	CI	0	0
Huycke[78]	1987	1	CI	1	1
Hirata[73]	1987	1	CI	1	0
Kapoor[74]	1989	1	CI	1	0
Pedersen[70]	1989	1	CI/VD	1	1
Tamura[79]	1990	1	CI	1	1
Grubb[75]	1992	24	VD	24	0
Sneddon[72]	1993	5	VD	5	5
Sakaguchi[76]	1995	10	VD	5	0
Calkins[77]	1995	17	VD	17	1
Tse[71]	1995	2	CI	2	2
Kosinski[121]	1996	1	VD	1	1
Total		70		64	13

See text for details. CI = Cardioinhibitory; VD = Vasodepressor; ETT = exercise tolerance test.

vasodepressor or mixed subtype. Exercise testing and head-up tilt table testing has been used to evaluate both exertional and postexertional types of neurocardiogenic syncope.

Some investigators have reported a concordance between exercise testing and head-up tilt table testing in the evaluation of exercise-related neurocardiogenic syncope (Table 4).[63,65,66,68,69] In 1989, Pedersen et al[70] described a patient with neurocardiogenic syncope induced after an exercise test and during head-up tilt table testing. In 1995, Tse and Lau[71] described two cases of exercise-associated asystole in which symptoms were reproduced by exercise testing and head-up tilt table testing with isoproterenol. Sneddon et al[72] reported five cases of exercise-induced vasodepressor syncope that was reproduced by exercise testing and head-up tilt table testing.

Other investigators however, have demonstrated a discordance between exercise testing and head-up tilt table testing.[73,74] In several series, the investigators claimed that exercise-related syncope was due to neurocardiogenic mechanisms; however, exercise testing failed to reproduce the symptoms. In a study of 24 young athletes with recurrent syncope during exercise, Grubb et al[75] reported that exercise testing did not reproduce symptoms, whereas head-up tilt table testing induced syncope in 79% of the patients. In another series of 10 patients with syncope related to exertion in the absence of structural heart disease, exercise testing did not produce syncope or hypotension in the 5 subjects in whom it was employed; however, head-up tilt table testing produced symptomatic hypotension-bradycardia in 9 of the 10 patients.[76] In 1995, Calkins et al[77] described a series of 17 patients without significant structural heart disease and exercise-induced vasodepressor syncope. Only one patient developed presyncope that occurred after exercise testing, while all patients had a positive head-up tilt table test. In 35±9 months (range 20 to 50 months) of follow-up, no sudden deaths were reported in this series.

Treatment for exercise-associated neurocardiogenic syncope has been described. Pharmacological pretreatment with either propranolol or atropine may prevent postexercise syncope.[78] Other patients have even been treated successfully with permanent pacing,[74] although pacing alone may not prevent exercise-related hypotension.[79] Deconditioning in the athlete may also result in improved symptoms in some patients. It may be necessary for some individuals who experience exertion-related syncope to avoid strenuous exercise altogether.

The diagnosis of exercise-associated neurocardiogenic syncope should be considered only after a thorough evaluation has excluded structural heart disease and arrhythmias. The diagnosis of exercise-induced neurocardiogenic syncope would be most secure if an exercise test can clearly reproduce the clinical scenario with documentation of hypotension and/or bradycardia.

Sinus Bradycardia

Asymptomatic resting bradycardia and short sinus pauses are common in the trained athlete and do not need treatment. Exercise testing is appropriate for patients with sinus pauses >3 seconds in length, sinoatrial exit block, or suspected sick sinus syndrome. The purpose of the testing is to determine whether the sinus rate increases appropriately with activity.

Chronotropic incompetence (a less than expected increase in heart rate prompted by exercise) has been linked to an increase in all-cause mortality and cardiac events.[80,81]

Atrial Flutter

During exercise the ventricular rate during atrial flutter may be quite rapid. Indeed, the rate may be so fast as to result in hemodynamic collapse, particularly if there is 1:1 conduction via the atrioventricular

(AV) node.[82,83] An exercise test or ambulatory monitoring is recommended for the athlete with atrial flutter, in order to evaluate the ventricular response during exercise. In addition, an evaluation for underlying structural heart disease should be conducted.

Once the patient is treated with medications, exercise testing may also be useful to demonstrate whether or not adequate control of the ventricular rate has been achieved. Rapid ventricular rates may be seen in subjects with enhanced AV nodal conduction and has been documented to be a rare cause of cardiac arrest. Because of the potential for 1:1 conduction through the AV node, the 26th Bethesda Conference requires that the ventricular rate while in atrial flutter and on medications to slow the ventricular response be similar to an appropriate sinus tachycardia rate for participation in only low-intensity sports (Table 3).

Atrial Fibrillation, Sinus Node Reentry, and Atrial Tachycardia

It is important that ventricular rates be controlled during exercise in patients with such rhythms as atrial fibrillation or atrial tachycardias so as to prevent hemodynamically induced symptoms such as lightheadedness, presyncope, or syncope. The ventricular rate in patients with atrial fibrillation is usually less difficult to control pharmacologically than is the ventricular rate in atrial flutter. However, in many patients with atrial tachycardias, the risk of 1:1 conduction during exercise should be considered. Exercise testing has a role in confirming adequate rate control in these conditions. In the absence of structural heart disease athletes with these atrial arrhythmias may participate in all competitive sports if their ventricular rates, with or without medication, are similar to an appropriate sinus tachycardia during exertion. Ambulatory monitoring may be an alternative to exercise testing in this situation (Table 3).

Nonparoxysmal Atrioventricular Junctional Tachycardia

The task force of the 26th Bethesda Conference recommends an exercise test as part of the evaluation of patients with nonparoxysmal AV junctional tachycardia. If there is no structural heart disease and if the ventricular rate is controlled during exercise, competition in all competitive sports is usually permitted.

Supraventricular Tachycardia

While paroxysmal supraventricular tachycardias are common and may frequently be induced by exercise, they are only rarely associated with sudden death in the absence of ventricular preexcitation. Such tachycardias may occur in patients and athletes with and without structural heart disease. Exercise testing may reproduce exercise-induced symptoms such as palpitations.[84] In addition, an exercise test may be used to evaluate the rate of supraventricular tachycardias during exercise. Exercise testing may also assess the ability of medical therapy to prevent recurrence of exercise-induced arrhythmias (Table 3).

Ventricular Preexcitation (Wolf–Parkinson–White Syndrome)

Ventricular preexcitation is associated with a small risk of sudden death, most likely due to very rapid conduction down the accessory pathway during atrial fibrillation, causing ventricular fibrillation. Patients with ventricular preexcitation who suffer cardiac arrest have been shown by electrophysiologic studies to have preexcited R-R intervals in atrial fibrillation of <250 milliseconds or antegrade refractory periods of the accessory pathway <250 milliseconds.[85]

Exercise testing has a relatively limited role in the risk stratification of patients with ventricular preexcitation.[86–88] Exercise testing may be used to evaluate the effects of exercise on the refractory period of the accessory pathway and to demonstrate the partial reversal of the protective effects of antiarrhythmics in the control of the ventricular response to atrial fibrillation.[89–91] The sensitivity (of placing a patient into the high-risk group) of persistent preexcitation during exercise testing is high (80%) but its specificity is low (28.6%).[92] The gradual catecholamine-induced shortening of the conduction time through the AV node may result in a gradual decrease in the degree of preexcitation during exercise testing. Sudden loss of preexcitation during exercise may identify individuals who are at lower risk of sudden death.[57]

The 26th Bethesda Conference recommends exercise testing as part of the evaluation of the athlete with ventricular preexcitation. In the presence of symptoms (palpitations, presyncope, syncope), the electrical properties of the accessory pathway, including the induction of atrial fibrillation, determined at electrophysiologic study are used in the stratification of the risks for the athlete and in the determination of eligibility for competitive sports.

Premature Ventricular Complexes

Premature ventricular complexes are quite common in the athlete. In one study, premature ventricular contractions occurred in 18% to 60% of athletes.[93] Premature ventricular contractions are not usually the result of structural heart disease. With exercise, premature ventricular complexes may increase or decrease in frequency. Most athletes do not experience hemodynamic-related symptoms from premature ventricular complexes. If symptoms such as impaired consciousness, fatigue, or dyspnea are associated with an increased frequency of premature ventricular complexes during exercise, participation in competitive sports should be limited, as recommended by the 26th Bethesda Conference (Table 3).

Ventricular Tachycardia, Ventricular Flutter, and Ventricular Fibrillation

The most important issue regarding ventricular tachycardia for the prognosis of the patient is the presence of structural heart disease. In the presence of structural heart disease, ventricular tachycardia is potentially life-threatening. While electrophysiologic testing has a central role in the evaluation and management of patients with these conditions, exercise testing may have an adjunctive role in demonstrating the suppression of ventricular tachycardia by medication. The 26th Bethesda Conference guidelines suggest that moderate and high-intensity competition is contraindicated for patients with ventricular tachycardia and structural heart disease. On the other hand, the report suggests that the athlete without structural heart disease who has been free from recurrence of ventricular tachycardia for 6 months and who cannot have ventricular tachycardia induced by exercise testing or at electrophysiologic study may participate in competitive sports (Table 3).

In the small subset of athletes with incidentally discovered asymptomatic nonsustained monomorphic slow ventricular tachycardia but without underlying structural heart disease, exercise testing may be used to confirm that ventricular tachycardia is not worsened with exercise. This select group of athletes is not felt to be at increased risk for sudden cardiac death and may be permitted to participate in all competitive sports.

Exertion frequently precipitates several types of ventricular tachycardias. Arrhythmogenic right ventricular dysplasia typically presents with a left bundle/variable axis morphology.[94,95] Right ventricular outflow tract ventricular tachycardia presents with a left bundle/inferior axis morphology and is amenable to radiofrequency ablation.[96] Idiopathic left ventricular tachycardia presents with a right bundle/left axis morphology, and is also amenable to radiofrequency ablation.[97,98]

Ventricular fibrillation usually occurs in the setting of underlying structural heart disease and is infrequently reproduced by exercise testing. In a series of 19 patients with ventricular fibrillation and no structural heart disease, exercise testing only produced ventricular tachycardia in 2 patients. Even in the absence of structural heart disease, patients with ventricular fibrillation have a high incidence of arrhythmia recurrence.[99] Patients who have symptomatic, rapid, nonsustained episodes of polymorphic ventricular tachycardia (even with a normal QTc interval and without significant structural heart disease) have recently been reported to have a poor prognosis.[100] In this series, nonsustained polymorphic ventricular tachycardia during exercise testing was seen in 4 of the 8 patients tested.

First-Degree Atrioventricular Block

First-degree AV block is not uncommon in athletes; in the asymptomatic athlete it does not warrant further evaluation.[101] However, exercise testing may play a role in the evaluation of individuals with a PR interval >0.3 seconds. In such patients, the 26th Bethesda Conference would permit participation in competitive sports if the PR interval does not prolong with exertion (Table 3).

Type I Second-Degree Atrioventricular Block

While type I second-degree AV block (Wenckebach) is not uncommon in the highly trained athlete, exercise testing is believed to be important in its evaluation. If the Wenckebach remains stable or disappears with exercise, no restrictions are placed on the athlete who is free of structural heart disease. In the rare case that the block worsens with exertion, further evaluation and permanent pacing may be indicated.

Congenital Complete Heart Block

Exercise testing plays a role in the evaluation of patients with congenital complete AV block. According to the guidelines established by the 26th Bethesda Conference, an athlete with congenital complete heart block may participate in all competitive sports if the athlete is free of:

(1) structural heart disease; (2) symptoms; or (3) exercise-induced ventricular ectopy. In addition, the athlete must have a narrow QRS escape that is faster than 40 beats per minutes and that increases with exercise. If a pacemaker is implanted because of symptoms, arrhythmias, or chronotropic incompetence of the escape rhythm, then an exercise test is indicated to determine whether the paced rate increases appropriately.

Type II Second–Degree Atrioventricular Block and Acquired Complete Heart Block

The 26th Bethesda Conference does not discuss the role of exercise testing in athletes with type II second-degree heart block or acquired complete heart block. Pacer insertion is required before participation in competitive sports for either of these conditions. It seems reasonable to perform an exercise test as part of an evaluation for structural heart disease.

The development of bradyarrhythmias with exertion is uncommon. However, there are several recent reports of this phenomenon. In each case, a resting ECG showed 1:1 AV conduction and an exercise test provoked AV block. In 1988, Peller et al[102] described three patients with exercise-related symptoms of either fatigue, dizziness, or syncope. Exercise testing produced symptomatic second-degree (type II) AV block or advanced AV block. All three patients improved with permanent pacing. In 1989, Ozder et al[103] described a patient with a 2-year history of exertional syncope. At exercise testing, symptomatic AV block developed. The patient was treated with pacing and had relief of her symptoms. In 1992, Reig et al[104] described a patient with dizziness upon walking that was documented to be due to 2:1 and advanced AV block. Therefore, exercise testing would certainly seem to be appropriate for the evaluation of exertional symptoms, and symptomatic bradycardia from AV block will rarely be discovered.

Complete Bundle Branch Block

The 26th Bethesda Conference recommends an exercise test as part of the evaluation of athletes with either right or left bundle branch block. If no higher degree of AV block develops and no symptoms are present, participation in all sports is permitted. Invasive electrophysiologic study in addition to stress testing is suggested for younger athletes with left bundle branch block. Exercise-induced bundle branch block is frequently rate-dependent. If coronary artery disease is absent, the prognosis is good.[105,106]

Long QT Syndrome

The recommendations of the 26th Bethesda Conference exclude athletes with long QT syndrome from competitive sports. Exercise testing has been performed in studies that compared the results in control patients with the results in patients with established long QT syndrome. In most forms of congenital long QT syndrome, the QTc lengthens with exercise.[107-109] In some patients with the congenital long QT syndrome, resting T and U waves are normal and abnormalities such as lengthening of the QT interval or the appearance of U waves are only noted with exercise or with other provocative measures. In the bradycardia-dependent congenital long QT syndrome, the QTc normalizes with exercise.[110] Thus, exercise testing may assist in the diagnosis of patients with the long QT syndrome.

Congenital Heart Disease

The 26th Bethesda Conference recommends selective exercise testing for competitive athletes with congenital heart disease. The exercise test quantifies exercise tolerance, evaluates the patient for the development of exercise-induced arrhythmias, and allows examination of hemodynamic alterations. The following paragraphs provide a review of the suggestions of the 26th Bethesda Conference. Frequently, these guidelines are based primarily on clinical judgment because adequate data from clinical series or clinical trials are limited.

Athletes with congenital heart disorders may exhibit important hemodynamic and arrhythmic findings during exercise testing (Table 5). Patients with severe left ventricular outflow obstruction (such as may occur in congenital valvular aortic stenosis, discrete subaortic stenosis, or supravalvular aortic stenosis) have findings that reflect impaired ability to increase cardiac output with exertion. Therefore, in the setting of vasodilatation induced by exercise, patients with left ventricular outflow obstruction may experience hypotension and syncope. Early in the course of congenital aortic stenosis, there may be an increase in cardiac output and pressure gradient with exercise; such individuals may remain asymptomatic during exercise.[111] Subendocardial ischemia from elevated intramyocardial forces may be an important factor in the development of ventricular fibrillation and sudden death in patients with advanced aortic stenosis.[112]

In the patient with severe aortic stenosis, exercise testing should not be performed, and strenuous physical activity should be avoided. Athletic participation is more controversial in patients with mild and moderate aortic stenosis. Symptomatic patients should probably avoid strenuous athletics. Exercise testing may be valuable in the evaluation of the asymptomatic patient with mild to moderate left ventricular outflow tract obstruction. The 26th Bethesda Conference suggests that asymptomatic athletes with moderate aortic stenosis be permitted to participate in limited sports and that athletes with mild aortic stenosis be permitted to participate in all sports if an exercise test is free of ischemia, arrhythmias, abnormal blood pressure response, or abnormal exercise tolerance.

Table 5
Congenital Heart Disease*

Disorder	Role of Exercise Test
Atrial septal defect, untreated	Not indicated
Atrial septal defect, closed	Indicated if pulmonary hypertension, symptomatic arrhythmias, or myocardial dysfunction
Ventricular septal defect, untreated	Not indicated unless pulmonary hypertension
Ventricular septal defect, closed	Not indicated unless pulmonary hypertension
Patent ductus arteriosus, untreated	Not indicated unless pulmonary hypertension
Patent ductus arteriosus, closed	Not indicated unless pulmonary hypertension
Pulmonic valve stenosis, untreated	Not indicated
Pulmonic valve stenosis, treated	Not indicated
Congenital aortic valve stenosis, untreated	Indicated in mild AS to assess exercise tolerance Indicated in moderate AS to assess ischemia, arrhythmias, exercise tolerance, exercise duration, and blood pressure response Not indicated in severe AS
Congenital aortic valve stenosis, treated	Indicated in mild AS to assess exercise tolerance Indicated in moderate AS to assess ischemia, arrhythmias, exercise tolerance, exercise duration, and blood pressure response Not indicated in severe AS
Coarctation of the aorta, untreated	Indicated to assess severity of obstruction, peak systolic blood pressure with exercise

Table 5 (continued)

Disorder	Role of Exercise Test
Coarctation of the aorta, treated	Indicated to assess peak systolic blood pressure
Elevated pulmonary resistance	Indicated if pulmonary artery peak systolic pressure >40 mm Hg
Ventricular dysfunction after cardiac surgery	Not indicated
Cyanotic congenital cardiac disease, unoperated	Individualized
Postoperative palliated cyanotic congenital heart disease	Indicated to assess working capacity
Postoperative tetralogy of Fallot	Indicated to assess rhythm abnormality
Transposition of great arteries, Postoperative Mustard or Senning	Indicated to assess functional capacity
Congenitally corrected transposition of the great arteries	Indicated to assess for arrhythmias
Postoperative arterial switch for transposition of the great arteries	Indicated to assess for functional capacity and arrhythmias
Postoperative Fontan operation	Indicated to assess exercise tolerance and oxygen saturation
Ebstein's anomaly	Indicated to assess arrhythmias following surgical repair
Congenital coronary anomalies	Indicated after operation to assess for ischemia
Marfan syndrome	Not indicated

*Adapted from Reference 1. AS = aortic valve stenosis.

Exercise testing is recommended for athletes with coarctation of the aorta. If mild coarctation is present, a normal exercise test is required before participation in all competitive sports can be recommended. The 26th Bethesda Conference suggests that an athlete with mild coarctation of the aorta should have a normal exercise test, including a peak systolic blood pressure ≤230 mm Hg, before participating in all sports. After correction of coarctation of the aorta, exercise testing is required; the patient must have a normal systolic blood pressure at rest and at peak exercise in order to be allowed to participate in competitive sports.

In patients with acyanotic heart disease and left-to-right shunts, exercise may transiently reverse the direction of the shunt. In uncomplicated atrial septal defect, the response of ejection fraction to exercise may be abnormal but usually does not result in a failure to increase blood pressure.[113] Athletes with atrial septal defects, ventricular septal defects, or a small patent ductus arteriosus without pulmonary hypertension can participate in sports and exercise testing is not required.

Exercise testing has an important role in many patients following surgical repair of cyanotic congenital heart disease. After correction of tetralogy of Fallot, an exercise test free of rhythm abnormalities is required before athletic participation is permitted. A normal exercise test is required after surgical repair of transposition of the great arteries before participation in restricted levels of competitive sports can be considered. For patients who have palliation of their condition with the Fontan operation, near normal exercise tolerance on exercise testing is required before participation in low or moderate static sports. After surgical correction of severe Ebstein's anomaly, an exercise test free of arrhythmias is required as part of the preparticipation evaluation. For the occasional patient who has congenitally corrected transposition of the great arteries without associated abnormalities, an exercise test free of arrhythmias is required as part of the evaluation before the patient can participate in all competitive sports.

Exercise testing is said to have a low sensitivity for detecting coronary artery anomalies.[114] Thallium scintigraphy has been used to detect ischemia due to coronary arteriovenous fistulas.[115–117] After surgical correction for congenital coronary anomalies, an exercise test free of ischemia is required before an individual can be permitted to participate in competitive sports.

Acquired Valvular Heart Disease

According to the 26th Bethesda Conference, exercise testing should be used selectively to evaluate patients with acquired valvular heart disease (Table 1). In athletes with mitral stenosis, exercise testing may be used to assess the maximal pulmonary artery systolic pressure during exercise by using either Doppler echocardiography or cardiac catheterization. If the pulmonary artery systolic pressure is equal to or greater than 80 mm Hg at rest or during exercise, participation in competitive athletics is not permitted at any level. If the pulmonary artery systolic pressure is between 50 and 80 mm Hg at rest or during exercise, only low dynamic competitive sports are allowed. Exercise testing is not recommended for the athlete with mitral regurgitation except in the presence of atrial fibrillation; an exercise test should confirm that ventricular rates are not excessive. In patients with mild or moderate aortic stenosis, exercise testing is used to evaluate exercise capacity, electrocardiographic changes, arrhythmias, and blood pressure response. The results of the exercise test help determine the athlete's eligibility for athletics. Exercise testing to the level of exertion at competition may be useful in assessing functional capacity in athletes with mild aortic insufficiency. Athletes with tricuspid stenosis may compete in all competitive sports if they are asymptomatic at exercise testing to the level of exertion of their sport. After valve replacement, repair, or valvuloplasty, exercise testing to the level of exertion expected in competition can be helpful to assess exercise capacity.

Pericarditis

The 26th Bethesda Conference excludes athletes with active pericarditis from participation in competitive sports. Prior to returning to sport activity, an evaluation that includes an exercise test is recommended (Table 2).

Conclusions

Exercise testing may simulate the hemodynamic and arrhythmic changes that occur with athletic activity. Exercise testing plays an important role in the evaluation of the athlete with exertional symptoms or with many known cardiovascular disorders. Exercise testing has limited positive predictive value when used for screening asymptomatic athletes from the general population, but exercise testing may be reasonable for subgroups of athletes at substantially increased risk of coronary artery disease.

References

1. Maron BJ, Mitchell JH. 26th Bethesda Conference: Recommendations for Determining eligibility for competition in athletes with cardiovascular abnormalities. *J Am Coll Cardiol* 1994;24:845–899.
2. Maron BJ, Thompson PD, Puffer JC, et al. Cardiovascular preparticipation screening of competitive athletes. *Circulation* 1996;94:850–856.

3. Vatner SF, Higgins CB, White S, et al. The peripheral vascular response to severe exercise in untethered dogs before and after complete heart block. *J Clin Invest* 1971;50:1950.
4. Guyton AC. The relationship of cardiac output and arterial pressure control. *Circulation* 1981;64:1079.
5. Rothe CF. Physiology of venous return: An unappreciated boost to the heart. *Arch Intern Med* 1986;146:977.
6. Epstein SE, Beiser GD, Stampfer M, et al. Characterization of the circulatory response to maximal upright exercise in normal subjects and patients with heart disease. *Circulation* 1967;35:1049.
7. Epstein SE, Robinson BF, Kahler RL, Braunwald E. Effects of beta-adrenergic blockade on the cardiac response to maximal and submaximal exercise in man. *J Clin Invest* 1965;44:1745.
8. Robinson BF, Epstein SE, Kahler RL, Braunwald E. Circulatory effects of acute expansion of blood volume: Studies during maximal exercise and at rest. *Circ Res* 1966;19:26.
9. Sheffield LT. Exercise stress testing. In Braunwald E (ed): *Heart Disease.* Philadelphia: W.B. Saunders Co.; 1992:224.
10. Stone PH, Turi ZG, Muller JE, et al. Prognostic significance of the treadmill exercise test performance 6 months after myocardial infarction. *J Am Coll Cardiol* 1986;8:1007.
11. Ellestad MH. *Stress Testing. Principles and Practice.* Philadelphia: F.A. Davis Company; 1986.
12. Sheffield LT, Maloof JA, Sawyer JA, Roitman D. Maximal heart rate and treadmill performance of healthy women in relation to age. *Circulation* 1967;57:79.
13. Pina IL, Balady GJ, Hanson P, et al. Guidelines for clinical exercise testing laboratories. *Circulation* 1995;91:912–921.
14. Pate RR, Blair SN, Durstine JL, et al. *Guidelines for Exercise Testing and Prescription/American College of Sports Medicine.* Philadelphia: Lea and Febiger; 1991:314.
15. Schlant R, Friesinger G, Leonard J, et al. Clinical competence in exercise testing: A statement for physicians from the ACP/ACC/AHA task force on clinical privileges in cardiology. *Ann Intern Med* 1987;107:588–589.
16. Fletcher GF, Froelicher VF, Hartley LH, et al. Exercise standards: A statement for health professionals from the American Heart Association. *Circulation* 1990;82:2286–2322.
17. Waller BF, Roberts WC. Sudden death while running in conditioned runners aged 40 years or over. *Am J Cardiol* 1980;45:1292–1300.
18. Maron BJ, Roberts WC, McAllister HA, et al. Sudden death in young athletes. *Circulation* 1980;62:218–229.
19. Maron BJ, Epstein SE, Roberts WC. Causes of sudden death in competitive athletes. *J Am Coll Cardiol* 1986;7:204–214.
20. Maron BJ, Shirani J, Poliac LC, et al. Sudden death in young competitive athletes. *JAMA* 1996;276:199–204.
21. Liberthson RR. Sudden death from cardiac causes in children and young adults. *N Engl J Med* 1996;334:1039–1044.
22. Burke AP, Farb A, Virmani R, et al. Sports-related and non-sports-related sudden cardiac death in young adults. *Am Heart J* 1991;121:568–575.
23. Riley CP, Oberman A, Sheffield LT. Electrocardiographic effects of glucose ingestion. *Arch Intern Med* 1972;130:703–707.
24. Kawai C, Hultgren HN. The effect of digitalis upon the exercise electrocardiogram. *Am Heart J* 1964;68:409.

25. Diamond GA, Forrester JS. Analysis of probability as an aid in the clinical diagnosis of coronary-artery disease. *N Engl J Med* 1979;300: 1350–1358.
26. Rifkin RD, Hood WB. Bayesian analysis of electrocardiographic exercise stress testing. *N Engl J Med* 1977;297:681–686.
27. Beleslin BB, Ostojic M, Stepanovic J, et al. Stress echocardiography in the detection of myocardial ischemia. *Circulation* 1994;90:1168–1176.
28. Berman DS, Hachamovitch R, Kiat H, et al. Incremental value of prognostic testing in patients with known of suspected ischemic heart disease: A basis for optimal utilization of exercise technetium-99m sestamibi myocardial perfusion single-photon emission computed tomography. *J Am Coll Cardiol* 1995;26:639–647.
29. Vaduganathan P, He Z-X, Raghavan C, et al. Detection of left anterior descending coronary artery stenosis in patients with left bundle branch block: Exercise, adenosine or dobutamine imaging? *J Am Coll Cardiol* 1996;28:543–550.
30. Mayo Clinic Cardiovascular Working Group on Stress Testing. Cardiovascular stress testing: A description of the various types of stress tests and indications for their use. *Mayo Clin Proc* 1996;71:43–52.
31. Ling LH, Pellikka PA, Mahoney DW, et al. Atropine augmentation in dobutamine stress echocardiography: Role and incremental value in a clinical practice setting. *J Am Coll Cardiol* 1996;28:551–557.
32. Epstein SE, Maron BJ. Sudden death and the competitive athlete: Perspectives on preparticipation screening studies. *J Am Coll Cardiol* 1986; 7:220–229.
33. Bruce RA, DeRouen TA, Hossack KF. Value of maximal exercise tests in risk assessment of primary coronary heart disease events in healthy men. *Am J Cardiol* 1980;46:371–378.
34. McHenry PL, O'Donnell J, Morris SN, Jordan JJ. The abnormal exercise electrocardiogram in apparently healthy men: A predictor of angina pectoris as an initial coronary event during long term follow-up. *Circulation* 1984;70:547–551.
35. Thompson PD. The cardiovascular complications of vigorous physical activity. *Arch Intern Med* 1996;156:2297–2302.
36. Maron BJ, Poliac LC, Roberts WO. Risk for sudden cardiac death associated with marathon running. *J Am Coll Cardiol* 1996;28:428–431.
37. Thompson PD, Funk EJ, Carleton RA, Sturner WQ. Incidence of death during jogging in Rhode Island from 1975 through 1980. *JAMA* 1982; 247: 2535–2538.
38. Willich SN, Lewis M, Arntz HR, et al. Physical exertion as a trigger of acute myocardial infarction. *N Engl J Med* 1993;329:1684–1690.
39. Mittleman MA, Maclure M, Toefler GH, et al. Triggering of acute myocardial infarction by heavy physical exertion: Protection against triggering by regular exertion. *N Engl J Med* 1993;329:1677–1683.
40. Siscovick DS, Weiss NS, Fletcher RH, Lasky T. The incidence of primary cardiac arrest during vigorous exercise. *N Engl J Med* 1984;311:874–877.
41. Havranek EP, Dunbar DN. Exertional syncope caused by left main coronary artery spasm. *Am Heart J* 1992;123:792–794.
42. Kato H, Ichinose E, Yoshioka F, et al. Fate of coronary artery aneurysms in Kawasaki disease: Serial coronary angiography and long-term follow-up study. *Am J Cardiol* 1982;49:1758–1766.
43. Burns JC, Shike H, Gordon JB, et al. Sequelae of Kawasaki disease in adolescents and young adults. *J Am Coll Cardiol* 1996;28:253–257.

44. Morales AR, Romanelli R, Boucek RJ. The mural left anterior descending coronary artery, strenuous exercise and sudden death. *Circulation* 1980; 62:230–237.

45. Waller BF, Catellier MJ, Clark MA, et al. Cardiac pathology in 2007 consecutive forensic autopsies. *Clin Cardiol* 1992;15:760–765.

46. Corrado D, Thiene G, Cocco P, Frescura C. Non-atherosclerotic coronary artery disease and sudden death in the young. *Br Heart J* 1992;68: 601–607.

47. Feld H, Guandanino V, Hollander G, et al. Exercised-induced ventricular tachycardia in association with a myocardial bridge. *Chest* 1991; 99: 1295–1296.

48. Botvinick EH, Dae MW, Krishnan R, Ewing S. Hypertrophic cardiomyopathy in the young: Another form of ischemic cardiomyopathy? *J Am Coll Cardiol* 1993;22:805–807.

49. Dilsizian V, Bonow RO, Epstein SE, Fananapazir L. Myocardial ischemia detected by thallium scitntigraphy is frequently related to cardiac arrest and syncope in young patients with hypertrophic cardiomyopathy. *J Am Coll Cardiol* 1993;22:796–804.

50. von Dohlen TW, Prisant LM, Frank MJ. Significance of positive or negative thallium-201 scintigraphy in hypertrophic cardiomyopathy. *Am J Cardiol* 1989;64:498–503.

51. Udelson JE, Bonow RO, O'Gara PT, et al. Verapamil prevents silent myocardial perfusion abnormalities during exercise in asymptomatic patients with hypertrophic cardiomyopathy: Assessment with thallium-201 emission computed tomography. *Circulation* 1989;79:1052–1060.

52. Stoddard MF, Prince CR, Dillon S, et al. Exercise-induced mitral regurgitation is a predictor of mormid events in subjects with mitral valve prolapse. *J Am Coll Cardiol* 1995;25:693–699.

53. Levine RA. Exercise induced regurgitation in mitral valve prolapse: Is it a new disease. *J Am Coll Cardiol* 1995;25:700–702.

54. Wilson NV, Meyer BM. Early prediction of hypertension using exercise blood pressure. *Prev Med* 1981;10:62–68.

55. Dlin RA, Hanne N, Silverberg DS, Bar-Or O. Follow-up of normotensive men with exaggerated blood pressure response to exercise. *Am Heart J* 1983;106:316–320.

56. Sung RJ, Lauer MR. Exercise-induced cardiac arrhythmias. In Zipes DP, Jalife J (eds): *Cardiac Electrophysiology From Cell to Bedside.* Philadelphia: W.B. Saunders Company; 1995:1013–1023.

57. Josephson ME, Schibgilla VH. Athletes and arrhythmias: Clinical considerations and perspectives. *Eur Heart J* 1996;17:498–509.

58. Wolff LJ, Brodsky MA. Arrhythmias in athletes. In Podrid PJ, Kowey PR (eds): *Cardiac Arrhythmia Mechanism, Diagnosis and Management.* Baltimore: Williams and Wilkins; 1995:1175–1187.

59. Committe on Sports Medicine and Fitness. Cardiac dysrhythmias and sports. *Pediatrics* 1995;95:786–788.

60. Driscoll DJ, Edwards WD. Sudden unexpected death in children and adolescents. *J Am Coll Cardiol* 1985;5:118B–121B.

61. Kramer MR, Drori Y, Lev B. Sudden death in young soldiers, high incidence of syncope prior to death. *Chest* 1988;93:345–347.

62. Boudoulas H, Weisler AM, Lewis PR, Warren JV. The clinical diagnosis of syncope. *Curr Probl Cardiol* 1982;7:1–40.

63. Benditt DG, Lurie KG, Adler SW, Sakaguchi S. Rationale and methodology of head-up tilt table testing for evaluation of neurally mediated (car-

dioneurogenic) syncope. In Zipes DP, Jalife J (eds): *Cardiac Electrophysiology From Cell to Bedside.* Philadelphia: W.B. Saunders Company; 1995: 1115–1129.

64. Driscoll DJ, Jacobsen SJ, Porter CJ, Wollan PC. Syncope in children and adolescents. *J Am Coll Cardiol* 1997;29:1039–1045.
65. Kapoor W. Evaluation and outcome of patients with syncope. *Medicine* 1990;69:160–175.
66. Benditt DG, Ferguson DW, Grubb BP, et al. Tilt table testing for assessing syncope. *J Am Coll Cardiol* 1996;28:263–275.
67. Schlesinger A. Life-threatening "vagal reaction" to physical fitness test. *JAMA* 1973;226:1119.
68. Ebert TJ, Denahan T. Hemodynamic response of high fit runners during head upright tilt testing to syncope. *Proceedings from the American Autonomic Society Annual Scientific Session.* Nashville, TN; 1993. Abstract.
69. Frederick S, Kosinski D, Grubb BP, et al. Comparison of aerobic capacity, parasympathetic modulation, and orthostatic tolerance in athletes. *Clin Auton Res* 1995;5:334. Abstract.
70. Pedersen WR, Janosik DL, Goldenberg IF, et al. Post-exercise asystolic arrest in a young man without organic heart disease: Utility of head-up tilt testing in guiding therapy. *Am Heart J* 1989;118:410–413.
71. Tse H-F, Lau C-P. Exercise-associated cardiac asystole in persons without structural heart disease. *Chest* 1995;107:572–576.
72. Sneddon JF, Scalia G, Ward DE, et al. Exercise induced vasodepressor syncope. *Br Heart J* 1993;71:554–557.
73. Hirata T, Yano K, Okui T, et al. Asystole with syncope following strenuous exercise in a man without organic heart disease. *J Electrocardiol* 1987;20: 280–283.
74. Kapoor WN. Syncope with abrupt termination of exercise. *Am J Med* 1989;87:597–599.
75. Grubb BP, Temesy-Armos PN, Samoil D, et al. Tilt table testing in the evaluation and management of athletes with recurrent exercise-induced syncope. *Med Sci Sports Exerc* 1992;25:24–28.
76. Sakaguchi S, Shultz JL, Remole SC, et al. Syncope associated with exercise, a manifestation of neurally mediated syncope. *Am J Cardiol* 1995;75: 476–481.
77. Calkins H, Seifert M, Morady F. Clinical presentation and long term follow-up of athletes with exercise-induced vasodepressor syncope. *Am Heart J* 1995;129:1159–1164.
78. Huycke EC, Card HG, Sobol SM, et al. Postexertional cardiac asystole in a young man without organic heart disease. *Ann Intern Med* 1987; 106:844–845.
79. Tamura Y, Onodera O, Kodera K, et al. Atrial standstill after treadmill exercise test and unique response to isoproterenol infusion in recurrent postexercise syncope. *Am J Cardiol* 1990;65:533–535.
80. Lauer MS, Okin PM, Larson MG, et al. Impaired heart rate response to graded exercise prognostic implications of chronotropic incompetence in the Framingham Study. *Circulation* 1996;93:1520–1526.
81. Ellestad MH. Chronotropic incompetence. The implications of heart rate response to exercise. (Compensatory parasympathetic hyperactivity?) *Circulation* 1996;93:1485–1487.
82. Robertson CE, Miller HC. Extreme tachycardia complicating the use of disopyramide in atrial flutter. *Br Heart J* 1980;44:602.

83. Waldo AL. Atrial flutter: Mechanisms, clinical features, and management. In Zipes DP, Jalife J (eds): *Cardiac Electrophysiology From Cell to Bedside*. Philadelphia: W.B. Saunders Company; 1995:666–681.

84. Yeh S-J, Lin F-C, Wu D. The mechanism of exercise provocation of supraventricular tachycardia. *Am Heart J* 1989;117:1041–1049.

85. Klein GJ, Bashore TM, Sellers TD, et al. Ventricular fibrillation in the Wolf-Parkinson-White syndrome. *N Engl J Med* 1979;301:1080–1085.

86. Bricker JT, Porter CJ, Garson A, et al. Exercise testing in children with Wolf-Parkinson-White syndrome. *Am J Cardiol* 1985;55:1001–1004.

87. Sharma AD, Yee R, Guiraudon G, Klein GJ. Sensitivity and specificity of invasive and noninvasive testing for risk of sudden death in Wolf-Parkinson-White syndrome. *J Am Coll Cardiol* 1987;10:373–381.

88. Gaita F, Giustetto F, Riccardi R, et al. Stress and pharmacologic tests as methods to identify patients with Wolf-Parkinson-White syndrome at risk of sudden death. *Am J Cardiol* 1989;64:487–490.

89. Auricchio A, Auricchio U, Chiariello L. Partial reversal by exercise of protective effect in atrial fibrillation inducibility in patients with an accessory atrioventricular connection: Comparison between flecainide and propafenone. *Giornale Italiano Di Cardiologia* 1994;24:131–136.

90. Auricchio A. Reversible protective effect of propafenone or flecainide during atrial fibrillation in patients with an accessory atrioventricular connection. *Am Heart J* 1992;124:932–937.

91. Chimenti M, Li Bergolis M, Moizi M, et al. Comparison of isoproterenol and exercise tests in asymptomatic subjects with Wolf-Parkinson-White syndrome. *PACE* 1992;15:1158–1166.

92. Daubert C, Ollitrault J, Descaves C, et al. Failure of the exercise test to predict the antegrade refractory period of the accessory pathway in Wolf-Parkinson-White syndrome. *PACE* 1988;11:1130–1138.

93. Jelinek MV, Lown B. Exercise stress testing for exposure of cardiac arrhythmia. *Prog Cardiovasc Dis* 1974;16:497–522.

94. Fontaine G, Guiraudon G, Frank R, et al. Stimulation studies and epicardial mapping in ventricular tachycardia: Study of mechanisms and selection for surgery. In Kulbertus HE (ed): *Reentrant Arrhythmias*. Lancaster: MTP Press; 1977:334–350.

95. Fontaine G, Fontaliran G, Lascault G, et al. Arrhythmogenic right ventricular dysplasia. In Zipes DP, Jalife J (eds): *Cardiac Electrophysiology From Cell to Bedside*. Philadelphia: W.B. Saunders Company; 1995:754–769.

96. Klein HS, Shih H, Hackett FK, et al. Radiofrequency catheter ablation of ventricular tachycardia in patients without structural heart disease. *Circulation* 1992;85:1666–1675.

97. Belhasson B, Rotmensch HH, Laniado S. Response to recurrent sustained ventricular tachycardia to verapamil. *Br Heart J* 1981;46: 679–682.

98. Nagagawa H, Beckman KJ, McClelland JH, et al. Radiofrequency catheter ablation of idiopathic left ventricular tachycardia guided by a Purkinje potential. *Circulation* 1993;88:2978–2979.

99. Wever EFD, Hauer RNW, Oomen A, et al. Unfavorable outcome in patients with primary electrical disease who survived an episode of ventricular fibrillation. *Circulation* 1993;88:1021–1029.

100. Eisenberg SJ, Scheinmen MM, Dullet NK, et al. Sudden cardiac death and polymorphous ventricular tachycardia in patients with normal QT intervals and normal systolic function. *Am J Cardiol* 1995;75:687–692.

101. Bjornstad H, Storstein L, Meen HD, Hals O. Electrocardiographic findings of heart rate and conduction times in athletic students and sedentary subjects. *Cardiology* 1993;83:258–267.
102. Peller OG, Moses JW, Klingfield P. Exercise-induced atrioventricular block: Report of three cases. *Am Heart J* 1988;115:1315–1317.
103. Ozder AB, Kucukoglu S, Dogar H, et al. Exercised-induced AV block. *Am Heart J* 1989;117:1407–1408.
104. Reig J, Domingo E, Reguant J, Corrons J. Orthostatic and exercise-induced advanced nodal atrioventricular block. *Chest* 1992;102:970–972.
105. Hertzeanu H, Shiner ARJ, Kellermann J. Exercise dependent complete left bundle branch block. *Eur Heart J* 1992;13:1447–1451.
106. Moran JF, Scurlock B, Henkin R, Scanlon PJ. Exercise-induced bundle branch block. *J Electrocardiol* 1992;25:229–235.
107. Shimizu W, Ohe T, Kurita T, Shimomura K. Differential response of QTU interval to exercise, isoproterenol, and atrial pacing in patients with congenital long QT syndrome. *PACE* 1991;14:1966–1970.
108. Weintraub RG, Gow RM, Wilkinson JL. The congenital long QT syndromes in childhood. *J Am Coll Cardiol* 1990;16:674–680.
109. Vincent GM, Jaiswal D, Timothy KW. Effects of exercise in heart rate, QT, QTc, QT/QS2 in the Romano-Ward inherited long QT syndrome. *Am J Cardiol* 1991;68:498–503.
110. Tobe TJ, de Langen CD, Bink-Boelkens MT, et al. Late potentials in a bradycardia-dependent long QT syndrome associated with sudden death during sleep. *J Am Coll Cardiol* 1992;19:541–549.
111. Kveselis DA, Rocchini AP, Rosenthal A, et al. Hemodynamic determinants of exercise-induced ST-segment depression in children with valvular aortic stenosis. *Am J Cardiol* 1985;55:1133.
112. Friedman WF, Pappelbaum SJ. *Indications for hemodynamic evaluation and surgery in congenital aortic stenosis. Pediatr Clin North Am* 1971; 18:1207.
113. Bonow RO, Borer JS, Rosing DR, et al. Left ventricular functional reserve in adult patients with atrial septal defect: Pre and post operative studies. *Circulation* 1981;63:1315.
114. Chu E, Cheitlin MD. Diagnostic considerations in patients with suspected coronary artery anomalies. *Am Heart J* 1993;126:1427–1438.
115. Glynn TP, Fleming RG, Haist JL, Huntman RK. Coronary arteriovenous fistula as a cause for reversible thallium-201 perfusion defect. *J Nucl Med* 1994;35:1808–1810.
116. Kawakami K, Shimada T, Yamada S, et al. The detection of myocardial ischemia by thallium-201 myocardial scintigraphy in patients with multiple coronary arterioventricular connections. *Clin Cardiol* 1991;14: 975–980.
117. Gupta NC, Beauvais J. Physiologic assessment of coronary artery fistula. *Clin Nucl Cardiol* 1991;16:40–42.
118. Rasmussen V, Haunso S, Skagen K. Cerebral attacks due to excessive vagal tone in heavily trained persons. *Acta Med Scand* 1978;204: 401–405.
119. Fleg JL, Assante AVK. Asystole following treadmill exercise in a man without organic heart disease. *Arch Intern Med* 1983;143:1821–1822.
120. Yerg JE, Seals DR, Hagberg JM, Ehsani EE. Syncope secondary to ventricular asystole in an endurance athlete. *Clin Cardiol* 1985;9:220–222.
121. Kosinski D, Grubb BP, Kip K, Hahn H. Exercise-induced neurocardiogenic syncope. *Am Heart J* 1996;132:451–452.

Part II

Strategies for Identification and Response

8

Noninvasive Imaging Techniques to Assess Cardiac Disease in the Athlete

J. Gregory Corrodi, MD and
James E. Udelson, MD

Sudden death in a young athlete is a tragic event that has significant effects on our society. It is therefore logical that every effort should be made to identify those individual athletes who are at increased risk of sudden death, for the purpose of addressing potentially reversible structural or electrical abnormalities or possibly precluding participation in athletic activity.

While this may seem a straightforward objective, the logistics of universal screening of all competitive athletes is complex, given the number of athletes, the very low prevalence of cardiovascular disease, the frequent absence of prodromal symptoms, the imprecision of available diagnostic testing, as well as the economic impact of such testing.

It has been estimated that there are more than 5 million young people involved in competitive athletics at the high school, college, and professional levels in the United States.[1] It has also been estimated that cardiovascular abnormalities probably account for a combined prevalence of approximately 0.2% in the athletic population.[2] These abnormalities can be broadly categorized into myocardial abnormalities (of which hypertrophic cardiomyopathy [HCM] is the most common),

From Estes NAM, Salem DN, Wang PJ (eds). *Sudden Cardiac Death in the Athlete.*
Armonk, NY: Futura Publishing Co., Inc.; ©1998.

coronary artery abnormalities (including congenital anomalies as well as coronary artery disease [CAD]), congenital heart disease, and arrhythmia/ conduction system abnormalities.[2,3] The majority of these abnormalities are difficult to diagnose by routine history and physical examination; therefore, various diagnostic imaging tests have been studied to improve disease detection in asymptomatic athletes. While echocardiography is the most widely used imaging technique recommended for those with suspected structural heart disease, several other imaging modalities such as myocardial perfusion imaging, electron beam (ultrafast) computed tomography scanning, and magnetic resonance (MR) imaging may be useful in selected cases.

Before discussing the utility of these imaging modalities in selected structural abnormalities associated with sudden cardiac death in the athletic population, it is useful to review the implications of diagnostic testing in the screening of such a population with a very low prevalence of disease.

Bayes' Theorem and the Prevalence of Disease

Performance characteristics of a test to detect disease are often expressed in terms of the sensitivity and specificity of the test to detect or rule out disease, particularly in the initial reports of a new testing modality. Sensitivity is defined as the proportion of subjects with disease in whom the test is positive, and specificity as the proportion of subjects without disease in whom the test is negative. These performance characteristics, however, fail to take into account numerous influences on the test itself. These influences include the prevalence of the disease in the population being studied, the "conservativeness" or "aggressiveness" with which the test results or images are interpreted as normal or abnormal, and finally, the selection of patients from among those undergoing the noninvasive imaging test to have the "gold standard" test, particularly when it involves an invasive procedure such as coronary arteriography.

When at test that has a certain sensitivity and specificity to detect or rule out disease is applied to a population, the predictive value of a positive or negative result for correctly identifying the disease in question is related to the prevalence of the disease in the population being studied. This statistical principle was first described by Bayes in 1763.[4] This concept can be illustrated by a diagram relating the probability of coronary disease following testing (the post-test likelihood of disease) to the pretest probability of CAD in an individual (based on age, gender, and symptoms), this latter attribute being analogous to the prevalence of disease in a population (Figure 1).[5–7] The sensitivity and specificity of the test in question will influence the positive and negative

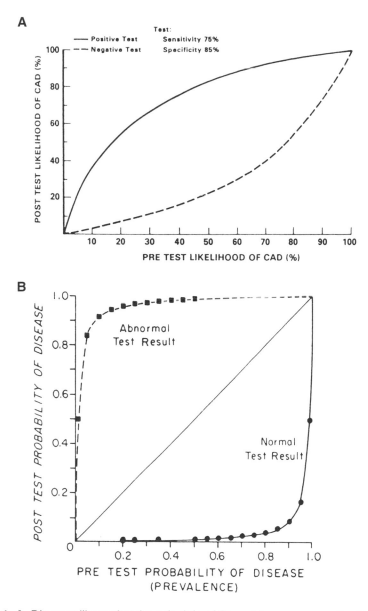

Figure 1. A. Diagram illustrating the principle of Bayes' theorem regarding the influence of disease prevalence on the predictive values of tests. For this test in question, a sensitivity of 75% with a specificity of 85% results in the positive and negative predictive curves (post-test likelihood of CAD, y-axis) for any given pretest likelihood (x-axis). Reprinted from Reference 5, with permission. **B.** If the sensitivity and specificity of the tests are increased to 99% and 99%, respectively, the predictive value curves change accordingly such that the predictive value of a positive test is higher across all disease prevalences, as is the predictive value of a negative test. Reprinted from Reference 6, with permission.

predictive value curves, such that for any pretest likelihood of coronary disease (or the assumed prevalence of disease in a population), the post-test probability of disease, given a positive or negative test, can then be estimated. As is clear from the diagram in Figure 1, Panel A, the predictive value of a positive test is relatively low in the lower prevalence range, and similarly, the predictive value of a negative test for ruling out disease is low at a high prevalence of disease, at sensitivity and specificity values commonly associated with noninvasive imaging tests. Figure 2 illustrates this type of analysis for a test with both a low sensitivity and high specificity (Panel A) as well as a test with a high sensitivity but low specificity (Panel B).[6,7]

This concept, and the implications for screening a population for a low prevalence disease state, can be best illustrated by a hypothetical example in which the same test is used to evaluate two different populations for the presence of coronary artery disease. The test in question has a sensitivity of 90% and a specificity of 90%, which generally

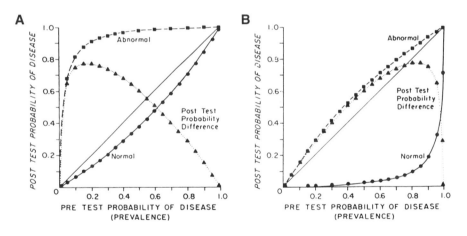

Figure 2. Predictive value curves for tests with varying sensitivity and specificity. **A.** Predictive value curves for a test with a low sensitivity (40%) and a high specificity (99%), as well as the post-test probability difference representing the difference between the positive (abnormal) and negative (normal) predictive curves at each level of pretest probability. In this setting, an *abnormal* test carries a very high predictive value for coronary artery disease (CAD) at most levels of pretest probability of CAD, while a normal test is less useful for ruling out disease. The peak point on the post-test probability curve (here at approximately 20% pretest probability) represents the disease prevalence at which the test being evaluated provides the greatest degree of discrimination between the presence and absence of disease. Reprinted from Reference 6, with permission. **B.** Predictive value curves for an abnormal or a normal test are given for a test with a high sensitivity (99%) and a low specificity (40%). Here, a *negative* or *normal* test is quite useful for ruling out disease across the whole range of disease prevalence, while a positive test has a relatively low predictive value for disease. Reprinted from Reference 6, with permission.

would be considered a very precise test to detect or rule out disease. The first group consists of 1000 50-year-old men with a history of atypical chest pain who would be estimated to have a prevalence of CAD of approximately 50%.[8] As illustrated in Table 1, this test would have a positive predictive value of 90% and a negative predictive value of 90% in this population. If we now study a second group of 1000 asymptomatic young men with a prevalence of CAD of only 1% using the same test, very different results for positive and negative predictive values are calculated (see Table 2). In this population with a very low prevalence of disease, the same test has a positive predictive value of only 8% and a negative predictive value of 99.9%. In this population a negative test would be very helpful in excluding disease, however 92% of positive tests would be false-positives. This concept has important implications in that those with positive tests would likely be subject to further potentially invasive and more risky testing. Moreover, the economic implications of this type of testing in a large population, and the subsequent testing to further evaluate the presence of disease, might be enormous.

The use of Bayesian analysis suggests that the results of noninvasive testing for the determination of the presence or absence of cardiac disease result in a spectrum or continuum of probabilities rather than a correct or incorrect decision that coronary disease is present or absent. The sensitivity and specificity of a test are incomplete descriptors of its

Table 1
Influence of Moderate Disease Prevalence on Predictive Values in a Test with 90% Sensitivity and 90% Specificity

1000 Patients; Prevalence of CAD 50%

	CAD (500)	No CAD (500)
Positive Test	450 (True Positive)	50 (False Positive)
Negative Test	50 (False Negative)	450 (True Negative)

PPV = TP/TP+FP = 450/450+50 = 90%
NPV = TN/TN+FN = 450/450+50 = 90%

CAD = coronary artery disease; PPV = positive predictive value; TP = true positive; FP = false positive; NPV = negative predictive value; TN = true negative; FN = false negative.

Table 2
Influence of Very Low Disease Prevalence on Predictive Values
in a Test with 90% Sensitivity and 90% Specificity

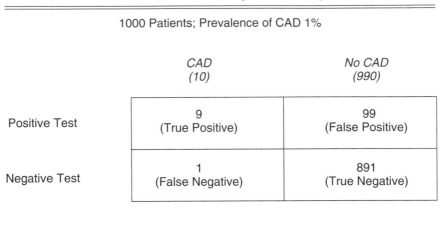

1000 Patients; Prevalence of CAD 1%

	CAD (10)	No CAD (990)
Positive Test	9 (True Positive)	99 (False Positive)
Negative Test	1 (False Negative)	891 (True Negative)

PPV = TP/TP+FP = 9/9+99 = 8%
NPV = TN/TN+FN = 891/891+1 = 99.9%

CAD = coronary artery disease; PPV = positive predictive value; TP = true positive; FP = false positive; NPV = negative predictive value; TN = true negative; FN = false negative.

potential performance when applied to different populations; the prevalence of disease in the population of interest must be taken into account.

The Asymptomatic Patient and Screening for Coronary Artery Disease

The discussion regarding the performance characteristics and predictive values of a test in a low prevalence population would suggest, as previously illustrated, that screening an asymptomatic population for the presence of CAD in order to consider early intervention or preclude athletic activity would result in many false-positive examinations. In a population with low prevalence of disease, it is likely that of all the positive test results, a much higher percentage would be false-positive than true-positive. For the general population, then, screening with noninvasive tests is likely to be a cost-ineffective procedure.

There are important subpopulations of subjects, however, in whom the detection of potential underlying asymptomatic coronary disease is compelling, including airline pilots, military personnel, as well as potentially, the competitive athlete. As would be expected, the predictive values for exercise testing with electrocardiography alone, or in conjunction with myocardial perfusion imaging, are relatively low in an asymptomatic low prevalence population.

Myocardial Perfusion Imaging

Several published reports have examined the use of noninvasive testing strategies to detect CAD in low prevalence populations. Uhl and colleagues[10] have shown that exercise thallium imaging by use of quantitative analysis performed well as a secondline screening procedure once initial screening was performed with exercise electrocardiogram (ECG). In a series of 191 asymptomatic airforce crewmen (mean age 41) who had abnormal exercise ECGs done as part of routine evaluation, exercise thallium imaging and coronary angiography were subsequently performed. Fourteen of 150 patients with minimal or no coronary artery disease were found to have perfusion abnormalities on exercise thallium imaging (specificity 90%), while 39 of the 41 patients with significant CAD (defined as >50% stenosis by angiography) were found to have perfusion abnormalities (sensitivity 95%) (see Table 3). This calculated to a predictive value of a positive myocardial perfusion scan of 74%, compared to 21% for the exercise ECG. These results again reflect the workings of Bayes' theorem, as the pretest probability of coronary disease in the population undergoing thallium imaging was higher than the whole population undergoing exercise ECG. Once the asymptomatic air crewmen had a positive ECG, their prior probability of coronary disease rose accordingly, and thallium imaging was applied in a more selected, higher prevalence population.[11] Thus, screening a selected asymptomatic population for disease with scintigraphic techniques is likely to result in a relatively low predictive value, but a more favorable predictive value when compared to exercise ECG. In populations in whom there is a compelling reason to screen for CAD, it appears that exercise radionuclide techniques may be best applied in a sequential fashion following risk factor analysis and exercise electrocardiography.[11]

Table 3
Thallium Scintigraphy in Asymptomatic Airforce Crewmen

Thallium Scintigrams	Normal Coronary Arteries	Minimal Coronary Artery Disease	Significant Coronary Artery Disease*
Abnormal	4	10	39
Normal	131	5	2

*Defined as >50% stenosis by angiography.
Modified from Reference 10. Reprinted with permission.

This illustrates an important concept in testing a low prevalence population, that is, the use of sequential application of Bayes' theorem in multiple testing procedures. In the study of asymptomatic airforce crewmen, only subjects with positive exercise ECGs subsequently underwent thallium scintigraphy. While the disease prevalence in the original population was very low, the disease prevalence of the selected subjects undergoing thallium imaging was intermediate, as all had positive exercise ECGs. This enhanced the usefulness of the imaging procedure, as illustrated by the markedly higher positive predictive value compared to exercise ECG alone.

This concept can be used to incorporate all of the elements of testing, such as the results of the exercise electrocardiogram and the radionuclide scintigraphic results. In this way, a pretest probability is determined from the clinical data, and a post-test probability is formulated from the results of the exercise electrocardiographic data (often referred to as the post-ETT probability). To interpret the probability of disease based on the scintigraphic data the determined probability from the clinical evaluation and the exercise ECG results then become the pretest probability of disease (ie, post-ETT probability = prescan probability) when interpreting the scintigraphic results.[5,9]

A similar principle was illustrated by Schwartz et al[12] who studied 845 asymptomatic military airmen undergoing coronary angiography as a consequence of abnormal noninvasive tests including exercise ECG, exercise radionuclide imaging, calcification on coronary artery fluoroscopy, ventricular ectopy on exercise ECG or ambulatory ECG monitoring, or new left bundle branch block on resting ECG. Patients were risk stratified according to age and cholesterol levels. The prevalence of CAD in the overall group was 16.9% based on angiographic results. Across all risk groups, the negative predictive value of thallium stress testing remained high (81% to 97%) while the positive predictive value was low (8% to 43%) (see Table 4). Classifying the airmen by age and cholesterol status allowed selection of the group with optimal predictive values. This study again demonstrates the potential caveats, strengths, and limitations of screening a population with a low prevalence of disease.

The low overall specificity (46%) and positive predictive value (25%) of thallium imaging in the study by Schwartz et al[12] is in contrast to the data using a similar test in a similar population from the earlier study of Uhl and colleagues (specificity 90%, positive predictive value 74%).[9] This discrepancy illustrates another important issue in assessing test performance, which has been described as "post-test referral bias."[10] In the Schwartz study, *only* subjects with abnormal noninvasive tests were sent on for coronary angiography, used as the gold standard for disease. The very large majority of this low prevalence

Table 4

Performance of Thallium Scintigraphy for Detecting CAD in Asymptomatic Men

Age (years)	Cholesterol Ratio	Sensitivity	Specificity	Positive Predictive Value	Negative Predictive Value
<45	<4.5	75% (9/12)	47% (89/189)	8% (9/109)	97% (89/92)
	4.5–6.0	83% (19/23)	46% (65/114)	20% (19/95)	94% (65/69)
	>6.0	82% (23/28)	46% (28/61)	41% (23/56)	85% (28/33)
>45	<4.5	75% (6/8)	48% (26/54)	18% (6/34)	93% (26/28)
	4.5–6.0	88% (23/26)	47% (27/57)	43% (23/53)	90% (27/30)
	>6.0	84% (16/19)	36% (13/36)	41% (16/39)	81% (13/16)

CAD = coronary artery disease. Modified from Reference 12. Reprinted with permission.

population had normal tests (the vast majority of whom did *not* have disease) and were *not* subjected to the gold standard test, coronary angiography. As there was no angiographic information to confirm the absence of disease, this large number of "true-negative" subjects was not included in the specificity calculation (true-negative/true-negative + false-positive). Adding the large number of true-negatives to both the numerator and denominator of the equation would significantly improve the specificity calculation. This problem arises when the test whose performance is being assessed (thallium imaging) against a gold standard is *itself* used to select patients to undergo the gold standard test. In the study by Uhl et al,[10] *all* subjects with abnormal exercise ECGs underwent *both* thallium imaging and coronary angiography, removing the post-test referral bias from the assessment of the performance of thallium imaging, and resulting in higher specificity and positive predictive value, as a more appropriate true-negative rate was used.

Electron Beam Computed Tomography

A number of studies have shown a correlation between coronary artery calcification and the presence and extent of atherosclerotic coronary artery disease.[13–17] This has led some to suggest that imaging techniques that detect coronary artery calcium may be potential screening tools for detecting coronary artery disease. Fluoroscopy is an easily performed and inexpensive noninvasive test that has shown only moderate sensitivity and specificity for the presence of coronary artery disease via the detection of coronary calcium.[18]

Ultrafast or electron beam computed tomography (EBCT) is a more recently developed technique which uses an electron gun and a stationary tungsten "target" rather than a standard x-ray tube to generate x-rays.[19] This design permits very rapid scanning times such that the entire test can be completed within 10 to 15 minutes.[19] EBCT has been advocated because of its higher contrast and spatial resolution, which may account for its reported greater sensitivity for detecting coronary calcification compared to fluoroscopy (90% versus 52% in one study).[20] The rapid, thin-slice image acquisition which can be done during a breath hold, the three-dimensional image registration, and the lack of need for intravenous contrast make it conceptually attractive for detecting and quantifying coronary artery calcium (see Figure 3).[21]

A number of investigators have examined the potential clinical utility of using EBCT as a noninvasive screening tool for the detection of coronary artery disease (see Table 5).[19] Tanenbaum et al[22] retrospectively studied 54 patients referred for both coronary angiography as well as EBCT of the heart for clinical indications. The finding of coronary artery calcification had a sensitivity of 88% and a specificity of

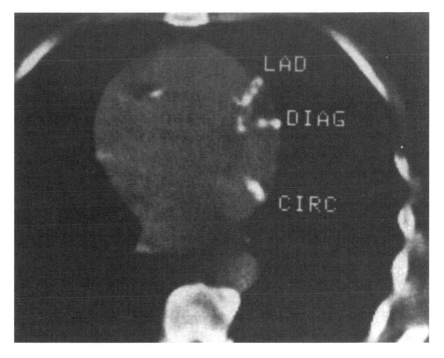

Figure 3. Electron beam computed tomography of the heart demonstrating coronary artery calcium in the left anterior descending (LAD), diagonal (DIAG), and left circumflex (CIRC) coronary arteries. The top of the image is anterior and the bottom is posterior. Reprinted from Reference 22, with permission.

100% for the detection of significant coronary artery disease, defined as luminal narrowing greater than 70%. However, this study population had a very high prevalence of coronary artery disease of 80%.

Several other investigators have studied EBCT in populations with a more moderate prevalence of coronary artery disease.[23–28] Breen et al[23] performed EBCT on 100 patients under 60 years of age who were referred for angiography, and found a sensitivity of 100% for the presence of any coronary calcium in predicting those with significant CAD (>50% stenosis), although they found a specificity of only 47%.[23] With use of EBCT, Budoff and coworkers[28] examined 710 patients also referred for clinically indicated coronary angiography, and reported similar findings with a sensitivity of 95% for the prediction of significant CAD (>50% stenosis) with a specificity of 44%. Specificity increased as the calcium score increased (as described by other investigators)[20,29] as well as when the number of calcified vessels increased.[28] Kaufmann et al[25] analyzed five quantitative measures of coronary artery calcium to determine which best correlated with the presence or absence as well as the severity of angiographically defined

Table 5
Predicting CAD with Electron Beam Computed Tomography

Author	Ref #	CAD Criteria*	N	Prevalence of CAD	Age (mean)	Sensitivity	Specificity	PPV	NPV
Tanenbaum	22	>70%	54 (36M, 18W)	80%	54	88%	100%	100%	69%
Breen	23	>50%	100 (91M, 9F)	47%	47	100%	47%	62%	100%
Fallavollita	24	>50%	106 (78M, 28F)	56%	44	85%	45%	66%	70%
Kaufmann	25	>50%	160 (133M, 27F)	40%	49	86%	81%	75%	90%
Rumberger	26	>50%	139 (89M, 50F)	47%	52	99%	62%	57%	97%
Devries	27	>70%	140 (70M, 70F)	43%	56	97%	41%	55%	94%
Budoff	28	>50%	710 (456M, 254F)	60%	56	95%	44%	72%	84%

CAD = coronary artery disease; M = males; F = females; PPV = positive predictive value; NPV = negative predictive value.
*Degree of angiographic stenosis used to define significant CAD. Modified from Reference 19. Reprinted with permission.

CAD. These investigators found that the quantity of coronary artery calcium, regardless of its method of measurement, strongly related to the severity of CAD. With use of the best cutpoint of calcific area for discriminating between patients with and without angiographically significant coronary artery disease, EBCT had a sensitivity of 86% and specificity of 81%.

Several investigators also examined the ability of coronary artery calcium to predict even minimal angiographic coronary artery narrowing as opposed to only more advanced, obstructive disease.[23,25,27,28] In all studies, sensitivities were slightly lower (range 81% to 94%) and specificities higher (range 54% to 86%) when compared to the prediction of obstructive coronary artery disease.

The effect of a subject's sex on the diagnostic accuracy of EBCT-detected coronary artery calcification has also been investigated. Budoff and coworkers[28] found similar sensitivities for the prediction of significant CAD in men and women (94% and 96%, respectively), but slightly higher specificity in women (39% versus 49%). Rumberger et al[26] showed similar results with sensitivities of 98% and 100% and specificities of 57% and 66% in men and women, respectively. Devries and colleagues[27] also found no significant differences in sensitivity and specificity on the basis of gender alone, although there was a suggestion of a lower sensitivity in younger women (under 60 years of age) compared with men of a similar age or older women.[27] This finding, however, was not statistically significant.

It has been suggested that the low specificity in some of these studies, as well as the high sensitivity, may be related to the age of the subjects, as the extent of coronary calcium clearly increases with age in pathologic studies even in the absence of significant obstructive atherosclerotic coronary artery disease.[20,30] Indeed Budoff et al[28] found a sensitivity of only 68% and a specificity of 74% in patients under 40 years of age. In contrast, sensitivity was 99% and specificity only 34% in patients older than 50 years old. In patients under 50 years of age, Fallavollita and colleagues[24] found coronary calcification to have a sensitivity of 85% with a specificity of 45%. The sensitivity to detect single-vessel disease was lower, at 75%.

As observed from a summary of studies that examined EBCT for detection of coronary artery disease (see Table 5), the absence of coronary calcium as detected by EBCT indicates a low likelihood of significant coronary artery obstruction in the populations studied. However, these series looked only at patients referred for coronary angiography for clinical reasons, and most patients were symptomatic. As highlighted by the recently published American Heart Association (AHA) Medical/Scientific Statement on coronary artery calcification[19] and as discussed earlier in this chapter, predictive values are based on prior probability and may be less optimal when applied to a young, asymptomatic population with a much lower prevalence of disease. There are very limited data evaluating the significance of coronary artery calcium as detected by EBCT in an asymptomatic population. A recent study by Arad et al[31] followed 1173 asymptomatic subjects (mean age 53) either self-referred or referred by physicians for EBCT for screening purposes. Cardiovascular events, which included cardiac death, nonfatal myocardial infarctions, revascularization procedures, and stroke occurred in 1.5% of the group over a 19-month follow-up. Total calcium scores were significantly higher in those with events compared to those without events. Using a calcium score cutpoint previously determined by the same investigators to be suggestive of significant coronary artery stenosis,[32] the sensitivity for predicting future cardiovascular events was 50% with a specificity of 95%. The NPV was high at 99% with a PPV of only 14%. However, of the small number of subjects experiencing a cardiac event over follow-up (18), as many had negative EBCT (9) as positive EBCT (9), based on the sensitivity of 50%. Lower calcium score cutpoints improved sensitivity but resulted in lower specificity. The NPV remained high (>99%) at all cutpoints, however the PPV was consistently low (5% to 14%). These data suggest a correlation between coronary calcium and future coronary events, although they also once again illustrate the limitation of screening a low prevalence population, as most positive tests would be false-positive.

The use of EBCT as a screening tool for coronary artery disease has many potential advantages in that it is noninvasive, requires no preparation or discontinuation of medicine, requires minimal patient cooperation, is relatively inexpensive, and gives rapidly available results.[19] However, data regarding use of EBCT in a low-risk, asymptomatic population are very limited. Further studies are needed to better define long-term risk of cardiovascular events in a very low-risk population with evidence of coronary artery calcium, as well as to better define the degree of calcification that portends an increased risk. As previously discussed, one must also consider the implications of a high percentage of false-positive test results when screening a very low-prevalence population. The recently published AHA Medical/Scientific Statement on coronary artery calcification concludes that, at this point, there are insufficient data to warrant the use of coronary artery calcium screening in low-risk asymptomatic subjects.[19]

Congenital Coronary Artery Anomalies

Congenital coronary anomalies have been shown to be associated with an increased risk of sudden death in young previously asymptomatic subjects.[3,33–35] The presence of congenital coronary anomalies in the adult population has been estimated to be 0.6% to 1.2% of patients undergoing angiography.[36,37] Several reviews of cases of coronary anomalies appear to document an increased risk of sudden death associated with anomalous origin of the left main coronary artery from the right coronary cusp,[33–35] and from anomalous origin of the right coronary artery from the left coronary cusp,[35] where the coronary artery courses between the aorta and the pulmonary artery. Sudden death appeared to occur more commonly in younger patients[34,35] and was often associated with physical exertion.[34,35] While the majority of patients were asymptomatic, a significant number did have symptoms prior to their event. In a review of 20 case reports of sudden death due to anomalous coronary arteries in young patients, Liberthson et al[34] reported that 20% of patients had symptoms of exertional chest pain, syncope, or ventricular tachycardia prior to their event. Taylor and colleagues[35] reviewed 242 cases of coronary anomalies from the Armed Forces Institute of Pathology registry and found that 38% of patients who died suddenly had symptoms prior to their death.

A number of potential mechanisms have been proposed to explain sudden death in the setting of anomalous origin of a coronary artery: "squeezing" of the coronary artery between the aorta and pulmonary artery during exercise,[38,39] an anatomically smaller coronary artery resulting in decreased coronary reserve,[39,40] "kinking" of the artery,[40] and "flaplike" closure of an abnormal coronary artery orifice resulting from stretching of the artery during exercise.[33] All of these proposed mechanisms imply that myocardial ischemia plays an integral role in the pathogenesis of sudden death in these patients. They also suggest that exercise myocardial perfusion imaging may be useful in its detection.

Indeed, there have been reports of exercise-induced thallium perfusion defects in patients with anomalous coronary arteries that have resolved following coronary bypass surgery.[34] To date there have been no large registries with consistent data on detecting ischemia by noninvasive imaging techniques, and no studies focusing on long-term prognosis and differences between those patients with and without ischemia. Thus, the sensitivity of myocardial perfusion imaging (or other noninvasive techniques) to detect the presence of congenital coronary anomalies cannot be stated with certainty.

Imaging Techniques in Hypertrophic Cardiomyopathy

HCM is a primary myocardial abnormality characterized by a hypertrophied and nondilated left ventricle that exists in the absence of a coexisting disease capable of producing the same degree of left ventricular hypertrophy (LVH).[41] It occurs in approximately 0.2% of the general population[42] and is strongly associated with the occurrence of sudden death.[43] Several series have shown HCM to be the most common cardiac cause of sudden death in the young athlete.[44,45] The annual mortality in people with HCM has been estimated to be between 1% and 6%,[46] with 40% of deaths occurring during or immediately following vigorous physical activity.[47] These data on annual mortality, however, are based predominantly on reports from large referral centers. It has been suggested that among community-based HCM patients, annual mortality is significantly lower.[48]

While the diagnosis of HCM is readily made by echocardiography, the identification of those patients at higher (or lower) risk of sudden death presents a dilemma. There are few clinical predictors of sudden death, with the majority of HCM patients who die suddenly being symptom free or minimally symptomatic prior to their death.[43,46,47] A history of syncope or a strong family history of sudden death appears to correlate with increased risk, while arrhythmias are likely to be the precipitating factor.[43,46] Maron et al[49] and McKenna and coworkers[50] independently reported an increased risk of sudden death in asymptomatic patients who were found to have nonsustained ventricular tachycardia on ambulatory electrocardiographic monitoring. In the 169 patients studied, the presence of ventricular tachycardia conferred an 8% per year risk of sudden death over a 3-year period compared with less than a 1% per year risk in those without ventricular tachycardia.

The frequent occurrence of chest pain in patients with HCM suggests a possible contribution of myocardial ischemia to the pathogenesis of this disease. There is convincing evidence that regional myocardial ischemia does indeed occur and may be responsible for chest pain. Pasternac and colleagues[51] and Cannon et al[52] both demonstrated induction of chest pain with rapid atrial pacing in patients with HCM accompanied by objective evidence of myocardial ischemia, including ST segment depression on ECG, increased coronary venous lactate concentration, and increased LV end-diastolic pressure. Autopsy studies have also shown evidence of intramyocardial fibrosis and scarring suggestive of prior ischemic injury.[53–55] Several mechanisms have been proposed to explain these findings, including systolic compression of large intramyocardial coronary arteries,[56] the presence of abnormally narrowed small intramural coronary arteries within the thickened myocardium,[57] and inadequate capillary density with respect to the increased muscle mass.[58]

A number of investigators, using thallium as a perfusion tracer, have demonstrated the presence of exercise-induced perfusion defects on planar and single-photon emission–computed tomography (SPECT) imaging, consistent with the possibility of myocardial ischemia.[59–63] Similar results have been reported with other radionuclide perfusion agents such as Tc99m-sestamibi.[64] Perfusion defects have been detected in both patients with a history of angina as well as in those who are asymptomatic. O'Gara et al[62] found reversible thallium defects on SPECT imaging in 58% of symptomatic patients as well as 56% of completely asymptomatic HCM patients. A significant minority of patients had fixed or irreversible thallium defects suggestive of prior infarction, supported by the finding of abnormal resting left ventricular ejection fraction in these patients.[62] These findings suggest that myocardial ischemia may play an important role in the pathogenesis and natural history of HCM even in the asymptomatic individual.

A subsequent investigation by Udelson and coworkers[63] confirmed and extended these data, demonstrating myocardial perfusion abnormalities after exercise thallium imaging in 52% of young asymptomatic or minimally symptomatic HCM patients. These investigators also reported that this "silent" myocardial ischemia was a dynamic process, as improvement in exercise myocardial perfusion abnormalities was seen in 71% of patients who were treated with verapamil, with ischemia completely prevented in the majority (Figure 4).

The presence of myocardial ischemia not only plays a role in the pathogenesis of HCM, but also may have important prognostic significance. von Dohlen et al[65] studied 28 patients with HCM and found 39%

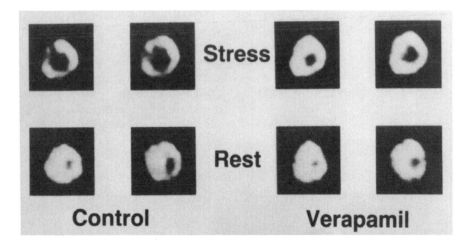

Figure 4. Short-axis tomograms obtained immediately after maximal treadmill exercise (top) and after 3 hours of rest (bottom) in an 18-year-old asymptomatic man with hypertrophic cardiomyopathy. Under control conditions (left), reversible septal and inferoposterior perfusion defects develop during exercise and are improved at rest. There is also apparent cavity dilatation induced by exercise. During oral verapamil (right), myocardial perfusion and apparent cavity dilatation are improved during exercise. Reprinted from Reference 63, with permission.

to have perfusion abnormalities on stress thallium imaging, consistent with the earlier reports.[59-64] Sixty-four percent of the patients with positive scans had nonsustained ventricular tachycardia on 24-hour ambulatory electrocardiographic monitoring, suggesting the possibility of a higher risk course. None of the 17 patients with normal perfusion on thallium imaging were found to have ventricular tachycardia.

Further evidence of the potential prognostic importance of myocardial ischemia emerges from the report by Dilsizian and colleagues[66] who by use of ambulatory electrocardiographic monitoring, exercise thallium scintigraphy, and invasive electrophysiologic studies, studied 15 high-risk HCM patients with a history of syncope or cardiac arrest as well as 8 patients with only a family history of sudden cardiac death. Of those patients with a history of impaired consciousness, only 40% had a history of angina, only 20% had ventricular tachycardia on 24- to 72-hour ambulatory ECG monitoring, and only 27% had inducible sustained ventricular tachycardia on programmed electrical stimulation. In contrast, all 15 patients with a history of impaired consciousness were found to have myocardial ischemia on exercise thallium imaging. Of those patients without a history of syncope or cardiac arrest, only 37% were found to have evidence of myocardial ischemia, while none had ventricular tachycardia on either ambulatory ECG monitoring or electrophysiologic testing and only 1 of 8 had a history of angina (Table 6). These data demonstrate that evidence of exercise-induced myocardial ischemia, as imaged by thallium scintigraphy, is frequently observed in patients with a history of cardiac arrest or syncope. In this study inducible ischemia was more closely associated with a history of cardiac arrest or syncope than was ambulatory ECG monitoring or invasive electrophysiologic testing. Eight of the patients with a history of impaired consciousness were subsequently treated with verapamil or a combination of verapamil and β-blocker. Seven of the eight patients showed improvement in regional

Table 6
Prevalence of Myocardial Ischemia and Inducible Ventricular Tachycardia in Young Patients with Hypertrophic Cardiomyopathy

	Ischemia (TI–201 SPECT)	Inducible VT (EP Study)
History of cardiac arrest or syncope	15/15 (100%)*	4/15 (27%)
Family history of cardiac arrest	3/8 (37%)*	0/8 (0%)

*P<0.01; TI = thallium; SPECT = single-photon emission computed tomography; VT = ventricular tachycardia; EP = electrophysiologic;
Modified from Reference 64. Reprinted with permission.

thallium uptake on subsequent exercise perfusion imaging. Follow-up data over a mean period of 23 months identified recurrent events in 4 of the original 15 patients with a history of impaired consciousness. Three of these events correlated with missed or discontinued doses of verapamil or β-blocker. In contrast, only 1 of the 8 patients without an initial history of impaired consciousness had a subsequent event, and he had evidence of inducible ischemia on exercise thallium imaging.

The above data suggest that the presence of myocardial ischemia in patients with HCM may identify a subgroup of patients who are at high risk of sudden death. These studies also demonstrate that myocardial ischemia in HCM is a dynamic process which can be altered with medical therapy, implying the potential for risk reduction in the subgroup of patients with this condition. Unfortunately, to this point there have been no large long-term studies focusing on prognosis based on perfusion imaging results, and it cannot be said with certainty that the absence of ischemia portends a very low risk of sudden death. It does appear that there may be a low-risk subgroup, as Maron and Klues[67] have described in a series of 14 highly competitive, elite athletes with HCM who have competed and survived without episodes of syncope or cardiac arrest despite years of repeated intense physical activity. While the 26th Bethesda Conference recommendation for patients with the diagnosis of HCM is to refrain from competitive athletics,[1] it is conceptually possible that by defining populations on the basis of current concepts of pathophysiology (including myocardial ischemia) and genetic predisposition, a very-low–risk group may be identified and allowed to participate, while the "not-low–risk" group may be identified in an symptomatic state and intervened upon appropriately.

Imaging Techniques in Right Ventricular Dysplasia

Right ventricular (RV) dysplasia is a rare myopathic disorder of the right ventricle characterized by fibro-fatty replacement of the myocardium.[68–70] The etiology is unknown, though there is often a genetic predisposition.[68–70] Patients with RV dysplasia are at risk for severe ventricular arrhythmias and sudden death[68–70]; this disorder accounted for 3% of sudden deaths in young competitive athletes in one series.[44] The 26th Bethesda Conference recommendation, therefore, is for these patients to refrain from competitive athletics once a diagnosis is established.[1]

The diagnosis of RV dysplasia can be definitively made by histologic specimen demonstrating transmural fibro-fatty replacement of myocardium.[68] The diagnosis obviously cannot be made in this way in clinical practice, thus the use of endomyocardial biopsy has been advocated.[71] However, the patchy nature of the fibro-fatty deposits which infrequently involve the intraventricular septum make the sensitivity as well as specificity of the biopsy technique of questionable reliability.[72]

Various imaging modalities have therefore been examined for detection of structural abnormalities consistent with RV dysplasia. Because of the variability in the clinical expression of RV dysplasia, the Arrhythmogenic Right Ventricular Dysplasia (ARVD) Task Force of the European Society of Cardiology has proposed standardizing the diagnostic criteria to include major and minor factors.[68] Structural abnormalities including severe dilatation and functional impairment of the right ventricle with no (or only mild) left ventricular impairment, localized right ventricular aneurysms (akinetic or dyskinetic areas with diastolic bulging), and severe segmental dilatation of the right ventricle as detected by various imaging modalities are considered as major criteria in the diagnosis.[68]

The most widely used, and what has traditionally been felt to be the most reliable, imaging modality for the diagnosis of RV dysplasia has been contrast angiography during right heart catheterization.[73] Multiple angiographic abnormalities have been proposed to be suggestive of RV dysplasia, including increased end-diastolic volume, reduced RV ejection fraction, diastolic bulges, localized akinetic or dyskinetic areas, and morphological abnormalities of the anterior wall ("*pile d'assiettes*").[73–75] While contrast angiography is often used as the reference standard, there are several noninvasive techniques that have gained increasing acceptance.

Manyari and coworkers[76] compared radionuclide angiography with contrast angiography in 44 patients suspected of having RV dysplasia. These investigators reported exercise RV ejection fraction, abnormal RV wall motion score greater than 1 during exercise, or RV/LV end-diastolic volume ratio greater than 1.8 to have sensitivities and negative predictive values of 100% (see Table 7). It was therefore concluded that noninvasive imaging with radionuclide angiography can be used to exclude the diagnosis of RV dysplasia without resorting to invasive techniques.

Le Guludec and colleagues[77] reported similar results in a prospective comparison between contrast and radionuclide angiography. In a study of 73 patients presenting with ventricular tachycardia of right ventricular origin, there was diagnostic concordance of 93% between the two techniques. Using contrast angiography as the reference standard, radionuclide angiography had a sensitivity of 94%, specificity of 90% positive predictive value, of 96% and negative predictive value of 86% for the diagnosis of RV dysplasia. Other investigators have suggested that the specificity of this technique can be increased by confirmation of the persistence of RV wall motion abnormalities during exercise.[78]

Table 7
Radionuclide Angiographic and Echocardiographic Measurements in the Identification of Patients with Right Ventricular Dysplasia

Criteria for Abnormality*	Sensitivity	Specificity	Positive Pred. Value	Negative Pred. Value
Rest RVEF<42%	93%	90%	81%	96%
Exercise RVEF<50%	100%	90%	81%	100%
Rest RV WMS>1	93%	97%	93%	97%
Exercise RV WMS>1	100%	97%	93%	100%
RV Dysfunction based on ANY of above criteria	100%	87%	78%	100%
RV Dilatation based on any of 6 Echo criteria#	100%	90%	82%	100%

RV = right ventricle; RVEF = right ventricular ejection fraction; WMS = wall motion score; Echo = echocardiographic.
*Criteria for abnormality were calculated a priori from the 95th percentile and the group mean ±1.645 times the standard deviation of a normal population (n = 40).
#Criteria for abnormality include RV end-diastolic diameter (EDD) >25mm, RV end-systolic diameter (ESD) >24mm, RV/LV EDD >0.5, RV/LV ESD >0.7, RV/LV end-diastolic volume >1.5, RV/LV end-systolic volume >18.
Modified from Reference 76. Reprinted with permission.

While both contrast and radionuclide angiography can accurately demonstrate morphological and functional abnormalities in the right ventricle, the newer radiologic techniques of MR imaging and ultrafast or EBCT may provide this information as well as additional information about the structure of the ventricular wall.

Magnetic Resonance Imaging in Right Ventricular Dysplasia

Blake et al[79] initially described the typical appearance of RV dysplasia as seen on MR imaging as high signal intensity distributed diffusely and transmurally in the right ventricular myocardium, representing fatty infiltration. However, given the variable nature of the disease, occasionally areas of high signal intensity were focal, and sometimes there was only extreme thinning of the ventricular wall.[79] Auffermann and colleagues[80] studied MR imaging in 36 patients with RV dysplasia diagnosed by the presence of ventricular tachycardia with LBBB morphology, repolarization abnormalities on ECG, characteristic abnormalities on right ventricular contrast angiography, and characteristic endomyocardial biopsy findings. In this study regional function abnormalities of the RV depicted by MR corresponded to contrast angiographic findings in 86% of patients. The MR findings were poorly specific, however, as focal functional abnormalities were also seen in 9 of 11 control subjects. Additionally, signal intensity changes in the myocardium of the right ventricle on MR imaging were visible in 22% of patients corresponding to fatty replacement as demonstrated by biopsy.

Ricci and colleagues[81] prospectively studied MR imaging in 15 patients with RV dysplasia and 15 patients with dilated cardiomyopathy. Akinetic or dyskinetic RV segments were detected in 11 of 15 patients with RV dysplasia by MR. There was an 88.5% correlation between MR and echocardiography in the assessment of regional and global RV function. An abnormal signal intensity pattern was found on MR in 8 of 15 RV dysplasia patients (see Figure 5). There were no areas of akinesis or dyskinesis and no abnormal signal intensity patterns seen in the 15 patients with dilated cardiomyopathy. One patient with RV dys-

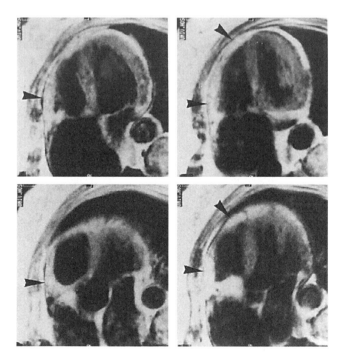

Figure 5. Magnetic resonance imaging in right ventricular dysplasia. Four axial slices in which high signal intensity (seen as white), presumably due to fatty infiltration, extends from the pericardial layer (arrowheads) to the endocardium of the right ventricular free wall. Reprinted from Reference 81, with permission.

plasia subsequently underwent cardiac transplantation. The distribution of fatty infiltration as seen by MR imaging correlated well with the anatomic specimen.

These studies show MR imaging to be a potentially useful technique for morphological and functional assessment of the right ventricle, while additionally giving structural information about the ventricular wall. MR imaging has certain advantages in that it is noninvasive, it can give a three-dimensional depiction of the ventricle, and it can demonstrate the distribution of fatty infiltration in the myocardium.[79–81] However, these results also show that the findings are not highly sensitive, and may have poor specificity. Moreover, there are certain technical limitations to the MR technique, such as poor resolution in certain aspects of the RV and the requirement of sinus rhythm for imaging.[80,81] With these caveats, MR imaging may provide important information to assist in the diagnosis of RV dysplasia in association with other techniques,[68] and may be useful in serial follow-up evaluation.

Electron Beam Computed Tomography Imaging in Right Ventricular Dysplasia

EBCT is a noninvasive imaging modality which may provide information regarding morphological and structural abnormalities of the right ventricle. EBCT provides superior spatial resolution compared with conventional CT and therefore can be used to acquire high-quality images of the beating heart.[82] Characteristic findings gathered from a small group of patients with RV dysplasia have included abundant epicardial adipose tissue, conspicuous low attenuation trabeculations, scalloped appearance of the RV free wall, and intramyocardial fat deposits.[83] Tada et al[84] studied EBCT findings in a group of 14 patients with RV dysplasia (diagnosed by the presence of RV wall motion abnormalities, fatty and fibrous infiltration of the RV myocardium, and recurrent ventricular tachycardia with LBBB morphology) and compared those findings with 16 patients with right ventricular abnormalities without RV dysplasia, as well as with 13 controls. These investigators confirmed the findings of the earlier study,[83] with abundant epicardial adipose tissue in 86%, conspicuous low attenuation trabeculations in 71%, scalloped appearance of the RV free wall in 79%, and intramyocardial fat deposits in 50% of the 14 patients with RV dysplasia (see Figure 6). Eighty-six percent of RV dysplasia patients had either conspicuous trabeculations with low attenuation, scalloped appearance of the RV free wall, or intramyocardial fat deposits. None of these four characteristic findings were observed in the two control groups. Thus, based on this relatively small group of patients, EBCT appears to provide reasonable sensitivity and specificity for the detection of RV dysplasia. In patients with RV dyspla-

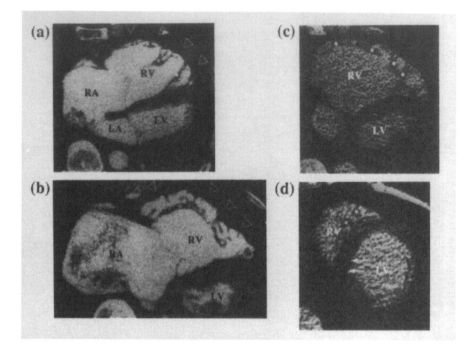

Figure 6. Electron beam computed tomography in right ventricular dysplasia. Panels **A** through **D** represent serial transverse volume-mode scans obtained at end-systole during the administration of contrast medium. Abundant epicardial adipose tissue (Δ in panels **A** and **B**), an enlarged right ventricle with scalloped surface of the free wall (seen best in panels **A** through **C**), conspicuous trabeculations with low attenuation (* in panels **A, C,** and **D**), and myocardial fat deposits (arrow in panel **D**) are all seen. RA = right atrium; LA = left atrium; RV = right ventricle; LV = left ventricle. Reprinted from Reference 84, with permission.

sia the localization of fatty infiltration may have important clinical implications, as Tada et al demonstrated electrophysiologic abnormalities corresponding to the areas of presumed adipose tissue replacement (as depicted by EBCT) in 86% of the patients with RV dysplasia.[84]

Analogous to MR imaging, EBCT has certain potential advantages over contrast and radionuclide angiography in that it gives both functional and morphological information, as well as an assessment of the degree and extent of fatty infiltration of the myocardium. From the as yet limited data in the literature, specificity to rule out RV dysplasia may potentially be higher with EBCT compared to MR imaging. EBCT has certain advantages over MR imaging in that it is less costly and less subject to motion artifact. It has certain disadvantages to more conventional techniques because of its limited availability and limited data to support its use. To date there are no long-term studies of any of these imaging techniques in relation to prognosis in RV dysplasia.

However, the three-dimensional potential for imaging a structure like the RV with its complex spatial anatomy, and the potential ability to image both functional and structural abnormalities, suggest that MR imaging and perhaps particularly EBCT may play an important role in the detection of RV dysplasia, as well as ruling-out that diagnosis in the setting of clinical suspicion.

Conclusions

This chapter illustrates that nonechocardiographic imaging techniques such as myocardial perfusion imaging, EBCT, and magnetic resonance imaging may play a role in the evaluation of young, asymptomatic athletes for cardiac disease. In considering these imaging techniques, it is important to understand the unique characteristics of the specific test, its performance characteristics, and the information that it provides with regards to a particular disease entity. As this application of these technologies is by definition an application in a low prevalence population, the principles of Bayes' theorem must be accounted for when interpreting the test results. These techniques may be most optimally applied when clinical suspicion has raised the possibility that cardiac disease may be present in an athlete.

References

1. Maron BJ, Mitchell JH. 26th Bethesda Conference: Revised eligibility recommendations for competitive athletes. *J Am Coll Cardiol* 1994;24: 848–899.
2. Maron BJ, Thompson PD, Puffer JC, et al. Cardiovascular Preparticipation Screening of Competitive Athletes. *Circulation* 1996;94:850–856.
3. Liberthson RR. Sudden death from cardiac causes in children and young adults. *N Engl J Med* 1996;334:1039–1044.
4. Bayes T. An essay toward solving a problem in the doctrine of chance. *Philos Trans R Soc Lond* 1763;53:370.
5. Epstein SE. Implications of probability analysis on the strategy used for noninvasive detection of coronary artery disease. Role of single or combined use of exercise electrocardiographic testing, radionuclide cineangiography and myocardial perfusion imaging. *Am J Cardiol* 1980;46: 491–499.
6. Hamilton GW, Trobaugh GB, Ritchie JL, et al. Myocardial imaging with thallium-201: An analysis of clinical usefulness based on Bayes' theorem. *Semin Nucl Med* 1978;8:358–364.
7. Udelson JE, Leppo JA. Single photon myocardial perfusion imaging and exercise radionuclide angiography in the detection of coronary artery disease. In Murray IPC, Ell PJ (eds): *Nuclear Medicine in Clinical Diagnosis and Treatment*. London: Churchill Livingstone; 1994:1129–1156.
8. Diamond GA, Forrester JS. Analysis of probability as an aid to the clinical diagnosis of coronary artery disease. *N Engl J Med* 1979;300: 1350–1358.

9. Rozanski A, Berman DS. The efficacy of cardiovascular nuclear medicine exercise studies. *Semin Nucl Med* 1987;17:104–120.
10. Uhl GS, Kay TN, Hickman JR. Computer-enhanced thallium scintigrams in asymptomatic men with abnormal exercise tests. *Am J Cardiol* 1981;48:1037–1043.
11. Uhl GS, Froelicher V. Screening for asymptomatic coronary artery disease. *J Am Coll Cardiol* 1983;1:946–955.
12. Schwartz RS, Jackson WG, Celio PV, et al. Accuracy of exercise thallium-201 myocardial scintigraphy in asymptomatic young men. *Circulation* 1993;87:165–172.
13. Blankenhorn DH, Stern D. Calcification of the coronary arteries. *AJR* 1959;81:772–777.
14. Frink RJ, Achor RWP, Brown AL, et al. Significance of calcium of the coronary arteries. *Am J Cardiol* 1970;26:241–247.
15. McCarthy JH, Palmer FJ. Incidence and significance of coronary artery calcification. *Br Heart J* 1974;36:499–506.
16. Rifkin RD, Parisi AF, Folland E. Coronary calcification in the diagnosis of coronary artery disease. *Am J Cardiol* 1979;44:141–147.
17. Rumberger JA, Simons DB, Fitzpatrick LA, et al. Coronary artery calcium area by electron-beam computed tomography and coronary atherosclerotic plaque area: A histopathologic correlative study. *Circulation* 1995;92:2157–2162.
18. Loecker TH, Schwartz RS, Cotta CW, et al. Fluoroscopic coronary artery calcification and associated coronary disease in asymptomatic young men. *J Am Coll Cardiol* 1992;19:1167–1172.
19. Wexler L, Brundage B, Crouse J, et al. Coronary artery calcification: Pathophysiology, epidemiology, imaging methods, and clinical implications. A statement for health professionals from the American Heart Association. *Circulation* 1996;94:1175–1192.
20. Agatston AS, Janowitz WR, Hildner FJ, et al. Quantification of coronary artery calcium using ultrafast computed tomography. *J Am Coll Cardiol* 1990;15:827–832.
21. Rumberger JA, Sheedy PF, Breen JF, et al. Electron beam computed tomography and coronary artery disease: Scanning for coronary artery calcification. *Mayo Clin Proc* 1996;71:369–377.
22. Tanenbaum SR, Kondos GT, Veselik KE, et al. Detection of calcific deposits in coronary arteries by ultrafast computed tomography and correlation with angiography. *Am J Cardiol* 1989;63:870–871.
23. Breen JF, Sheedy PF, Schwartz RS, et al. Coronary artery calcification detected with ultrafast CT as an indication of coronary artery disease. *Radiology* 1992;185:435–439.
24. Fallavollita JA, Brody AS, Bunnell IL, et al. Fast computed tomography detection of coronary calcification in the diagnosis of coronary artery disease: Comparison with angiography in patients <50 years old. *Circulation* 1994;89:285–290.
25. Kaufmann RB, Peyser PA, Sheedy PF, et al. Quantification of coronary artery calcium by electron beam computed tomography for determination of severity of angiographic coronary artery disease in younger patients. *J Am Coll Cardiol* 1995;25:626–632.
26. Rumberger JA, Sheedy PF, Breen JF, et al. Coronary calcium, as determined by electron beam computed tomography, and coronary disease on arteriogram: Effect of patient's sex on diagnosis. *Circulation* 1995; 91:1363–1367.
27. Devries S, Wolfkiel C, Fusman B, et al. Influence of age and gender on the

presence of coronary calcium detected by ultrafast computed tomography. *J Am Coll Cardiol* 1995;25:76–82.

28. Budoff MJ, Georgiou D, Brody A, et al. Ultrafast computed tomography as a diagnostic modality in the detection of coronary artery disease. *Circulation* 1996;93:898–904.

29. Wong ND, Vo A, Abrahamson D, et al. Detection of coronary artery calcium by ultrafast computed tomography and its relation to clinical evidence of coronary artery disease. *Am J Cardiol* 1994;73:223–227.

30. Janowitz WR, Agatston AS, Kaplan G, et al. Differences in prevalence and extent of coronary artery calcium detected by ultrafast computed tomography in asymptomatic men and women. *Am J Cardiol* 1993; 72:247–254.

31. Arad Y, Spadaro LA, Goodman K, et al. Predictive value of electron beam computed tomography of the coronary arteries: 19-month follow-up of 1173 asymptomatic subjects. *Circulation* 1996;93:1951–1953.

32. Guerci AD, Spadaro LA, Popma JJ, et al. Electron beam tomography of the coronary arteries: Relationship of coronary calcium score to arteriographic findings in asymptomatic adults. *Am J Card Imaging* 1995;9:5. Abstract.

33. Cheitlin MD, DeCastro CM, McAllister HA. Sudden death as a complication of anomalous left coronary origin from the anterior sinus of Valsalva: A not-so-minor congenital anomaly. *Circulation* 1974;50:780–787.

34. Liberthson RR, Dinsmore RE, Fallon JT. Aberrant coronary artery origin from the aorta: Report of 18 patients, review of literature and delineation of natural history and management. *Circulation* 1979;59:748–754.

35. Taylor AJ, Rogan KM, Virmani R. Sudden cardiac death associated with isolated congenital coronary artery anomalies. *J Am Coll Cardiol* 1992; 20:640–647.

36. Kimbiris D, Iskandrian AS, Segal BL, et al. Anomalous aortic origin of coronary arteries. *Circulation* 1978;58:606–615.

37. Cieslinski G, Rapprich B, Kober G. Coronary anomalies: Incidence and importance. *Clin Cardiol* 1993;16:711–715.

38. Cohen LS, Shaw LD. Fatal myocardial infarction in an 11-year-old boy associated with a unique coronary artery anomaly. *Am J Cardiol* 1967;19: 420–423.

39. Benson PA, Lack AR. Anomalous aortic origin in the left coronary artery: Report of two cases. *Arch Pathol* 1968;86:214–216.

40. Jokl E, McClellan JT, Williams WC, et al. Congenital anomaly of the left coronary artery in young athletes. *Cardiology* 1966;49:253–258.

41. Maron BJ, Epstein SE. Hypertrophic cardiomyopathy: A discussion of nomenclature. *Am J Cardiol* 1979;43:1242–1244.

42. Maron BJ, Gardin JM, Flack JM, et al. Prevalence of hypertrophic cardiomyopathy in a general population of young adults. Echocardiographic analysis of 4111 subjects in the CARDIA Study. Coronary artery risk development in (young) adults. *Circulation* 1995;92:785–789.

43. Maron BJ, Fananapazir L. Sudden death in hypertrophic cardiomyopathy. *Circulation* 1992;85(suppl 1):I57–I63.

44. Maron BJ, Shirani J, Poliac L, et al. Sudden death in young competitive athletes: Clinical, demographic, and pathological profiles. *JAMA* 1996; 276:199–204.

45. Maron BJ, Thompson PD, Puffer JC, et al. Cardiovascular preparticipation screening of competitive athletes: A statement for health professionals from the Sudden Death Committee (Clinical Cardiology) and Congenital Cardiac Defects Committee (Cardiovascular Disease in the Young), American Heart Association. *Circulation* 1996;94:850–856.

46. Maron BJ, Cecchi F, McKenna WJ. Risk factors and stratification for sudden cardiac death in patients with hypertrophic cardiomyopathy. *Br Heart J* 1994;72(suppl):S13–S18.

47. Maron BJ, Roberts WC, Epstein SE. Sudden death in hypertrophic cardiomyopathy: A profile of 78 patients. *Circulation* 1982;65:1388–1394.

48. Spirito P, Chiarella F, Carratino L, et al. Clinical course and prognosis of hypertrophic cardiomyopathy in an outpatient population. *N Engl J Med* 1989;320:749–755.

49. Maron BJ, Savage DD, Wolfson JK, et al. Prognostic significance of 24 hour ambulatory electrocardiographic monitoring in patients with hypertrophic cardiomyopathy: A prospective study. *Am J Cardiol* 1981; 48: 252–257.

50. McKenna WJ, England D, Doi YL, et al. Arrhythmia in hypertrophic cardiomyopathy. I: Influence on prognosis. *Br Heart J* 1981;46:168–172.

51. Pasternac A, Noble J, Streulens Y, et al. Pathophysiology of chest pain in patients with cardiomyopathies and normal coronary arteries. *Circulation* 1982;65:778–788.

52. Cannon RO, Rosing DR, Maron BJ, et al. Myocardial ischemia in patients with hypertrophic cardiomyopathy: Contribution of inadequate vasodilator reserve and elevated left ventricular pressures. *Circulation* 1985;71: 234–243.

53. Roberts WC, Ferrans VJ. Pathologic anatomy of the cardiomyopathies. Idiopathic dilated and hypertrophic types, infiltrative types, and endomyocardial disease with and without eosinophilia. *Hum Pathol* 1975;6: 287–342.

54. St. John Sutton MG, Lie JT, Anderson KR, et al. Histopathological specificity of hypertrophic obstructive cardiomyopathy. Myocardial fibre disarray and myocardial fibrosis. *Br Heart J* 1980;44:433–443.

55. Maron BJ, Epstein SE, Roberts WC. Hypertrophic cardiomyopathy and transmural myocardial infarction without significant atherosclerosis of the extramural coronary arteries. *Am J Cardiol* 1979;43:1086–1102.

56. Pichard AD, Meller J, Teichholz LE, et al. Septal perforator compression (narrowing) in idiopathic hypertrophic subaortic stenosis. *Am J Cardiol* 1977;40:310–314.

57. Maron BJ, Wolfson JK, Epstein SE, et al. Intramural ("small vessel") coronary artery disease in hypertrophic cardiomyopathy. *J Am Coll Cardiol* 1986;8:545–547.

58. Maron BJ, Bonow RO, Cannon RO, et al. Hypertrophic cardiomyopathy: Interrelations of clinical manifestations, pathophysiology, and therapy. *N Engl J Med* 1987;316:780–789.

59. Rubin KA, Morrison J, Padnick MB, et al. Idiopathic hypertrophic subaortic stenosis: Evaluation of anginal symptoms with thallium-201 myocardial imaging. *Am J Cardiol* 1979;44:1040–1045.

60. Pitcher D, Wainwright R, Maisey M, et al. Assessment of chest pain in hypertrophic cardiomyopathy using exercise thallium-201 myocardial scintigraphy. *Br Heart J* 1980;44:650–656.

61. Hanrath P, Mathey D, Montz R, et al. Myocardial thallium-201 imaging in hypertrophic obstructive cardiomyopathy. *Eur Heart J* 1981;2:177–185.

62. O'Gara PT, Bonow RO, Maron BJ, et al. Myocardial perfusion abnormalities in patients with hypertrophic cardiomyopathy: Assessment with thallium-201 emission computed tomography. *Circulation* 1987;76:1214–1223.

63. Udelson JE, Bonow RO, O'Gara PT, et al. Verapamil prevents silent myocardial perfusion abnormalities during exercise in asymptomatic patients with hypertrophic cardiomyopathy. *Circulation* 1989;79:1052–1060.

64. Dilsizian V, Smeltzer WR, Dextras R, et al. Regional thallium abnormalities in hypertrophic cardiomyopathy: Myocardial ischemia or disturbed cellular active cation uptake? *Circulation* 1990;82:III-9. Abstract.

65. von Dohlen TW, Prisant LM, Frank MJ. Significance of positive or negative thallium-201 scintigraphy in hypertrophic cardiomyopathy. *Am J Cardiol* 1989;64:498-503.

66. Dilsizian V, Bonow RO, Epstein SE, Fananapazir L. Myocardial ischemia detected by thallium scintigraphy is frequentlyy related to cardiac arrest and syncope in young patients with hypertrophic cardiomyopathy. *J Am Coll Cardiol* 1993;22:796-804.

67. Maron BJ, Klues HG. Surviving competitive athletics with hypertrophic cardiomyopathy. *Am J Cardiol* 1994;73:1098-1104.

68. McKenna WJ, Thiene G, Nava A, et al. Diagnosis of arrhythmogenic right ventricular dysplasia/cardiomyopathy. *Br Heart J* 1994;71:215-218.

69. Dalal P, Fufisic K, Hupart P, et al. Arrhythmogenic right ventricular dysplasia: A review. *Cardiology* 1994;85:361-369.

70. Basso C, Thiene G, Corrado D, et al. Arrhythmogenic right ventricular cardiomyopathy: Dysplasia, dystrophy, or myocarditis? *Circulation* 1996;94:983-991.

71. Angelini A, Basso C, Nava A, et al. Endomyocardial biopsy in arrhythmogenic right ventricular cardiomyopathy. *Am Heart J* 1996;132:203-206.

72. Strain J. Adiposc dysplasia of the right ventricle: Is endomyocardial biopsy useful? *Eur Heart J* 1989;10(suppl D):84-88.

73. Chiddo A, Gaglione A, Bortone A, et al. Right ventricular dysplasia: Angiographic study. *Eur Heart J* 1989;10(suppl D):42-45.

74. Daubert C, Descaves C, Foulgoc JL, et al. Critical analysis of cineangiographic criteria for diagnosis of arrhythmic right ventricular dysplasia. *Am Heart J* 1988;115:448-459.

75. Daubert C, Druelles P, Foulgoc JL, et al. Benefits and limits of selective right ventricular cineangiography in arrhythmogenic right ventricular dysplasia. *Eur Heart J* 1989;10(suppl D):46-48.

76. Manyari DE, Duff HJ, Kostuk WJ, et al. Usefulness of noninvasive studies for diagnosis of right ventricular dysplasia. *Am J Cardiol* 1986;57:1147-1153.

77. Le Guludec D, Slama MS, Frank R, et al. Evaluation of radionuclide angiography in diagnosis of arrhythmogenic right ventricular cardiomyopathy. *J Am Coll Cardiol* 1995;26:1476-1483.

78. Bruzzone F, Borziani S, Clavario P, et al. Right ventricular dysplasia: Radioisotopic angiography. *Eur Heart J* 1989;10(suppl D):37-41.

79. Blake LM, Scheinman MM, Higgins CB. MR features of arrhythmogenic right ventricular dysplasia. *AJR* 1994;162:809-812.

80. Auffermann W, Wichter T, Breithardt G, et al. Arrhythmogenic right ventricular disease: MR imaging vs angiography. *AJR* 1993;161:549-555.

81. Ricci C, Longo R, Pagnan L, et al. Magnetic resonance imaging in right ventricular dysplasia. *Am J Cardiol* 1992;70:1589-1595.

82. Boyd DP, Farmer DW. Cardiac computed tomography. In Collin SM, Skorton DJ (eds): *Cardiac Imaging and Imaging Processing.* New York, NY: McGraw-Hill; 1986:68-87.

83. Hamada S, Takamiya M, Ohe T, et al. Arrhythmogenic right ventricular dysplasia: Evaluation with electron-beam CT. *Radiology* 1993;187:723-727.

84. Tada H, Shimizu W, Ohe T, et al. Usefulness of electron-beam computed tomography in arrhythmogenic right ventricular dysplasia: Relationship to electrophysiological abnormalities and left ventricular involvement. *Circulation* 1996;94:437-444.

9

Public Access to Defibrillation:

Response to Emergencies at Athletic Events—Economic, Training, and Cost Implications

Richard O. Cummins, MD, MPH, MSc
and Mary Fran Hazinski, RN, MSN

Introduction

Effective resuscitation of any victim of sudden cardiac arrest is most likely to occur when a system is in place to ensure that basic and advanced life support are promptly provided by trained personnel. This system of response in the community has been labeled a "Chain of Survival" by the American Heart Association (AHA),[1] and includes prompt activation of the emergency medical services (EMS) system, bystander cardiopulmonary resuscitation (CPR), early defibrillation, and advanced cardiac life support (ACLS).[2] Within the past several years, the AHA has advocated further development of this chain to include "Public Access Defibrillation," with defibrillation provided by first responders to the scene of a cardiac arrest.[3,4] This chapter presents the application of these concepts to any response to sudden cardiac collapse at athletic

From Estes NAM, Salem DN, Wang PJ (eds). *Sudden Cardiac Death in the Athlete.* Armonk, NY: Futura Publishing Co., Inc.; ©1998.

events, emphasizing the need for development of an organized system of response to these emergencies. It describes a project in progress to evaluate the cost of training National Collegiate Athletic Association (NCAA) Division I team physicians and athletic trainers in the use of automatic external defibrillators (AEDs), including issues of training cost and skill retention. Finally, it addresses practical issues of such training, including legal and liability issues, and cost-effectiveness.

Cardiac Emergencies in Sports

Cardiac emergencies in sports may occur in a variety of settings. These variations must be considered when designing a response system. First, more than two thirds of the reported episodes of sudden cardiac arrest occur among football or basketball players; therefore, it would be logical to focus system response on these two sports. Second, more than half of these emergencies occur during training sessions, rather than during actual competition.[5] Team athletic trainers rather than team physicians are most likely to be present during these practice sessions. Approximately one third of episodes of sudden cardiac arrest in athletes do occur during or immediately after a team competition, when a team physician is most likely to be present.[5] Finally, cardiac emergencies may also develop among spectators attending the athletic event.[4] In fact, the probability/frequency of such emergencies can generally be predicted based on the attendance at the event.

An ideal system of response to sudden cardiac arrest in athletes should include ready availability of an AED at the sites of training and competition for both football and basketball teams. In order to ensure maximal application of any AED, its use cannot be restricted to team physicians, but should be extended to athletic trainers, who will be present during all team training and competitive sessions. Finally, cardiac arrest among spectators should be anticipated, and training of personnel planned accordingly.

The Chain of Survival Concept

The Chain of Survival is a widely used metaphor to describe the critical actions that should occur in response to cardiac emergencies.[1,6–10] The concept is straightforward: an EMS system response to cardiac arrest must be organized with multiple divisions; each of these divisions requires separate attention and separate programs. Weaknesses in any one link will condemn a system to poor survival rates. There are four links in the chain of survival as described by the AHA[1,10]:

- Early access
- Early CPR
- Early defibrillation
- Early advanced life support

The Early Access Link

Early access begins the chain of survival. The purpose of this first "link" is to get trained help to the victim as quickly as possible. When cardiac arrest or collapse occurs, someone must recognize a medical emergency and activate the EMS system. Delays may occur in recognition of the emergency, decision to make the 911 call, location of the telephone, and placement of call. The early access link can be strengthened through public education, specifically education of those individuals most likely to witness a cardiac arrest. In addition, an efficient emergency communication system must exist. Educational programs developed by the AHA attempt to inform the public of local emergency access numbers.

The Early Cardiopulmonary Resuscitation Link

The second link in the chain of survival is immediate bystander CPR. This CPR should begin as soon as a cardiac arrest is identified and the EMS system has been activated. Early CPR is extremely important because it buys time for the cardiac arrest patient.[11] It produces sufficient blood flow to maintain central nervous system and myocardial viability.

Basic CPR must be started as soon as possible and must be followed quickly by defibrillation, intubation, and cardiovascular medications. When CPR is started early, the victim is more likely to be in ventricular fibrillation (VF) (rather than asystole) when a monitoring unit arrives at his or her side.[12] Several studies suggest that CPR prolongs the duration of VF, prolonging the interval during which defibrillation may be effective.[13–15] Finally, defibrillation is more likely to convert the victim's rhythm to one producing spontaneous circulation if CPR is provided immediately after collapse.[12]

The Early Defibrillation Link

The rationale for early defibrillation emerges from data that demonstrate that almost 85% of persons with ambulatory, out-of-hospital primary cardiac arrest experience ventricular arrhythmias during the early minutes after they collapse. A principle of early defibrillation holds that the professional rescuer who arrives first at the scene of a cardiac arrest should carry and be trained to operate a defibrillator.[16] With few exceptions, the defibrillator used should be an AED.

The purpose of early defibrillation is to reestablish a normal spontaneous rhythm in the heart. Many recent developments should reduce the time to defibrillation. Use of AEDs by the first responding emergency personnel such as police,[17,18] use of automatic defibrillators by "community responders" (ie, people whose usual occupation or training would not require responding to emergencies),[4,19] and "home defibrillation programs" for high-risk patients[19,20] should all shorten the time between collapse and defibrillation.

Although defibrillation was considered part of ACLS care in the past, early defibrillation has now achieved such importance that it stands by itself as a separate link in the chain of survival.

The Early Advanced Cardiac Life Support Link

For many victims of sudden cardiac death, CPR and defibrillation do not achieve or sustain resuscitation. The unique interventions of the early ACLS link—intubation and intravenous medications—may be necessary to maximize the chances of survival.[21] In the United States, ACLS for victims of prehospital cardiac arrest is generally provided by paramedics. In other countries, ACLS is provided by either nurses or emergency physicians.[8] Although early defibrillation alone produces a considerable proportion of all survivors of cardiac arrest, intubation and intravenous medications are also important. These interventions are thought to not only promote the return of a spontaneous rhythm and circulation, but to also stabilize and maintain patients during the immediate postresuscitation period. Early ACLS may also aid in restoration of circulation to people suffering from non-VF rhythms.

Automatic External Defibrillators

The new technology of AEDs has revolutionized the approach to out-of-hospital cardiac arrest.[22] These devices attach to the patient through remote defibrillator pads. The defibrillation pads are dual-function, enabling both rhythm assessment and delivery of electrical shocks. The devices analyze a sampling from or variety of characteristics of the surface electrocardiogram (ECG) signal, including amplitude, frequency, and morphology. All AEDs employ a simple four-step operation[23]:

- Step one, turn the power on
- Step two, attach the device to the patient through the adhesive defibrillator pad

- Step three, press the analyze control
- Step four, press the shock control

AEDs contain both audio and light prompts that direct the user through the steps of operation. New devices contain audio prompts that also instruct the operator to perform all the steps of basic CPR. Additional recent technological innovations include use of biphasic defibrillation wave forms and extremely long shelf-life batteries.[24-26] These innovations have enabled the development of small, light, inexpensive AEDs with long shelf lives, low maintenance, and self-monitoring functions.

From a conceptual perspective, a strong chain of survival is established as the key to improving outcomes from sudden cardiac death. Early defibrillation is considered the most important link in a strong chain of survival. AEDs are considered the key to providing a strong early defibrillation link.

Public Access Defibrillation Concept

The concept of public access defibrillation has received a great deal of publicity over the past several years.[3,4] In its simplest form, public access defibrillation means bystander-initiated defibrillation. This means the witness to most out-of-hospital cardiac arrests (the bystander) will be trained to operate defibrillators, and that defibrillators will be immediately available to the bystander.[23] Public access defibrillation means performance of defibrillation by *trained,* nontraditional emergency responders. Such nontraditional responders include police, security personnel, ski patrollers, administrators for large assembly areas, team physicians, athletic trainers, aircraft flight attendants, ferry boat crew members, gate keepers at gated communities, watchmen at high-rise apartment complexes, and personnel employed at remote work site areas such as the merchant marines and oil rigs.

It is important to recognize that the public access defibrillation concept is not similar to the "public telephone concept." The public telephone concept, in the opinion of these authors, is invalid. People who use a public telephone have never been trained specifically to use those devices. The public telephone concept also contends that the first time an emergency responder needs to use the device will be the first time the responder has actually seen the device.

The public access defibrillation concept, in reality, is founded on the "fire extinguisher" principle. Large fire extinguishers in public buildings constitute specialized equipment that is widely available but used only by specially trained operators. These specially trained operators are required to have review at regular intervals, and regular maintenance of their skills.

The fire extinguisher concept is based on Occupatioanl Safety and Health Administration (OSHA) fire extinguisher regulations (29CFR 1910.157).

Employers shall provide portable fire extinguishers, and shall mount, locate, and identify them so they are readily accessible to employees. . . (C) (1). . . shall also provide an educational program to familiarize employees with the general principles of fire extinguisher use. . . (G) (1). . . shall provide the education upon initial employment and annually thereafter (G) (2).

These regulations convey the intent of the fire extinguisher concept: specialized equipment provided to specifically trained operators with regular review and maintenance.

Public Access Defibrillation: Results from Public Assemblies and Sporting Events

One good example of the application of the concept of public access defibrillation to large public assemblies comes from the experience at Expo '86. This World's Fair was conducted in Vancouver, British Columbia in the summer of 1986. Eighteen million visitors attended Expo '86 over a 5-month period. Security personnel were trained to use AEDs, which were available at specially marked refreshment stands. When an emergency occurred, security personnel were dispatched to retrieve the AED and respond to the victim in cardiac arrest. If the victim demonstrated absence of pulse, breathing, and consciousness, the security personnel attached the device to the victim and followed the protocols. In the summer of 1986, there were six cardiac arrests, producing a rate of 1 cardiac arrest per 3 million visitors. In all six of these cardiac arrests, the device was properly attached, and the rhythm was properly assessed. Two of these victims demonstrated ventricular fibrillation. The AED assessed the rhythm correctly, delivered a shock, and restored the spontaneous circulation. Both of these VF arrest survivors were awake and talking by the time of the ambulance transport to the hospital.[27]

Cardiac Arrest at Seattle, Washington Sporting Events

Dr. Leonard Cobb at the University of Washington has meticulously tracked the cardiac arrests treated by Seattle paramedics stationed at athletic events at the Kingdome in the City of Seattle, and at Husky Stadium on the campus of the University of Washington. Dr. Cobb reports an incident of 1 cardiac arrest per 2 million attendees at these athletic events. Calculating the average number of event attendees and the average duration of the sporting events yields an incidence of 1 cardiac arrest per 1000 patient years. Surprisingly, this incidence is approximately the same as observed in most United States communities: one cardiac arrest per year per thousand people. A survival rate of 67% has been reported for victims in VF treated by the paramedics on the scene.[4] This yields a life-saved rate of 1 life per 3.7 million attendees.

The Qantas Airlines Medical Response Program

Another example of public access defibrillation comes from the Qantas Cardiac Arrest Program.[28] Several publications have appeared, raising concerns about in-flight medical emergencies[29] and even deaths[30] during commercial air travel. The medical directors of Qantas airlines have reported the results of their innovative program to supply AEDs to 53 B-747 and B-767 aircraft flying international routes for Qantas Airlines.[28] The medical director of the program was responsible for training all 370 flight service directors. In some settings, the AEDs were placed in air terminals. During the course of the study (1991 to 1994) there were seven aircraft diversions and 29 cardiac arrests. This was a rate of 87 deaths per million flights, or 0.72 deaths per million passengers. The results of the program from September 1991 to December 1994 were impressive. There were 29 cardiac arrests in this period. Sixteen of these arrests occurred on board aircraft. Four of these cardiac arrest patients were in VF. The device correctly assessed the rhythm and delivered defibrillatory shocks to all four patients in VF. Two individuals were discharged alive to home. During the time of the study, there were 13 cardiac arrests on the ground in the terminal. Eleven of these people were in VF, and the device correctly assessed and delivered shocks to all 11 of these VF patients. Three of these patients were discharged alive to home.

Automatic External Defibrillators
for Team Physicians and Trainers

In early 1997, a project began at Vanderbilt University in collaboration with the HeartStream Corporation (manufacturers of the ForeRunner Automatic External Defibrillator; Seattle, Washington). This project was designed to apply the public access defibrillation concept to athletic events through education of team physicians and team trainers. This project was undertaken to answer the following questions:

How quickly can team physicians and trainers learn to use AEDs? How long will they remember the skill? Will they be able to perform automatic external defibrillation at the moment of an actual cardiac emergency? Will such a program save lives and how much will it cost?

The Vanderbilt SPE-AED project began with a survey of NCAA Southeastern Conference (SEC) athletic teams. There are 12 SEC teams: Alabama, Arkansas, Auburn, Florida, University of Georgia, Kentucky, Louisiana State University, Mississippi, Mississippi State, South Carolina, University of Tennessee, and Vanderbilt University. The survey was conducted by telephone, and sought to determine whether the team possessed a defibrillator, and if so, what type (automatic versus manual)? The survey asked where the defibrillators were located during practice and during games. The survey contained questions about the number of people trained in AED use, and who was authorized to use the defibrillator. In addition, there were inquiries regarding CPR training by team physicians and trainers.

Preliminary results from this study indicate that most team physicians worked within the specialty of sports medicine, with the majority specializing in orthopedics. There were, however, team physicians who were specialized in family practice, internal medicine, dentistry, and osteopathy. Most of the team physicians had not participated in an ACLS course within the last 3 years. The only physicians who had obtained ACLS Provider status within recent years were those who recently graduated from a residency program.

Six of the 12 teams had purchased defibrillators; 5 had purchased AEDs and 1 purchased a manual defibrillator several years ago. The teams with defibrillators include: Alabama, Auburn, University of Georgia, Louisiana State University, University of South Carolina, and Vanderbilt University. Specific defibrillators purchased included: Physio-Control (Redmond, WA), SurVivaLink (Minnetonka, MN), Laerdal Heart Start (Laerdal Medical Company, Wappinger Falls, NY), and Heartstream (Seattle, WA). SEC athletic teams without defibrillators include: Arkansas, Florida, Kentucky, Mississippi, Mississippi State, and the University of Tennessee.

All SEC teams had certified athletic trainers (CATs) in place. All CATs are required to complete training in basic life support every 2 years. Most of these trainers were also familiar with AEDs, and some were trained in their use.

- Arkansas: 2 of 11 CATs were trained in AED use
- Auburn: all CATs were trained in AED use
- Georgia: all CATs were trained in AED use
- LSU: 1 out of 11 CATs was trained in AED use
- South Carolina: half of the CATs were trained in AED use

• Vanderbilt: used a manual defibrillator, and only MDs were authorized to deliver a shock

The Vanderbilt SPE-AED project is currently in progress. The project provides a brief training period of team physicians and athletic trainers with review of CPR and training in the use of AED use. The AED training requires<30 minutes and can be incorporated into a regular AHA Heart Saver course. Since all CATs had been current with basic lifesaving (BLS) skills, the AED training consistently required <1 hour. Upon completion of the course, team physicians and athletic trainers are videotaped responding to a simulated cardiac arrest with a mannequin. The videotaping is performed within 1 hour of the initial training. Responders are asked to enter a room where a person has had a cardiac arrest. The patient (a life-size mannequin), a telephone, and an automatic defibrillator are located in the room. The subjects are filmed executing the protocols that they had been trained to follow earlier that day. The videotapes are sent to a collaborative research team at the University of Washington, where they are graded in the following dimensions: CPR skills, sequence of AED use, time to first defibrillation, and a safety score.

The study addresses the issue of whether these responders would successfully defibrillate a patient who was in VF in a timely fashion, and without posing a danger to themselves or bystanders. The videotapes are examined for contact between the operator and the patient during shock delivery, and for whether the device is operated in such a manner that a defibrillator shock would be delivered to people in VF.

Skill retention is addressed by a follow-up video made using a scenario performed approximately 6 weeks to 6 months after the initial training session. Team trainers receive a brief explanation: *Do you remember that training you had X weeks ago? Well, let's pretend that the person in the next room has had a cardiac arrest. Would you please enter the room and execute the protocols you learned at the initial course?* A videotape is made of this performance and graded in a standard fashion outlined above.

The Vanderbilt SPE-AED project is due for completion in late 1997. A number of observations already possible from this project are particularly relevant to the themes of the Keystone Conference:

1. While a number of NCAA Division II teams are aware of automatic external defibrillators and have gone so far as to actually purchase one of these devices, many teams have failed to develop a response system.
2. Issues of who should be trained and authorized to use the device have not yet been consistently addressed.

3. Location of the devices during practice, during competition, and during actual public attendance at competitions is inconsistent. Devices locked in offices or stored separate from the team cannot be accessed in a timely fashion.
4. Response plans for use during road trips have not been addressed.
5. Seasonal sports overlaps have not been addressed. For example, in most locations basketball competition begins prior to the end of football season. The availability of a response team and defibrillator are not sorted out on occasions when these sports occur simultaneously.

The above questions can be addressed through establishment of a response system. These authors strongly recommend that national organizations such as National Association of Athletic Trainers place the issue of response to cardiac emergencies high on their agendae. AEDs are being purchased and placed with Division I teams, as well as with professional teams. Preliminary data suggest that these teams lack a coordinated response system or plan. Protocols should be developed regarding placement, storage, retrieval, and use of these devices. In addition, the sequence of actions to be followed when an athlete collapses on the field during competition in a public stadium must be spelled out and practiced. It is recommended that certified athletic trainer associations, as well as team physician organizations, address this topic in a consensus guideline manner.

The AHA continues to address these issues pertaining to the interface between public bystander defibrillation and organized EMS system defibrillation.[3,23,26] More and more, EMS systems will respond in a rapid fashion with automatic external defibrillators, and will find that a bystander has already initiated defibrillation with an appropriate public access defibrillator. The AHA will address these issues to assure a smooth interaction and interface between these various tiers of an emergency response. These concepts are consistent with the AHA's promotion of a strong chain of survival.

Will Public Access Defibrillation Applied to Sports Teams and Athletic Competitions Work?

This question requires specific information in regards to the incidence of sudden death in athletes. The interested reader is referred to other chapters in this volume. Informed observers are aware that success in the arena of public access defibrillation requires facing the "cascade of multiple probabilities." In other words, for a successful resuscitation program to occur, a sequence of events of varying probabilities must all occur:

- The cardiac arrest must be witnessed, and the witness to the cardiac arrest must respond appropriately.
- The witness must be aware of the availability of and location of an automatic external defibrillator, must properly retrieve the device, and must properly operate the device.
- The cardiac rhythm of the arrest victim must be either VF or ventricular tachycardia.
- The device must assess the rhythm correctly, charge, and deliver a shock.
- Following a shock, the postshock rhythm must restore spontaneous circulation and establish effective perfusion.
- Patients with a restored heartbeat must survive to hospital admission.
- Patients who are admitted must survive to hospital discharge
- Patients who are discharged alive should be neurologically intact, with a reasonable longevity.

Presently, probability estimates can be attached to each of these steps with reasonable accuracy. It is known that automatic external defibrillators will assess the rhythm correctly and deliver a shock to ventricular defibrillation within accuracy approaching 95% to 99%.[26] The AHA is initiating a CPR-D program nationally to incorporate training in the use of automatic external defibrillators into basic CPR training.[23] However, the key first links in the chain of survival must be performed by the bystander, who must recognize the cardiac arrest, activate the EMS system, begin CPR, and use an AED.

Is Public Access Defibrillation— Applied to the Sports Arena—Legal?

In all states, defibrillators are considered "medical devices." Consequently, they are regulated by health practice and medical device acts. AEDs are "legal" if they are purchased under the authority of a physician. It is a simple matter, however, for the team physician or someone representing a medical authority to appoint a trainer for the AED instruction and to confirm the protocols that will be followed. The team physician or university medical authority then must sign a "prescription" for the people trained. In practice throughout the United States, many EMS personnel have assumed responsibility for AED training. All follow the AHA protocols for early defibrillation. Upon completion of training by an EMS trainer, a physician signs a course completion card which functions, in effect, as the "prescription" for the device to be used.

Liability Issues

No discussion of public access defibrillation would be complete without consideration of liability questions. Manufacturers of medical devices assume product liability risk and build in mechanisms for addressing these product liability claims. Defibrillators, in particular, are intended for use in life-or-death situations. While there are deaths associated with defibrillators, such deaths are almost never due to defibrillators. The American medical climate is such that there will be inevitable wrongful death lawsuits. The vast majority of these find no merit in the allegations of incorrect function of the defibrillator.

In some situations institutional risk management authorities are opposed to the use of public access defibrillation in their institution. Most of these concerns are unrealistic and based on a mandate to avoid exposure to any liability risk. Most innovative leaders on this topic, such as medical directors for police defibrillation programs, recognize that there is no way of guaranteeing "zero liability risk." The reality is that most liability lawsuits are dismissed with a determination of no merit. Nevertheless, institutions and medical directors should be prepared to, on occasion, undergo the inconvenience and personal disruption of our American litigation system.

For the actual user of the AED, there is virtually no liability. Most AED users are agents of a larger institution, and are not at individual risk. The major requirement is that the AED user uses the device per training instructions and per product protocol. It is possible for an AED user to use the device in a totally frivolous and capricious manner. Misadventures are always possible, but extremely unlikely.

Will Creation of a Team AED Response System be Cost-Effective?

Cost-effectiveness estimates are always an exercise in speculation. Cost is measured in dollars, and effectiveness is measured in the total number of lives saved, or the total life-years saved. For example, a 25-year-old college athlete who is saved and lives for 40 more years represents 40 life-years saved, as well as one single life saved. In addition, many people now recommend adjusting the estimate for effects on quality of life. The actual number of lives saved will be revealed by future surveillance research.[31] One could argue that the quality of response for survivors resuscitated with early CPR-D could be much higher than with our current systems. For example, a young athlete collapsing in arrhythmic arrest, in most locations, is treated no sooner than 8 to 10 minutes following the collapse. Public access defibrillation applied to this situation would provide defibrillation many minutes sooner. Improved neurological outcomes would be expected. Finally, no cost-effectiveness argument would be complete without an awareness that preparation for a proper response will decrease litigation risk. It is far better to invest resources into proper preparation and never use the device, than it is to avoid the initial investment, only to be faced with a large wrongful death litigation at some point in the future.

Another issue in regards to cost-effectiveness is the concept of incremental cost and incremental effectiveness. Incremental cost means how much more do we have to pay now, over and above what we currently pay? Incremental lives saved means, how many more lives will we save compared to the number we currently save? These questions must be addressed by every site considering adding public access defibrillation to sports teams.

In reality, a team AED program would require very little additional or incremental cost. CPR training is now required for all certified athletic trainers, so there would be no additional cost associated with CPR training. Defibrillation training can be easily incorporated into basic CPR training, using CPR-D curricula already developed by the AHA.[23] Therefore, no incremental cost associated with defibrillation training should occur. Additional personnel cost would be minimal because the AED training would focus only on persons already employed.

The price of AEDs has decreased dramatically in recent years. Devices are now available for less than $3000. The success of this technology, with increased volume of sales and increased competition, will serve to further reduce the cost.

Summary: What Does the Future Hold?

This is an interesting area of sports medicine. Innovations in technology are actually driving innovations in practice. The widespread availability, low cost, small size, and long shelf life with minimum maintenance are making early defibrillation available in settings never before dreamed possible. Team physicians and athletic trainers who have taken on the responsibility of providing the best care possible to athletes and spectators, are coming to accept the need for CPR training and for training in the use of AEDs. It is fortunate, indeed, that the incidence of these tragic events is low. However, low frequency of occurrence is not an argument for lack of preparedness. The cost of this training and technology is decreasing so fast that any argument that benefit is not worth the cost cannot be sustained in the late 1990s. Team physicians and team trainers are imminently qualified and capable of responding with this state-of-the-art intervention.

The Vanderbilt SPE-AED project is demonstrating that skills are easy to acquire and easy to retain. If this and other projects obtain positive results, it will be incumbent upon national organizations to look closely at their responsibilities to the individuals and organizations that they serve. These authors predict that some day athletic trainers responding to rare events on the field, and more frequent events in the bleachers, will become standard practice. AEDS hanging conveniently on the wall, ready for immediate use, will be as common as the adhesive tape dispenser and the ice pack.

References

1. Cummins RO, Ornato JP, Thies W, et al. Improving survival from cardiac arrest: The "chain of survival" concept. *Circulation* 1991;83:1832–1847.
2. Guidelines for cardiopulmonary resuscitation and emergency cardiac care. Emergency Cardiac Care Committee and Subcommittees, American Heart Association. Part IX. Ensuring effectiveness of communitywide emergency cardiac care [see comments]. *JAMA* 1992;268(16):2289–2295.
3. Weisfeldt M, Kerber R, McGoldrick RP, et al. Public access defibrillation: A statement for healthcare professionals from the American Heart Association Task Force on Automatic External Defibrillation. *Circulation* 1995; 92:2763.
4. Weisfeldt M, Kerber R, McGoldrick RP, et al. American Heart Association report on the Public Access Defibrillation Conference, December 8–10, 1994. *Circulation* 1995;92:2740–2747.
5. Maron B, Shirani J, Poliac LC, et al. Sudden death in young competitive athletes: Clinical, demographic, and pathological profiles. *JAMA* 1996;276: 199–204.
6. Cummins R. The "chain of survival" concept: How it can save lives. *Heart Dis Stroke* 1992;1:43–45.
7. Cummins RO. Emergency medical services and sudden cardiac arrest: The "chain of survival" concept. *Annu Rev Public Health* 1993;14:313–333.
8. Cummins R, Graves J. The chain of survival in Europe: EMS systems compared to USA systems. In Skinner D (ed): *Textbook of Emergency Medicine.* Cambridge: Churchill-Livingstone; 1995.
9. Kaye W, Mancini M, Giuliano K, et al. Strengthening the in-hospital chain of survival with rapid defibrillation by first responders using automated external defibrillators: Training and retention issues. *Ann Emerg Med* 1995;25:163–168.
10. Montgomery WH. Prehospital cardiac arrest: The chain of survival concept. *Ann Acad Med Singapore* 1992;21(1):69–72.
11. Cummins RO, Eisenberg MS. Prehospital cardiopulmonary resuscitation: Is it effective? *JAMA* 1985;253:2408–2412.
12. Cummins RO, Eisenberg MS, Hallstrom AP, Litwin PE. Survival of out-of-hospital cardiac arrest with early initiation of cardiopulmonary resuscitaiton. *Am J Emerg Med* 1985;3:114–118.
13. Brown C, Michael D, Griffith R, et al. The effect of bystander CPR on the

median frequency of the ventricular fibrillation ECG signal. *Ann Emerg Med* 1992;21:461–462. Abstract.

14. Joslyn SA, Pomrehn PR, Brown DD. Survival from out-of-hospital cardiac arrest: Effects of patient age and presence of 911 Emergency Medical Services phone access. *Am J Emerg Med* 1993;11(3):200–206.

15. Swor R, Boji B, Cynar M, et al. Bystander vs EMS First Responder CPR: Initial rhythm and outcome in witnessed non-monitored out-of-hospital cardiac arrest. *Acad Emerg Med* 1995;2:494–498.

16. Kerber R, Members of Emergency Cardiac Care Committee. Statement on early defibrillation from the American Heart Association. *Circulation* 1991;83:2233.

17. Mosesso VJ, Davis E, Carlin R, et al. Use of automated defibrillators by police first-responders for treatment of out-of-hospital cardiac arrests. *Ann Emerg Med* 1993;22:920. Abstract.

18. White R, Asplin B, Bugliosi T, Hankins D. High discharge survival rate after out-of-hospital ventricular fibrillation with rapid defibrillation by police and paramedics. *Ann Emerg Med* 1996;28:480–485.

19. Cummins RO, Schubach JA, Litwin PE, Hearne TR. Training lay persons to use automatic external defibrillators: Success of initial training and one-year retention of skills. *Am J Emerg Med* 1989;7(2):143–149.

20. Eisenberg MS, Moore J, Cummins RO, et al. Use of the automatic external defibrillator in home of survivors of out-of-hospital ventricular fibrillation. *Am J Cardiol* 1989;63:443–446.

21. Cummins R (ed). *1994 Textbook of Advanced Cardiac Life Support, 3rd Edition*. Dallas: American Heart Association; 1994.

22. Cummins R. From concept to standard-of-care? Review of the clinical experience with automated external defibrillators. *Ann Emerg Med* 1989;18:1269–1275.

23. Stapleton E, Hazinski M, Cummins R. Automated external defibrillation. In Hazinski M, Chandra N (eds): *Basic Life Support for Healthcare Providers*. Dallas: American Heart Association; 1997:9/1–9/17.

24. Bardy G, Gliner B, Kudenchuk P, et al. Truncated biphasic pulses for transthoracic defibrillation. *Circulation* 1995;91:1768–1774.

25. Bardy G, Marchlinski F, Sharma A, et al. Multicenter comparison of truncated biphasic shocks and standard damped sine wave monophasic shocks for transthoracic ventricular fibrillation. *Circulation* 1996;94:2507–2514.

26. Kerber R, Becker L, Bourland J, et al. Automatic external defibrillators for public access defibrillation: Recommendations for specifying and reporting arrhythmia analysis, algorithm performance, incorporating new waveforms, and enhancing safety. *Circulation* 1997;95:1677–1682.

27. Weaver WD, Cobb LA, Hallstrom AP. Considerations for improving survival from out-of-hospital cardiac arrest. *Ann Emerg Med* 1986;15:1181–1186.

28. O'Rourke M, Donaldson E. An airline cardiac arrest programme. *Circulation* 1994;90(4, pt 2):I–287.

29. Cummins RO, Schubach JA. Frequency and types of medical emergencies among commercial air travelers. *JAMA* 1989;261(9):1295–1299.

30. Cummins RO, Chapman PJ, Chamberlain DA, et al. In-flight deaths during commercial air travel. How big is the problem? [see comments] *JAMA* 1988;259(13):1983–1988.

31. Cummins R, Hein K, Larsen M, et al. What is the health-related "quality-of-life" of survivors of sudden out-of-hospital cardiac arrest? *Circulation* 1996;94(suppl):2079.

10

Race and Gender Considerations in Sudden Death in the Athlete

Richard Allen Williams, MD

Introduction

Are the race and the sex of the competitive athlete important factors to consider when looking at sudden cardiac death (SCD)? Are there significant differences in incidence of SCD between black and white athletes? Why is there such a great disparity between males and females in the occurrence of this phenomenon? Is there enough evidence to establish black race and male sex as risk factors for SCD in competitive athletes?

These questions and others regarding race and gender are addressed in this chapter. It is important to attempt to find answers to these questions in order to provide direction for future initiatives and also to give some guidance and perspective to the clinician who will examine an athlete either during a preparticipation physical or after an acute event has occurred. Toward these ends, information obtained from a comprehensive literature review are analyzed, as are accounts gathered from newspaper reports, investigations personally conducted by the author, and reports from the Armed Forces Institute of Pathology and the National Center for Catastrophic Sports Injury Research (NCCSIR). The focus in this chapter is on SCD in the young athlete un-

From Estes NAM, Salem DN, Wang PJ (eds). *Sudden Cardiac Death in the Athlete.* Armonk, NY: Futura Publishing Co., Inc.; ©1998.

der 30 years of age who participates in organized sports at the high school, college, and professional levels.

Background of Sudden Cardiac Death in Blacks

It is now well recognized that there is a different disease profile in Blacks than in Whites,[1] and that the race of a patient must be taken into account when the clinician attempts to evaluate and treat various medical conditions. It is known, for instance, that certain diseases tend to predominate in Blacks, whereas others are more commonly found in Whites. Cardiovascular conditions resulting in sudden death that are seen more frequently in Blacks include left ventricular hypertrophy,[2] sarcoidosis,[3] and coronary disease.[4-8] Left ventricular hypertrophy is found primarily in association with hypertension and has been determined to be a risk factor for SCD.[9,10] This must be distinguished from a condition described by Topol et al,[11] which they termed *hypertensive hypertrophic cardiomyopathy;* the latter is seen principally in elderly black females and may involve sudden death. SCD is the most common form of death in patients with cardiac sarcoidosis, about two thirds of whom are black.[12] Coronary artery disease presents an interesting situation in which the prevalence of the condition is greater in Whites but the incidence of SCD is higher in Blacks.[13] For instance, in a 1984 study involving 2275 subjects in Charleston, South Carolina, Keil and Associates[14] found that the rate of SCD in black males was three times higher than in white males. Other studies that have demonstrated what appears to be a paradox include the Hagstrom study[15] in Nashville, Tennessee (1971) and the Oalmann investigation[16] in New Orleans (1971); the latter report showed a fivefold higher rate of SCD in black males as opposed to white males in the 30- to 44-year age category, and there was a 47% higher rate in black males as opposed to white males in those who were 45 to 64 years of age, despite a higher proportion of deaths assigned to coronary heart disease.

Another entity that deserves brief consideration here but is not thought of as a cardiac condition is sickle cell trait. There are several studies in the literature[17-22] of death during exertion in individuals with sickle cell trait; and isolated instances of sudden death in athletes with this disorder have been reported. It is thought that the mechanism of death in cases related to heavy physical effort such as in athletes and in military recruits involves dehydration and low oxygen tension, leading to sickling of erythrocytes, as well as exertional rhabdomyolysis. One report contains seven cases of the latter condition, which was found in nontraumatic sports deaths; all seven individuals were African Americans with sickle cell trait.[23] This disorder therefore must be considered when the risk for death among athletes is discussed, particularly in regards to black athletes. However, it must be acknowledged at the same time that there must be thousands of individuals with sickle cell trait who participate in competitive sports and never have become ill from this disorder, and it seems wise not to create special screening or precautionary measures for athletes who may have sickle cell trait.

Sudden Cardiac Death in Black Athletes

This is an area which has not been well investigated because SCD has not been regarded as having an inordinate or different representation in the African American population. First of all, no demographic evidence exists that Blacks in general have a higher prevalence of conditions that have been found to predispose to SCD in young athletes, such as hypertrophic cardiomyopathy (HCM) and coronary artery anomalies. There is also no indication that a genetic predilection exists in Blacks for these conditions. However, information is beginning to evolve that strongly suggests that black athletes may indeed suffer a disproportionate amount of the SCD that occurs in competitive sports.

Media reports of SCD episodes provided an early suggestion that black athletes were dying in disproportionate numbers. Between 1975 and 1990, the author, who noted the appearance of a string of SCD reports in small black newspapers in the Los Angeles area, collected, reviewed, and analyzed clinical and autopsy data on 24 black athletes[24] who had died under various circumstances (Table 1). The distribution of deaths was about equal for football and basketball, with three fatalities occurring in track athletes. Most of the autopsies showed the presence of HCM; other diseases represented were coronary artery anomalies, Marfan syndrome with aortic rupture, and idiopathic concentric left ventricular hypertrophy. All except two were male, the age range was 13 to 28 years (average age 18.7), and all died either during vigorous physical activity or immediately thereafter. Toxicological studies were performed in all cases and showed no evidence of illicit or performance-enhancing drugs. An example of the cases cited is that of R.C., who had competed in organized sports at high school, college, and professional levels but was unable to continue his sports career because of hypertension. He subsequently became a physical education instructor at a junior college, and while running wind sprints with his track students, suddenly collapsed and died. Autopsy revealed a huge heart, weighing 630 grams, which demonstrated hypertrophy of the lower third of the intraventricular septum. Microscopic analysis showed severe diffuse myocardial fibrosis. Fourteen years later, R.C.'s 17-year-

Table 1
Media-Reported Deaths of Young Black Athletes

Name of Athlete	Age	Year	Sport
Edward D. Bell	16	1975	Football
George W. Stewart	20	1975	Football
Stanley Neal	16	1979	Football
Isam Maynard	–	1979	Football
James Barber	16	1979	Football
Jim O'Brien	17	1979	Football
J. V. Cain	28	1979	Football
Hayword Harris	–	1980	Football
Greg Pratt	20	1983	Football
Paul Cunningham	–	1983	Football
Kevin Copeland	17	1989	Football
Ellis Files	19	1974	Basketball
Owen Brown	22	1976	Basketball
Eddie Brooks	13	1976	Basketball
Antonio Britt	–	1981	Basketball
Loen Richardson	–	1981	Basketball
Arturo Brown	–	1982	Basketball
Hank Gathers	23	1990	Basketball
Tony Penny	23	1990	Basketball
Weston Hatch	17	1990	Basketball
Ron Copeland	28	1975	Track
Freeman Miller	21	1980	Track
Kimberly Howling	13	1990	Track
Flo Hyman	31	1986	Volleyball

Revised from Reference 24, with permission.

old son, K.C., a stand-out high school football star in Los Angeles, collapsed and died during a football game in which he was participating. Postmortem examination revealed HCM.

In 1980, Maron et al[25] published a report on sudden death in young US athletes, citing HCM as the most common cause. In that retrospective study, approximately 30% of the decedents were African American, but no speculation was entertained about the apparent disproportionate representation of Blacks in this group. In 1988, the first article in the medical literature to suggest that there may be a special problem in Blacks related to SCD and HCM appeared as a three-part special report by Lubell.[26] Hypertensive left ventricular hypertrophy was also cited as a cause of SCD in Blacks who engage in vigorous exercise. A following report in 1990 by Thomas and Cantwell,[27] in the same journal, *The Physician and Sportsmedicine,* contained a series of case reports on SCD occurring in basketball players. There were four cases, all during the same year, and three were found to have HCM on postmortem examination, while a third black player died of an ischemia-related arrhythmia caused by an anomalous coronary artery. The death of the one white athlete was due to arrhythmias associated with severe aortic stenosis and moderately advanced coronary atherosclerosis.

The next study of sports-related SCD was performed by Burke et al[28] in 1991 as a retrospective analysis of 34 young athletes (mean age 24 years). In this group in which individuals were matched for age, sex, and race with a non-sports-related cohort, African Americans had a greater likelihood of dying from HCM than did Whites. Of the 8 cases of HCM, 6 athletes were black and 2 were white (Table 2). Overall, of the 34 exercise-related sudden cardiac deaths, 15 were in Blacks and 19 were in Whites; 3 individuals were female, only 1 of whom, a swimmer, had HCM. In this study, it is of interest that the Blacks whose deaths were exercise related were younger than the Whites (mean ages 23.5 years versus 27.2 years, respectively), and the incidence of HCM was higher in the exercising Blacks, although the incidence of HCM in those Blacks and Whites whose deaths were non-sports–related was similar. This information regarding the differences in SCD between Blacks and Whites with HCM is important: inasmuch as approximately one half of the cases of SCD in young athletes under age 30 that are due to HCM should be genetically influenced in an autosomal dominant manner, equal racial distribution of deaths would be expected. Such a result occurred in the sedentary individuals in this study, but as was observed, the racial distribution was skewed in the exercising group, which showed more Blacks dying from HCM. Does vigorous exercise serve more as a "trigger" for SCD in Blacks with HCM than in Whites? Although the numbers of cases in this study are small, this is

Table 2
Exercise-Related Deaths: Distribution of Race/Sports

Cause of death (n)	Black	White	Sport
Severe atherosclerosis (9)	1	9	Running (5) Other (4)
Hypertrophic cardiomyopathy (8)	6	2	Basketball (7) Swimming (1)
Anomalous coronary arteries (4)	2	2	Basketball (2) Basketball (1) Soccer (1)
Others (13)	6	7	Basketball (5) Running (4) Other (4)

From Reference 28, with permission.

an intriguing question that is posed by the data, and it indicates an area which merits future investigation.

Another study on sudden death in young competitive athletes by Maron et al[29] in 1996, indicated a higher prevalence of HCM in African Americans than in Caucasians. In an analysis of clinical, demographic, and pathologic profiles involving a total of 134 sudden deaths due to cardiovascular causes, HCM, the most common cause of SCD, was found to predominate in Blacks (48%) over Whites (26%). Furthermore, of the 14 individuals with possible HCM (hearts with some morphological features consistent with but not diagnostic of HCM), the 17 persons with anomalous origin of the coronary arteries, and the 6 athletes with ruptured aortic aneurysm, most of the decedents were black. No deaths in Blacks were reported from aortic valve stenosis or arrhythmogenic right ventricular dysplasia. This study may be considered pivotal for two reasons: (1) it is the first one involving a sizeable number of cases to show a grossly disproportionate incidence of SCD in black athletes compared to Whites; and (2) it suggests that the three principle causes of SCD in young athletes (HCM, anomalous coronary arteries, and aortic rupture) occur more commonly in Blacks.

Mueller et al[30] conducted a similar investigation of 160 nontraumatic deaths in high school and college athletes based on data collected by the NCCSIR. These data showed that of 136 athletes whose cause of death could be determined, 78 (57.4%) were white and 52 (38%) were black (Table 3). The racial breakdown for those with HCM roughly paralleled these figures: of 56 athletes with HCM, 33 (59%)

Table 3
Characteristics of 136 High School and College Athletes Experiencing Nontraumatic Sports Death, July 1983–June 1993

Characteristic	Total	Male	Female
Number of athletes	136	124	12
Race-no. (%)			
Caucasian	78 (57.4%)	69 (55.6%)	9 (75%)
African American	52 (38%)	49 (39.5%)	3 (25%)
Hispanic	3 (2.2%)	3 (2.4%)	0
Asian	1 (0.7%)	1 (0.8%)	0
Puerto Rican	1 (0.7%)	1 (0.8%)	0
Native American	1 (0.7%)	1 (0.8%)	0
Activity at time of collapse-no. (%)			
Practice	83 (61%)		
Competition	53 (39%)		

From Reference 30, with permission.

were white and 20 (36%) were black. Although the disparity between the two racial groups regarding HCM and SCD is not as great as in the Maron study cited above, there is still a disproportionate representation of black individuals.

Sudden Cardiac Death in Female Athletes

As previously stated, HCM should be equally distributed among males and females. In the subpopulation of young athletes dying from this disorder before age 30, males have been found to predominate in overwhelming numbers in all studies conducted thus far, in which the genders of the individuals analyzed have been reported. As an example, the study by Burke cited above examined 34 individuals; only 3 (9%) were women, and only 1 of these had HCM (Table 4). In the 1995 report by Van Camp et al[23] in which 160 nontraumatic deaths in college and high school athletes occurring between 1983 and 1993 were analyzed, 146 were males (90%) and 14 were females (10%). The authors also derived an estimated death rate for males and females involved in nontraumatic sports fatalities, and determined that the death rate for high school and college males was 7.47 per million athletes per year, versus 1.44 for females—a more than fivefold higher rate of nontraumatic sports deaths for males ($P<0.0001$). Football was the principle sport involved in the male deaths (67 cases), followed by basketball (37 cases), track (10 cases), and wrestling (9 cases) (Table 5). For females, basketball was the main sport (5 cases) followed by swimming (3 cases) (Table 6).

Cardiovascular causes of death were determined for 100 of the 160 individuals; HCM was the most frequently found cause (51 cases, 51%) (Table 7). Of those with HCM, 50 were male (98%) and only 1 was female (2%). Five additional cases, all males, were classified as probable HCM because they did not meet the strict criteria for this disorder. In the study by Maron et al[29] cited earlier on 134 young competitive athletes with SCD, there were 14 females (10%); only 2 had HCM. Of the 24 cases referred to above, which were collected and analyzed by the author, only 2 were females (10%).

These data concerning the frequency of SCD in women indicate that the death rate for female athletes is about 10% of all cases, and the incidence of HCM in those who expire during competitive sports is 2% to 5%. This shows a vast difference between the sexes in the outcomes of vigorous physical activity. Indeed, the small number of females who die during competitive sports raises the question of whether there should be any great concern for the female athlete's safety during competition. Before a conclusion such as this is reached, however, further investigation and collection of data on women athletes must be accomplished.

Table 4
Causes Of Death, Sports-Versus Non–Sports-Related

	Sports-Related		Non–sports-Related	
n	34	(5%)	656	(95%)
Age (yr, mean)	26		32	
Sex				
Male	31	(91%)	501	(76%)
Female	3	(9%)	155	(24%)
Race				
White	19	(56%)	368	(56%)
Black	15	(44%)	281	(43%)
Asian			7	(1%)
Cause of death	*n*	Percent	*n*	Percent
Severe atherosclerosis (CHD)	9	26	307	47**
Hypertrophic cardiomyopathy	8	24*	20	3.0
Idiopathic LV hypertrophy	3	9	42	6.4
Unknown (tunnel)	6(2)	18	104 (7)	16
Anomalous coronary artery	4	12	8	1.2
Mocarditis	2	6	31	4.5
Right ventricular dysplasia	1	3	0	0
SH with LV hypertrophy	0	0	31	4.7
Aortic dissection	0	0	17	2.6
Cardiac sarcoidosis	0	0	13	2.0
Aortic stenosis	0	0	12	1.8
Floppy mitral valve	0	0	11	1.7
Other	1	3	60	9.1

CHD = Coronary heart disease; LV = left ventricular; SH = systemic hypertension.
*Statistically significant increase over total and age- and sex-matched control whites.
**Statistically significant increase over total blacks, but not with age- and sex-matched controls.
Other differences were not statistically significant. From Reference 28, with permission.

There has been speculation that perhaps females are somehow protected from SCD during intense physical exertion. Pelliccia et al[31] have shown that elite female athletes do not demonstrate significant increases in left ventricular wall thickness, which they found to be within normal limits in their echocardiographic study of 600 highly trained Italian females who were preparing for the Olympic games between 1986 and 1993. In addition, when the measurement for left ventricular cavity dimension and wall thickness in these athletes was compared to

Table 5
Nontraumatic Sports Deaths In Male High School And College Athletes, July 1983–June 1993

Fall Sports		Total Deaths	Estimated Athletes Participating*	Estimated Death Rates per Million Athletes per Year
Cross-Country	High School	3	1,552,413	1.93
	College	1	138,873	7.2
Field Hockey	High School	0	290	0
	College	0	0	0
Football	High School	53	9,449,220	5.61
	College	14	690,219	20.28
Soccer	High School	6	2,108,958	2.85
	College	1	246,085	40.6
Water Polo	High School	0	92,055	0
	College	1	16,175	61.82

Spring Sports		Total Deaths	Estimated Athletes Participating*	Estimated Death Rates per Million Athletes per Year
Baseball	High School	5	4,107,505	1.22
	College	2	389,339	5.14
Golf	High School	0	1,196,635	0
	College	0	112,722	0
Lacrosse	High School	0	180,393	0
	College	1	54,478	18.36
Tennis	High School	1	1,336,764	0.75
	College	0	123,737	0
Track	High School	9	4,296,343	2.09
	College	1	272,263	3.67

Table 5 (continued)

Winter Sports		Total Deaths	Estimated Athletes Participating*	Estimated Death Rates per Million Athletes per Year
Basketball	High School	28	5,112,448	5.48
	College	9	259,364	34.7
Gymnastics	High School	0	50,286	0
	College	0	8,007	
Ice Hockey	High School	1	229,655	4.35
	College	1	43,823	22.82
Swimming	High School	0	832,919	0
	College	1	98,797	10.2
Volleyball	High School	0	140,384	0
	College	0	9,747	0
Wrestling	High School	9	2,397,129	3.75
	College	0	102,388	0

Total		Total Deaths	Estimated Athletes Participating*	Estimated Death Rates per Million Athletes per Year
	High School	115	33,083,397 / 1.9** = 17,412,314	6.60
	College	31	2,566,017 / 1.2** = 2,138,348	14.50
	High School And College	146	19,550,662	7.47

*Athletes counted once for every year of participation and for each sport in which they participated.

**Estimation of the total number of athletes participating in high school and college sports requires division by estimated number of participated in by athletes per year (1.9 for high school athletes and 1.2 for college athletes–see Methods). This estimate is then used to calculate the estimated death rates for the high school, college, and combined high school and college groups.

From Reference 23, with permission.

Table 6
Nontraumatic Sports Deaths In Female High School
And College Athletes, July 1983–June 1993

		Total Deaths	Estimated Athletes Participating*	Estimated Death Rates per Million Athletes per Year
Fall Sports				
Cross country	High School	1	1,023,646	0.98
	College	0	105,953	0
Field hockey	High School	0	491,274	0
	College	0	51,991	0
Football	High School	0	844	0
	College	0	0	–
Soccer	High School	1	1,052,873	0.95
	College	1	84,530	11.83
Water polo	High School	0	9,006	0
	College	0	0	–
Winter Sports				
Basketball	High School	4	3,907,849	1.02
	College	1	213,010	4.69
Gymnastics	High School	0	288,506	0
	College	0	17,043	0
Ice hockey	High School	0	698	0
	College	0	0	–
Swimming	High School	3	852,480	3.52
	College	0	95,277	0
Volleyball	High School	0	2,884,819	0
	College	0	188,317	0
Wrestling	High School	0	1,494	0
	College	0	0	–
Spring Sports				
Golf	High School	0	323,767	0
	College	0	12,547	0
Lacrosse	High School	0	87,167	0
	College	0	29,466	0
Softball	High School	0	2,500,642	0
	College	0	199,629	0
Tennis	High School	0	1,246,627	0
	College	1	108,913	9.18
Track	High School	2	3,312,021	0.60
	College	0	175,321	0

Table 6 (continued)

		Total Deaths	Estimated Athletes Participating*	Estimated Death Rates per Million Athletes per Year
Total	High School	115	18,001,713	
			1.9**	
			9,474,586	1.16
	College	31	1,281,997	
			1.2**	
			1,068,331	2.81
	High School And College	146	10,542,917	1.33

*Athletes counted once for every year of participation and for each sport in which they participated.

**Estimation of the total number of athletes participating in high school and college sports requires division by estimated number of participated in athletes per year (1.9 for high school athletes and 1.2 for college athletes-see Methods). This estimate is then used to calculate the estimated death rates for the high school, college, and combined high school and college groups. From Reference 23, with permission.

those for 738 male athletes, the cavity size and thickness were significantly less in the women than in the men (11% less for the cavity dimensions and 23% less for the wall thickness measurements). It was also noted that left ventricular wall thickness in female athletes was only 6 to 12 mm and thus offered no confusion with the measurements usually seen in HCM. It is therefore easier to differentiate the female athlete's heart, with its physiologic adaptations, from that of an individual with HCM. This is not always the case with males, where there may be overlap in measurement and blurring of distinctions on the echocardiogram.

Some studies have also suggested that the male-female difference in cardiac response to physical training may be a result of androgen-mediated changes in cardiac protein synthesis that affect males.[32] Research in rodents has demonstrated a cardiac "sexual dimorphism" presumably due to testosterone.[33]

One must also consider that woman athletes may have lower death rates because they are less exposed as a group to intense physical exercise and are less involved in competitive sports; this may therefore create a bias in favor of fewer deaths in women as compared to men. At this point, we must acknowledge the fact that there is a vast gender difference in SCD rates, and admit that the reasons for this difference are not completely known. Perhaps the causes will be revealed as research in this fascinating area continues.

Table 7
Causes Of Nontraumatic Sports in Deaths
In High School And College Athletes

Nontraumatic Sports Deaths	Total (N = 136)	Male (N = 124)	Female (N = 12)
Athletes with cardiovascular conditions	100[*,2]	92[*,2]	8
Hypertrophic cardiomyopathy	51[†,3]	50[†,3]	1
Probable hypertrophic cardiomyopathy	5	5	0
Coronary artery anomaly	16[*,†]	14[*,†]	2
Myocarditis	7[4]	7[4]	0
Aortic stenosis	6	6	0
Dilated cardiomyopathy	5	5	0
Atherosclerotic coronary artery disease	3	2	1
Aortic rupture	2	2	0
Cardiomyopathy-nonspecific	2[4]	2[4]	0
Tunnel subaortic stenosis	2[5]	2[5]	0
Coronary artery aneurym	1	0	1
Mitral valve prolapse	1	1	0
Right ventricular cardiomyopathy	1	0	1
Ruptured cerebellar arteriovenous malformation	1	0	1
Subarachnoid hemorrhage	1	0	1
Wolff-Parkinson-White syndrome	1[3]	1[3]	0
Athletes with noncardiovascular conditions	30[*]	27[*]	3
Hyperthermia	13	12	1
Rhabdomyolysis and sickel cell trait	7[*]	6[*]	1
Status asthmaticus	4	3	1
Electrocution due to lightning	3	3	0
Amold-Chiari II malformation	1	1	0
Aspiration-blood-GI bleed	1	1	0
Exercise-induced anaphylaxis	1	1	0
Athletes with cause of death undetermined	7	6	1

[*]One male athlete had a cardiovascular condition (coronary artery anomaly) and a noncardiovascular condition (rhabdomyolysis and sickle cell trait).

[2]Five male athletes had multiple cardiovascular conditions.

[3]One male had hypertrophic cardiomyopathy and Wolff-Parkinson-White syndrome.

[†]Three male athletes had hypertrophic cardiomyopathy and a coronary artery anomaly.

[4]One male athlete had myocarditis and a nonspecific cardiomyopathy.

[5]One male athlete had hypoplasia of the aortic arch associated with tunnel subaortic stenosis.

From Reference 23, with permission.

Conclusions

In regard to young African American athletes, the data presented above indicate that they may be at increased risk of SCD, especially from HCM. This should be taken fully into consideration in all deliberations on the subject of SCD in athletes. Although it is true that not enough is known about the denominator, ie, how many black individuals in competitive athletics or in the general population are at risk, and although there seems to be a preponderance of black athletes involved in certain competitive sports such as basketball and football where the highest number of deaths occur, the evidence suggests that there is a disproportionate impact of SCD upon the subgroup of African American athletes. More data collection will help to clarify this situation, and further research focused on the African American athlete should help to explain why this increased risk exists.

Future iterations of the Bethesda Conference on Cardiovascular Abnormalities in the Athlete[34,35] and of the recommendations from the American Heart Association concerning cardiovascular preparticipation screening of competitive athletes[36] should place greater emphasis on the unusual profile of the black athlete and devise more focused methods of pursuing this mystery.

In regard to gender differences in SCD prevalence, important lessons can be learned through a search for the putative protective mechanism which appears to lower the risk for women of dying from athletic participation. As we learn more about how females avoid SCD, perhaps we will be inclined to reverse the question that Professor Henry Higgins posed in *My Fair Lady:* "Why can't a woman be more like a man?"

References

1. Williams RA (ed). *Textbook of Black-Related Diseases*. New York: McGraw-Hill; 1975:381.
2. Gordon T, Kannel WB. Premature mortality from coronary heart disease. The Framingham Study. *JAMA* 1971;215:1617.
3. Roberts WC, McAllister HA, Ferrans VJ. Sarcoidosis of the heart: A clinicopathologic study of 35 necropsy patients (group I) and review of 78 previously described necropsy patients (group II). *Am J Med* 1977;63:38.
4. Friedman M, Manwaring JH, Rosenman RH, et al. Instantaneous and sudden deaths. Clinical and pathological differentiation in coronary artery disease. *JAMA* 1973;225:1319.
5. Gillum RF. Coronary artery disease in black populations: Mortality and morbidity. *Am Heart J* 1982;104:839–851.
6. Williams RA. Coronary artery disease in blacks. In Hall WD, Saunders E, Shulman NB (eds): *Hypertension in Blacks: Epidemiology, Pathophysiology and Treatment*. Chicago: Year Book Medical Publishers; 1985:71–82.
7. Shapiro S, Weinblatt E, Frank CW, et al. Incidence of coronary heart disease in a population insured for medical care (HIP). *Am J Public Health* 1969;59(suppl 2):1–101.
8. Gillum RF, Liu KC. Coronary heart disease mortality in United States blacks, 1940–1978: Trends and unanswered questions. *Am Heart J* 1984; 108:728–732.
9. Savage DD, Garreson RJ, Castelli WP, et al. Echocardiographic left ventricular hypertrophy in the general population is associated with in-

creased 2-year mortality, independent of standard coronary risk factors—The Framingham study. *AHA Council Cardiovasc Epidemiol Newslett* 1985;37:33.

10. McLenachan JM, Henderson E, Morris KI, et al. Ventricular arrhythmias in patients with hypertensive left ventricular hypertrophy. *N Engl J Med* 1987;317:787.
11. Topol EJ, Traill TA, Fortuin NJ. Hypertensive hypertrophic cardiomyopathy of the elderly. *N Engl J Med* 1985;312:277.
12. Porter GH. Sarcoid heart disease. *N Engl J Med* 1960;263:1350.
13. Kuller L, Lillienfield A, Fisher R. Epidemiological study of sudden and unexpected deaths due to arteriosclerotic heart disease. *Circulation* 1966; 34(6):1056–1068.
14. Keil JE, Loadholt CB, Weinrich MC, et al. Incidence of coronary heart disease in blacks in Charleston, South Carolina. *Am Heart J* 1984;108: 779–786.
15. Hagstrom RM, Federspiel CF, Ho YC. Incidence of myocardial infarction and sudden death from coronary heart disease in Nashville, Tennessee. *Circulation* 1971;44:884–890.
16. Oalmann MC, McGill HL, Strong JP. Cardiovascular mortality in a community: Result of a survey in New Orleans. *Am J Epidemiol* 1971;94:546.
17. Kark JA, Posey DM, Schumacher HR, et al. Sickle-cell trait as risk factor for sudden death in physical training. *N Engl J Med* 1987;317:781–787.
18. Koppes GM, Daley JJ, Coltman CA, et al. Exertion-induced rhabdomyolysis with acute renal failure and disseminated intravascular coagulation in sickle cell trait. *Am J Med* 1977;63:313.
19. Phillips M, Robinovits M, Higgins JR, et al. Sudden cardiac death in Air Force recruits: A 20-year review. *JAMA* 1986;256:2696.
20. Jones SR, Binder RA, Nonowho EM Jr. Sudden death in sickle cell trait. *N Engl J Med* 1970;282:323.
21. Diggs LW. The sickle cell trait in relation to the training and assignment of duties in the Armed Forces. III. Hyposthenuria, hematuria, sudden death, rhabdomyolysis, and acute tubular necrosis. *Aviat Space Environ Med* 1984;55:358.
22. Death of an athlete with sickle cell trait. *Med World News* 1974;15:44.
23. Van Camp SP, Bloor CM, Mueller FO, et al. Nontraumatic sports death in high school and college athletes. *Med Sci Sports Exerc* 1995;27:641–647.
24. Williams RA. Sudden cardiac death in blacks, including black athletes. In Saunders E (ed): *Cardiovascular Diseases in Blacks*. Philadelphia: F.A. Davis Company; 1991; 309.
25. Maron BJ, Roberts WC, McAllister HA, et al. Sudden death in young athletes. *Circulation* 1980;62:218–229.
26. Lubell A. Special report: Blacks and exercise. *Physician Sportsmed* 1988; 16:162.
27. Thomas RJ, Cantwell JD. Sudden death during basketball games. *Physician Sportsmed* 1990;19:75.
28. Burke AP, Farb V, Virmani R, et al. Sports-related and non-sports-related sudden cardiac death in young adults. *Am Heart J* 1991;121:568–575.
29. Maron BJ, Shirani J, Poliac LC, et al. Sudden death in young competitive athletes: Clinical, demographic, and pathological profiles. *JAMA* 1996; 276:199–204.
30. Mueller FO, Cantu RC, Van Camp SP. Catastrophic injuries in high school and college sports. Unpublished monograph, with permission.

31. Pelliccia A, Maron BJ, Calasso F, et al. Athlete's heart in women. Echocardiographic characterization of highly trained elite female athletes. *JAMA* 1996;276:211–215.
32. McGill HC, Anselmo VC, Buchanan JM, et al. The heart is a target for androgen. *Science* 1980;207:775–777.
33. Koenig H, Goldstone A, Lu CY. Testosterone-mediated sexual dimorphism of the rodent heart. *Circ Res* 1982;50:782–787.
34. Mitchell JH, Maron BJ, Epstein SE. 16th Bethesda Conference: Cardiovascular abnormalities in the athlete: Recommendations regarding eligibility for competition. *J Am Coll Cardiol* 1985;6(6):1186–1232.
35. Maron BJ, Mitchell JH. 26th Bethesda Conference: Recommendations for determining eligibility for competition in athletes with cardiovascular abnormalities. *J Am Coll Cardiol* 1994;24(4):845–899.
36. Maron BJ, Thompson PD, Puffer JC, et al. Cardiovascular preparticipation screening of competitive athletes. A statement for health professionals from the Sudden Death Committee (Clinical Cardiology) and Congenital Cardiac Defects Committee (Cardiovascular Disease in the Young), American Heart Association. *Circulation* 1996;94:850–856.

11

Triggers of Sudden Cardiac Death in the Athlete

Geoffrey H. Tofler, MD

Introduction

Episodes of sudden death that occur during physical exercise exert an impact far beyond their numbers. In part, this is because athletes are generally regarded as the most healthy individuals in society. Also, in the eyes of the public, deaths that occur during exercise appear to contradict recommendations regarding the cardioprotective effect of regular physical activity.[1] The case for cardioprotection is based in part on large population studies such as that by Blair and colleagues.[2,3] In an observational cohort study among 32,421 men and women, Blair and colleagues found that low fitness (the lowest quintile of exercise duration on a treadmill) was an independent predictor of mortality both among men (relative risk [RR] 1.52; 95% confidence interval [CI], 1.28 to 1.82) and women (RR 2.10; 95% CI, 1.36 to 3.21).[2] Beneficial physiologic effects, including lower blood pressure and cholesterol levels, reduced platelet aggregability, and improved fibrinolytic activity, have also been associated with regular exercise.[4]

Since sudden cardiac death events typically occur without warning and are often unwitnessed, the rigorous study of their precipitants has been limited. Thus, although anecdotal cases of sudden death at the time of physical exertion have long been recognized, until recently there has been relatively little systematic analysis of triggering activities.

From Estes NAM, Salem DN, Wang PJ (eds). *Sudden Cardiac Death in the Athlete.* Armonk, NY: Futura Publishing Co., Inc.; ©1998.

When considering the triggers of sudden cardiac death in the athlete, it is important to make the distinction between younger athletes (typically <35 years), in whom the underlying substrate is often congenital, and older athletes (>35 years), in whom coronary artery disease is by far the most common underlying condition.[5]

Circadian Variation of Sudden Cardiac Death

The presence of a circadian variation of disease onset supports the role of physical exertion as a trigger of acute cardiovascular disease.[6] The first large study to demonstrate a circadian pattern of sudden cardiac death was a retrospective analysis of deaths that occurred in Massachusetts in 1983.[7] From 26,798 mortality records, 2203 individuals had out-of-hospital sudden cardiac death occurring within 1 hour of symptom onset. The time of death in this population peaked from 9 AM to 11 AM, with a smaller secondary peak from 5 PM to 6 PM (Figure 1).[7] A weakness of this study—its reliance on death certificates for determination of cause and time of death—was addressed in a subsequent analysis of the well-characterized Framingham Heart Study population. Charts of 2458 individuals were reviewed, of whom 264 (11% of the total) fit the definition of sudden cardiac death (unexpected

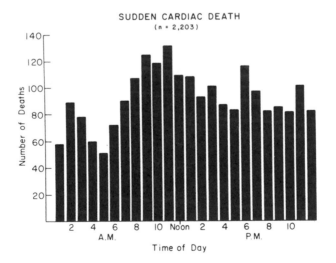

Figure 1. The time of day of out-of-hospital sudden cardiac death for individuals dying in Massachusetts in 1983. A statistically significant ($P<0.001$) circadian rhythm is present with a primary peak between 7 AM and 11 AM and a secondary peak between 5 PM and 6 PM. Reproduced from Reference 7, Circulation, 1987, American Heart Association, with permission.

death within 1 hour from symptom onset).[8] If the exact time of death could not be determined (for example, if an individual was found dead in bed), the probability of death was evenly distributed over the period during which the death could have occurred (for example, between midnight and 6 AM). Even with this assumption, which decreased the likelihood of detection of a morning peak, the frequency of onset of sudden cardiac death was low at night and demonstrated a sharp morning increase between 6 AM and 9 AM. This temporal pattern was present among men and women, as well as among older and younger individuals. In a prospective study, Levine and coworkers[9] found similar results among all patients seen for out-of-hospital cardiac arrests by the City of Houston Emergency Medical Services. Harmonic regression analysis of the 1019 primary cardiac arrests occurring over a 1-year period clearly demonstrated a significant peak in the morning hours between 8 AM and noon. Undoubtedly, part of the increased morning frequency of sudden cardiac death would be secondary to the increased morning risk of myocardial ischemia and infarction. In addition, however, there is abundant evidence of a primary increase in arrhythmia during the morning. For example, in 164 ambulatory patients studied over 3 consecutive days by use of 24-hour Holter monitoring, Canada et al[10] showed that ventricular premature beats have a trough during the night and a peak during daytime hours in parallel with sympathetic nervous system arousal. Twidale and colleagues[11] observed in 68 patients with sustained ventricular tachycardia that the peak incidence of episodes occurred between 10 AM and noon. Recently Gillis and coworkers[12] reported that the circadian pattern of premature beats was absent in patients with prior infarction and severe left ventricular dysfunction as well as in patients receiving β-blocker therapy. Since these subgroups have altered autonomic activity, these data support a role for the autonomic nervous system in the causation of the morning peak of arrhythmias.

Recent data suggest that sudden cardiac death is more closely related to awakening and onset of morning activities than merely time of day. Willich and coworkers[13] identified 101 cases of sudden death in which informants witnessed the event or could provide clear data about it. Adjustment for individual time of awakening demonstrated a relative risk of sudden cardiac death during the 3 hours after awakening of 2.6 (95% CI 1.6, 4.2) compared to the risk at other times of the day.[13]

These data suggest that the onset of morning activities increase the risk of disease onset. For the subjects discussed above for whom the morning was the peak period of risk, the underlying condition in the vast majority of cases was coronary artery disease. In contrast, when Maron and colleagues[14] examined the time of sudden death in young competitive athletes, 63% of deaths occurred between 3 PM and 9 PM, corresponding to the time of main athletic activity. Ciampricotti[15] also found a peak incidence of sudden death of athletic associated sudden deaths in the afternoon.

Physical Activity as a Trigger of Sudden Cardiac Death

Many of the initial studies examining the association of physical activity with sudden cardiac death relied on case series. While they can provide valuable insights into mechanism, these studies are subject to biases including selection bias and lack of control data. To establish that exertion is a trigger of sudden death, it is more powerful to determine that the rate of sudden cardiac death is elevated during periods of exercise compared with periods of rest. This has now been done in several case-control studies. In a population-based evaluation in Rhode Island, the incidence of cardiovascular deaths during jogging was compared with the incidence during sedentary activity.[16] Although only 12 cases of sudden cardiac death during jogging were recorded over a 6-year period, the age-adjusted relative risk was 7, versus the estimated rate during sedentary activities. A study in Seattle compared 133 married men without a history of prior heart disease who died suddenly with a random sample of married men living in the same area.[17] Among men with low levels of regular physical activity (<20 minutes per week), the relative risk of sudden death occurring during jogging was 56. The relative risk was reduced to 4 among those individuals who exercised more than 140 minutes per week. Vouri reported that the risk of sudden cardiac death during cross-country skiing was 4.5 compared with the risk during sedentary activities.[18] In this study, the relative risk of sudden death was greater for strenuous competitive exercise than for nonstrenuous exercise.

These studies, which establish that physical exercise is a trigger for sudden death, particularly among sedentary individuals, are consistent with and are supported by data from nonfatal myocardial infarction. In the 3339 patients that entered into the Thrombolysis in Myocardial Infarction (TIMI II) Trial, moderate or marked physical activity occurred at onset of infarction in 18.5% of the cases.[19] These findings are consistent with the hypothesis that myocardial infarction may be triggered by external factors, because moderate or marked activity would have constituted a proportionately much smaller percentage of the 24-hour day. A limitation of these data—the lack of control information—has been addressed by the case-crossover study design developed by Maclure and Mittleman.[20,21] With use of this study design, the relative risk of infarction following a specific activity can be calculated as the frequency of the activity during a designated hazard period compared with the frequency of the activity during a comparable 2-hour

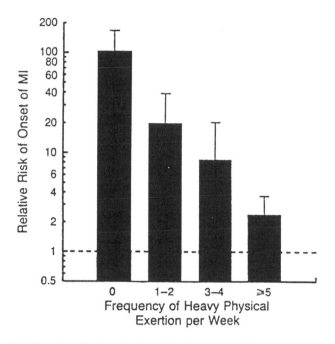

Figure 2. Modification of the relative risk of myocardial infarction by usual frequency of heavy exertion. Reproduced from Reference 21, with permission.

period 24 to 26 hours prior to infarction. Using this method, heavy exertion (estimated to be >6 metabolic equivalents [METS]) produced a 5.4-fold increase in risk (95% CI, 2.6 to 11.1) of infarction in the subsequent 1 hour.[21] The frequency of exercise was an important modifier, such that for sedentary individuals the relative risk was 105, whereas in those who exercised more than five times per week, the relative risk was only doubled (Figure 2). Among athletes under 35 years of age, sudden death during competitive sport or practice sessions is an significant mode of death. Thus, although the absolute risk in any individual is very low, there is a considerable likelihood that a death that occurs in an athlete will occur in relation to sporting activity.

Prodromal Symptoms

To prevent sudden death during athletic activity, it is attractive to speculate that prodromal symptoms can be used to identify subjects at high risk. Northcote and colleagues[22] studied the circumstances surrounding 60 sudden deaths associated with squash playing. Since the mean age of the population was 46 years, coronary artery disease was by far the principle underlying cause—in 51 cases. Forty-five (75%) of those who died had reported prodromal symptoms, the most common of which was chest pain (25%). Increasing fatigue was noted in 12 subjects, excessive breathlessness was noted in 6 subjects. Risk factors were also relatively common; 25 were smokers, 18 had a family history of premature myocardial infarction (<55 years), while 14 had hypertension. In a study of mainly football players in South Africa, Opie[23] also found that prodromal symptoms were common in those who died of sports-related sudden cardiac death. Of 18 individuals who sustained fatal heart attacks either during or after sport, 9 had prior chest pain or pressure, and 4 had complained of tiredness or exhaustion. Denial of prodromal symptoms may also be common in such individuals.[24] Despite the large number of marathon runners recently evaluated by Maron et al, the small number of runners dying with sudden cardiac death (n=4) limited evaluation of prodromal symptoms. None of the four reported prior symptoms.[25]

Psychological Factors

Although the role of mental stress in triggering sudden cardiac death in athletes has not been studied with the rigor of physical exertion, psychological factors appear to play a significant contributory role in many cases of sudden cardiac death; either by triggering the fatal event or by resulting in a delay in responding to premonitory symptoms. Of the 18 heart attacks reported by Opie,[23] psychological factors were thought to have been important in eight sportsmen. For example, one jogger had a heart attack 7 years previously, which he "fought by running" up to 7 miles a day, and he died while running. In one case, a tennis player was club champion and was defending his title against a much younger player. Because he was determined to win, he continued to play despite symptoms, and died shortly afterwards. A champion rugby player had "passed out" in the changing room 3 weeks before he died, but he ignored medical advice not to play again. A referee left the field with chest pain and was advised to go to the hospital immediately, but he insisted on first taking a shower, during which he died. In the Northcote study of squash players, 12 of the 60 subjects were considered to be competitive, ambitious, hard driving, and perfectionist; 13 were thought to be very aggressive; 2 to be very competitive; and 1 to be obsessive about fitness.[22] Acute psychological or emotional stress might have contributed to death in 4 of the 60 cases.

Viral Infection

The role of viral infection as a potentiating factor in sudden cardiac death associated with physical exertion has not been well studied.

In a study of young Finnish conscripts, Koskenvuo[26] identified that in one third of sudden deaths (15 of 45), onset occurred during near-maximal or maximal physical exertion. In 4 of the 15 men, death had occurred soon after vaccination. The authors suggested that strenuous exertion may be risky for up to 2 weeks after vaccination. In the Northcote study, 4 of the 60 subjects had a recent upper respiratory infection.[22] While the role of viral infection in sudden death requires further study, it has been associated with an increase in nonfatal myocardial infarction.[27] Furthermore, the 60% increase in cardiac deaths during winter months may be related in part to viral illness.[28] Infections have been associated with a prothrombotic state.[29]

Absolute Risk of Physical Exertion

The clinical significance of physical exertion as a trigger of infarction can only be determined by consideration of absolute risks for the population and, more specifically, for the individual. Population studies from Seattle and King County (Washington) indicate that 15% of sudden cardiac deaths occur while the victim is engaged in leisure time physical activity. Of these sudden deaths, 6% occur during vigorous exercise, while 9% occur during less intense physical activities such as walking.[17] Because of the large number of sudden deaths per year, 6% represents thousands of potentially preventable deaths. While the total annual number of deaths is large, the risk to the individual is very small. Siscovick and colleagues[17] estimated that the absolute risk of sudden cardiac death during vigorous exercise was 1 per 20,000 exercise sessions per year. The incidence rates of sudden cardiac death among joggers at the Aerobics Institute in Dallas and among marathon runners in South Africa have been reported to be in the range of 3 to 4 per 20,000 joggers or runners per year.[30,31] These data fit with estimates for nonfatal myocardial infarction. If the average hourly risk for a 50-year-old, nonsmoking, nondiabetic male is 1 in 1 million, a sixfold increase in risk will result in a 6 per 1 million risk; still very small.

Nonetheless, since the relative risk is higher in sedentary individuals and the absolute risk is higher in individuals with known cardiovascular disease or risk factors, a medical evaluation and supervised stress test prior to embarking on an exercise program is recommended.

What is a Trigger?

When considering the issue of triggering, it is helpful to consider a trigger to be the final component cause that is sufficient to produce disease onset. A trigger can be readily recognized, particularly when its latent period is short (ie, onset of disease occurs immediately or shortly after the activity).[32] There may be other component causes that are present in a particular individual. One possible schema is described in Figure 3. When considering the mechanism, it is also important to consider the role of extrinsic and intrinsic contributions. Although sudden death is ultimately an electrical event, multiple factors may play a role in its pathogenesis. Figure 4 indicates how heavy physical activity may lead to sudden death. This figure illustrates how a triggering event produces physiologic responses, designated as acute risk factors, that increase myocardial susceptibility to a lethal arrhythmia. For example, acute hemodynamic, hemostatic, and vascular tone changes, as well as neurophysiologic variation may occur.[6] These physiologic responses may lead to sudden death by three pathways. First, in the presence of coronary stenosis, an increase in myocardial oxygen demand or a decrease in oxygen supply may lead to myocardial ischemia and a lowering of the threshold for ventricular arrhythmia. Second, the physiologic responses may act directly on an abnormal and susceptible myocardium or electrical substrate (due to prior infarction, hypertrophy, or electrical abnormalities such as accessory pathways) to decrease the threshold for arrhythmias. Third, in the presence of a vulnerable atherosclerotic plaque, the acute physiologic changes may precipitate plaque injury and thrombosis, causing transient ischemia and reperfusion episodes or myocardial infarction and thereby lowering the threshold for ventricular arrhythmias and sudden death. Onset occurs

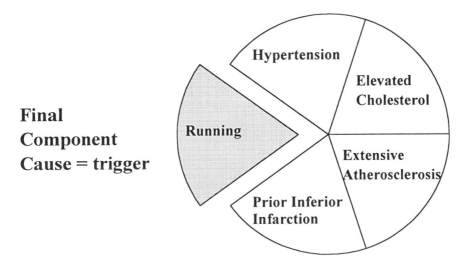

Figure 3. The trigger and component causes that may produce sudden cardiac death in a specific individual. Component causes differ in each individual. See the text for discussion.

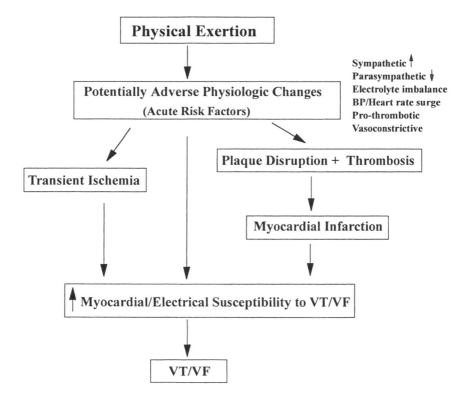

Figure 4. Mechanisms by which physical exertion may trigger sudden cardiac death. VT = ventricular tachycardia; VF = ventricular fibrillation. See the text for a detailed discussion.

when a vulnerable but not necessarily stenotic atherosclerotic plaque disrupts in response to hemodynamic stresses. The extent of pro-thrombotic and vasoconstrictive forces then plays an important role in determining whether the thrombus that forms at the site of a disrupted plaque will completely occlude the lumen of the affected artery. During heavy physical exertion, the sympathetic nervous system is activated and both cardiac output and blood pressure increase. Heavy exertion has been shown to acutely activate platelet function in patients with prior myocardial infarction and in sedentary individuals, but not in healthy volunteers. On the other hand, heavy exertion has been shown to increase fibrinolytic activity. The net effect of these opposing forces on thrombus formation may be important in determining the probability of disease onset. Frequently the mechanism is the same as for myocardial infarction, where plaque rupture and thrombosis occurs, leading to myocardial necrosis and acute electrical instability. Ciampricotti[33] presented an excellent example of acute plaque rupture and thrombosis occurring in an individual following a tennis game. This led to ventricular fibrillation.

In the United States, hypertrophic cardiomyopathy is the most common condition associated with sudden death in young athletes.[14] Although studies have not demonstrated a causal relationship, it is possible that the Valsalva maneuver or epinephrine surges associated with sporting activity may increase subaortic obstruction and predispose to sudden death. In anomalous origin of the coronary artery, vigorous exercise may lead to an alteration of the angle of take off and to ischemia. With vigorous activity, a fall in plasma potassium level and high levels of catecholamines may lower the threshold to ventricular fibrillation. In aortic stenosis, inappropriate vasodilation with exertion may lead to a fall in blood pressure.

While physical exertion has been the principle trigger identified in sports-related sudden death, it is likely that psychological stress plays an important contributing role in many cases. Verrier et al,[34] using a dog model of partial coronary stenosis, demonstrated that exposure to adverse stimuli reduced the threshold for ventricular arrhythmias during ventricular stimulation. Even without direct stimulation of the heart, stress increases the myocardial electrical instability, particularly in the presence of ischemia. Although substantial animal data support the causal association of increased sympathetic drive and sudden death, the clinical evidence is more limited. Engel,[35] reviewing the circumstances of death in 170 individuals, speculated that the common denominator associated with sudden death was emotional arousal (happiness, fear, and anger). Arrhythmias associated with the long QT syndrome further support the link between mental stress, autonomic nervous system, arrhythmias, and sudden death. Syncope or cardiac arrest precipitated by emotional or physical stress is a reported clinical presentation of patients with this syndrome.[36]

Although the exact mechanism by which mental stress leads to arrhythmias and sudden cardiac death is not fully understood, the autonomic nervous system seems to play a major role in this process.[37] Besides surges in catecholamines, it is likely that psychological stress releases substances such as thrombin, thromboxane, and adenosine diphosphate, which enhance platelet aggregation, alter the rheologic properties of the blood, and change both coronary blood flow and the electrical properties of the heart. Autonomic activity may exert its harmful effect by predisposing to arrhythmias (by enhancing baseline and triggered automaticity, reentrant circuits, and hypokalemia) and precipitating ischemia. Evidence suggests that sympathetic hyperactivity increases the risk of life-threatening arrhythmias, especially in the setting of myocardial ischemia, whereas increased vagal activity exerts a protective antifibrillatory effect. Studies in animals show that direct stimulation of the sympathetic nervous system with drugs or electrical probes can evoke ventricular fibrillation and a variety of ventricular arrhythmias. Blockade of sympathetic stimulation with pharmacological or surgical sympathectomy reduces the profibrillatory influence of diverse types of stress or ischemia.[38] In dogs with experimental myocardial infarction, Schwartz et al[39] demonstrated that vagal stimulation initiated shortly after onset of coronary occlusion exerts a protective effect against ventricular fibrillation. The protective effects achieved by β-adrenergic blocking agents, both in experimental and clinical studies, further support the important role of the autonomic nervous system in the genesis of arrhythmias and sudden cardiac death. Heart rate variability (HRV), which provides a measure of sympathetic/parasympathetic balance, is an important and independent predictor of SCD in patients with coronary artery disease.[40] Depressed HRV, representing a depressed cardiac vagal tone, is associated with increased mortality after myocardial infarction. HRV also exhibits a circadian rhythm with the lowest values in the morning.[41] The increased adrenergic tone and the withdrawal of vagal tone in the morning may create an interval with a lower threshold for malignant arrhythmias. Emotional stress may also produce an autonomic imbalance characterized by sympathetic predominance. In a spectral analysis of the HRV obtained during laboratory mental stress, Pagani et al[37] showed an increase in the low-frequency (ie, the sympathetic tone) and a decrease in the high-frequency (ie, the vagal tone) power spectra.

Future Directions

Although physical exertion has been identified as a trigger of sudden death in the athlete, it is largely unknown why the arrhythmia occurs on one particular day as opposed to another day of apparent equal physical exertion. In older individuals, added influences might be progression of atherosclerosis with a greater degree of stenosis, increased plaque vulnerability, or a silent or unrecognized infarction. In younger individuals, a recent clinical or subclinical viral illness, increased psychological stress, drug use or some other cause of endothelial dysfunction, or hypercoagulability may be contributors. Prospective epidemiologic studies will be helpful in unraveling some of these contributing factors. Individuals with implantable cardioverter defibrillators provide an exciting opportunity to study the role of potential triggering activities. A circadian rhythm of defibrillator discharges has been reported paralleling that of sudden cardiac death.[42,43] Genetic studies also provide promise of identification of individuals who may be at increased risk of a stress-related sudden death.

While research from the epidemiologic to the basic molecular level is needed, it is important to stress the value of addressing known risk factors such as cigarette smoking and drug use. Similarly, although studies clearly establish that heavy physical exertion is a trigger of acute cardiovascular disease, a perspective is needed that emphasizes the extremely low risk to the individual subject, and the protective effect of regular exertion. In sedentary individuals, particularly those with cardiac risk factors, a stress test prior to embarking on a fitness program is justified. In certain high-risk subgroups, such as those with coronary heart disease, the use of aspirin and β-blockers is beneficial. Although several studies have demonstrated that β-blockers can prevent sudden death and nonfatal myocardial infarction, the mechanism of the beneficial effect remains to be clearly established. The Beta-Blocker Heart Attack Trial (BHAT) showed that the major reduction in sudden death among those receiving β-blockade occurred during the morning hours of increased adrenergic activity.[44] For prevention, it is important for athletes and their coaches to recognize prodromal symptoms and maintain vigilance for what may be atypical presentations. The often strong psychological overlay and tendency to minimize symptoms must also be addressed. From a public health perspective, recognition of the role of physical exertion as a trigger of sudden death or of acute psychological stress in spectators leads to consideration of the cost-benefit of providing external defibrillators at sporting events.

References

1. NIH consensus development panel on physical activity and cardiovascular health. Physical activity and cardiovascular health. *JAMA* 1996;276: 241–246.
2. Blair SN, Kampert JB, Kohl HW, et al. Influences of cardiorespiratory fitness and other precursors on cardiovascular disease and all-cause mortality in men and women. *JAMA* 1996;276:205–210.
3. Blair SN, Kohl HW, Paffenbarger RS, et al. Physical fitness and all-cause mortality: A prospective study of healthy men and women. *JAMA* 1989; 262:2395–2401.
4. Curfman GD. The health benefits of exercise: A critical reappraisal. *N Engl J Med* 1993;328:574–576.
5. McManus BM, Waller BF, Graboys TB, et al. Exercise and sudden death— Part 1. *Curr Probl Cardiol* 1981;6:1–89.
6. Muller JE, Tofler GH, Stone PH. Circadian variation and triggers of onset of acute cardiovascular disease. *Circulation* 1989;79:733–743.
7. Muller JE, Ludmer PL, Willich SN, et al. Circadian variation in the frequency of sudden cardiac death. *Circulation* 1987;75:131–138.
8. Willich SN, Levy D, Rocco MB, et al. Circadian variation in the incidence of sudden cardiac death in the Framingham Heart Study population. *Am J Cardiol* 1987;60:801–806.
9. Levine RL, Pepe PE, Fromm RE, et al. Prospective evidence of a circadian rhythm for out-of-hospital cardiac arrests. *JAMA* 1992;267:2935–2937.

10. Canada WB, Woodward W, Lee G, et al. Circadian rhythm of hourly ventricular arrhythmia frequency in man. *Angiology* 1983;34:274–282.
11. Twidale N, Taylor S, Hekkle WF, et al. Morning increase in the time of onset of sustained ventricular tachycardia. *Am J Cardiol* 1989;64:1204–1206.
12. Gillis AM, Peters RW, Mitchell LB, et al. Effects of left ventricular dysfunction on the circadian variation of ventricular premature complexes in healed myocardial infarction. *Am J Cardiol* 1992;69:1009–1014.
13. Willich SN, Goldberg RJ, Maclure M, et al. Increased onset of sudden cardiac death in the first three hours after awakening. *Am J Cardiol* 1992;70:65–68.
14. Maron BJ, Shirani J, Poliac LC, et al. Sudden death in young competitive athletes. *JAMA* 1996;276:199–204.
15. Ciampricotti R, El Gamal M, Relik T. Clinical and angiographic findings of patients with acute ischemic syndromes during and after sport. *Am Heart J* 1990;120:1267–1278.
16. Thompson PD, Funk EJ, Carleton RA, Sturner WQ. Incidence of death during jogging in Rhode Island from 1975 through 1980. *JAMA* 1982;247:2535–2538.
17. Siscovick DS, Weiss NS, Fletcher RH, Lasky T. The incidence of primary cardiac arrest during vigorous exercise. *N Engl J Med* 1984;311:874–877.
18. Vouri I. The cardiovascular risks of physical activity. *Acta Med Scand Supp* 1984;711:205–214.
19. Tofler GH, Muller JE, Stone PH, et al. Modifiers of timing and possible triggers of acute myocardial infarction in the TIMI II population. *J Am Coll Cardiol* 1992;20:1049–1055.
20. Maclure M. The case-crossover design: A method for studying transient effects on the risk of acute events. *Am J Epidemiol* 1991;133:144–153.
21. Mittleman MA, Maclure M, Tofler GH, et al. Triggering of acute myocardial infarction by heavy physical exertion. Protection against triggering by regular exertion. Determinants of myocardial infarction onset study investigators. *N Engl J Med* 1993;329:1677–1683.
22. Northcote RJ, Flannigan C, Ballantyne D. Sudden death and vigorous exercise—a study of 60 deaths associated with squash. *Br Heart J* 1986;55:198–203.
23. Opie LH. Sudden death and sport. *Lancet* 1975;1:263–266.
24. Northcote RJ, Evans ADB, Ballantyne D. Sudden death in squash players *Lancet* 1984;1:148–151.
25. Maron BJ, Poliac LC, Roberts, WO. Risk for sudden cardiac death associated with marathon running. *J Am Coll Cardiol* 1996;28:428–431.
26. Koskenvuo K. Sudden death among Finnish conscripts. *Br Med J* 1976;2:1413–1415.
27. Ruben FL. Prevention and control of influenza. *Am J Med* 1987;82(suppl 6A):31–34.
28. Ornato JP, Siegel L, Craren EJ, Nelson N. Increased incidence of cardiac death attributed to acute myocardial infarction during winter. *Coron Artery Dis* 1990;1:199–203.
29. Stout RW, Crawford V. Seasonal variation in fibrinogen concentrations among elderly people. *Lancet* 1991;338:9–13.
30. Gibbons LW, Cooper KH, Meyer BM, et al. The acute cardiac risk of strenuous exercise. *JAMA* 1980;244:1799–1801.
31. Noakes TD, Opie LH, Rose AG. Marathon running and immunity to coronary heart disease: Fact versus fiction. *Clin Sports Med* 1984;3:527–543.

32. Rothman KJ. Induction and latent periods. *Am J Epidemiol* 1981;114: 253–259.
33. Ciampricotti R, El Gamal M. Recurrent myocardial infarction and sudden death after sport. *Am Heart J* 1989;117:188–191.
34. Verrier RL, Hagestad EL, Lown B. Delayed myocardial ischemia induced by anger. *Circulation* 1987;75:249–254.
35. Engel GL. Sudden and rapid death during psychological stress: Folklore or folk wisdom? *Ann Intern Med* 1971;74:771–782.
36. Schwartz PJ, Zaza A, Locati E, Moss AJ. Stress and sudden death: The case of the long QT syndrome. *Circulation* 1991;83(suppl II):70–80.
37. Pagani M, Mazzuero G, Ferrari A, et al. Sympathovagal interaction during mental stress: A study using spectral analysis of heart rate variability in healthy control subjects and patients with a prior myocardial infarction. *Circulation* 1991;83(suppl II):43–51.
38. Verrier RL, Lown B. Effects of left stellectomy on enhanced cardiac vulnerability induced by psychological stress. *Circulation* 1977;56(suppl III):80–88.
39. Schwartz PJ, La Rovere MT, Vanoli E. Autonomic nervous system and sudden cardiac death: Experimental basis and clinical observations for post-myocardial infarction risk stratification. *Circulation* 1992;85(suppl I): 77–91.
40. Kleiger RE, Miller JP, Bogger JT, Moss AJ, and the Multicenter Post-Infarction Research Group. Decreased heart rate variability and its association with increased mortality after acute myocardial infarction. *Am J Cardiol* 1987;59:256–262.
41. Huikuri HV, Linnaluoto MK, Seppanen T, et al. Circadian rhythm of heart rate variability in survivors of cardiac arrest. *Am J Cardiol* 1992;70: 610–615.
42. Lampert R, Rosenfeld L, Batsford W, et al. Circadian variation of sustained ventricular tachycardia in patients with coronary artery disease and implantable cardioverter-defibrillators. *Circulation* 1994;90:241–247.
43. Tofler GH, Gebara OCE, Mittleman MA, et al. Morning peak in ventricular tachyarrhythmias detected by time of implantable cardioverter/defibrillator therapy. *Circulation* 1995;92:1203–1208.
44. Peters RW, Muller JE, Goldstein S, et al. Propranolol and the morning increase in the frequency of sudden cardiac death (BHAT Study). *Am J Cardiol* 1989;63:1518–1520.

Part III

Arrhythmias in the Athlete:
Evaluation and Management

12

The Approach to the Athlete with Wolff-Parkinson-White Syndrome:

Risk of Sudden Cardiac Death

Andrew D. Krahn, MD, FRCPC, FACC,
George J. Klein, MD, FRCPC, FACC, and
Raymond Yee, MD, FRCPC, FACC

Introduction

In 1930 Wolff, Parkinson, and White first described young healthy individuals prone to paroxysmal tachycardia, whose resting electrocardiogram (ECG) showed a shortened PR interval with widening of the QRS complex (Wolff-Parkinson-White syndrome [WPW]).[1] The shortening of the PR interval associated with a slurred upstroke of the QRS complex (delta wave) was originally described in a case report by Wilson[2] 15 years previously. Since that time, knowledge of WPW has grown substantially and now includes a pathologic description of the accessory pathway responsible for the electrocardiographic manifestations, an appreciation of the classic atrioventricular (AV) accessory pathway and its variants, and the development of invasive techniques used to induce arrhythmias and characterize and eliminate the accessory pathway.

From Estes NAM, Salem DN, Wang PJ (eds). *Sudden Cardiac Death in the Athlete.*
Armonk, NY: Futura Publishing Co., Inc.; ©1998.

WPW in an athlete may present with a broad range of symptoms, from the asymptomatic athlete with preexcitation on a routine ECG to the athlete resuscitated from a cardiac arrest. This broad spectrum of presentations warrants different intensities of investigation and therapy based on their risk and benefit. The decision to intervene with pharmacological therapy or potentially curative radiofrequency catheter ablation is based on assessment of clinical presentation, the perceived risk of sudden death in the athlete, and an estimate of risk of morbidity and mortality from the proposed intervention.

What is an Athlete?

Recent years have seen heightened public awareness of arrhythmias in prominent professional athletes. Although the term *athlete* brings these high-visibility individuals to mind, the term includes a broad spectrum of abilities with varying frequency and intensity of physical activity. There is a commonly held belief that sudden death or life-threatening arrhythmias are more common in athletes, and that strenuous exercise will enhance the probability of events. Anecdotal reports have clearly linked fatal arrhythmias to physical activity in a small number of individuals. In WPW patients, this concern is understandable since exercise is associated with an increased adrenergic state which is known to shorten refractoriness in the accessory pathway and which may increase atrial and ventricular irritability.[3–5] Although exercise may trigger arrhythmias or nonarrhythmic fatal events in older athletes with structural heart disease, there is little evidence to support this belief in young patients with structurally normal hearts. Since there is no evidence per se that exercise increases the frequency or severity of symptoms in WPW, there is little practical difference between the approach to the "athletic" and the "nonathletic" WPW patient.

Clinical Presentation

The athlete with preexcitation may present in 1 of 5 ways (Table 1). Recent heightened awareness of risk for sudden death in athletes has increased the intensity of surveillance for the potential substrate for arrhythmias. A routine ECG may demonstrate preexcitation in an asymptomatic athlete (Figure 1). The athlete may also present with paroxysmal tachycardia symptoms (which may or may not be documented by ECG) with preexcitation noted on a routine ECG. Symptoms are usually caused by atrioventricular reentrant tachycardia (AVRT) (see below). Syncope or presyncope may also occur, with or without reported palpitations, with preexcitation on the resting ECG. Tachycardia symp-

Table 1
Clinical Presentations in Wolff-Parkinson-White Syndrome

Presentation
Asymptomatic athlete with preexcitation on routine electrocardiogram
Paroxysmal tachycardia symptoms with preexcitation on electrocardiogram
Syncope with preexcitation on routine electrocardiogram
Irregular palpitations with atrial fibrillation on electrocardiogram
Ventricular fibrillation arrest

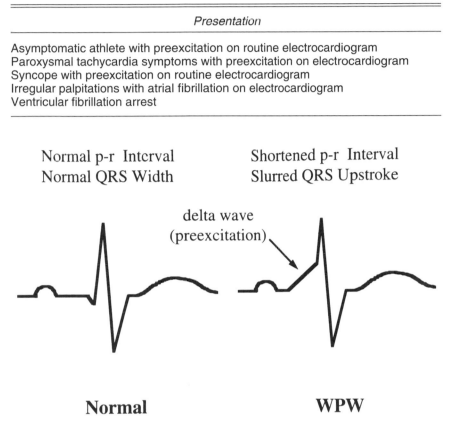

Figure 1. Schematic drawing of the normal electrocardiogram (left) and the classic electrocardiographic findings or preexcitation seen in Wolff-Parkinson-White syndrome (WPW). Note the shortened PR interval and the widened QRS complex resulting from a slurred upstroke (delta wave).

toms may be described as irregular palpitations with documented atrial fibrillation with a preexcited QRS complex. Finally, WPW may present after resuscitation from hemodynamically significant preexcited atrial fibrillation or a ventricular fibrillation (VF) arrest.

Arrhythmias

Arrhythmias in athletes with the WPW pattern on ECG may be one of two types. The stereotypical presentation is AVRT, a reciprocating tachycardia involving the AV node in one limb and the accessory pathway in the other. The most common variant involves antegrade conduction over the AV node and retrograde conduction over the accessory pathway (termed *orthodromic AVRT;* Figure 2). Much less common is antidromic tachycardia where the activation sequence is reversed, and even less common is tachycardia involving two accessory pathways. The rate of AVRT is typically 150 to 250 bpm. This is usually associated with palpitations and lightheadedness, but is infrequently associated with syncope and is very rarely life threatening.

The second form of arrhythmia involves conduction of an atrial arrhythmia over the accessory pathway (and the AV node). This includes conduction of atrial tachycardia, atrial fibrillation, and atrial flutter. The rate of these tachycardias reflects the rate of the underlying atrial rhythm and the refractory characteristics of the accessory pathway and the AV node. For example, atrial flutter is seldom associated with 1:1 conduction over the normal AV node, but may present with 1:1 conduction over an accessory pathway with rates as high as 350 bpm. This wide-complex regular tachycardia is easily mistaken for monomorphic ventricular tachycardia (Figure 3). Atrial fibrillation may be associated with a very rapid ventricular response if the refractory period of the accessory pathway is short (Figure 4). The rapid ventricular stimulation resulting from preexcited atrial fibrillation may result in degeneration to VF (Figure 5). This is the accepted mechanism by which sudden

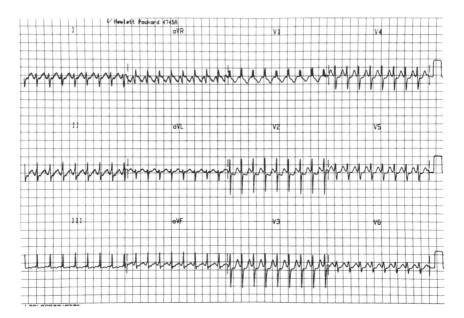

Figure 2. Twelve-lead electrocardiogram of orthodromic atrioventricular reentrant tachycardia.

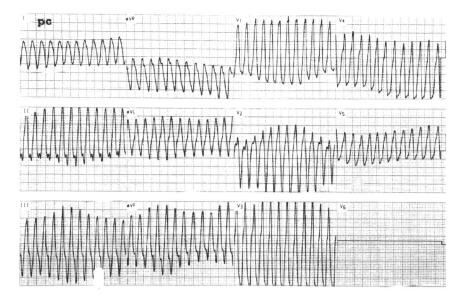

Figure 3. Twelve-lead electrocardiogram of atrial flutter with 1:1 conduction over an accessory pathway.

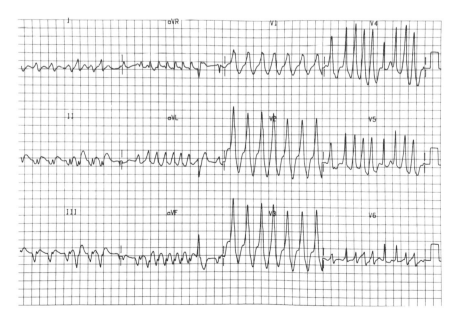

Figure 4. Twelve-lead electrocardiogram of atrial fibrillation demonstrating an irregular ventricular response with variable degrees of preexcitation. The minimum preexcited RR interval seen in the left precordial leads (V$_4$) measured 200 milliseconds.

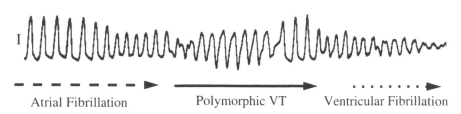

| Atrial Fibrillation | Polymorphic VT | Ventricular Fibrillation |

Figure 5. Rhythm strip of preexcited atrial fibrillation degenerating to polymorphic ventricular tachycardia (VT) and subsequent ventricular fibrillation.

death occurs in patients with WPW. Atrial fibrillation may result from primary atrial pathology or as a secondary tachycardia initiated by AVRT (so-called tachycardia-induced tachycardia). In WPW patients with retrograde conduction only (concealed), AVRT may occur but atrial fibrillation is not conducted anterogradely over the accessory pathway and, hence, is not associated with risk for degeneration to VF and sudden death.

Arrhythmia Substrate

The accessory pathway is an abnormal myocardial connection between the atria and the ventricles that allows conduction from the atrium to the ventricle (anterograde), from the ventricle to the atrium (retrograde), both directions, or neither direction (Figure 6). In WPW with antegrade conduction, the ventricle is activated by fusion over the AV node and over the accessory pathway. This results in early myocardial activation at the site of the accessory pathway insertion, followed by combined His-Purkinje and accessory pathway activation. This process results in the classic electrocardiographic finding of preexcitation with a shortened PR interval and a slurred upstroke to the QRS complex (delta wave) (Figure 7). The location of the accessory pathway can be estimated based on the vector of the delta wave, although the precise location requires accurate intracardiac recordings. When an accessory pathway conducts in the retrograde direction only, it is termed *concealed* because there is no evidence of it on the resting ECG. Discussion of the less common variants of preexcitation involving pathways connecting the atria to various components of the AV node and His-Purkinje system, and connections within the AV node, His-Purkinje system, and ventricular myocardium will not be discussed further in this chapter, but have not generally been linked to sudden death.

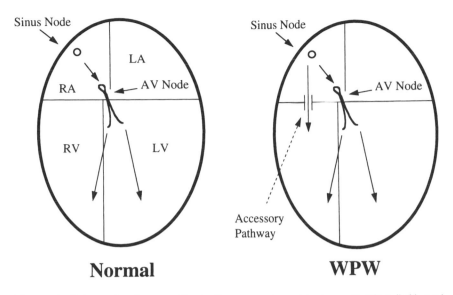

Normal　　　　　　　　**WPW**

Figure 6. Schematic diagram illustrating normal ventricular activation (left) and preexcitation over an accessory pathway in Wolff-Parkinson-White syndrome (WPW) (right). RA = right atrium; LA = left atrium; AV = atrioventricular; RV = right ventricle; LV = left ventricle.

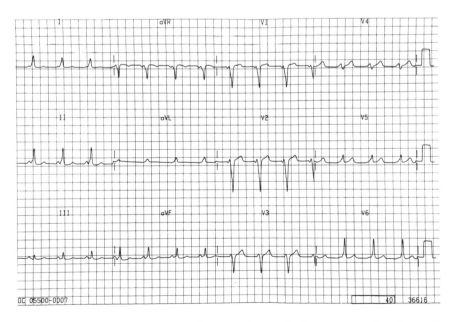

Figure 7. Twelve-lead electrocardiogram demonstrating preexcitation in a 28-year-old male with a right lateral accessory pathway.

Risk of Sudden Death

The risk of sudden death in WPW is difficult to determine. Autopsy series of young individuals with sudden cardiac death suggest a low incidence of WPW (symptomatic or asymptomatic) recognized prior to death.[6] In one series of 29 competitive athletes who died suddenly, none of them were found to have WPW.[7] A second series found pathologic evidence of an accessory pathway in 2 of 17 athletes who died suddenly, although 1 athlete had a "nodoventricular" pathway, the significance of which was speculative.[8] Prior to the era of catheter ablation, the estimated prevalence of WPW was 1.2 to 3.1 cases per 1000.[9–14] This implies that roughly 500,000 Americans have WPW (antegrade preexcitation), suggesting that the overall risk of sudden death is low. Guize et al[10] reported on 151 cases of WPW in a population study of 138,048 subjects, and reported only 1 sudden death in 695 person-years of follow-up. Berkman and Lamb[15] described 128 cases of WPW followed at least 5 years without any reported sudden deaths. Flensted-Jensen et al[16] reported on 47 cases of WPW, 29 of whom had palpitations. The overall mortality compared to a population-wide mortality rate was increased twofold, but none of the deaths were attributed to an arrhythmia. Leitch et al[17] followed 75 asymptomatic WPW patients for a median of 4.3 years. There were no sudden deaths in 348 patient-years of follow-up. In 19 men with preexcitation noted on ECG who were part of a cohort of 3983 pilots followed over a 40-year period in the Manitoba Follow-up Study, sudden death that may have been attributed to WPW was not seen during 28 ± 4 years of follow-up after preexcitation was noted.[14] Although the number of cases is small, the duration of follow-up is consistent with a low risk for sudden death. Thus the overall risk of sudden death in a population of WPW patients is likely to be very low.

The population-based approach to assessing risk suggests that the overall risk of sudden death in WPW is low. Although this approach is useful for estimating risk, it can be difficult to apply to individual athletes who are concerned about the safety of ongoing participation, particularly those athletes with an unusually high intensity of exercise. In addition, clinical judgment can be influenced by the public prominence of the athlete and the attendant pressure to manage the athlete's accessory pathway aggressively. By examining the issue from another perspective, several authors have characterized patients with WPW presenting with hemodynamically unstable preexcited atrial fibrillation or VF.[4,18,19] Retrospective data on WPW patients who presented with VF compared to a control population of WPW patients without VF demonstrated that VF patients had a higher prevalence of both AVRT and atrial fibrillation, a shorter minimum preexcited RR interval in atrial fibrillation (SRR Prx AF, often abbreviated SRR; 180 versus 240 mil-

Table 2
Clinical and Investigative Characteristics of High- and Low-Risk
Patients with Wolff-Parkinson-White Syndrome

Low Risk
Intermittent preexcitation on electrocardiogram or ambulatory monitoring
Abrupt loss of preexcitation during exercise testing
Asymptomatic
Single accessory pathway
Accessory pathway antegrade effective refractory period ≥350 ms
Shortest RR interval during atrial fibrillation ≥250 ms

"Higher" Risk*
History of syncope
History of atrial fibrillation and atrioventricular reentrant tachycardia
History of hemodynamically significant atrial fibrillation or resuscitated ventricular fibrillation
Multiple accessory pathways
Accessory pathway antegrade effective refractory period <350 ms
Shortest RR interval during atrial fibrillation <250 ms (<200 ms highest risk)

*The absolute risk remains low, but risk is increased compared to the "low" risk group.

liseconds), a shorter mean RR interval in atrial fibrillation (269 versus 340 milliseconds), and a higher incidence of multiple accessory pathways.[4,18,19] An SRR less than 250 milliseconds was found in all 24 WPW patients with VF in the series by Klein et al,[18] with 19 of the 24 SRRs less than 200 milliseconds versus 26 of 73 non-VF controls. These data suggest that an SRR ≤200 milliseconds is sensitive but not specific. The accessory pathway effective refractory period (ERP) appears to be less useful in differentiating VF patients from others.[4,18] Although the mean ERP was different between groups, there was more overlap of values compared to use of the SRR. As a result of these studies, an SRR Prx AF ≥250 milliseconds is considered a low-risk pathway, ≤200 milliseconds is considered high risk, and values between 200 and 250 milliseconds are considered intermediate. An accessory pathway antegrade ERP ≥350 milliseconds can be used as a marker for low risk , although it is a less than ideal surrogate for the SRR (Table 2).

Investigations

Noninvasive Testing

The resting ECG typically detects preexcitation. Further ECGs or ambulatory monitoring are unlikely to yield further insights into risk.

The one exception to this is the detection of intermittent preexcitation (Figure 8). This finding is related to a poor margin of safety for conduction over the accessory pathway, which implies a long refractory period, a slow ventricular response in atrial fibrillation, and low risk for sudden death.[20] When intermittent conduction is noted, it is important to rule out normalization of the QRS that is not related to conduction failure in the accessory pathway, such as change in autonomic tone resulting in shortening of conduction in the AV node without loss of conduction in the accessory pathway. This finding is more likely when preexcitation is subtle. The QRS will also normalize during junctional rhythms or with junctional extrasystoles, and may normalize after a ventricular ectopic as a result of retrograde penetration into the accessory pathway, resulting in antegrade refractoriness. If these causes of normalization are excluded, intermittent preexcitation implies an extremely low risk for sudden death.

Exercise testing may also be used to assess athletes with WPW. If abrupt loss of the delta wave is seen during exercise, accessory pathway refractoriness can be estimated.[4,20,21] Loss of preexcitation must be abrupt and associated with a change in the pattern of repolarization. Multiple ECG lead monitoring during exercise facilitates detection of loss of preexcitation. Loss of preexcitation during exercise usually implies a low-risk pathway, obviating further investigations in the asymptomatic

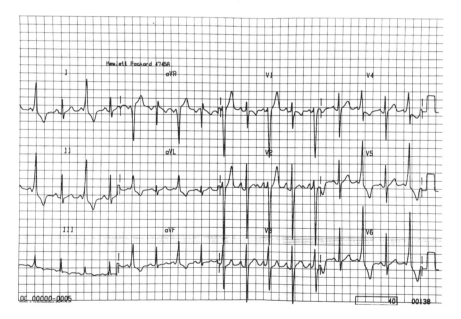

Figure 8. Twelve-lead electrocardiogram demonstrating intermittent preexcitation. Note the alternating normalization of the slurred upstroke of the QRS complex.

athlete. Unfortunately, enhancement of AV node conduction with exercise often results in progressive normalization of the QRS, making conduction over the accessory pathway difficult to assess in most individuals and negating the ability to accurately determine refractoriness.[22]

Pharmacological challenge of accessory pathway conduction with class I antiarrhythmics has been evaluated based on the premise that pathways with short refractory periods will be less affected than those with long refractory periods. Wellens et al[23] found that intravenous procainamide resulted in transient normalization of the preexcited QRS complex. There was a low incidence of QRS normalization in pathways with an ERP less than 270 milliseconds. Boahene et al[24] concluded that the effect of procainamide on accessory pathway conduction was dose-dependent. Loss of preexcitation at lower doses corresponded with a longer ERP. A cutoff point of 550 mg of intravenous procainamide yielded a sensitivity of 60% and a specificity of 89% for identification of patients at low risk (SRR Prx AF >250 milliseconds). Unfortunately, although loss of preexcitation at the extremes of the dose-response curve is obviously useful in determining risk, response in the intermediate doses is not necessarily reassuring. Fananapazir et al[25] found a statistically significant but poor correlation between response to intravenous procainamide and the SRR Prx AF. Preexcitation was lost (suggesting a low-risk pathway) in 33% of patients with an SRR less than 260 milliseconds, including two patients with a history of VF. Fananapazir et al[25] concluded that procainamide infusion was ineffective for identifying patients with WPW who are at risk for sudden death. Noninvasive testing is appealing in asymptomatic athletes with preexcitation, but is seldom used in symptomatic patients, since it represents an imperfect surrogate for induction of arrhythmias and measurement of refractoriness, which are obtained with electrophysiologic (EP) testing.

Electrophysiologic Testing

EP testing involves transvenous insertion of intracardiac catheters that permit measurement of conduction times and performance of programmed stimulation to induce arrhythmias and assess refractoriness. Atrial fibrillation is induced with atrial burst pacing or extrastimuli to assess ventricular response rate and determine the SRR Prx AF. Although the surface ECG provides a rough idea of the location of an accessory pathway, intracardiac electrogram recording is required to accurately locate the accessory pathway.

EP testing is indicated in athletes who present with a cardiac arrest, preexcited atrial fibrillation, or exercise-induced symptoms suggestive of tachycardia. This procedure is currently most often performed in conjunction with catheter ablation of the accessory pathway (see below). EP testing is also indicated in athletes with documented arrhythmias that do not occur during exercise, to determine the nature of the arrhythmia substrate and aid in the decision regarding optimal therapy. The role of EP testing is least clear in asymptomatic athletes with WPW who do not demonstrate abrupt loss of preexcitation during exercise testing. Leitch et al[17] performed EP testing in 75 asymptomatic WPW patients and followed them for a median of 4.3 years. Thirty-one percent of patients had an SRR Prx AF less than 250 milliseconds; it was less than 200 milliseconds in only 11%. There were no sudden deaths in 348 patient-years of follow-up. Leitch et al[17] concluded that EP testing was not useful in asymptomatic patients because the adverse event rate was so low. Despite its apparent poor predictive value in asymptomatic WPW patients, EP testing is often performed when there is a high degree of concern regarding the safety of the accessory pathway, such as in prominent professional athletes.

Pharmacological Therapy

Therapy for athletes with WPW is strongly influenced by the presence or absence of symptoms, the degree of concern on the part of the athlete or physician, and the risk of the proposed therapy. Drug therapy is usually effective but is accompanied by a small risk of worsening arrhythmias, and it may affect the athlete's performance. Since many antiarrhythmic drugs have negative inotropic properties, they may affect the high-performance athlete. In the context of a structurally normal heart (which is usually the case in WPW), class IC drugs such as flecainide or propafenone are usually effective and well tolerated with minimal effect on performance.

Catheter Ablation

Catheter ablation is performed after a diagnostic EP study when a clinical decision is reached to ablate the accessory pathway. The decision to proceed with ablation is based on the balance of the risk and the benefit of the procedure, and it must be tailored to the individual athlete. A deflectable catheter is placed at the site of the accessory pathway and radiofrequency energy is delivered to eliminate the culprit accessory pathway (Figure 9). This technique is effective in 80% to 95% of cases and is influenced by the number and location of accessory pathways and the experience and volume of the center involved.[26] Catheter ablation is associated with a 1% to 3% significant complication rate, including cardiac perforation and tamponade, AV node injury and pacemaker dependence, and pulmonary or systemic embolism, which may permanently affect the athlete's ability to participate.

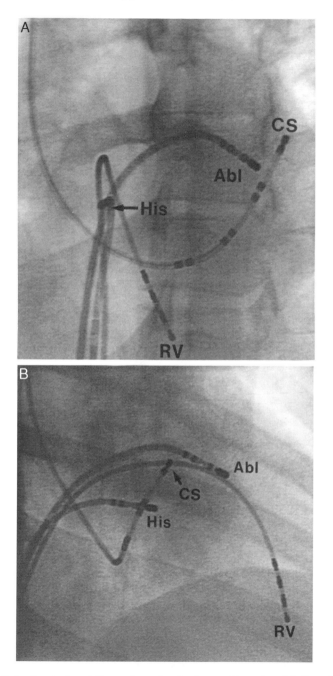

Figure 9. A. Left anterior oblique view of catheter positions for ablation of a left lateral accessory pathway. **B.** Right anterior oblique view of catheter positions for ablation of a left lateral accessory pathway. Abl = ablation catheter; His = His recording catheter; RV = right ventricular catheter; CS = coronary sinus catheter.

The potential complications of ablation are importantly related to the location of the accessory pathway. Right-sided accessory pathways which are not near the interatrial septum are associated with a very low risk of complications, and an attempt at catheter ablation is usually undertaken if there is any concern about the accessory pathway. Left-sided pathways are associated with a small risk of systemic embolism (of greatest concern is cerebrovascular accident), which is probably on the order of 1.5 per 1000.[26] In addition, left-sided ablation is associated with a small risk of aortic or mitral valve injury and coronary or femoral arterial injury. Finally, ablation of septal accessory pathways carries with it the risk of injury to the AV node. In one series of 114 posteroseptal accessory pathway ablations, three patients developed permanent AV block and pacemaker dependence with inferoposterior current application.[27] In all three cases AV block was preceded by junctional tachycardia. Although ablation of midseptal and anteroseptal accessory pathways is associated with a high success rate (80% to 90%),[26] the risk of AV node injury is reportedly on the order of 1% to 5%. A detailed description of the specific techniques used to minimize the risk of AV block is beyond the scope of this chapter. Clearly, an experienced operator with sound clinical judgment is required in this situation, particularly when AV node injury is career threatening to the athlete.

Conclusions

Consideration of WPW in an athlete is not substantially different than that for any other individual. Given all of the information regarding the range of clinical presentations in an athlete with WPW, the low but sporadic risk of sudden death, and the efficacy and risk of medical therapy or curative catheter ablation, the clinician must weigh the various components of the athlete's presentation and advise, diagnose, and treat. There is often more scrutiny of a given treatment strategy because of the belief that exercise may enhance the probability of sudden death, the potential publicity surrounding a high-profile athlete, and the interaction between the physician and regulatory bodies regarding safety of ongoing participation. One approach to this difficult problem is outlined in Figure 10. The symptomatic athlete should be offered curative therapy with catheter ablation. The asymptomatic athlete must weigh the low risk of life-threatening arrhythmia during follow-up with the relatively low but immediate risk of catheter ablation. In some individuals, the balance of career considerations with regulatory bodies and concern regarding the uncertainty of observational follow-up will make it more expedient to proceed with curative catheter ablation.

Athlete with WPW

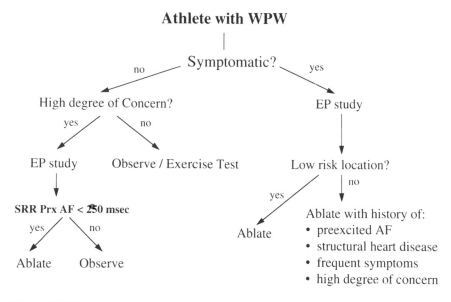

Figure 10. Management algorithm for the athlete with Wolff-Parkinson-White syndrome (WPW). EP = electrophysiology; SRR Prx AF = shortest preexcited RR interval in atrial fibrillation; AF = atrial fibrillation.

References

1. Wolff L, Parkinson J, White PD. Bundle branch block with short P-R interval in healthy young people prone to paroxysmal tachycardia. *Am Heart J* 1930;5:685–704.
2. Wilson FN. A case in which the vagus influenced the form of the ventricular complex of the electrocardiogram. *Arch Intern Med* 1915;16:1008–1027.
3. Gaita F, Giustetto C, Riccardi R, et al. Stress and pharmacologic tests as methods to identify patients with Wolff-Parkinson-White syndrome at risk of sudden death. *Am J Cardiol* 1989;64:487–490.
4. Sharma AD, Yee R, Guiraudon G, Klein GJ. Sensitivity and specificity of invasive and noninvasive testing for risk of sudden death in Wolff-Parkinson-White syndrome. *J Am Coll Cardiol* 1987;10:373–381.
5. Szabo TS, Klein GJ, Sharma AD, et al. Usefulness of isoproterenol during atrial fibrillation in evaluation of asymptomatic Wolff-Parkinson-White pattern. *Am J Cardiol* 1989;63:187–192.
6. Phillips M, Robinowitz M, Higgins JR, et al. Sudden cardiac deaths in air force recruits. A 20 year review. *JAMA* 1986;256(19):2696–2699.
7. Maron BJ, Epstein SE, Roberts WC. Causes of sudden death in competitive athletes. *J Am Coll Cardiol* 1986;7:204–214.
8. Corrado D, Thiene G, Nava A, et al. Sudden death in young competitive athletes: Clinicopathologic correlations in 22 cases. *Am J Med* 1990;89:588–596.
9. Soria R, Guize L, Chretien JM, et al. L'histoire naturelle de 270 cas de syndrome de Wolff Parkinson White dans une enquete de population generale. *Arch Mal Coeur* 1989;82:331–336.

10. Guize L, Soria R, Chaouat JC, et al. Prevalence et evolution du syndrome de Wolff Parkinson White dans une population de 138,048 sujets. *Ann Med Interne* 1985;136:474–478.
11. Sears GA, Manning GW. The Wolff Parkinson White pattern in routine electrocardiography. *Can Med Assoc J* 1962;87:1213–1217.
12. Averill KH, Fosmoe RJ, Lamb LE. Electrocardiographic findings in 67,375 asymptomatic subjects: Wolff Parkinson White syndrome. *Am J Cardiol* 1960;6:108–129.
13. Hiss RG, Lamb LE. Electrocardiographic findings in 122,043 individuals. *Circulation* 1962;25:947–961.
14. Krahn AD, Manfreda J, Tate RB, ᵣ t al. The natural history of electrocardiographic preexcitation in men. *ɪnn Intern Med* 1992;116:456–460.
15. Berkman NL, Lamb LE. The Wolff-Parkinson-White electrocardiogram. A follow-up study of five to twenty-eight years. *N Engl J Med* 1968;278:492–494.
16. Flensted-Jensen E. Wolff-Parkinson-White syndrome. A long-term follow-up of 47 cases. *Acta Med Scand* 1969;186:65–74.
17. Leitch JW, Klein GJ, Yee R, Murdock C. Prognostic value of electrophysiology testing in asymptomatic patients with Wolff-Parkinson-White pattern. *Circulation* 1990;82:1718–1723.
18. Klein GJ, Bashore TM, Sellers TD, et al. Ventricular fibrillation in the Wolff-Parkinson-White syndrome. *N Engl J Med* 1979;301:1080–1085.
19. Teo WS, Klein GJ, Guiraudon GM, et al. Multiple accessory pathways in the Wolff-Parkinson-White syndrome as a risk factor for ventricular fibrillation. *Am J Cardiol* 1991;67:889–891.
20. Klein GJ, Gulamhusein SS. Intermittent preexcitation in the Wolff-Parkinson-White syndrome. *Am J Cardiol* 1983;52:292–296.
21. Levy S, Broustet JP, Clementy J, et al. Syndrome de Wolff-Parkinson-White: Correlations entre l'exploration electrophysiologique et l'effect de l'epreuve d'effort sur l'aspect electrocardiographique de preexcitation. (Wolff-Parkinson-White syndrome: Correlation between the results of electrophysiologic investigation and exercise tolerance testing on the electrical aspect of preexcitation.) *Arch Mal Coeur* 1979;72:634–640.
22. Daubert C, Ollitrault J, Descaves C, et al. Failure of the exercise test to predict the anterograde refractory period of the accessory pathway in Wolff Parkinson White syndrome. *PACE* 1988;II:1130–1138.
23. Wellens HJJ, Braat S, Brugada P, et al. Use of procainamide in patients with the Wolff-Parkinson-White syndrome to disclose a short refractory period of the accessory pathway. *Am J Cardiol* 1982;50:1087–1089.
24. Boahene KA, Klein GJ, Sharma AD, et al. Value of a revised procainamide test in the Wolff-Parkinson-White syndrome. *Am J Cardiol* 1990;65: 195–200.
25. Fananapazir L, Packer DL, German LD, et al. Procainamide infusion test: Inability to identify patients with Wolff Parkinson White syndrome who are potentially at risk for sudden death. *Circulation* 1988;77(6): 1291–1298.
26. Scheinman MM. NASPE survey on catheter ablation. *PACE* 1995;18: 1474–1478.
27. Thakur RK, Klein GJ, Yee R, Krahn AD. The risk of AV nodal block during ablation of posteroseptal accessory pathways. *PACE* 1996;19(II):571.

13

Ventricular Arrhythmias

Mark S. Link, MD and N.A. Mark Estes III, MD

Introduction

Ventricular arrhythmias in the athlete are uncommon and can be associated with a wide spectrum of symptoms. Such arrhythmias can have variable prognostic significance. Although the incidence of sudden death in athletes under the age of 30 years is low, it increases in the older athlete due to the increased prevalence of coronary artery disease (CAD). Although few athletes are electrocardiographically monitored, most of the sudden deaths in athletes are thought to be due to ventricular arrhythmias. These sudden deaths in athletes, as well as those in nonathletes, are usually associated with structural heart disease. The diagnosis and treatment of ventricular arrhythmias in athletes is made more difficult by the rarity of these arrhythmias in this young healthy age group. In addition, major alterations in daily and competitive life are required when the diagnosis of ventricular arrhythmias or structural heart disease is made. In this chapter, the diagnosis and treatment of athletes with ventricular arrhythmias is discussed. This chapter also discusses the evaluation and treatment of athletes with ventricular premature beats and nonsustained and sustained ventricular arrhythmias, sudden death, and the importance of the cardiac substrate in which these arrhythmias occur. Recommendations for participating in competitive athletics are based on the 26th Bethesda Conference on Recommendations for Determining Eligibility for Competition in Athletes with Cardiovascular Abnormalities.[1]

From Estes NAM, Salem DN, Wang PJ (eds). *Sudden Cardiac Death in the Athlete.* Armonk, NY: Futura Publishing Co., Inc.; ©1998.

Incidence and Predisposing Factors

Of the approximately 300,000 sudden deaths that occur in this country, only a small percentage are in the young. It is estimated that 20 to 30 young competitive athletes die suddenly each year. In a review of nine studies on sudden death in young patients including athletes and nonathletes, Liberthson[2] found an incidence of 1.3 to 8.5 deaths in 100,000 patient-years. However, under-reporting may be significant. It is generally thought that most cases of sudden death in the young are due to ventricular arrhythmias. Yet, there is little direct evidence of ventricular arrhythmias causing sudden death, as these young healthy athletes are rarely electrocardiographically monitored at the time of death. In a referred population of 16 athletes who survived cardiac arrest, 2 were found to have the long QT syndrome (LQTS), 5 had Wolff-Parkinson-White syndrome (WPW), 8 had ventricular tachycardia (VT) or ventricular fibrillation (VF), and 1 athlete had atrial fibrillation with heart block.[3] Substantial clinical observations indicate that sudden death is arrhythmic in patients with hypertrophic cardiomyopathy (HCM), arrhythmogenic right ventricular dysplasia (ARVD), idiopathic dilated cardiomyopathy (IDCM), the LQTS, and CAD. However, it is also clear that there may be factors other than ventricular arrhythmias that cause sudden death. In HCM, sudden death has also been reported with supraventricular arrhythmias.[4] In IDCM, sudden death has been reported to be due to bradyarrhythmias or secondary to electromechanical dissociation in up to 50% of patients.[5]

It is unusual for sudden death to occur in the absence of structural heart disease. In 158 young competitive athletes with sudden death, Maron et al[6] found a cardiovascular cause in 134 (85%). Of the 134 athletes with a cardiovascular cause of death, structural heart disease was found in 97%. The most common structural heart disease was HCM (certain in 36%, possible in 10%). Coronary artery anomalies accounted for 24% of the structural heart disease. Aortic stenosis, dilated cardiomyopathy, myocarditis, ARVD, CAD, and congenital heart disease accounted for most of the remaining cases. In Europe, a higher incidence of ARVD is seen. In European series of sudden death in the athlete, ARVD is the most common structural heart disease found.[7] It is not clear why there is a difference in the prevalence of ARVD and HCM in North America and Europe. Ventricular arrhythmias in the setting of congenital heart disease such as Ebstein's anomaly, tetralogy of Fallot, and other stenotic or regurgitant valvular heart disease also indicate a higher risk of life-threatening arrhythmic events in the athlete.[8] IDCM and acute myocarditis are also rare causes of sudden death. In older athletes, CAD is more prevalent and accounts for a higher frequency of sudden death.

The incidence of exercise-induced arrhythmias varies by structural heart disease. In ARVD[9] and right ventricular outflow tract VT[10] arrhythmias are frequently provoked by exertion. In HCM, arrhythmias and sudden death are associated with exertion in approximately half of the patients.[11] In CAD, vigorous exercise is associated with up to a sevenfold risk of sudden death and acute myocardial infarction (Figure 1).[12] However, the long-term benefit of exercise in lowering the risk of sudden cardiac death and myocardial infarction is also well established.[13] In the review of idiopathic VF by Viskin and Belhassen,[14] 15% of the patients had their VF while exercising.[14] In the LQTS, exercise (particularly swimming) has been reported as a trigger for sudden death and syncope.[15] In patients with congenital abnormalities of the coronary arteries, nearly all deaths are associated with exertion.[16]

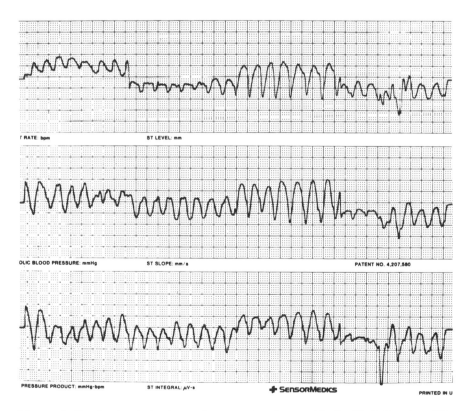

Figure 1. Twelve-lead electrocardiogram showing ventricular fibrillation in a 53-year-old male with coronary artery disease undergoing an exercise tolerance test.

Evaluation of Athletes with Possible
Cardiac Arrhythmias (Table 1)

This section is a discussion of the evaluation of athletes with possible cardiac arrhythmias. This evaluation is not the routine screening that the American Heart Association recommends,[17] but is an evaluation performed because of symptoms in an athlete that may be arrhythmic in origin. The evaluation of athletes is not dissimilar from that of other patients with possible symptoms and signs of arrhythmic disease. The key elements of the evaluation include the symptoms, the presence or absence of structural heart disease, and the family history. As a general rule, the severity of the symptoms is related to the risk of ventricular arrhythmias and sudden death. For example, resuscitated sudden death is more concerning than syncope, which is more con-

Table 1
Evaluation of the Athlete With Ventricular Arrhythmias

Evaluation	Emphasis
History	Symptoms Syncope Family history of sudden death/cardiac disease
Physical exam	Change of murmurs with Valsalva, squatting Marfanoid stature
Electrocardiogram	QT_c in the LQTS Epsilon wave, inverted anterior T waves in ARVD Pseudoinfarct pattern in HCM
Holter/Event monitor	Quantitate arrhythmias Correlative symptoms with arrhythmias
Exercise testing	Exercise-induced symptoms and arrhythmias
Echocardiogram	Assess for HCM RV, LV valvular disease
MRI	If ARVD suspected
Cardiac catheterization	As indicated, consider RV gram
EP evaluation	As indicated, sensitivity lower in patients without CAD

QT_c = corrected QT interval; LQTS = Long QT Syndrome; ARVD = arrhythmogenic right ventricular dysplasia; HCM = hypertrophic cardiomyopathy; RV = right ventricle; LV = left ventricle; EP = electrophysiologic; MRI = magnetic resonance imaging; CAD = coronary artery disease

cerning than presyncope, which is more concerning than palpitations. Sudden onset of syncope or syncope at peak exercise are also more troubling than gradual onset of syncope or syncope that is orthostatic or situational in nature. Injury secondary to syncope is also concerning. Frequent episodes of presyncope and lightheadedness are less likely to be ventricular in origin than occasional episodes of syncope. Those athletes with cardiac symptoms that are worrisome should, at a minimum, receive a resting 12-lead electrocardiogram (ECG) and an echocardiogram. If the athlete is over age 35, an evaluation for cardiac ischemia should also be considered.

An assessment for structural heart disease is of paramount importance in the evaluation of athletes with possible cardiac symptoms. In the absence of structural heart disease there are very few symptoms that are concerning for an increased risk of sudden death. The one clear exception is for those patients with resuscitated sudden death and no structural heart disease. Most other patients who are at risk for sudden death have evidence of structural heart disease that can be diagnosed by an ECG, an echocardiogram, and an exercise stress test in patients over 35 years old.

Also important in the evaluation of athletes is the family medical history. HCM, LQTS, CAD, and even some varieties of ARVD and IDCM are genetic in origin. Therefore, the presence of early sudden death or hereditary cardiac abnormality in the family of an athlete should prompt a thorough cardiac work-up, regardless of the presenting symptoms.

In addition to ECGs, echocardiograms, and exercise tests, 24-hour Holter monitors can be useful in those patients with frequent or reproducible symptoms. Those athletes with intermittent symptoms may be best evaluated with a continuous loop monitor. These monitors continuously record a 1- to 3-minute segment of a surface ECG. Pushing a button on the loop monitor freezes the tape, and therefore the previous few minutes of the event are recorded. In athletes thought to be of high risk, more invasive testing including a cardiac catheterization and an electrophysiologic study (EPS) may be warranted.

The differential diagnosis of a wide complex tachycardia deserves some mention. The three diagnostic possibilities include a supraventricular tachycardia with a preexisting or rate-related conduction block, an arrhythmia involving an accessory pathway (atrioventricular reentry and atrial fibrillation), and an arrhythmia of ventricular origin. Clues pointing to the diagnosis of a supraventricular arrhythmia or an accessory pathway include association of a P wave and the QRS complex, a typical bundle branch pattern or typical WPW pattern, and the absence of structural heart disease. In addition, if the ventricular response is irregular, atrial fibrillation is most often the cause. Clues pointing toward an arrhythmia of ventricular origin include dissociation of the P wave and QRS complex, a QRS duration wider than 150 milliseconds, the presence of fusion beats, and the presence of structural heart disease. Most episodes of wide complex tachycardia are ventricular in origin.[18] When there is doubt, episodes of wide-complex tachycardia are treated as ventricular. Treatment with cardioversion, lidocaine, or procainamide will not harm patients with supraventricular arrhythmias, but treatment of ventricular arrhythmias with verapamil often has dire consequences.[18] Adenosine may prove to be useful in the differential diagnosis of wide-complex tachycardias, but presently it should be used judiciously.[19]

Electrophysiologic Observations (Table 2)

Ventricular stimulation is often performed in patients with symptoms consistent with ventricular arrhythmias or in those patients who survive sudden death and ventricular arrhythmias. However, the interpretation of ventricular stimulation must be taken in context with

Table 2
Value of Programmed Stimulation in Patients With Spontaneous Sustained Ventricular Tachycardia

Condition	Sensitivity	Specificity
Normal Heart	+	+++
HCM	++	++
CAD	++++	++++
Anomalous CAD	−	−
ARVD	+++	+++
LQTS	−	−
IDCM	++	++
Idiopathic LV VT	+++	+++
Idiopathic RV VT	+++	+++

− = no utility; + = poor utility; ++ = fair utility; +++ = good utility; ++++ = excellent utility; HCM = hypertrophic cardiomyopathy; CAD = coronary artery disease; ARVD = arrhythmogenic right ventricular dysplasia; LQTS = Long QT syndrome; IDCM = idiopathic cardiomyopathy; LV = left ventricle; VT = ventricular tachycardia; RV = right ventricle.

other clinical features. In these young patients with a diagnosis other than CAD, especially, the presenting clinical syndrome, spontaneous arrhythmias, and underlying organic heart disease are as important as the results of ventricular stimulation. The method of ventricular stimulation varies from laboratory to laboratory but, as a rule, consists of 1 to 3 extrastimuli given in the right ventricular apex and/or outflow tract at shorter and shorter cycle lengths until refractoriness is observed. These extrastimuli are given in sinus rhythm and after a paced drive train.

There are many factors that relate to sensitivity, specificity, and predictive value of ventricular stimulation. The first and probably most important determinant of sensitivity is the presence of structural heart disease. Ventricular stimulation is of highest sensitivity in patients with CAD. In CAD patients with spontaneous sustained VT, ventricular stimulation provokes VT in up to 95% of patients.[20,21] Of the highest specificity is the induction of sustained monomorphic VT. The induction of VT is rarely seen except in those patients who have previously had VT or whose risk of VT in follow-up is quite high.[21] However, the significance of induced nonsustained VT and VF is less well established. Many authorities claim that the induction of VF is only significant in those patients presenting with a cardiac arrest.[22]

In comparison with patients with CAD, sensitivities and specificities are much lower in patients with HCM, IDCM, ARVD, and congenital heart disease.[23] In the largest series of EPS in HCM patients, 230 patients underwent an EPS evaluation. In these patients, selected only on the basis of a diagnosis of HCM and not presenting with complaints, sustained ventricular arrhythmias were induced in 36%. Polymorphic VT was much more common (3 to 1) than monomorphic VT (Figure 2).[24] Of the patients presenting with sudden death, a ventricular arrhythmia was induced in 66%. Inducibility in patients with asymptomatic HCM was 30%. Inducible ventricular arrhythmias predicted a higher incidence of cardiac arrest in follow-up, especially in those patients presenting with symptoms of impaired consciousness. However, 3 of the 17 patients (all 3 presented with syncope or sudden death) with a subsequent cardiac arrest did not have inducible ventricular arrhythmias.[24] Other investigators have found no difference in the incidence of inducible arrhythmias (22%) in those patients with HCM with and without symptoms of syncope or sudden death.[25] These investigators also found that polymorphic VT or VF was three times as common as monomorphic VT. It appears that EPS in HCM is most useful in patients presenting with syncope or cardiac arrest. However, even if these patients are noninducible, the risk of sudden death remains high, especially in those with previous syncope or sudden death. The use of EPS for screening asymptomatic HCM patients appears to be quite limited.

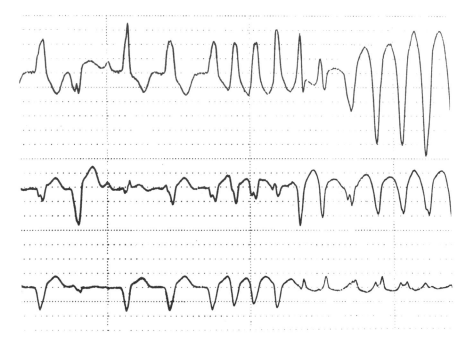

Figure 2. Leads I, II, and V₁ of a 39-year-old male with hypertrophic cardiomyopathy undergoing an electrophysiologic evaluation. With sensed triple extrastimuli the induction of polymorphic ventricular tachycardia, a response commonly seen in patients with hypertrophic cardiomyopathy, is seen. This patient presented with presyncope and had reproducible polymorphic ventricular tachycardia at his electrophysiologic evaluation.

In patients with ARVD presenting with a ventricular arrhythmia, a ventricular arrhythmia can be induced in 70% to 80% (Figure 3).[26,27] In these patients, inducibility at EPS increases the risk of subsequent sudden death.[28] However, the use of EPS in ARVD patients who are asymptomatic is undefined at present.

In patients with no structural heart disease, the sensitivity and specificity of EPS varies depending on the classification of the arrhythmic disorder. Patients with idiopathic right ventricular outflow tract tachycardia (also referred to as repetitive monomorphic VT) are often difficult to induce with ventricular premature stimuli.[10,29] With the addition of isoproterenol and rapid ventricular pacing, ventricular arrhythmias can be induced in 60% to 70% of these patients. It is believed that the mechanism of this tachycardia is triggered activity and not reentry. Conversely, patients with idiopathic left ventricular VT are readily inducible with ventricular stimulation (Figure 4).[30] This tachycardia is usually verapamil-sensitive and thought to be due to

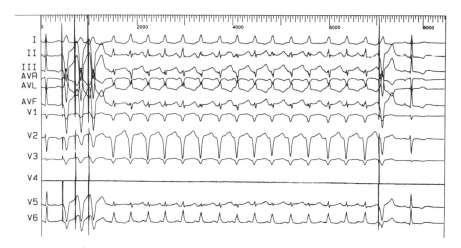

Figure 3. Induction of ventricular tachycardia in a 33-year-old female with arrhythmogenic right ventricular dysplasia. Note the left bundle morphology and the termination of the ventricular tachycardia with a single paced beat. This patient presented with a cardiac arrest during skiing.

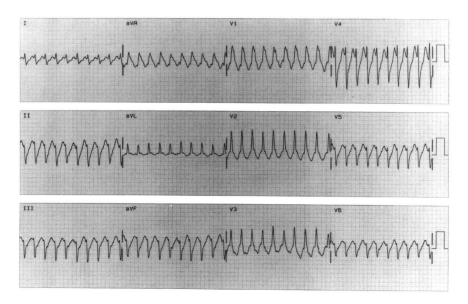

Figure 4. Twelve-lead surface electrocardiogram during electrophysiologic evaluation of a 47-year-old female with idiopathic left ventricular tachycardia. Note the right bundle morphology and inferior axis of the ventricular tachycardia. This patient presented with presyncope for several years. Ventricular tachycardia was found during Holter monitoring.

reentry. In patients with idiopathic VF, ventricular stimulation produces VF or polymorphic VT in 40% to 70%.[14,31,32] In several studies,[25,31,32] even those patients who were noninducible had a high incidence of recurrence. Induced monomorphic VT is rare is this disorder.

In patients with IDCM who present with spontaneous ventricular arrhythmias, ventricular arrhythmias can be induced in 60% to 70%.[33–35] In patients without previous clinical arrhythmias, ventricular arrhythmias can be induced in 10% to 40%[36,37]; however, the predictive value of inducible arrhythmias is poor. In most series, patients without inducible arrhythmias have the same risk of subsequent sudden death as those who are inducible.[33,35,37] In a review of 377 patients with IDCM who were undergoing EPS, noninducibility did not have a strong negative predictive value. These noninducible patients have an incidence of sudden death nearly equal (approximately 70%) to those patients with an induced arrhythmia.[23] As in HCM, EPS in IDCM has a poor predictive value and cannot be relied on to predict future events.

Data on the use of EPS in patients with congenital heart disease are limited. While the occurrence of ventricular arrhythmias and sudden death in patients with repaired tetralogy of Fallot ranges from 1% to 7%, the use of EPS in this situation and with other congenital heart disease is unclear (Figure 5).[38] In patients with the LQTS, programmed electrical stimulation is of very limited value and, currently, is rarely employed.[39] Catecholamine infusions and exercise testing have been used to evaluate those patients with suspected LQTS. In patients with the LQTS, catecholamine infusions and exercise paradoxically increase the QTc interval.[40]

In summary, EPS is a useful tool to evaluate symptoms, prognosticate future events, and guide treatment in athletes with CAD. However, as many athletes with documented ventricular arrhythmias, survived sudden death, or symptoms consistent with cardiac arrhythmias have a diagnosis other than CAD, one can see the limitations of ventricular stimulation in these patients. In these other conditions, EPS is most useful in ARVD and idiopathic VT (either right ventricular outflow tract or idiopathic left VT). It is especially useful in the ablation of VT in patients with no structural heart disease. EPS may also play a role in the prognostication and treatment of patients with HCM and IDCM, but with its limited sensitivity and specificity, the results of EPS in these conditions cannot be used solely to guide treatment. In athletes with congenital heart disease, EPS is also probably useful, but data on EPS in this group are limited. EPS currently plays no role in the LQTS.

EPS is usually indicated for those athletes with resuscitated sudden death. In addition, athletes with syncope and structural heart disease usually undergo EPS. However, the results of EPS in athletes

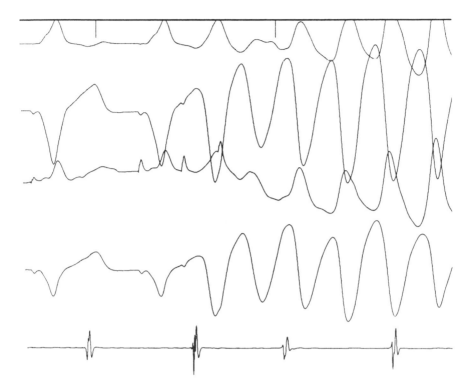

Figure 5. Induction of polymorphic ventricular tachycardia in a 19-year-old football player with corrected transposition of the great arteries and Ebstein's anomaly. This patient presented with syncope and received an implantable cardioverter defibrillator. In 1 year of follow-up, the patient has had one nonsustained arrhythmic event.

without CAD must not be taken in isolation from the clinical event, familial history, and other factors.

Treatment of the Athlete with Ventricular Arrhythmias (Tables 3, 4, and 5)

Treatment options for ventricular arrhythmias include antiarrhythmic agents, ablation, and implantable cardioverter defibrillators (ICDs). Antiarrhythmic drugs are increasingly becoming feared as the potential for proarrhythmia and increased risk of sudden death is being realized.[41] In the young athlete, side effects and the possibility of a lifetime of therapy also limit antiarrhythmic drug use. Currently, very few ventricular tachyarrhythmias are curable and the lifetime risk of sudden cardiac death remains high.

Table 3
Risk Stratification of the Athlete With Ventricular Arrhythmias for Sudden Death

Condition	FMH of SCD	Syncope	>10 VPB/hr	SMVT	LVEF <40%	VT/VF at EPS	Abn SAECG	dec HRV	Bradycardia
Normal Heart									
HCM	✓	✓		✓					
CAD		✓	✓	✓	✓	✓	✓	✓	
Anomalous CAD									
ARVD		✓		✓		✓	✓		
LQTS	✓	✓		✓					✓
IDCM		✓		✓	✓	✓			
Idiopathic LV VT									
Idiopathic RV VT									

HCM = hypertrophic cardiomyopathy; CAD = coronary artery disease; ARVD = arrhythmogenic right ventricular dysplasia; LQTS = Long QT syndrome; IDCM = idiopathic cardiomyopathy; LV = left ventricle; VT = ventricular tachycardia; RV = right ventricle; FMH = family medical history; SCD = sudden cardiac death; VPB = ventricular premature beat; SMVT = sustained monomorphic VT; LVEF = left ventricular ejection fraction; VF = ventricular fibrillation; EPS = electrophysiologic study; SAECG = signal-averaged electrocardiogram; dec = decreased; HRV = heart rate variability; Abn = abnormal.

Table 4

Clinical Features, Treatment Options, and Recommendations for Athletic Participation for Athletes With Ventricular Arrhythmias

Condition	SCD Risk	Electrocardiogram	VT Morphology	Treatment Options	Athletic Competition
Normal Heart	−	N1	RB/LB	AAD RFA	After 3 months
HCM	+	pseudoinfarct	VF RB/LB	BB, AAD Myectomy ICD	Low intensity
CAD	+	Q waves Ischemic changes	VF RB/LB	AAD ICD Surgery	Low intensity
Anomalous CAD	+	N1	VF	CABG	No restriction after CABG, if no inducible ischemia
ARVD	+	T wave inversions RBBB Epsilon wave	LB	AAD RFA ICD	Low intensity
LQTS	+	Long QT$_c$	Torsades de pointes	BB PPM, ICD Sympathectomy	Low intensity
IDCM	+	IVCD LBBB	RB/LB	AAD ICD	Low intensity
Idiopathic LV VT	−	N1	RB/LAD	RFA	After 3 months
Idiopathic RV VT	−	N1	LB/RAD	RFA	After 3 months

Modified for Cardiac Arrhythmias and Electrophysiologic Observations in the Athlete, in *The Athlete and Heart Disease*. Edited by RA Williams. Lippincott-Raven: In press. For abbreviations see Table 3. In addition, N1 = normal; RB = right bundle; LB = left bundle; AAD = antiarrhythmic drugs; RFA = radiofrequency ablation; BB = beta-blocking agents; ICD = implantable cardioverter def brillator; CABG = coronary artery bypass surgery; PPM = permanent pacemaker; IVCD = intraventricular conduction delay; LBBB = left bundle branch block; LAD = left axis deviation; RAD = right axis deviation.

Table 5
Clinical Features, Treatment Options, Recommendations for
Athletic Participation for Athletes with Ventricular Arrhythmias

Arrhythmia	Symptoms	Treatment Options*	Athletic Competition
VPB	None Palpitations Fatigue Presyncope	No therapy Reassurance BB AAD	No restrictions
NSVT	None Palpitations Fatigue Presyncope Syncope	No therapy Reassurance BB AAD	No SHD-No restrictions SHD-low intensity
Sustained VT/VF	Palpitations Syncope Sudden death	No SHD-RFA SHD-AAD, ICD	No restrictions if RFA and no SHD Otherwise, low intensity

*Individualized decision based on symptoms, SHD, and risk stratification. For abbreviations see Tables 3 and 4; in addition SHD = structural heart disease.

The risk of sudden death is low for those patients with no underlying heart disease and idiopathic left VT or right ventricular outflow tract VT.[42] In these patients without structural heart disease, cure rates with radiofrequency ablation approach 90%.[43,44] Thus, radiofrequency ablation is an ideal treatment for the athlete with no structural heart disease and VT. Nonsustained VT and frequent premature ventricular contractions, even if exercise induced, do not increase the risk of subsequent sudden death.[45–47] Athletes who have no structural heart disease and a history of VT that is without recurrence for 6 months (regardless of treatment) are allowed to participate in competitive athletics without restriction.[48]

Those survivors with idiopathic VF, however, have a high incidence of recurrent sudden death.[31] Although there are limited data regarding these patients, the risk of recurrent arrhythmic death appears to be high, even with antiarrhythmic agents.[31,49] Treatment with ICDs in these patients is associated with a high incidence of appropriate ICD shocks and a low mortality rate.[31,50] Therefore, ICD therapy is recommended in patients with idiopathic VF. Competitive athletics in patients with ICDs is limited to low-intensity athletics.[48]

On the other hand, in patients with underlying organic heart disease, cure of the underlying disease and thus of their predisposition to ventricular arrhythmias is unlikely. Catheter ablation in ventricular arrhythmias in the presence of heart disease is currently investigational and cannot be relied on to protect against sudden death.[43] According to the Bethesda Conference, only low-intensity competitive athletics are permitted in athletes with structural heart disease and sustained ventricular arrhythmias, without regard to the method of treatment.[48]

In the athlete with HCM, risk factors for sudden cardiac death include family history of sudden death,[11] presentation with syncope or sudden death,[11,24] and inducible ventricular arrhythmias.[11,24] Spontaneous nonsustained VT as a risk factor for sudden death is controversial and may not be an independent factor.[51,52] Strategies for the treatment of HCM include β-blockers, antiarrhythmic agents, myectomy, permanent pacemakers, and ICDs.[53] Myectomy may decrease the risk of sudden cardiac death, but does not eliminate it.[54] The same can be said of β-blockers, amiodarone, and pacemakers. Indeed, implantation of the ICD is the surest way to prevent sudden cardiac death in the patient with HCM. An ICD should be offered to those athletes with HCM who survive sudden death. For others thought to be at high risk based on family medical history of sudden death or inducible ventricular arrhythmias, an ICD may be appropriate. For patients with a lower risk of sudden death, an ICD is an option but it is not universally agreed upon. Competitive athletics should be prohibited for most individuals with HCM.[55]

ARVD patients with inducible VT at EPS, drug failure during serial testing, irregular antiarrhythmic drug intake, previous cardiac arrest, and presence of late potentials on signal-averaged ECGs are at increased risk for ventricular arrhythmias.[28] Many patients with ARVD meet one of these criteria. Risk factors for sudden cardiac death include presentation with syncope[56] and markedly depressed right ventricular function.[26] Furthermore, ARVD is a progressive disease and the patient's risk of sudden cardiac death may increase with time.[26,57,58] Options for treatment of ARVD include antiarrhythmic agents, ablation, and ICDs; however, as ARVD is a likely progressive disease, treatments effective at one point may become ineffective later in time.[26,57] Radiofrequency ablation is often acutely successful but recurrences of VT are common and sudden death is described.[58–60] Sotalol is thought to be particularly effective in ARVD patients.[61] Current opinions of the optimal treatment for these patients vary, but in those of sufficiently high risk for sudden death, an ICD should be considered.[9,56] Moderate- and high-level competitive athletics are contraindicated in view of the frequent provocation of arrhythmias with exercise.[48]

Although some studies have shown an increased risk of sudden death in IDCM in patients with nonsustained VT and inducible arrhythmias, the most important risk factor is the degree of left ventricular dysfunction.[62] The presence of syncope may also increase the risk of sudden death.[63] In the patient with IDCM, class I antiarrhythmic agents are rarely effective and are possibly toxic. Thus, class I antiarrhythmic agents should generally be avoided. β-blockers are probably effective and should be prescribed to all patients who can tolerate them. Amiodarone may have the highest efficacy of all antiarrhythmic agents for life-threatening ventricular arrhythmias in this condition.[64] However, the optimal place of amiodarone and ICD therapy has yet to be determined (Figure 6).[65] Because angiotensin-converting enzyme (ACE) inhibitors lower the risk of all-cause mortality and possibly even sudden death, they should be given to all patients who can tolerate them.

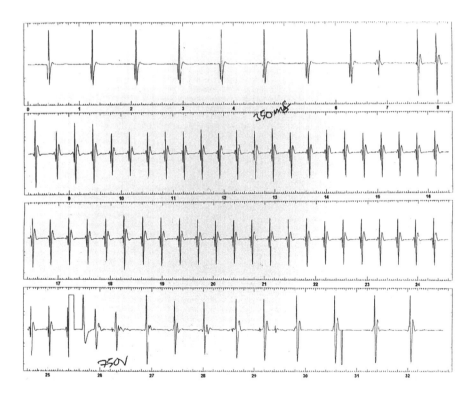

Figure 6. Continuous intracardiac tracing from a 37-year-old male with idiopathic dilated cardiomyopathy and an implantable cardioverter defibrillator (ICD). This tracing demonstrates ventricular tachycardia at a cycle length of 350 milliseconds (170 bpm) initiating in the top right panel. This ventricular tachycardia continues for 17 seconds while the ICD recognizes the rhythm and charges its capacitors. In the lower panel the ventricular tachycardia is terminated by a shock from the defibrillator. This patient presented with syncope but was noninducible at his electrophysiologic evaluation.

Patients with IDCM and spontaneous sustained ventricular arrhythmias should avoid competitive athletics of moderate or high intensity.[48]

Patients with the LQTS are at increased risk of sudden death if there is a family history of sudden death, if they personally have had syncope or sudden cardiac death, or if bradycardia is present (Figure 7).[40,66] β-blockers should be an initial therapy for all patients with the LQTS. Permanent pacemakers should be used when bradycardia

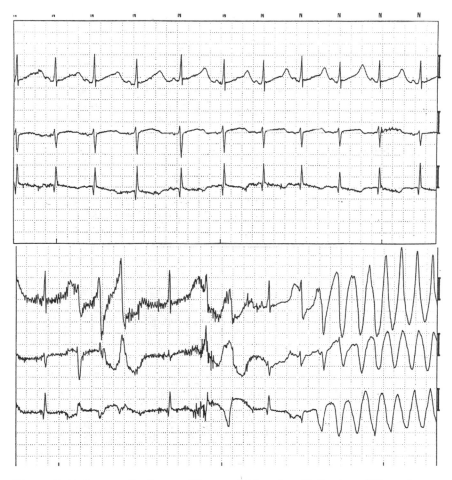

Figure 7. Holter monitor from a 15-year-old female with the long QT syndrome. The upper panel demonstrates markedly abnormal T wave prolongation. In the bottom panel severe bradycardia is followed by the initiation of torsade de pointes. This patient presented with frequent episodes of presyncope and syncope. A Holter monitor and surface electrocardiogram confirmed the diagnosis of the long QT syndrome.

occurs with β-blocker therapy or when symptoms recur with use of β-blockers. More controversial treatments include ganglionectomy and ICD therapy.[15,67]

A number of risk factors for sudden death have been defined for patients with CAD.[41] These include >10 premature ventricular contractions per hour, nonsustained and sustained VT, inducible VT, low left ventricular ejection fraction, abnormal signal-averaged ECG, and decreased heart rate variability. In patients with CAD and ventricular arrhythmias, EPS is more predictive of response to antiarrhythmic therapy. However, even patients made noninducible by an antiarrhythmic agent have a yearly sudden death incidence of 5% to 10%.[41] Class I agents currently have little role in the management of arrhythmias in these patients. Amiodarone has proven to be more effective than conventional agents in the prevention of sudden death. Currently, ICDs may offer the best protection against sudden death. However, whether ICDs or amiodarone prolong life is being tested in three major randomized trials, the results of which are still pending.[68] Ventricular resection of the arrhythmic focus in selected patients with aneurysms and VT is another option with a high incidence of cure and a relatively low mortality.[69] In athletes with CAD and ventricular arrhythmias, only low-intensity competitive athletics are permitted.[48]

There are no clear risk factors for sudden death in anomalous coronary arteries. Most of the deaths that occur with anomalous coronary arteries occur with exertion. Unfortunately, there are rarely warning symptoms of syncope or lightheadedness. If an athlete has been diagnosed with anomalous coronary arteries, surgical therapy should be considered.[8] If revascularization is undertaken and the patient has no inducible myocardial ischemia a return to competitive athletics can be allowed.[8]

In regard to other congenital heart diseases, it is predominantly those patients with tetralogy of Fallot in whom ventricular arrhythmias are seen.[70] The risk of ventricular arrhythmias increases with longer follow-up and may reach 25%.[71] An increased risk of ventricular arrhythmias and sudden death has been reported in those patients with markedly elevated right ventricular pressures and in those patients with an inducible ventricular arrhythmia at EPS.[70] Treatment options for these patients include antiarrhythmic agents, radiofrequency ablation,[72] and the ICD.

Conclusions

The evaluation of athletes with symptoms consistent with ventricular arrhythmias remains a rare but important facet of sports cardiology. The diagnosis of ventricular arrhythmias can frequently end an athletic career. In the evaluation of the athlete, the severity and description of the symptoms are important. Symptoms that are more severe (resuscitated sudden death and syncope) and symptoms that are associated with exertion or injury are more concerning than light-headedness, palpitations, and symptoms that are situational or orthostatic. Athletes who are at risk for sudden death almost universally have structural heart disease. The few exceptions include those athletes with WPW, the LQTS, and idiopathic VF. Electrophysiologic evaluation is especially useful for those athletes with CAD, ARVD, and VT not associated with structural heart disease. Cure of sustained ventricular arrhythmias is presently only possible in those patients with VT and no structural heart disease. The majority of athletes with sustained ventricular arrhythmias are not curable and need more invasive treatment. Thus, in most of these patients, competitive athletics of moderate and high intensity are restricted.

References

1. 26th Bethesda Conference: Recommendations for Determining Eligibility for Competition in Athletes with Cardiovascular Abnormalities. Bethesda, MD. *J Am Coll Cardiol* 1994; Vol. 24.
2. Liberthson RR. Sudden death from cardiac causes in children and young adults. *N Engl J Med* 1996;334:1039–1044.
3. Furlanello F, Bertoldi A, Bettini R, et al. Life threatening tachyarrhythmias in athletes. *PACE* 1992;15:1403–1411.
4. Madariaga A, Carmona JR, Mateas FR, et al. Supraventricular arrhythmia as the cause of sudden death in hypertrophic cardiomyopathy. *Eur Heart J* 1994;15:134–137.
5. Luu M, Stevenson WG, Stevenson LW, et al. Diverse mechanisms of unexpected cardiac arrest in advanced heart failure. *Circulation* 1989;80:1675–1680.
6. Maron BJ, Shirani J, Poliac LC, et al. Sudden death in young competitive athletes: Clinical, demographic, and pathologic profiles. *JAMA* 1996;276:199–204.
7. Corrado D, Thiene G, Nava A, et al. Sudden death in young competitive athletes: Clinicopathologic correlations in 22 cases. *Am J Med* 1990;89:588–596.
8. Graham TP Jr, Bricker JT, James FW, Strong WB. Task force 1: Congenital heart disease. *J Am Coll Cardiol* 1994;24:867–873.
9. Link MS, Wang PJ, Haugh CJ, et al. Arrhythmogenic right ventricular dysplasia: Clinical results with implantable cardioverter defibrillators. *J Intervent Cardiovasc Electrophysiol* 1997;1:41–48.
10. Buxton AE, Waxman HL, Marchlinski FE, et al. Right ventricular tachycardia: Clinical and electrophysiologic characteristics. *Circulation* 1983;68:917–927.
11. Maron BJ, Fananapazir L. Sudden cardiac death in hypertrophic cardiomyopathy. *Circulation* 1992;85(suppl I):I57–I63.
12. Thompson PD. The cardiovascular complications of vigorous physical activity. *Arch Intern Med* 1996;156:2297–2302.

13. Wight JN, Salem D. Sudden cardiac death and the athlete's heart. *Arch Intern Med* 1995;155:1473–1480.
14. Viskin S, Belhassen B. Idiopathic ventricular fibrillation. *Am Heart J* 1990;120:661–671.
15. Roden DM, Lazzara R, Rosen M, et al. Multiple mechanisms in the long-QT syndrome: Current knowledge, gaps, and future directions. *Circulation* 1996;94:1996–2012.
16. Maron BJ. Triggers for sudden cardiac death in the athlete. *Cardiol Clin* 1996;14:195–210.
17. Maron BJ, Thompson PD, Puffer JC, et al. Cardiovascular preparticipation screening of competitive athletes. *Circulation* 1996;94:850–856.
18. Stewart RB, Bardy GH, Greene HL. Wide complex tachycardia: Misdiagnosis and outcome after emergent therapy. *Ann Intern Med* 1986;104:766–771.
19. Sharma AD, Klein GJ, Yee R. Intravenous adenosine triphosphate during wide QRS complex tachycardia: Safety, therapeutic efficacy, and diagnostic utility. *Am J Med* 1990;88:337–343.
20. Brugada P, Green M, Abdollah H, Wellens HJJ. Significance of ventricular arrhythmias initiated by programmed ventricular stimulation: The importance of the type of ventricular arrhythmia induced and the number of premature stimuli required. *Circulation* 1984;69:87–92.
21. Bigger JT, Reiffel JA, Livelli FD, Wang PJ. Sensitivity, specificity, and reproducibility of programmed ventricular stimulation. *Circulation* 1986;73(suppl II):II73–II78.
22. Prystowsky EN. Electrophysiologic-electropharmacologic testing in patients with ventricular arrhythmias. *PACE* 1988;11:225–251.
23. Anderson KP, Mason JW. Clinical value of cardiac electrophysiological studies. In Zipes DP, Jalife J (eds): *Cardiac Electrophysiology*. Philadelphia: W.B. Saunders Co.; 1995:1133–1150.
24. Fananapazir L, Chang AC, Epstein SE, McAreavey D. Prognostic determinants in hypertrophic cardiomyopathy. *Circulation* 1992;86:730–740.
25. Kuck KH, Kunze KP, Nienaber CA, Costard A. Programmed electrical stimulation in hypertrophic cardiomyopathy. Results in patients with and without cardiac arrest or syncope. *Eur Heart J* 1988;9:177–185.
26. Peters S, Reil GH. Risk factors of cardiac arrest in arrhythmogenic right ventricular dysplasia. *Eur Heart J* 1995;16:77–80.
27. Wichter T, Martinez-Rubio A, Kottkamp H, et al. Reproducibility of programmed ventricular stimulation in arrhythmogenic right ventricular dysplasia/cardiomyopathy. *Circulation* 1996;94(suppl 1):1–626.
28. Wichter T, Haverkamp W, Martinez-Rubio A, Borggrefe M. Long-term prognosis and risk-stratification of arrhythmogenic right ventricular dysplasia/cardiomyopathy. *Circulation* 1995;92:I–97. Abstract.
29. Rahilly GT, Prystowsky EN, Zipes DP, et al. Clinical and electrophysiologic findings in patients with repetitive monomorphic ventricular tachycardia and otherwise normal electrocardiogram. *Am J Cardiol* 1982;50:459–468.
30. Ohe T, Shimomura K, Aihara N, et al. Idiopathic sustained left ventricular tachycardia: Clinical and electrophysiologic characteristics. *Circulation* 1988;77:560–568.
31. Wever EF, Hauer RN, Oomen A, et al. Unfavorable outcome in patients with primary electrical disease who survived an episode of ventricular fibrillation. *Circulation* 1993;88:1021–1029.
32. Meissner MD, Lehmann MH, Steinman RT, et al. Ventricular fibrillation

in patients without significant structural heart disease: A multicenter experience with implantable cardioverter-defibrillator therapy. *J Am Coll Cardiol* 1993;21:1406–1412.

33. Milner PG, DiMarco JP, Lerman BB. Electrophysiological evaluation of sustained ventricular tachyarrhythmias in idiopathic dilated cardiomyopathy. *PACE* 1988;11:562–568.

34. Liem LB, Swerdlow CD. Value of electropharmacologic testing in idiopathic dilated cardiomyopathy and sustained ventricular tachyarrhythmias. *Am J Cardiol* 1988;62:611–616.

35. Poll DS, Marchlinski FE, Buxton AE, Josephson ME. Usefulness of programmed stimulation in idiopathic dilated cardiomyopathy. *Am J Cardiol* 1986;58:992–997.

36. Das SK, Morady F, DiCarlo L, et al. Prognostic usefulness of programmed ventricular stimulation in idiopathic dilated cardiomyopathy without symptomatic ventricular arrhythmias. *Am J Cardiol* 1986;58: 998–1000.

37. Turitto G, Ahuja RK, Caref EB, El-Sherif N. Risk stratification for arrhythmic events in patients with nonischemic dilated cardiomyopathy and nonsustained ventricular tachycardia: Role of programmed ventricular stimulation and the signal-averaged electrocardiogram. *J Am Coll Cardiol* 1994;24:1523–1528.

38. Perry JC, Garson A. Arrhythmias following surgery for congenital heart disease. In Zipes DP, Jalife J (eds): *Cardiac Electrophysiology*. Philadelphia: W.B. Saunders Co.; 1995:838–848.

39. Bhandari AK, Shapiro W, Morady F, et al. Electrophysiologic testing in patients with the long QT syndrome. *Circulation* 1985;71:63–71.

40. Jackman WM, Friday KJ, Anderson JL, et al. The long QT syndromes: A critical review, new clinical observations and a unifying hypothesis. *Prog Cardiovasc Dis* 1988;31:115–172.

41. Link MS, Homoud M, Foote CB, et al. Antiarrhythmic drug therapy of ventricular arrhythmias: Current perspectives. *J Cardiovasc Electrophysiol* 1996;7:653–670.

42. Brooks R, Burgess JH. Idiopathic ventricular tachycardia. *Medicine* 1988; 67:271–294.

43. Klein LS, Miles WM. Ablative therapy for ventricular arrhythmias. *Prog Cardiovasc Dis* 1995;37:225–242.

44. Calkins H, Kalbfleisch SJ, El-Atassi R, et al. Relation between efficacy of radiofrequency catheter ablation and site of origin of idiopathic ventricular tachycardia. *Am J Cardiol* 1993;71:827–833.

45. Kennedy HL, Whitlock JA, Sprague MK, et al. Long-term follow-up of asymptomatic healthy subjects with frequent and complex ventricular ectopy. *N Engl J Med* 1985;312:193–197.

46. Busby MJ, Shefrin EA, Fleg JL. Prevalence and long-term significance of exercise-induced frequent or repetitive ventricular ectopic beats in apparently healthy volunteers. *J Am Coll Cardiol* 1989;14:1659–1665.

47. Kinder C, Tamburro P, Kopp D, et al. The clinical significance of nonsustained ventricular tachycardia: Current perspectives. *PACE* 1994;17: 637–664.

48. Zipes DP, Garson A. Task force 6: Arrhythmias. *J Am Coll Cardiol* 1994; 24:892–899.

49. Wellens HJJ, Lemery R, Smeets JL, et al. Sudden arrhythmic death without overt heart disease. *Circulation* 1992;85(suppl I):I92–I97.

50. Tung RT, Shen WK, Hammill SC, Gersh BJ. Idiopathic ventricular fibrillation in out-of-hospital cardiac arrest survivors. *PACE* 1994;17:1405–1412.
51. Spirito P, Rapezzi C, Autore C, et al. Prognosis of asymptomatic patients with hypertrophic cardiomyopathy and nonsustained ventricular tachycardia. *Circulation* 1994;90:2743–2747.
52. McKenna WJ, Sadoul N, Slade AKB, Saumarez RC. The prognostic significance of nonsustained ventricular tachycardia in hypertrophic cardiomyopathy. *Circulation* 1994;90:3115–3117.
53. Wigle ED, Rakowski H, Kimball BP, Williams WG. Hypertrophic cardiomyopathy: Clinical spectrum and treatment. *Circulation* 1995;92:1680–1692.
54. Seiler C, Hess OM, Schoenbeck M, et al. Long-term follow-up of medical versus surgical therapy for hypertrophic cardiomyopathy: A retrospective study. *Circulation* 1991;17:634–642.
55. Maron BJ, Isner JM, McKenna WJ. Task force 3: Hypertrophic cardiomyopathy, myocarditis and other myopericardial diseases and mitral valve prolapse. *J Am Coll Cardiol* 1994;24:880–885.
56. Marcus FI, Fontaine G. Arrhythmogenic right ventricular dysplasia/cardiomyopathy: A review. *PACE* 1995;18:1298–1314.
57. Corrado D, Basso C, Camerini F, et al. Is arrhythmogenic right ventricular dysplasia/cardiomyopathy a progressive heart muscle disease? A multicenter clinico-pathologic study. *Circulation* 1995;92:I–470.
58. Shoda M, Kasanuki H, Ohnishi S, Umemura J. Recurrence of new ventricular tachycardia after successful catheter ablation in patients with an arrhythmogenic right ventricular dysplasia. *Circulation* 1992;86:I–580.
59. Asso A, Farre J, Zayas R, et al. Radiofrequency catheter ablation of ventricular tachycardia in patients with arrhythmogenic right ventricular dysplasia. *J Am Coll Cardiol* 1995;25:315A.
60. Leclercq JF, Chouty F, Cauchemez B, et al. Results of electrical fulguration in arrhythmogenic right ventricular disease. *Am J Cardiol* 1988; 62:220–224.
61. Witcher T, Borggrefe M, Haverkamp W, et al. Efficacy of antiarrhythmic drugs in patients with arrhythmogenic right ventricular disease. *Circulation* 1992;86:29–37.
62. Borggrefe M, Block M, Breithardt G. Identification and management of the high risk patient with dilated cardiomyopathy. *Br Heart J* 1994; 72(suppl):S42–S45.
63. Middlekauff HR, Stevenson WG, Stevenson LW, Saxon LA. Syncope in advanced heart failure: High risk of sudden death regardless of origin of syncope. *J Am Coll Cardiol* 1993;21:110–l 16.
64. Dec GW, Fuster V. Idiopathic dilated cardiomyopathy. *N Engl J Med* 1994; 331:1564–1575.
65. Borggrefe M, Chen X, Martinez-Rubio A, et al. The role of implantable cardioverter defibrillators in dilated cardiomyopathy. *Am Heart J* 1994; 127:1145–1150.
66. Moss AJ. Prolonged QT-interval syndromes. *JAMA* 1986;256:2985–2987.
67. Tan HL, Hou CJY, Lauer MR, Sung RJ. Electrophysiologic mechanisms of the long QT interval syndromes and torsade de pointes. *Ann Intern Med* 1995;122:701–714.
68. Estes NAM III. Clinical strategies for use of the implantable cardioverter defibrillator: The impact of current trials. *PACE* 1996;19:1011–1015.
69. Rastegar H, Link MS, Foote CB, et al. Perioperative and long-term results with mapping-guided subendocardial resection and left ventricular endoaneurysmorrhaphy. *Circulation* 1996;94:1041–1048.

70. Stevenson WG, Klitzner T, Perloff JK. Electrophysiologic abnormalities. In Perloff JK, Child JS (eds): *Congenital Heart Disease in Adults*. Philadelphia: W.B. Saunders; 1991:259–295.
71. Joffe J, Georgakopoulos D, Celermajer DS, et al. Late ventricular arrhythmia is rare after early repair of tetralogy af Fallot. *J Am Coll Cardiol* 1994;23:1146–1150.
72. Goldner BG, Cooper R, Blau W, Cohen TJ. Radiofrequency catheter ablation as a primary therapy for treatment of ventricular tachycardia in a patient after repair of tetralogy of Fallot. *PACE* 1994;17:1441–1446.

Right Ventricular Dysplasia:

Evaluation and Management in Relation to Sports Activities

Frank I. Marcus, MD

Description of the Disease

Arrhythmogenic right ventricular dysplasia (ARVD) is a familial disease in which the free wall of the right ventricle is partially or almost entirely replaced by fat.[1,2] The remaining muscle fibers are interspersed with fatty tissue, providing a substrate for ventricular arrhythmias. The left ventricle is usually not involved but may be minimally or moderately affected. Typically, ARVD occurs in young adults, particularly in men. At least 80% of ARVD patients are diagnosed before age 40. The physical examination is usually not remarkable in young patients. There may be prominence of the left precordium consistent with right ventricular enlargement. A chest x-ray may show minimal cardiac enlargement or, in the advanced stage, marked cardiomegaly.

In young normal individuals the T wave in lead V_1 is usually upright but may be flat; however, it is almost always upright in lead V_2. In patients with ARVD who have symptomatic arrhythmias, the electrocardiogram (ECG) usually shows T wave inversion in leads V_1 and V_2 that can extend to V_6.[3] Of particular importance in screening for ARVD is the observation that there is prolongation of the QRS complex in lead V_1, V_2, or V_3, due to parietal block.[4] In a series of 50 cases of

From Estes NAM, Salem DN, Wang PJ (eds). *Sudden Cardiac Death in the Athlete.* Armonk, NY: Futura Publishing Co., Inc.;©1998.

ARVD compared with an age- and sex-matched control group, the diagnosis of ARVD could be determined by ECG with 84% sensitivity and 100% specificity if the QRS duration in leads V_1, V_2, or V_3 was longer than 110 milliseconds and the T wave was negative in V_2.[4] Peters and colleagues[5] have indicated that a QRS duration ratio V_2+V_3/V_4+V_5 >1.2 is specific for this condition. Young athletes served as controls in this study. These same criteria distinguished patients with ARVD from those with right ventricular outflow tract tachycardia, provided that the QRS R/S transition occurred in V_3 or V_4.[6] Similar results were obtained in patients with incomplete right bundle branch block (RBBB) with T wave inversion in V_1. In patients with complete RBBB who have ARVD, 7 of 11 (64%) had a duration of the QRS complex in V_1, V_2, or V_3 longer by 52 ± 36 milliseconds than that in V_6, consistent with parietal block in addition to RBBB.[7] In six airline pilots with RBBB and no cardiac condition, this difference was 7 ± 10 milliseconds (Figure 1).

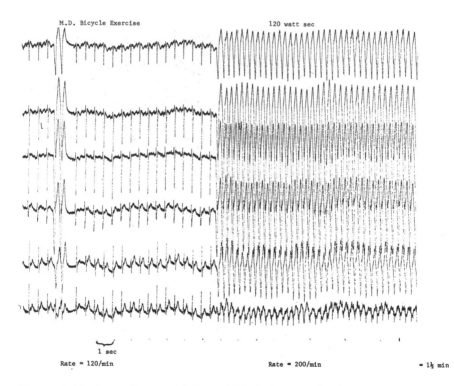

Figure 1. Electrocardiogram, V_1 through V_6 during exercise in a 21-year-old competitive cyclist with arrhythmogenic right ventricular dysplasia. There is one ventricular couplet of left bundle branch block configuration followed by the onset of sustained ventricular tachycardia of the same morphology at a rate of 200 bpm. The paper speed is 10 mm/s.

There are data to indicate that a longer QRS duration in V_1 through V_3 is associated with a greater risk of sudden death.[8,9]

A discreet wave (termed the *epsilon wave*) just beyond the QRS complex, particularly in V_1, may be observed in 5% to 30% of patients with ARVD. This represents potentials of small amplitude due to delayed right ventricular activation. The signal-averaged ECG is positive in approximately 70% of patients with ARVD who have a history of ventricular fibrillation or sustained ventricular tachycardia.[9] There appears to be a correlation of the degree of abnormality of the signal-averaged ECG with the extent of the right ventricular disease.[9,10] The signal-averaged ECG is normal in athletes without heart disease or ventricular arrhythmias.[11] Other noninvasive tests to confirm selective right ventricular enlargement or a decrease in right ventricular function are the echocardiogram, radionuclide angiography, and magnetic resonance imaging (MRI). The latter technique has the advantage of providing tissue characterization in addition to observing right and left ventricular volumes and wall motion abnormalities. It is increasingly being used to aid in the diagnosis of ARVD.[2,12]

The usual clinical presentation of ARVD is that of palpitations, nonsustained ventricular tachycardia, or sustained ventricular tachycardia. Uncommonly, sudden cardiac death may be the first manifestation of this condition.

Sudden Cardiac Death and Arrhythmogenic Right Ventricular Dysplasia

There is a marked variation in the reported incidence of sudden cardiac death due to ARVD. This may be due to study differences in the regional prevalence of the disease. In the Veneto region of Italy, of 60 sudden deaths in patients below age 35, 20% were due to right ventricular dysplasia.[13] None of the patients were diagnosed with this condition before death. In five, sudden death was the first sign of the condition. In seven, there was a history of palpitations or ventricular arrhythmias. Ten of these individuals died during exertion. Of 1000 individuals who died suddenly before age 65 and were examined at autopsy in Lyon, France, 50 cases (5%) had ARVD.[14] None of these 1000 patients had a medical cause of death due to homicide or recreational drug use and none had a history of cardiac disease. In contrast, only 3 of 547 individuals (0.55%) between the ages of 15 and 35 who died suddenly were found to have ARVD in an autopsy series reported from Maryland.[15] This marked difference in the incidence of sudden cardiac death due to ARVD in the various reports cited can be partly explained by the high prevalence of this condition in the Veneto region of Italy, but the 10-fold higher incidence of sudden death due to ARVD between Lyon, France and Maryland is difficult to explain on this basis. It is likely to be related to the lack of recognition of this disease by forensic pathologists. At autopsy, moderate or marked amount of epicardial fat in the free wall of the right ventricle can be normal.[16] In an autopsy study (performed in Olmstead County, MN) of 54 individuals who died suddenly between the ages of 20 and 40, adipose tissue comprising ≥75% of the right ventricular free wall was found in 9 (17%) of these individuals.[17] However, in 6 of the 9, the cause of death was determined to be other than ARVD. The forensic pathologist must differentiate a marked degree of adipose tissue in the free wall of the right ventricle from the fatty replacement of myocardial tissue in right ventricular dysplasia. The gross differentiation must be based on careful examination of diffuse right ventricular enlargement in the absence of left ventricular enlargement and/or aneurysmal bulges in the right ventricular wall. These latter findings can readily be missed unless specifically sought. The histological confirmation requires surviving strands of cardiac myocytes imbedded in fibrous tissue within fat.[18] It is hypothesized that the hearts in patients with right ventricular dysplasia are more susceptible to myocarditis, and it is not uncommon to see evidence of a superimposed myocarditis on the above described histological picture.[2,12]

It has been repeatedly observed that a majority of arrhythmic deaths due to ARVD occur during exertion (Figure 2). For example, in the report by Thiene et al,[13] 10 of the 12 patients with ARVD who died suddenly did so during exertion. These same investigators reported on the frequency of exercise-related sudden death in 182 consecutive individuals under age 35.[19] Eighteen of these 182 sudden deaths were due to ARVD; of these 8 (44%) were related to exercise. The incidence of exercise-related sudden death was significantly greater than that found in individuals who died of other causes, except for individuals who died due to an anomalous coronary artery. Therefore, it should be anticipated that ARVD would be well recognized as a cause of sudden cardiac death in athletes. In fact, this condition was the most common cause (6 of 17 cases) of arrhythmic death in young competitive athletes in the Veneto Region of Italy.[20] In a recent report by Maron,[21] 4 of 134 athletes who died suddenly (3%) had ARVD.[21] In one there was an associated myocarditis and in one there was also involvement of the left ventricle. In addition, it has been found that individuals with ARVD who perform intensive and regular sports activities have symptoms at a younger age and that palpitations, syncope, and sudden death are more frequent in the athletic group than in patients with ARVD who are not athletically inclined.[22] This higher incidence of arrhythmias during exertion may be due to several factors including increased cat-

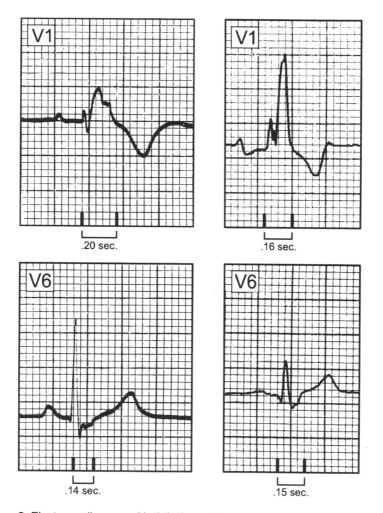

Figure 2. Electrocardiogram with right bundle branch block pattern is shown from a patient with arrhythmogenic right ventricular dysplasia (ARVD) (left) and from a patient with hypertension (right). In the patient with ARVD the difference in the duration of the QRS complex in V_1 and V_6 is 60 ms, while in the other patient it is 10 ms.

echolamines acting on a dilated right ventricle whose fibers are further stretched during exertion. Right ventricular dilatation may be further enhanced during exercise due to the fact that there is less of a decrease of pulmonary resistance than of peripheral vascular resistance.[23] The combination of these factors can result in exercise-induced ventricular tachycardia that can be extremely rapid. Since the rate of the tachycardia can exceed 200 bpm during exertion (Figure 1), it is understandable that ventricular fibrillation may ensue.

Since sudden cardiac death can be due to ARVD in a small but not insignificant number of athletes, how can this entity be detected? One approach may be based on the following observations: in a series of 10 victims with ARVD who died suddenly between the ages of 15 and 35 and who were not diagnosed while alive, ECGs obtained for unknown reasons prior to death showed that 8 had ECG changes.[24] All of the 8 individuals had T wave inversion in the anterior precordial leads, 3 had T wave inversion in V_1 and V_2 and 5 in V_1 through V_3. In 70%, the duration of the QRS complex was >110 milliseconds in the right precordial leads. The same group of investigators found that the majority of individuals with ARVD who died suddenly before age 35 had a history of palpitations, ventricular arrhythmias, or syncope.[13,20] Based on this information, one approach would be to screen athletes for a history of palpitations and/or symptoms suggestive of arrhythmias, such as near syncope. Since this condition is known to be genetic and is transmitted with the pattern of autosomal dominance with variable penetrance, a history of sudden death in immediate family members should be sought. If the individual has a suspicious clinical history, a 12-lead ECG could be obtained to look for T wave inversion in the anterior precordial leads and prolongation of the QRS in the right precordial leads. Further noninvasive investigation could then be performed on this selective population.

There must be increasing awareness of ARVD among pathologists as well as among radiologists who perform MRI examinations. In the former case, education must be directed toward recognition of the pathologic diagnosis of ARVD, and for the latter group, there must be standardization of the technique of MRI as well as its interpretation. This, in part, could be accomplished through educational efforts directed at these specialists. In addition, the natural history of this condition must be elucidated. Additional information on how to counsel family members of those diagnosed with ARVD is needed; particularly, information to help determine whether young family members can safely participate in sports or competitive athletics. Presently, it seems reasonable to suggest that family members who have a normal ECG and do not have nonsustained or sustained ventricular tachycardia on a 24-hour ambulatory ECG and during an exercise stress test can participate in sports. On the other hand, family members who are identified by echocardiogram as having ARVD and who have sustained or nonsustained ventricular tachycardia at rest or with exercise should not be permitted to engage in competitive sports.[25] In fact, their exercise should be markedly limited and treatment should be initiated either with a β-blocker or with sotalol.

ARVD registries were recently established in Europe and in the United States in an attempt to gather information to further answer the many questions that are still unresolved with regard to diagnosis, treatment, and prognosis of this condition.

References

1. Marcus FI, Fontaine GH, Guiraudon G, et al. Right ventricular dysplasia: A report of 24 adult cases. *Circulation* 1982;65:384–398.
2. Marcus FI, Fontaine GH. Arrhythmogenic right ventricular dysplasia/cardiomyopathy: A review. *PACE* 1995;18:1298–1314.
3. Fontaine G, Tsezana R, Lazarus A, et al. Troubles de la repolarisation et de la conduction intraventriculaire dans la dysplasie ventriculaire droite arhythmogene. *Ann Cardiol Angeiol* 1994;43:5–10.
4. Fontaine G, Umemura J, DiDonna P, et al. La duree des complexes QRS dans la dysplasie ventriculaire droite arythmogene. *Ann Cardiol Angeiol* 1993;42:399–405.
5. Peters S, Reil GH, McKenna WJ. Different ECG algorithms for the differentiation of arrhythmogenic right ventricle and athlete's heart. First International Symposium on Arrhythmogenic Right Ventricular Dysplasia—Cardiomyopathy. June 16–18, 1996; Paris, France.
6. Peters S, Weber B, Reil GH. Conventional electrocardiogram in arrhythmogenic right ventricular dysplasia-cardiomyopathy and idiopathic right ventricular outflow tract tachycardia. *Ann Nonvasive Cardiol* 1996;1(4): 400–404.
7. Fontaine G, Sohal P, Piot O, et al. Parietal block superimposed on right bundle branch block: A new ECG marker of right ventricular dysplasia. *J Am Coll Cardiol* 1997;29:(#2 suppl A):110A:934–954. Abstract.
8. Corrado D, Turrini P, Buja G, et al. Does "QT dispersion" in arrhythmogenic right ventricular cardiomyopathy reflect a ventricular conduction defect at risk of sudden arrhythmic death? First International Symposium on Arrhythmogenic Right Ventricular Dysplasia—Cardiomyopathy. June 16–18, 1996; Paris, France.
9. Oselladore L, Nava A, Turrini P, et al. Is signal averaged electrocardiography (SAECG) a useful method in diagnosing patients affected with arrhythmogenic right ventricular cardiomyopathy (ARVC)? First International Symposium on Arrhythmogenic Right Ventricular Dysplasia—Cardiomyopathy. June 16–18, 1996; Paris, France.
10. Mehta D, Goldman M, David O, et al. Value of quantitative measurement of signal-averaged electrocardiographic variables in arrhythmogenic right ventricular dysplasia: Correlation with echocardiographic right ventricular cavity dimensions. *J Am Coll Cardiol* 1996;28:713–719.
11. Biffi A, Ansalone G, Verdile L, et al. Ventricular arrhythmia and athlete's heart. *Eur Heart J* 1996;17:557–563.
12. Basso C, Thiene G, Corrado D, et al. Arrhythmogenic right ventricular cardiomyopathy; dysplasia, dystrophy, or myocarditis? *Circulation* 1996;94: 983–991.
13. Thiene G, Nava A, Corrado D, et al. Right ventricular cardiomyopathy and sudden death in young people. *N Engl J Med* 1988;318:129–133.
14. Loire R, Tabib A. Mort subite cardiaque inattendue, bilan de 1000 autopsies. *Arch Mal Coeur* 1996;89:13–18.
15. Goodin JC, Farb A, Smialek JE, et al. Right ventricular dysplasia associated with sudden death in young adults. *Mod Pathol* 1991;4:702–706.
16. Shirani J, Berezowski K, Roberts WC. Quantitative measurement of normal and excessive (Cor Adiposum) subepicardial adipose tissue: Its clinical

significance, and its effect on electrocardiographic QRS voltage. *Am J Cardiol* 1995;76:414–418.

17. Shen WK, Edwards D, Hammill SC, et al. Right ventricular dysplasia: A need for precise pathological definition for interpretation of sudden death. *J Am Coll Cardiol* 1994;34A:847–865. Abstract.
18. Fontaliran F, Fontaine G, Filette F, et al. Frontieres nosologiques de la dysplasie arythmogene: Variations quantitatives du tissu adipeux ventrciulaire droit normal. *Arch Mal Coeur* 1991;84:33–38.
19. Corrado D, Thiene G, Nava A, et al. Exercise-related sudden death in the young. *Eur Heart J* 1993;(suppl 368):P2006. Abstract.
20. Corrado D, Thiene G, Nava A, et al. Sudden death in young competitive athletes: Clinicopathologic correlations in 22 cases. *Am J Med* 1990;89: 588–596.
21. Maron BJ, Shirani J, Poliac LC, et al. Sudden death in young competitive athletes. *JAMA* 1996;276:199–204.
22. Daubert C, Vauthier M, Carre F, et al. Influence of exercise and sport activity on functional symptoms and ventricular arrhythmias in arrhythmogenic right ventricular disease. *J Am Coll Cardiol* 1994;34A:847–864. Abstract.
23. Douglas PS, O'Toole ML, Hiller WDB, et al. Different effects of prolonged exercise on the right and left ventricles. *J Am Coll Cardiol* 1990;15:64–69.
24. Buja GF, Corrado D, Turrini P, et al. Electrocardiographic features of arrhythmogenic right ventricular cardiomyopathy in young sudden death victims. First International Symposium on Arrhythmogenic Right Ventricular Dysplasia—Cardiomyopathy. June 16–18, 1996; Paris, France.
25. Scognamiglio R, Rahimtoola SH, Thiene G, et al. Concealed phase of familial arrhythmogenic right ventricular cardiomyopathy (ARVC): Early recognition and long-term follow-up. *J Am Coll Cardiol* 1997;29:(#2 suppl A):744–753.

Sudden Death in
The Athlete:

The European Perspective

**Domenico Corrado, MD, Cristina Basso, MD,
and Gaetano Thiene, MD**

Introduction

Most sudden deaths (SDs) in athletes are due to cardiovascular diseases.[1–10] Atherosclerotic coronary artery disease is the major pathologic substrate of SD in older athletes,[2,4,5] whereas a spectrum of conditions including cardiomyopathies,[3,6,7,11,12] congenital coronary artery anomalies,[13,14] mitral valve prolapse,[15] conduction system abnormalities,[16] myocarditis,[1,5,6] and aortic dissection[6,7] may cause sudden cardiac arrest in younger athletes (≤35 years of age). Early diagnosis of these cardiovascular disorders in athletes may reduce mortality by preventing potential fatalities during athletic training and competition. A systematic screening by preparticipation examination of individuals embarking in competitive sports has been advocated. However, the "culprit" diseases are clinically silent, and rarely are diagnosed or even suspected before death.[6,7] Therefore, controversy re-

This study was supported by the Juvenile Sudden Death Research Project of the Veneto Region, Venice, and by the National Council for Research, Target Project FATMA, Rome, Italy.

From Estes NAM, Salem DN, Wang PJ (eds). *Sudden Cardiac Death in the Athlete.* Armonk, NY: Futura Publishing Co., Inc.; ©1998.

mains over the cost-effectiveness of population-based preparticipation screening.[17,18]

On the basis of the data obtained from the prospective clinico-pathologic investigation on juvenile SD that has been carried out in the Veneto Region since 1979, this chapter addresses the differences in prevalence of cardiovascular causes of SD in young competitive athletes in the US and in Italy, the only country where a systematic preparticipation clinical screening is in practice.[19,20]

Sudden Death in Young Competitive Athletes: The North American Studies

Hypertrophic cardiomyopathy (HCM) has been implicated as the principle cause of sudden cardiac arrest on the athletic field in the US, where it accounts for about one third of fatal cases.[3,6,8-10] The second most frequent cardiovascular pathologic substrate is the congenital anomaly of coronary arteries.[3,6,10,13] Less common causes include atherosclerotic coronary artery disease, myocarditis, dilated cardiomyopathy, mitral valve prolapse, arrhythmogenic right ventricular cardiomyopathy (dysplasia) (ARVC), aortic valve stenosis, and the long QT syndrome.[3,6,8-10] Uncommon noncardiovascular pathologies that may precipitate SD consist mainly of cerebral aneurysm, sickle cell trait, and bronchial asthma.[8,10]

Hypertrophic Cardiomyopathy

Studies on SD in the athlete in North America have consistently shown that HCM is the most common pathologic substrate. Maron et al[3] evaluated the cause of SD in 29 highly conditioned competitive athletes (aged 13 to 30 years) and attributed 50% of sports-related cardiac fatalities to HCM. In the series by Waller and Roberts,[4] 22% of athletes who died suddenly during or shortly after competitive sports had HCM. Burke et al,[8] in a retrospective study comparing sports- versus non-sports-related SD, demonstrated that HCM was a leading cause of SD in the athlete (24% of cases); moreover, there was a statistically significant prevalence of HCM in fatal events that occurred during athletic competition as compared with non-exercise-related catastrophes. In the recent study carried out by the National Center for Catastrophic Sport Injury Research on the frequency and etiology of nontraumatic sports death in high school and college athletes in the US, HCM was the most common cause of death, occurring in 50 of 136 (37%) SD victims.[9]

HCM is a heart muscle disease, usually genetically transmitted and characterized by a hypertrophied, nondilated left ventricle in the

absence of predisposing diseases.[3,10] The familial form of HCM is genetically heterogeneous, and a number of mutations encoding for contractile proteins, such as β-myosin heavy chain, cardiac troponin T,
and α-tropomyosin, have been identified.[21–23]

Pathologic features of HCM include: cardiomegaly due to left ventricular hypertrophy that usually is "asymmetric" with disproportionate septal thickening; reduction in left ventricular chamber size with
increased myocardial "stiffness," which may critically impair diastolic
compliance and intramural coronary blood filling; and a subaortic septal "plaque" associated with a thickening of the anterior leaflet of the
mitral valve as the result of dynamic left ventricular outflow tract obstruction.[3,6,10] The histologic hallmark of the disease is the so-called
myocardial disarray, which consists of widespread bizarre and disordered arrangement of myocytes; the associated diffuse interstitial fibrosis is an acquired phenomenon, ascribed to a progressive disease of
the intramural coronary arteries, which show a dysplasia of the tunica
media with or without lumen obstruction (small vessel disease).[3,6,10]
Additional histologic signs of acute (contraction band and coagulative
necrosis) and/or healed (gross septal scars and/or extensive replacement fibrosis) acquired myocardial injury may be found in young athletes who died suddenly.[24,25]

Sudden cardiac arrest in athletes with HCM has been attributed to
primary ventricular arrhythmias[26,27] most likely arising from the dysplastic myocardium. The observation of acquired myocardial damage, either acute or in the setting of large septal scars, supports the hypothesis that myocardial ischemia intervenes in the natural history of the
disease and contributes to the arrhythmogenicity.[24,25,27] Other potential
mechanisms of syncope and cardiac arrest in HCM include paroxysmal
supraventricular arrhythmias,[28] atrioventricular (AV) block, and hypotension due to inappropriate vasodilator response to exercise.[29]

Anomalous Coronary Artery Origin

The anomalous origin of a coronary artery is the second most common pathologic condition that has been incriminated in sudden and unexpected cardiac arrest in North American athletes. The most frequent
anatomic findings consist of both (left and right) coronary arteries arising from either the right coronary sinus or the left coronary sinus.[30,31] In
both conditions, the anomalous coronary vessel, as it leaves the aorta,
shows an acute angle with the aortic wall and, thus, it usually runs between the aorta and the pulmonary trunk following an early aortic intramural course, with a "slit-like" lumen.[13,14] Pathologic examination
of the ventricular myocardium usually reveals signs of acute or healed
ischemic damage in the territory supplied by the anomalous coronary

vessel. Fatal myocardial ischemia has been related to exercise-induced aortic root expansion, which compresses the anomalous vessel against the pulmonary trunk and increases the acute angulation of the coronary take off, aggravating the slit-like shape of the lumen of the proximal intramural portion of the aberrant coronary vessel.[13,14,30,31] It is difficult to reproduce this mechanism of myocardial ischemia in a clinical setting, as shown by the occurrence of false-negative electrocardiogram (ECG) exercise testing in a young athlete who subsequently died suddenly from the aforementioned coronary anomaly.[13,14]

Sudden Death in the Athlete: The Veneto Region Experience

The Veneto Region of Northeastern Italy covers an area of 18.368 km^2, and has a population of 4,380,797 inhabitants, according to the 1991 Census; all residents are white and the population is ethnically homogeneous.

A prospective clinicopathologic study on SD in young people ($\leq$35 years of age) has been carried out in the Veneto Region of Italy since 1979. According to the study design,[12] all young people who died suddenly and were referred to each Collaborative Medical Center for autopsy underwent postmortem examination by the local pathologist or medical examiner. After extracardiac causes of death were excluded, the entire heart was forwarded to the Institute of Pathological Anatomy of the University of Padua for detailed morphological investigation. Circumstances surrounding fatal cardiac arrest and prior clinical history were investigated in each case. In the time interval from January 1979 to December 1995, 232 consecutive cases of juvenile sudden death were prospectively studied according to the above clinicopathologic protocol.

Forty-six (20%) SD victims were young competitive athletes (41 males and 5 females, mean age 23.6 years) who participated in a variety of sports: soccer (20 cases), basketball (5 cases), swimming (4 cases), cycling (3 cases), rugby, running, gymnastics, tennis, skiing, and judo (2 cases each), weight lifting, and volleyball (1 case each).

SD was sports related in 37 athletes (80%), and it occurred during (32 cases) or immediately after (5 cases) a competitive match. In 18 subjects (45%), SD was preceded by warning symptoms and/or ECG changes.

Autopsy findings are summarized in Table 1. HCM was an infrequent cause of sports-related SD. The more prevalent causes of SD during athletic competition included: ARVC (10 athletes, 22%); single-vessel premature coronary artery disease, affecting the proximal left

Table 1
Causes of Sudden Death in 46 Young Competitive Athletes
Veneto Region, Italy (1979–1995)

Cause	No. of Athletes	Cause	No. of Athletes
ARVC	10	Hypertrophic cardiomyopathy	1
Atherosclerotic CAD	9	Dilated cardiomyopathy	1
Nonatherosclerotic CAD	7	Dissecting aortic aneurysm	1
Conduction system abnormalities	4	Cerebral berry aneurysm	1
Mitral valve prolapse	4	Pulmonary thromboembolism	1
Myocarditis	3	Long QT syndrome	1
Cerebral embolism	2	Unexplained	1

ARVC = arrhythmogenic right ventricular cardiomyopathy; CAD = coronary artery disease.

anterior descending coronary artery with the morphological features of accelerated atherosclerosis (9 athletes, 17%); and congenital anomalies of coronary arteries (7 athletes, 15%). Other cardiovascular diseases occurring less frequently included: conduction system pathology (4 cases), myocarditis (3 cases), dilated cardiomyopathy, pulmonary thromboembolism, aortic rupture, and the long QT syndrome (1 case each). Death was due to an extracardiac cerebral cause in three athletes, and it remained unexplained in one.

Therefore, SD in young competitive athletes was related to the same pathologic substrates described in the other series, although the relative prevalence of causes of death differed from that previously reported. Unlike the US series, in the Italian study HCM was an uncommon cause of SD in the athlete, although it accounted for non-sports-related SD in the general young population with a prevalence similar to that found in the US.[32] Conversely, the Italian study showed a high prevalence of ARVC and premature atherosclerotic coronary artery disease as causes of sports-related SD.

Arrhythmogenic Right Ventricular Cardiomyopathy

ARVC is a heart muscle disorder that is characterized pathologically by fibro-fatty replacement of right ventricular myocardium.[7,12,33,34] The disease is often familial with an autosomal dominant pattern of inheritance, and its most frequent clinical presentation consists of arrhythmias of right ventricular origin (Figures 1 and 2) and SD.[7,12,33,34] Since the left ventricle is usually spared, cardiac performance may be normal, thus allowing young affected subjects to face strenuous exercise.

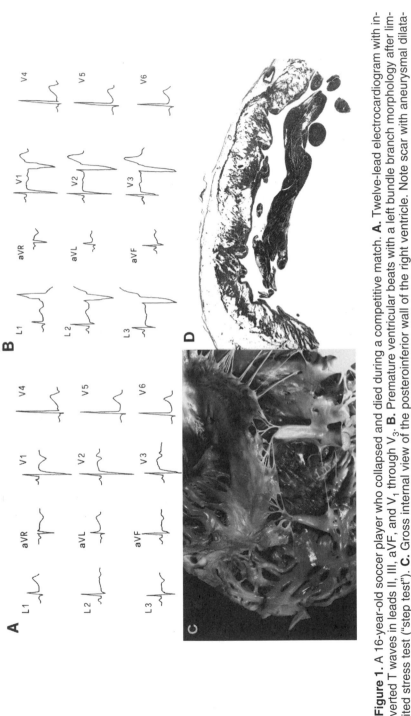

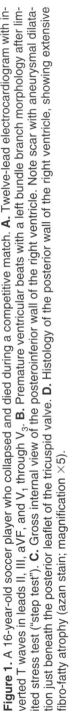

Figure 1. A 16-year-old soccer player who collapsed and died during a competitive match. **A.** Twelve-lead electrocardiogram with inverted T waves in leads II, III, aVF, and V₁ through V₃. **B.** Premature ventricular beats with a left bundle branch morphology after limited stress test ("step test"). **C.** Gross internal view of the posteroinferior wall of the right ventricle. Note scar with aneurysmal dilatation just beneath the posterior leaflet of the tricuspid valve. **D.** Histology of the posterior wall of the right ventricle, showing extensive fibro-fatty atrophy (azan stain; magnification ×5).

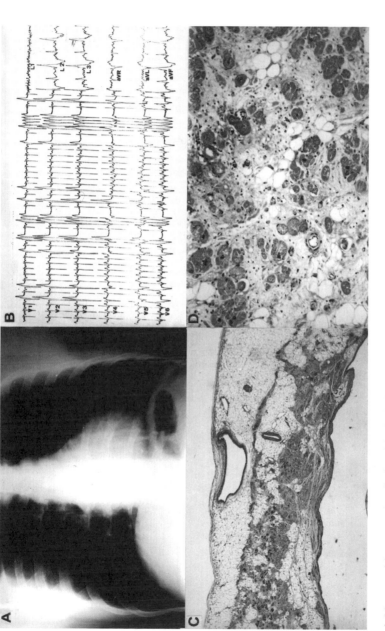

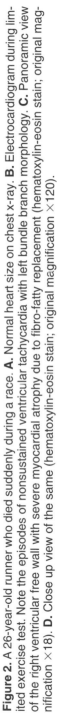

Figure 2. A 26-year-old runner who died suddenly during a race. **A.** Normal heart size on chest x-ray. **B.** Electrocardiogram during limited exercise test. Note the episodes of nonsustained ventricular tachycardia with left bundle branch morphology. **C.** Panoramic view of the right ventricular free wall with severe myocardial atrophy due to fibro-fatty replacement (hematoxylin-eosin stain; original magnification ×18). **D.** Close up view of the same (hematoxylin-eosin stain; original magnification ×120).

At macroscopic examination, the hearts of young competitive athletes who die suddenly from ARVC disclose only slight right ventricular dilatation, and massive transmural fibro-fatty replacement of the right ventricular (RV) musculature, which accounts for aneurysms (infundibular, inferior, and apical) (Figure 1), scarring fibrosis, and/or large areas of very thin, translucent wall.[7,12,34] This gross appearance of the RV allows definitive differential diagnosis from training-induced RV changes ("athlete's heart"), which usually consist of global RV enlargement.[35] Histologically, fibro-fatty atrophy of RV myocardium is often associated with signs of focal myocardial degeneration and necrosis, with patchy inflammatory infiltrates.[7,12,34] The fibrosis is of the replacement type and suggests a postnecrotic scarring process. The arrhythmogenicity of ARVC is reasonably explained by the widespread, irregular disruption of the RV myocardium and electrical wave front, with inhomogeneous conduction and activation from site to site, which predisposes to the onset of malignant reentrant ventricular tachyarrhythmias.[36]

The propensity for ARVC to precipitate "arrhythmic" sudden cardiac arrest during physical exercise is most likely linked to some hemodynamic and neurohumoral factors. Physical exercise has an opposite effect on the right and left ventricle and it results in acute disproportionate increase in RV afterload and cavity enlargement,[37] which in turn may elicit ventricular arrhythmias by "stretching" the diseased right ventricular musculature. Progression of the disease from the epicardium to the endocardium might account for a functional and/or structural sympathetic denervation (sympathetic nerve trunks travel in the subepicardial layer) with supersensitivity to catecholamines and enhanced arrhythmogenicity during sympathetic stimulation.[38]

Premature Atherosclerotic Coronary Artery Disease

Atherosclerotic coronary artery disease is the major cause of SD in adult and elderly exercising individuals.[2,4,5] Previous series in the US showed that premature coronary artery disease is an uncommon pathologic substrate of sports-related SD in young athletes.[3,6,8–10] Conversely, in the series of athletes investigated in the Veneto Region, atherosclerotic coronary artery disease appears to be an important cause of SD even in young competitive athletes.[7] Premature coronary atherosclerosis in young people and athletes exhibits distinctive pathologic features such as extent, site, and morphology of the obstructive atherosclerotic plaques.[7,39,40] In young athletes who die of coronary artery disease, SD is frequently the first manifestation of the disease in the absence of previous angina pectoris and/or myocardial infarction.[7,39,40] Coronary atherosclerosis is more often a "single-vessel disease" that distinctively affects the left anterior descending coronary artery; obstructive plaques are rarely complicated by acute thrombosis and are mostly fibrocellular due to a neointimal smooth muscle cell hyperplasia (so-called accelerated atherosclerosis) in the presence of a preserved tunica media[39,40] (Figure 3). These morphological features may result in abnormal hypervasoreactivity and may possibly precipitate cardiac arrest by vasospastic myocardial ischemia.[40] The identification of these young athletes at risk of ischemic cardiac arrest is a challenge due to the absence of risk factors and warning symptoms and the limitation of the stress test in detecting myocardial ischemia[7] (Figure 3).

Systematic Preparticipation Athletic Screening

The low prevalence of HCM in the series of young competitive athletes who died suddenly in the Veneto Region of Italy is likely to be related to the systematic clinical screening of all young people embarking in competitive athletic activity that has been in place for more than 20 years in this region. It has probably changed the natural prevalence of pathologic substrates of sports–related SD.[20] The preparticipation athletic screening includes familial and patient clinical history, physical examination, standard 12-lead ECG, and limited exercise test

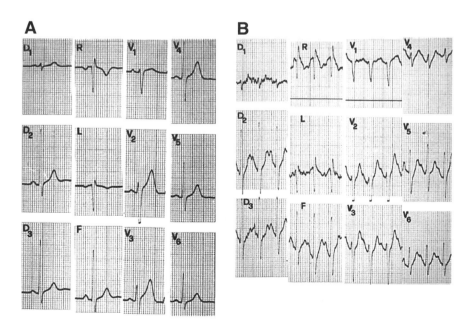

Figure 3. A 19-year-old basketball player who died suddenly during effort. **A.** Normal basal electrocardiogram (ECG). **B.** ECG during stress test showing neither ST-T abnormalities nor arrhythmias.

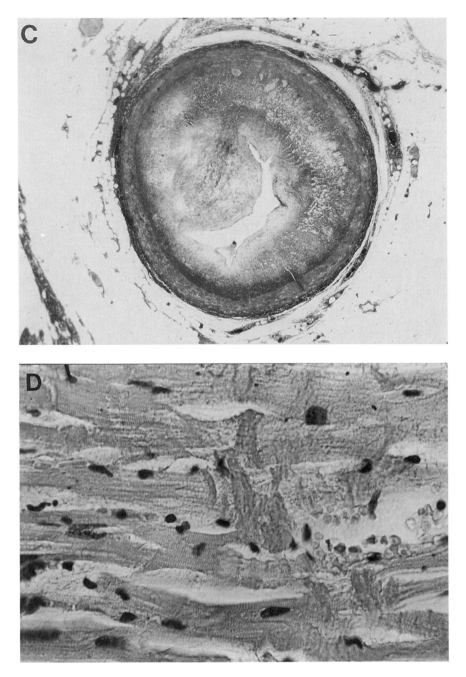

Figure 3. (continued) C. Cross section of the proximal left anterior descending coronary artery showing severely obstructive and predominantly fibrocellular plaque (azan stain; original magnification ×15). **D.** Contraction band necrosis in the myocardium of the anterior left ventricular free wall (hematoxylin-eosin stain; original magnification ×480).

(Montoye modified) on an annual basis.[20] Basal 12-lead ECG is reported to be very sensitive and it is abnormal in approximately 95% of patients with HCM.[18] Therefore, the above cardiovascular screening would be sensitive enough to identify pathologic symptoms, abnormal physical signs, and ECG changes and to lead to further study such as echocardiography. An ongoing investigation on data regarding the number of athletes with abnormalities detected on preparticipation screening and the causes of disqualification for competitive sport in the Veneto Region of Italy would definitively support the role of cardiovascular screening in the reduction of SDs from HCM. However, indirect evidence comes from the study in the US by Burke and colleagues[8] and from a similar study in the Veneto region of Italy,[32] both comparing sports–related versus non-sports-related SD in the young. The studies show a similar prevalence of HCM in non-sports-related SD in North America and Italy (3% versus 5%), but a strong difference in sports-related fatal events (24% versus 2%). The similar prevalence of HCM as a cause of non-sports–related SD in the nonathletic young population of the US and Italy strongly suggest a *selective* reduction of SD from HCM in competitive athletes who undergo systematic preparticipation screening.

Other factors that may explain the discrepancy between the Italian and previous North American series include the study design, the ethnic, geographic, and genetic background of the population examined, and the thoroughness of morphological investigation, as well as the interpretation of autopsy findings.

The Italian study was designed to prospectively investigate a consecutive series of SDs in young people that occurred in the Veneto Region, which is populated by a homogeneous white population. There have been no previous studies that have prospectively investigated a consecutive series of SDs in athletes that occurred in a well-defined geographic location with a homogeneous ethnic group. The milestone study by Maron et al[3] was predominantly retrospective and collected fatal cases from several locations in the US by several means such as news media reports of SD in athletes, hospital-based pathology registries, or medical examiner offices.[3]

Racial factors may influence the results, as evidenced by the study by Burke et al[8] which showed that Blacks who died during exercise had a greater incidence of HCM than Whites.

The high incidence of ARVC in the Italian series may be due to a genetic factor in the population of this region of Italy.[12] However, the concept of ARVC as a peculiar "Venetian disease" is misleading; there is growing evidence that ARVC is ubiquitous, is still largely underdiagnosed at both clinical and postmortem investigation, and accounts for significant arrhythmic morbidity and mortality, mostly in young people. Comparison of the results of the present investigation with previous findings of studies on SD in athletes in the US is most likely limited by the fact that ARVC is a clinicopathologic condition that was only recently discovered.[12,33]

The accuracy of autopsy and interpretation of pathologic findings may play a crucial role in the determination of the causes of SD. With studies of large series, autopsy investigation is usually performed by multiple examiners including local pathologists and medical examiners. In the present study, in order to obtain a higher level of confidence in the results, morphological examination of all hearts was performed by the same team of experienced cardiovascular pathologists according to a standard protocol. ARVC is rarely associated with cardiomegaly and usually spares the coronary arteries and the left ventricle, so that affected hearts may be erroneously diagnosed as normal hearts.[7,12,34] Therefore, in the past, a number of SDs in young competitive athletes, in which the routine pathologic examination disclosed a normal heart, may, in fact, have been due to an under-recognized ARVC.[12]

Prodromal Symptoms and Signs

In order to assess the efficacy and limitations of Italian preparticipation screening, pathologic findings were related to athlete clinical history and ECG recordings in an attempt to understand why the underlying disease had not been suspected during life at preparticipation screening. As reported in Table 2, athletes who died from ARVC had warning clinical histories and ECG signs, whereas athletes with coro-

Table 2
Prodromal Symptoms and Signs at
Preparticipation Athleting Screening
Veneto Region, Italy (1979–1995)

Clinical Prodroma:	ARVC 8/10 *(80%)*	Atherosclerotic CAD 2/9 *(22%)*	Congenital CAD 2/7 *(29%)*
Familial history for heart disease at risk of SD	2	–	–
Effort-induced palpitations	6	1	
Syncope	5	1	1
Chest pain	–	–	–
ST-T abnormalities	8	–	1
Ventricular arrhythmias	6	–	2

ARVC = arrhythmogenic right ventricular cardiomyopathy; CAD = coronary artery disease; SD = sudden death.

nary artery disease, both atherosclerotic and congenital, did not exhibit significant symptoms and ECG changes at preparticipation athletic screening.

The Italian study confirms that early identification of young subjects with coronary artery disease at preparticipation athletic screening is limited by the scarcity of warning signs and the low sensitivity of both basal and exercise ECG in detecting signs of myocardial ischemia in athletes with coronary atherosclerosis as well as in those with anomalous coronary artery. In screening large populations of apparently healthy individuals, the use of exercise ECG to induce myocardial ischemia is limited by its low predictive value and pretest probability.[41]

Unlike athletes with coronary artery diseases, athletes who died from ARVC often had a history of warning syncopal episodes as well as ECG signs such as inverted T waves in right precordial leads and ventricular arrhythmias with left bundle branch block morphology, which ranged from individual premature ventricular beats to sustained ventricular tachycardia. The affected young competitive athletes were not identified at preparticipation screening because ARVC is largely unrecognized as a pathologic substrate for risk of SD during sports. The ventricular arrhythmias, even nonsustained and sustained ventricular tachycardia, with left bundle branch pattern were considered idiopathic on apparently normal hearts, and the affected individuals were not investigated further. The Italian experience lends support to the proposal that with increased awareness of the symptoms, ECG features, and arrhythmias of ARVC, more athletes at risk may be identified and SD prevented. Therefore, the finding at preparticipation athletic screening of even a single premature ventricular beat with left bundle branch block morphology associated with right precordial T wave abnormalities on ECG, with or without a history of syncopal attacks, should raise the legitimate suspicion of an underlying ARVC. Definitive diagnosis of ARVC depends on specific evaluation by cross-sectional echocardiography,[42] nuclear magnetic resonance,[43] and in selected cases, by right ventricular angiography with endomyocardial biopsy.[44,45]

Conclusions

Systematic monitoring of SD in young people in the Veneto Region of Italy, a well-defined geographic area populated by a homogeneous ethnic group, where a systematic preparticipation athletic screening is in practice, have demonstrated that the relative prevalence of causes of SD in young competitive athletes differs from that previously reported in the US. HCM has been an uncommon cause of fatal events in athletes, most likely due to preparticipation clinical evaluations that seem to result in identification and disqualification of the affected subjects. Definitive evidence for the role of preparticipation screening in reducing SD can be provided by an ongoing investigation on data regarding the number of athletes with abnormalities detected on preparticipation screening and the causes of disqualification for competitive sport in the Veneto Region of Italy. ARVC, a poorly recognized clinicopathologic condition that may lead to sports-related cardiac arrest, was the most frequently encountered cardiovascular substrate. A significant subset of young athletes had premature atherosclerotic coronary artery disease which distinctively affected the proximal left anterior descending coronary artery. Unlike coronary artery diseases, both atherosclerotic and congenital, fatal ARVC may have been suspected at preparticipation athletic screening on the basis of arrhythmic prodromal symptoms and ECG signs.

References

1. Buddington RS, Stahl CJI, McAllister HA, et al. Sports, death and unusual heart disease. *Am J Cardiol* 1974;33:129.
2. Thompson PD, Stern MP, Williams P, et al. Death during jogging or running: A study of 18 cases. *JAMA* 1979;242:1265.
3. Maron BJ, Roberts WC, McAllister MA, et al. Sudden death in young athletes. *Circulation* 1980;62:218–229.
4. Waller BF, Roberts WC. Sudden death while running in conditioned runners aged 40 years or over. *Am J Cardiol* 1980;45:1292.
5. Virmani R, Robinowitz M, McAllister HA. Nontraumatic death in joggers. *Am J Med* 1982;72:874.
6. Maron BJ, Epstein SE, Roberts WC. Causes of sudden death in competitive athletes. *J Am Coll Cardiol* 1986;7:204.
7. Corrado D, Thiene G, Nava A, et al. Sudden death in young competitive athletes: Clinico-pathologic correlations in 22 cases. *Am J Med* 1990;89:588–596.
8. Burke AP, Farb A, Virmani R, et al. Sports-related and non-sports-related sudden cardiac death in young adults. *Am Heart J* 1991;12I:568.
9. Van Camp SP, Bloor CM, Mueller FO, et al. Non-traumatic sports death in high school and college athletes. *Med Sci Sports Exerc* 1995;27:641–647.
10. Maron BJ, Shirani J, Poliac LC, et al. Sudden death in young competitive athletes. Clinical demographics, and pathological profiles. *JAMA* 1996;276:199–204.
11. Maron BJ, Roberts WC, Epstein SE. Sudden death in hypertrophic cardiomyopathy: A profile of 78 patients. *Circulation* 1982;65:1388.
12. Thiene G, Nava A, Corrado D, et al. Right ventricular cardiomyopathy and sudden death in young people. *N Engl J Med* 1988;318:129–133.
13. Virmani R, Rogan K, Cheitlin MD. Congenital coronary artery anomalies: Pathologic aspects. In Virmani R, Forman MB (eds): *Nonatherosclerotic Ischemic Heart Disease*. New York: Raven Press; 1989:153.
14. Corrado D, Thiene G, Cocco P, Frescura C. Non-atherosclerotic coronary artery disease and sudden death in the young. *Br Heart J* 1992;68:601–607.
15. Topaz O, Edwards JE. Pathologic features of sudden death in children, adolescents, and young adults. *Chest* 1985;87:476–482.

16. Thiene G, Pennelli N, Rossi L. Cardiac conduction system abnormalities as a possible cause of sudden death in young athletes. *Hum Pathol* 1983;14:70–74.
17. Maron BJ, Bodison SA, Wesley YE, et al. Results of screening a large group of intercollegiate competitive athletes for cardiovascular disease. *J Am Coll Cardiol* 1987;10:1214–1221.
18. Maron BJ, Thompson PD, Puffer JC, et al. Cardiovascular preparticipation screening of competitive athletes. A statement for health professionals from the Sudden Death Committee (Clinical Cardiology) and Congenital Cardiac Defects Committee (Cardiovascular Disease in the Young), American Heart Association. *Circulation* 1996;94:850–856.
19. Legislation of October 26, 1971. 1099. Tutela Sanitaria delle Attività Sportive (Medical Protection of Athletic Activities). *Gazzetta Ufficiale* December 23, 1971:324.
20. Pelliccia A, Maron BJ. Preparticipation cardiovascular evaluation of the competitive athlete: Perspectives from the 30-year Italian experience. *Am J Cardiol* 1995;75:827–829.
21. Solomon SD, Jarcho JA, McKenna WJ, et al. Familial hypertrophic cardiomyopathy is a genetically heterogenous disease. *J Clin Invest* 1990;86:993–999.
22. Thierfelder L, Watkins H, MacRae C, et al. Alpha-tropomyosin and cardiac troponin T mutations cause familial hypertrophic cardiomyopathy: A disease of the sarcomere. *Cell* 1994;77:701–712.
23. Watkins H, Rosenzweig A, Hwang D-S, et al. Characteristics and prognostic implications of myosin missense mutations in familial hypertrophic cardiomyopathy. *N Engl J Med* 1992;326:1108–1114.
24. Basso C, Frescura C, Corrado D, et al. Congenital heart disease and sudden death in the young. *Hum Pathol* 1995;26:1065–1072.
25. Basso C, Corrado D, Nava A, Thiene G. Hypertrophic cardiomyopathy: Pathologic evidence of myocardial ischemic injury in young sudden death victims. *Circulation* 1996;94:I–427.
26. Mc Kenna WJ, Camm AJ. Sudden death in hypertrophic cardiomyopathy of patients at high risk. *Circulation* 1989;80:1489–1492.
27. Dilsizian V, Bonow RO, Epstein SE, et al. Myocardial ischemia detected by thallium scintigraphy is frequently related to cardiac arrest and syncope in young patients with hypertrophic cardiomyopathy. *J Am Coll Cardiol* 1993;22:796–804.
28. Krikler DM, Davies MJ, Rowland W, et al. Sudden death in hypertrophic cardiomyopathy associated accessory atrioventricular pathways. *Br Heart J* 1980;43:245–251.
29. Frenneaux MP, Counihan PJ, Caforio ALP, et al. Abnormal blood pressure response during exercise in hypertrophic cardiomyopathy. *Circulation* 1990;82:1995–2002.
30. Cheitlin MD, De Castro CM, McAllister HA. Sudden death as a complication of anomalous left coronary origin from the anterior sinus of Valsalva: A not so minor congenital anomaly. *Circulation* 1994;50:780–787.
31. Roberts WC, Siegel RJ, Zipes DP. Origin of the right coronary artery from the left sinus of Valsalva and its functional consequences: Analysis of 10 necropsy patients. *Am J Cardiol* 1982;49:863–868.
32. Corrado D, Thiene G, Nava A, et al. Sport-related sudden death in young people. *Circulation* 1993;88:I-51.
33. Marcus FI, Fontaine GH, Guiraudon G, et al. Right ventricular dysplasia: A report of 24 cases. *Circulation* 1982;65:384–398.

34. Maron BJ, Pelliccia A, Spirito P. Cardiac disease in young trained athletes. Insights into methods for distinguishing athlete's heart from structural heart disease, with particular emphasis on hypertrophic cardiomyopathy. *Circulation* 1995;91:1596–1601.

35. Basso C, Thiene G, Corrado D, et al. Arrhythmogenic right ventricular cardiomyopathy: Dysplasia, dystrophy, or myocarditis? *Circulation* 1996;94: 983–991.

36. Fontaine G, Frank R, Tonet JL, et al. Arrhythmogenic right ventricular dysplasia: A clinical model for the study of chronic ventricular tachycardia. *Jpn Circ J* 1984;48:515–538.

37. Douglas PS, O'Toole ML, Hiller WDB, Reichek N. Different effects of prolonged exercise on the right and left ventricles. *J Am Coll Cardiol* 1990;15: 64–69.

38. Wichter T, Hindricks G, Lerch H, et al. Regional myocardial sympathetic dysinnervation in arrhythmogenic right ventricular cardiomyopathy. *Circulation* 1994;89:667–683.

39. Corrado D, Thiene G, Pennelli N. Sudden death as the first manifestation of coronary artery disease in young people (≤35 years). *Eur Heart J* 1988; 9:139–144.

40. Corrado D, Basso C, Poletti A, et al. Sudden death in the young. Is coronary thrombosis the major precipitating factor? *Circulation* 1994;90: 2315–2323.

41. Schlant RC, Blomqvist CG, Brandenburg RO, et al. Guidelines for exercise testing . *J Am Coll Cardiol* 1986;8:725–738.

42. Nava A, Thiene G, Canciani B, et al. Familial occurrence of right ventricular dysplasia: A study of nine families. *J Am Coll Cardiol* 1988;12: 1222–1228.

43. Menghetti L, Basso C, Nava A, et al. Spin-echo nuclear magnetic resonance for tissue characterization in arrhythmogenic right ventricular cardiomyopathy. *Heart* 1997;76:467–470.

44. Daliento L, Rizzoli G, Thiene G, et al. Diagnostic accuracy of right ventricular ventriculography in arrhythmogenic right ventricular cardiomyopathy. *Am J Cardiol* 1990;66:741–745.

45. Angelini A, Basso C, Nava A, Thiene G. Endomyocardial biopsy in arrhythmogenic right ventricular cardiomyopathy. *Am Heart J* 1996;132: 203–206.

16

Hypertrophic Cardiomyopathy as a Cause of Sudden Death in the Young Competitive Athlete

Barry J. Maron, MD

The young highly conditioned competitive athlete projects the imagery of the healthiest facet of our society.[1] Nevertheless, youthful (or older) athletes may die suddenly, often during sports competition or training.[2–7] Such catastrophes are always unexpected events and while relatively uncommon, nevertheless convey a particularly tragic and devastating impact on the community. In particular, the fact that many such athletes may have performed at exceptionally high levels of excellence for long periods of time with severe cardiovascular malformations has intrigued investigators and the lay public for some time.

Over the past few years, the underlying cardiovascular diseases responsible for sudden death in trained athletes and others participating in sporting activities have been the subject of several reports, and a large measure of clarification has resulted.[1–7] Recognition that athletic field catastrophes may be due to a variety of detectable cardiovascular lesions has also stimulated intense interest in preparticipation screening[8] as well as issues related to the criteria for eligibility and disqualification from competitive sports.[9]

From Estes NAM, Salem DN, Wang PJ (eds). *Sudden Cardiac Death in the Athlete*. Armonk, NY: Futura Publishing Co., Inc.;©1998.

Definitions

A competitive athlete has been defined as one who participates in an organized team or individual sport that requires regular competition against others as a central component, places a high premium on excellence and achievement, and requires vigorous and intense training in a systematic fashion.[9] This definition is arbitrary, and many individuals may participate in "recreational" sports in a truly competitive fashion.

Causes of Sudden Death

Several studies have documented the cardiovascular diseases responsible for sudden death in young competitive athletes or youthful asymptomatic individuals with active lifestyles.[2-7] These structural abnormalities are independent of the normal physiologic adaptations in cardiac dimension evident in many trained athletes that usually consist of increased left ventricular end-diastolic cavity dimension or occasionally wall thickness.[10-12] Also, by convention, deaths attributable to conditions such as cerebrovascular accident, heat stroke, pulmonary disease, peripheral embolism, drug abuse, or commotio cordis were preferentially excluded from these studies.

It is also important to be cautious in assigning strict prevalence figures for the relative occurrence of various cardiovascular diseases in studies of sudden death in athletes; patient selection biases and other limitations unavoidably influence the acquisition of such data in the absence of a systematic national registry. Indeed, the available published studies differ with regard to methods used to document cardiovascular diagnosis, and were derived from a variety of data bases.

Even with these considerations in mind, it has nevertheless been demonstrated convincingly that the vast majority of sudden deaths in young athletes (<35 years) are due to a variety of primarily congenital cardiovascular diseases (over 20 in number) (Figure 1).[2] Indeed, virtually any such disease capable of causing sudden death in young people may potentially do so in young competitive athletes. It should be emphasized that while these diseases may be relatively common in young athletes dying suddenly, each is uncommon in the general population. Also, the lesions responsible for sudden death do not occur with the same frequency, with most responsible for ≤5% of all deaths (Figure 1).

Hypertrophic Cardiomyopathy

The single most common cardiovascular abnormality among the causes of sudden death in young athletes is hypertrophic cardiomy-

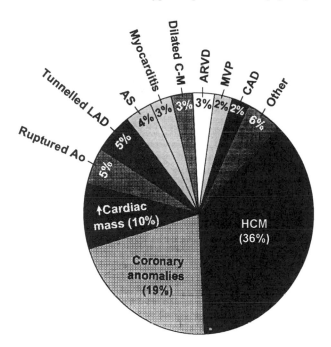

Figure 1. Causes of sudden cardiac death in young competitive athletes (median age, 17) based on systematic tracking of 158 athletes in the United States, primarily 1985 to 1995. In an additional 2% of the series, no evidence of cardiovascular disease sufficient to explain death was evident at autopsy. Ao = aorta; LAD = left anterior descending; AS = aortic stenosis; C-M = cardiomyopathy; ARVD = arrhythmogenic right ventricular dysplasia; MVP = mitral valve prolapse; CAD = coronary artery disease. HCM = hypertrophic cardiomyopathy. Adapted from Reference 2, with permission from the American Medical Association.

opathy (HCM),[2,3,5–7] usually in the nonobstructive form[13–15] (Figures 1–3) and with a prevalence in the range of 35%. HCM is a primary and familial cardiac malformation with heterogeneous expression, complex pathophysiology, and diverse clinical course for which several disease-causing mutations in genes encoding proteins of the cardiac sarcomere have been reported. HCM is a relatively uncommon malformation, occurring in about 0.2% (1 in 500) of the general population.[16]

Left ventricular hypertrophy has traditionally been regarded as the gross anatomic marker and, likely, the determinant of many of the clinical features and course in most patients with HCM.[13,14] Since the left ventricular cavity is usually small or normal in size, increased left ventricular mass is due almost entirely to an increase in wall thickness. Consequently, the clinical diagnosis of HCM has been based on the definition (by two-dimensional echocardiography) of the most characteristic morphological feature of the disease, ie, asymmetric thickening of

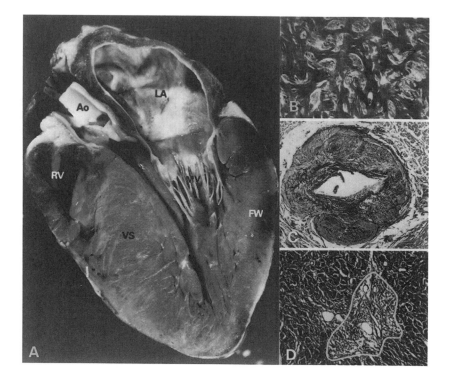

Figure 2. Morphological components of the disease process in hypertrophic cardiomyopathy (HCM), the most common cause of sudden death in young athletes. **A.** A gross heart specimen sectioned in a cross-sectional plane similar to that of the echocardiographic (parasternal) long axis; left ventricular wall thickening shows an asymmetric pattern and is confined primarily to the ventricular septum (VS), which bulges prominently into the left ventricular outflow tract. Left ventricular cavity appears reduced in size. **B, C,** and **D.** Histologic features characteristic of left ventricular myocardium in HCM. **B.** Septal myocardium shows a markedly disordered architecture with adjacent hypertrophied cardiac muscle cells arranged at perpendicular and oblique angles. **C.** An intramural coronary artery with thickened wall, due primarily to medial hypertrophy, and apparently narrowed lumen. **D.** Replacement fibrosis in an area of ventricular myocardium in the region of an abnormal intramural coronary artery. FW = left ventricular free wall; Ao = aorta; LA = left atrium; RV = right ventricle; MV = mitral valve.

Figure 3. Variability of patterns of left ventricular hypertrophy in patients with hypertrophic cardiomyopathy (HCM) shown in a composite of diastolic stop-frame images in parasternal short-axis plane. **A, B,** and **D.** Wall thickening is diffuse, involving substantial portions of ventricular septum and free wall. **A.** At papillary muscle level, all segments of the left ventricular wall are hypertrophied including posterior free wall (PW), but the pattern of thickening is asymmetric with the anterior portion of ventricular septum (VS) predominant and massive (ie, 50 mm). **B.** Here the hypertrophy is diffuse, involving three segments of left ventricle but with the posterior wall spared and thin (<10 mm; arrowheads) and with particularly abrupt changes in wall thickness evident (arrows). **C.** Marked hypertrophy is

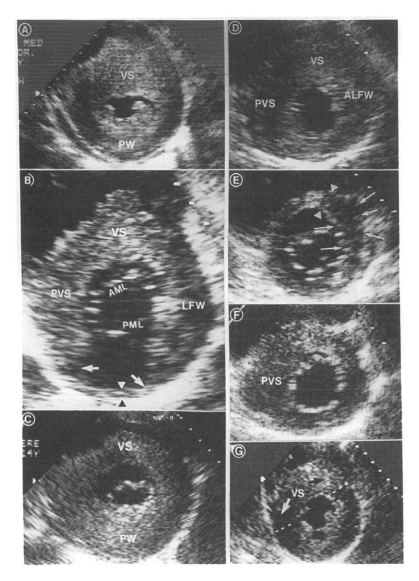

Figure 3. (*continued*) shown in a pattern distinctly different from **A, B,** and **D,** in which the thickening of *PW* is predominant and the ventricular septum is of near-normal thickness. **D.** Diffuse distribution of hypertrophy involving three segments of left ventricle similar to **B.** but without sharp transitions in the contour of the wall. **E.** Hypertrophy predominantly involving lateral free wall (arrows) and only a small portion of contiguous anterior septum (arrow heads). **F.** Hypertrophy predominantly of posterior ventricular septum (PVS), and to lesser extent the contiguous portion of anterior septum. **G.** Thickening involving anterior and posterior septum to a similar degree, but with sparing of the free wall. Calibration dots are 1 cm apart. AML = anterior mitral leaflet; LFW = lateral free wall; PML = posterior mitral leaflet; ALFW = anterolateral free wall. Reproduced from Reference 18, with permission from the American College of Cardiology.

the left ventricular wall associated with a nondilated cavity and in the absence of another cardiac or systemic disease capable of producing the magnitude of hypertrophy present (eg, systemic hypertension or aortic stenosis).[13,14,16–19] Because the nonobstructive form of HCM is predominant, the well-described clinical features of dynamic obstruction to left ventricular outflow, such as a loud systolic ejection murmur, systolic anterior motion of the mitral valve, or partial premature closure of the aortic valve, are not required for diagnosis.

While HCM may be suspected during preparticipation sports evaluations by the prior occurrence of exertional syncope, by a family history of the disease or of premature cardiac death, or by a loud heart murmur, such clinical features are relatively uncommon among all individuals affected by this disease. Consequently, standard screening procedures with only history and physical examination cannot be expected to reliably and consistently identify HCM.[8] One retrospective study showed that potentially lethal cardiovascular abnormalities, including HCM, were suspected by preparticipation history and physical in only 3% of high school and collegiate athletes who ultimately died suddenly of these diseases.[2]

In hospital- and outpatient-based patient profiles, sudden death in HCM has shown a predilection for young, asymptomatic, and healthy individuals and occurs frequently during moderate or severe exertion, similar to its demographic profile in athletic populations.[8] These observations support the generally accepted and prudent recommendation of the 26th Bethesda Conference to disqualify young competitive athletes with HCM from intense competitive sports.[9] Indeed, with a disease such as HCM in which there is a propensity for potentially lethal arrhythmias in some individuals, the stress of intense athletic training and competition (as well as associated alterations in blood volume, hydration, and electrolytes) probably increases the risk of sudden cardiac death in highly trained competitive athletes compared to nonathletes with this disease.[9]

Disease variables that appear to identify patients who are at greatly increased risk include: prior aborted cardiac arrest or sustained ventricular tachycardia; family history of multiple sudden or other premature HCM-related death (or identification) of a high-risk genotype; multiple repetitive nonsustained ventricular tachycardia on ambulatory Holter ECG; recurrent syncope; and possibly massive left ventricular hypertrophy.[15] The magnitude of the left ventricular outflow gradient has not been associated with an increased risk of sudden death, which may occur in both patients with subaortic obstruction and patients without subaortic obstruction.

Patients with HCM considered to be a particularly high risk for sudden death probably deserve aggressive preventive treatment, regardless of whether symptoms have intervened. The available therapeutic measures are the same as those used most frequently in coronary artery disease or dilated cardiomyopathy, ie, amiodarone administered in a relatively low maintenance dosage (200 to 300 mg per day) or use of the implantable cardioverter-defibrillator. The precise clinical criteria for choosing between these two treatment strategies have not been defined and randomized clinical data are not yet available. At present, a number of factors, such as the availability of advanced technology and cost-benefit considerations, may influence the choice. Furthermore, cultural differences in patient expectations and physician attitudes may have an important influence on the decision.

Based on both echocardiographic and necropsy analyses in large numbers of patients, it is apparent that the HCM disease spectrum is characterized by vast structural diversity with regard to the patterns and extent of left ventricular hypertrophy (Figure 3).[13,18,19] Indeed, virtually all possible patterns of left ventricular hypertrophy occur in HCM, and no single phenotypic expression can be considered "classic" or typical of this disease. Absolute thickness of the left ventricular wall varies greatly, although the average reported value is usually 21 to 22 mm.[18] Wall thickness is profoundly increased in many patients, including some showing the most severe hypertrophy observed in any cardiac disease; 60 mm is the most extreme wall thickness dimension reported to date.[19] On the other hand, the HCM phenotype is not invariably expressed as a particularly thickened left ventricle and some patients show only a mild increase of 13 to 18 mm; there are also a few genetically affected individuals with normal thicknesses (≤12 mm).[15]

The pattern of wall thickening is often strikingly heterogeneous, involving noncontiguous segments of the left ventricle (ie, with areas of normal thickness evident in between) or showing marked differences in wall thickness in contiguous segments. Transitions between thickened areas and regions of normal thickness are often sharp and abrupt, not infrequently creating right-angled contours of the wall. The variability in morphological expression of HCM is underlined by the fact that even first-degree relatives with the disease usually show great dissimilarity in the pattern of left ventricular wall thickening.[20]

Differential Diagnosis of Hypertrophic Cardiomyopathy and Athlete's Heart

In some young athletes, segmental hypertrophy of the anterior ventricular septum (wall thicknesses 13 to 15 mm), consistent with a relatively mild morphological expression of HCM, may be difficult to distinguish from the physiologic form of left ventricular hypertrophy, which is an adaptation to athletic training (ie, athlete's heart).[21] This distinction between athlete's heart[10–12,22] and cardiac disease has particularly important implications because in an effort to minimize risk, identification of cardiovascular disease in an athlete may be the basis for disqualification from competition.[9,21] By the same token, the improper diagnosis of cardiac disease in an athlete may lead to unnecessary withdrawal from athletics, thereby depriving that individual of the varied benefits of sports.

In asymptomatic individuals within this morphological "gray zone," the differential diagnosis between athlete's heart and HCM can be approached by clinical assessment and noninvasive testing (Figure 4).[21] While this distinction cannot be resolved with certainty in some athletes, careful analysis of several echocardiographic and clinical features permits this diagnostic differentiation in most.

Wall Thickness

In highly trained athletes, although the region of predominant left ventricular wall thickening always involves the anterior septum, the thicknesses of other segments of the wall are similar. In patients with

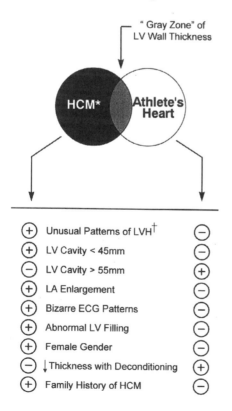

Figure 4. Chart showing criteria used to distinguish hypertrophic cardiomyopathy (HCM) from athlete's heart when the left ventricular (LV) wall thickness is within the shaded gray zone of overlap (13 to 15 mm), consistent with both diagnoses. *Assumed to be the nonobstructive form of HCM in this discussion, since the presence of substantial mitral valve systolic anterior motion would confirm, per se, the diagnosis of HCM in an athlete. †May involve a variety of abnormalities including heterogeneous distribution of left ventricular hypertrophy (LVH) in which asymmetry is prominent, and adjacent regions may be of greatly different thicknesses, with sharp transitions evident between segments; also, patterns in which the anterior ventricular septum is spared form the hypertrophic process and the region of predominant thickening may be in the posterior portion of septum or anterolateral or posterior free wall. ↓ indicates decreased; LA = left atrial. Reproduced from Reference 21, with permission from the American Heart Association.

HCM, while the anterior portion of the ventricular septum is usually the region of maximal wall thickening, the pattern of hypertrophy is often heterogeneous,[18,23] asymmetry is prominent, and areas other than the anterior septum may show the most marked thickening.[18,23] In addition, contiguous portions of the left ventricle often show strikingly different wall thicknesses, and the transition between such areas is often sharp and abrupt.

Cavity Dimension

An enlarged left ventricular end-diastolic cavity dimension (>55 mm) is present in more than one third of highly trained elite male athletes.[12,24] Conversely, the diastolic cavity dimension is small (usually <45 mm) in most patients with HCM, and is >55 mm only in those who evolve to the end-stage phase of the disease with progressive heart failure and systolic dysfunction.[25] Therefore, in some instances it is possible to distinguish the athlete's heart from HCM solely on the basis of left ventricular diastolic cavity dimension.[21] For example, a cavity >55 mm in an athlete with borderline wall thickness would constitute strong evidence against the presence of HCM; conversely, a cavity dimension <45 mm would be inconsistent with the athlete's heart. However, in those athletes in whom left ventricular cavity size falls between these extremes, this variable alone will not resolve the differential diagnosis.

Doppler Transmitral Waveform

Abnormalities of left ventricular diastolic filling have been identified noninvasively with pulsed Doppler echocardiography. Most patients with HCM, including those with relatively mild hypertrophy that could be confused with athlete's heart, show abnormal Doppler diastolic indices of left ventricular filling and relaxation independently of whether symptoms or outflow obstruction are present.[26]

On the other hand, trained athletes have invariably demonstrated normal left ventricular filling patterns.[21,27–34] Consequently, in an athlete suspected of having HCM, a distinctly abnormal Doppler transmitral flow-velocity pattern strongly supports this diagnosis, while a normal Doppler study is compatible with either HCM or athlete's heart.

Gender

Sex differences with regard to cardiac dimensions and left ventricular mass have been identified in trained athletes.[34–36] For example, female athletes rarely show left ventricular wall thicknesses ≥12 mm. Therefore, female athletes with wall thicknesses within the gray zone between athlete's heart and HCM[34] (in the presence of normal cavity size) are most likely to have HCM.

Regression of Left Ventricular Hypertrophy with Deconditioning

Serial echocardiographic examination demonstrating a decrease in cardiac dimensions and mass after a short period of athletic deconditioning can show increased left ventricular cavity size or wall thickness to be a physiologic consequence of athletic training.[37–39] For example, elite athletes with left ventricular hypertrophy may show reduction in wall thickness (of about 2 to 5 mm) with 3 months of deconditioning.[39] However, identification of such changes in wall thickness requires compliance from highly motivated competitive athletes to interrupt training, and also serial echocardiographic studies of optimal technical quality. An unequivocal decrease in left ventricular wall thickness with deconditioning is inconsistent with the presence of pathologic hypertrophy and HCM.

Familial Transmission and Genetics

The most definitive evidence for the presence of HCM in an athlete with increased wall thickness comes from the demonstration of the disease in a relative.[40–46] Therefore, for those athletes in whom the distinction between HCM and athlete's heart cannot be achieved definitively by other methods, one potential approach for resolving this diagnostic uncertainty is the echocardiographic screening of family members. Absence of HCM in a family, however, does not exclude HCM since the disease may be "sporadic" (ie, absent in relatives other than the index case), presumably as a result of de novo mutation.[43]

Recent advances in the understanding of the genetic alterations responsible for HCM raise the possibility of DNA diagnosis in athletes suspected of having this disease.[21,40–46] At present, mutations responsible for HCM have been identified in five genes located on chromosomes 14, 1, 11, 19, and 15; each of these genes encodes proteins of the sarcomere: β-myosin heavy chain, cardiac troponin T, myosin-binding protein-C, troponin-I and α-tropomyosin, respectively.[40–46] Thus, mutations of four different genes can cause HCM. This substantial genetic heterogeneity, and the expensive, time-intensive methodologies required, has made it extremely difficult at present to use the techniques of molecular biology for the purpose of resolving clinically the differential diagnosis between athlete's heart and HCM.

Other Diseases

In addition, frequently at autopsy hearts are encountered with increased mass (and wall thickness) and nondilated left ventricular cavity suggestive of HCM, but in which the objective morphological findings are not sufficiently striking to permit a definitive diagnosis of this disease.[2] It is uncertain whether some of these cases (often referred to as idiopathic left ventricular hypertrophy)[6] represent a mild morphological expression of HCM, or possibly unusual instances of athlete's heart with particularly marked physiologic left ventricular hypertrophy, and with deleterious consequences.

Less common causes of sudden death in young athletes[2-7] include myocarditis, dilated cardiomyopathy, Marfan syndrome with ruptured aorta, aortic valve stenosis, atherosclerotic coronary artery disease, the long QT syndrome, mitral valve prolapse, and arrhythmogenic right ventricular dysplasia. It has also been suggested that major coronary arteries tunneled within the left ventricular myocardium for part of their course constitute a potentially lethal anatomic variant that may cause sudden unexpected death during exertion in otherwise healthy young individuals.[2,47]

Occasionally, athletes who die suddenly demonstrate no evidence of structural cardiovascular disease, even after careful gross and microscopic examination of the heart. In such instances (about 2% of youthful athletic field deaths)[2] it may not be possible to exclude with certainty noncardiac factors (eg, drug abuse) as responsible for the catastrophe, or to determine whether careful inspection of the specialized conducting system and associated vasculature by means of serial sectioning (which is not part of the standard medical examiners' protocol) would have revealed occult but clinically relevant abnormalities. Obviously, while one can only speculate on the potential etiologies of such deaths, it is possible that some are due to either previously unidentified Wolff-Parkinson-White syndrome, a primary arrhythmia in the absence of cardiac morphological abnormalities, rare but known diseases in which structural cardiac abnormalities are characteristically lacking at necropsy such as long QT syndrome, or possibly exercise-induced coronary spasm or undetected segmental forms of right ventricular dysplasia.

Demographics

Based primarily on data assembled from broad-based United States populations,[2,3,5-7] a profile of young competitive athletes who die suddenly has emerged. Such athletes participated in a large number and variety of sports, the most frequent (approximately 70%) being basketball and football , probably reflecting the high participation level in these popular team sports, but probably also reflecting their intensity. The vast majority (approximately 90%) of athletic field deaths occur in men; the relative infrequency in women probably reflects a lower participation level, sometimes less intense levels of training, and the fact that certain diseases most commonly accountable for sudden death in athletes appear to occur somewhat less frequently in women (eg, HCM). Most athletes (approximately 60%) are of high school age at the time of death; however, other sudden deaths occur in young athletes who have achieved collegiate or even professional levels of competition.

The vast majority of athletes who incur sudden death, regardless of their particular underlying disease, had been free of cardiovascular symptoms during their lives and were not suspected to harbor cardiovascular disease. Sudden collapse usually occurs associated with exercise, predominantly in the late afternoon and early evening hours, corresponding to peak periods of competition and training, particularly in organized team sports such as football and basketball (Figure 5).[2,5] These observations substantiate that, in the presence of certain underlying structural cardiovascular diseases, physical activity represents a trigger and an important precipitating factor for sudden collapse on the athletic field. This predilection for sudden death late in the day is similar for athletes with HCM as well as athletes with other lesions. This observation in athletes with HCM contrasts strikingly with the findings in patients with HCM (who were *not* competitive athletes) in whom a bimodal pattern of circadian variability over the 24-hour day with regard to sudden death has been documented, in which a prominent early- to mid-morning peak is evident, similar to that described in patients with coronary artery disease (acute myocardial infarction and angina) (Figure 5).[48]

Although the majority of reported sudden deaths in competitive athletes have been in white males, a substantial proportion (>40%) are in African American athletes.[2] There is also evidence that HCM is an important cause of sudden death in young African American athletes and that such catastrophes appear to be significantly more common in black athletes compared to white athletes (Figure 6). This observation could, of course, be influenced by disproportionate participation rates with regard to racial groups and also selection biases in the reporting of cases. Nevertheless, the substantial occurrence of HCM-related sudden

---

Figure 5. Histograms showing hourly distribution of sudden cardiac death in 127 competitive athletes with hypertrophic cardiomyopathy (HCM) and with a variety of other predominantly congenital cardiovascular malformations (**A**), and in 94 nonathlete patients with HCM (**B**). **A.** *Athletes:* Time of death was predominantly

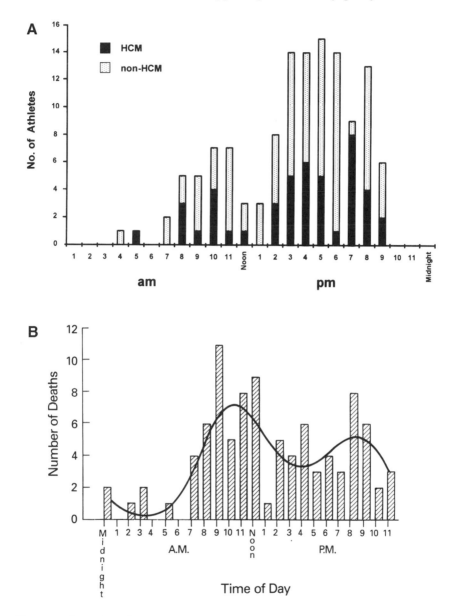

Figure 5. (continued) in the late afternoon and early evening, largely correspond-ing to the time of training and competition. Bold portions of the bars represent the hour of death for the athletes with HCM. Reproduced from Reference 2, with per-mission from the American Medical Association. **B.** *HCM:* In contrast, superim-posed line denotes a bimodal pattern for sudden death (double-harmonic model) with a prominent early peak between 7 AM and 1 PM and a secondary peak in the early evening, most evident between 8 PM and 10 PM. Reproduced from Reference 48, with permission from the Journal of American College of Cardiology.

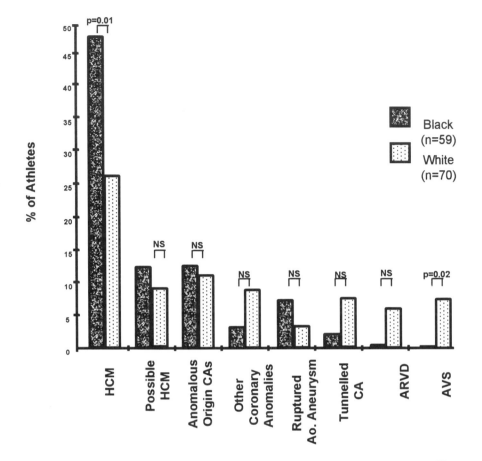

Figure 6. Impact of race on cardiovascular causes of sudden death in competitive athletes. "Possible HCM" denotes those hearts with some morphological features consistent with (but not diagnostic of) hypertrophic cardiomyopathy (HCM). Ao. = aortic; ARVD= arrhythmogenic right ventricular dysplasia; AVS = aortic valve stenosis; CA = coronary anomalies; HCM = hypertrophic cardiomyopathy. Reproduced from Reference 2, with permission from the American Medical Association.

death in young black male athletes contrasts sharply with the very infrequent reporting of black patients with HCM in hospital-based populations (particularly tertiary referral centers).[49,50] Therefore, in young black males, HCM is most frequently encountered when the disease results in sudden and unexpected death during competitive athletics.[50] These data emphasize the disproportionate access to subspecialty health care between the African American and white communities in the United States, which makes it less likely for young black males to receive a relatively sophisticated cardiovascular diagnosis such as HCM, compared to their white counterparts.[50] Consequently, it would appear that African American athletes with HCM are less likely to be disqualified from competition, to reduce their risk for sudden death, in accordance with the recommendations of the 26th Bethesda Conference.[9]

References

1. Maron BJ. Sudden death in young athletes: Lessons from the Hank Gathers affair. *N Engl J Med* 1993;329:55–57.
2. Maron BJ, Shirani J, Poliac LC, et al. Sudden death in young competitive athletes: Clinical, demographic and pathological profiles. *JAMA* 1996;276: 199–204.
3. Burke AP, Farb A, Virmani R, et al. Sports-related and non-sports-related sudden cardiac death in young athletes. *Am Heart J* 1991;121:568–575.
4. Corrado D, Thiene G, Nava A, et al. Sudden death in young competitive athletes: Clinicopathologic correlations in 22 cases. *Am J Med* 1990;39:588–596.
5. Van Camp SP, Bloor CM, Mueller FO, et al. Nontraumatic sports death in high school and college athletes. *Med Sci Sports Exer* 1995;27:641–647.
6. Maron BJ, Roberts WC, McAllister HA, et al. Sudden death in young athletes. *Circulation* 1980;62:218–229.
7. Liberthson RR. Sudden death from cardiac causes in children and young adults. *N Engl J Med* 1996;334:1039–1044.
8. Maron BJ, Thompson PD, Puffer JC, et al. Cardiovascular preparticipation screening of competitive athletes. *Circulation* 1996;94:850–856.
9. Maron BJ, Mitchell JH. 26th Bethesda Conference. Recommendations for determining eligibility for competition in athletes with cardiovascular abnormalities. *J Am Coll Cardiol* 1994;24:845–899.
10. Huston TP, Puffer JC, Rodney WM. The athletic heart syndrome. *N Engl J Med* 1985;313:24–32.
11. Maron BJ. Structural features of the athlete heart as defined by echocardiography. *J Am Coll Cardiol* 1986;7:190–203.
12. Pelliccia A, Maron BJ, Spataro A, et al. The upper limit of physiologic cardiac hypertrophy in highly trained elite athletes. *N Engl J Med* 1991; 324:295–301.
13. Maron BJ, Bonow RO, Cannon RO, et al. Hypertrophic cardiomyopathy: Interrelation of clinical manifestations, pathophysiology, and therapy. *N Engl J Med* 1987;316:780–789, 844–852.
14. Wigle ED, Sasson Z, Henderson MA, et al. Hypertrophic cardiomyopathy. The importance of the site and extent of hypertrophy. A review. *Prog Cardiovasc Dis* 1985;28:1–83.
15. Spirito P, Seidman CE, McKenna SJ, Maron BJ. The management of hypertrophic cardiomyopathy. *N Engl J Med* 1997;336:775–785.
16. Maron BJ, Gardin JM, Flack JM, et al. Assessment of the prevalence of hypertrophic cardiomyopathy in a general population of young adults: Echocardiographic analysis of 4111 subjects in the CARDIA Study. *Circulation* 1995;92:785–789.
17. Maron BJ, Roberts WC, Epstein SE. Sudden death in hypertrophic cardiomyopathy: A profile of 78 patients. *Circulation* 1982;65:1388–1394.
18. Klues HG, Schiffers A, Maron BJ. Phenotypic spectrum and patterns of left ventricular hypertrophy in hypertrophic cardiomyopathy: Morphologic observations and significance as assessed by two-dimensional echocardiography in 600 patients. *J Am Coll Cardiol* 1995;26:1699–1708.
19. Maron BJ, Gross BW, Stark SI. Extreme left ventricular hypertrophy. *Circulation* 1995;92:3748.

20. Ciró E, Nichols PF, Maron BJ. Heterogeneous morphologic expression of genetically transmitted hypertrophic cardiomyopathy: Two-dimensional echocardiographic analysis. *Circulation* 1983;67:1227–1233.
21. Maron BJ, Pelliccia A, Spirito P. Cardiac disease in young trained athletes: Insights into methods for distinguishing athlete's heart from structural heart disease with particular emphasis on hypertrophic cardiomyopathy. *Circulation* 1995;91:1596–1601.
22. Shapiro LM, Smith RG. Effect of training on left ventricular structure and function: An echocardiographic study. *Br Heart J* 1983;50:534–539.
23. Maron BJ, Gottdiener JS, Epstein SE. Patterns and significance of the distribution of left ventricular hypert ophy in hypertrophic cardiomyopathy: A wide-angle, two-dimensional e .hocardiographic study of 125 patients. *Am J Cardiol* 1981;48:418–428.
24. Spirito P, Pelliccia A, Proschan MA, et al. Morphology of the "athlete's heart" assessed by echocardiography in 947 elite athletes representing 27 sports. *Am J Cardiol* 1994;74:802–806.
25. Spirito P, Maron BJ, Bonow RO, Epstein SE. Occurrence and significance of progressive left ventricular wall thinning and relative cavity dilatation in patients with hypertrophic cardiomyopathy. *Am J Cardiol* 1987;60:123–129.
26. Maron BJ, Spirito P, Green KJ, et al. Noninvasive assessment of left ventricular diastolic function by pulsed Doppler echocardiography in patients with hypertrophic cardiomyopathy. *J Am Coll Cardiol* 1987;10:733–742.
27. Lewis JF, Spirito P, Pelliccia A, Maron BJ. Usefulness of Doppler echocardiographic assessment of diastolic filling in distinguishing "athlete's heart" from hypertrophic cardiomyopathy. *Br Heart J* 1992;68:296–300.
28. Colan SD, Sanders SP, MacPherson D, Borow KM. Left ventricular diastolic function in elite athletes with physiologic cardiac hypertrophy. *J Am Coll Cardiol* 1985;6:545–549.
29. Granger CB, Karuimeddini MK, Smith VE, et al. Rapid ventricular filling in left ventricular hypertrophy. I: Physiologic hypertrophy. *J Am Coll Cardiol* 1985;5:862–868.
30. Pearson AC, Schiff M, Mrosek D, et al. Left ventricular diastolic function in weight lifters. *Am J Cardiol* 1986;58:1254–1259.
31. Fagard R, Van den Brocke C, Bielen E, et al. Assessment of stiffness of the hypertrophied left ventricle of bicyclists using left ventricular inflow Doppler velocimetry. *J Am Coll Cardiol* 1987;9:1250–1254.
32. Finkelhor RS, Hanak IJ, Bahler RC. Left ventricular filling in endurance-trained subjects. *J Am Coll Cardiol* 1986;8:289–293.
33. Nixon JV, Wright AR, Porter TR, et al. Effects of exercise on left ventricular diastolic performance in trained athletes. *Am J Cardiol* 1991;68:945–949.
34. Pelliccia A, Maron BJ, Culasso F, et al. Athlete's heart in women: Echocardiographic characterization of highly trained elite female athletes. *JAMA* 1996;276:211–215.
35. Milliken MC, Stray-Gundersen J, Pesock RM, et al. Left ventricular mass as determined by magnetic resonance imaging in male endurance athletes. *Am J Cardiol* 1988;62:301–305.
36. Riley-Hagen M, Peshock RM, Stray-Gunersen J, et al. Left ventricular dimensions and mass using magnetic resonance imaging in female endurance athletes. *Am J Cardiol* 1992;69:1067–1074.
37. Ehsani AA, Hagberg JM, Hickson RC. Rapid changes in left ventricular dimensions and mass in response to physical conditioning and deconditioning. *Am J Cardiol* 1978;42:52–56.

38. Fagard R, Aubert A, Lysens R, et al. Noninvasive assessment of seasonal variations in cardiac structure and function in cyclists. *Circulation* 1983; 67:896–901.

39. Maron BJ, Pelliccia A, Spataro A, Granata M. Reduction in left ventricular wall thickness after deconditioning in highly trained Olympic athletes. *Br Heart J* 1993;69:125–128.

40. Maron BJ, Nichols PF, Pickle LW, et al. Patterns of inheritance in hypertrophic cardiomyopathy: Assessment by M-mode and two-dimensional echocardiography. *Am J Cardiol* 1984;53:1087–1094.

41. Watkins H, Conner D, Thierfelder L, et al. Mutations in the cardiac myosin binding protein-C gene on chromosome 11 cause familial hypertrophic cardiomyopathy. *Nat Genet* 1995;11:434–437.

42. Thierfelder L, Watkins H, MacRae C, et al. α-Tropomyosin and cardiac troponin T mutations cause familial hypertrophic cardiomyopathy: A disease of the sarcomere. *Cell* 1994;77:701–712.

43. Watkins H, Thierfelder L, Hwang D-S, et al. Sporadic hypertrophic cardiomyopathy due to de novo myosin mutations. *J Clin Invest* 1992;90: 1666–1671.

44. Watkins H, Rosenzweig A, Hwang D-S, et al. Characteristics and prognostic implications of myosin missense mutations in familial hypertrophic cardiomyopthy. *N Engl J Med* 1992;326:1108–1114.

45. Marian AJ, Roberts WC. Recent advances in the molecular genetics of hypertrophic cardiomyopathy. *Circulation* 1995;92:1336–1347.

46. Schwartz K, Carrier L, Guicheney P, Komajda M. Molecular basis of familial cardiomyopathies. *Circulation* 1995;91:532–540.

47. Morales AR, Romanelli R, Boucek RJ. The mural left anterior descending coronary artery, strenuous exercise and sudden death. *Circulation* 1980; 62:230–237.

48. Maron BJ, Kogan J, Proschan MA, et al. Circadian variability in the occurrence of sudden cardiac death in patients with hypertrophic cardiomyopathy. *J Am Coll Cardiol* 1994;23:1405–1409.

49. Maron BJ, Spirito P. Impact of patient selection biases on the perception of hypertrophic cardiomyopathy and its natural history. *Am J Cardiol* 1993;72:970–972.

50. Maron BJ, Poliac LC, Mathenge R. Hypertrophic cardiomyopathy as an important cause of sudden cardiac death on the athletic field in African-American athletes. *J Am Coll Cardiol* 1997;29(suppl A):462A. Abstract.

Part IV

Structural Heart Disease and Illicit Drug Use

17

Marfan Syndrome

Deeb N. Salem, MD and Richard D. Patten, MD

The Marfan syndrome is a heritable disorder of connective tissue that was first described in 1896 by a French physician who reported the classic skeletal manifestations in a 5-year-old girl.[1] The most notable historical figure who suffered from this genetic ailment was the 16th president of the United States, Abraham Lincoln.[2] The exact defect in protein synthesis or metabolism that causes Marfan syndrome is not entirely known, but evidence suggests that an abnormality of the cross linkage of both collagen and elastin may be the culprit.[3] Most patients with Marfan syndrome do not exhibit chromosomal abnormalities; however, there have been reports of enlarged or elongated satellites on chromosome 14, determined by the G-banding technique.[1] In addition, abnormalities on chromosome 15 have been noted. In fact, specific abnormalities in genes encoding microfibrillar proteins (called fibrillins) located on chromosome 15 have been discovered in patients with Marfan syndrome, suggesting a causative role of these connective tissue elements.[4] Marfan syndrome is inherited by a simple Mendelian autosomal dominant pattern, although as many as 15% of cases may be sporadic. Rare cases may carry an autosomal recessive inheritance pattern.[1,5] Most patients with Marfan syndrome who die prematurely do so as a result of the cardiovascular complications.

The prevalence of Marfan syndrome has been reported to be 4 to 6 per 100,000 people without racial or ethnic predilection.[5] The actual prevalence may be considerably greater because manifestations may extend from easily identifiable "classic" cases to those in relatively normal

From Estes NAM, Salem DN, Wang PJ (eds). *Sudden Cardiac Death in the Athlete.* Armonk, NY: Futura Publishing Co., Inc.; ©1998.

individuals. The diagnosis of the Marfan syndrome is based on the presence of the following: (1) family history; (2) ocular manifestations; (3) skeletal abnormalities; and (4) cardiovascular manifestations. In a patient with a positive family history, the diagnosis is confirmed if the patient exhibits characteristic manifestations in two of the three systems listed. In a patient without a family history of Marfan syndrome, a diagnosis is made if the patient manifests cardiovascular complications in addition to manifestations in one of the other systems (ie, ocular or skeletal).[6]

Most patients with Marfan syndrome (>80%) have a family history of the disease consistent with an autosomal dominant inheritance pattern.[5] The most common ocular manifestation is "ectopia lentis," displacement of the lens (usually upward), present in 50% to 80% of patients and usually found at the first detailed ophthalmic examination. In addition, increased axial length of the globe is common, as is a relatively flat cornea. These ocular features provide further objective measures for diagnosing the condition.[5]

The skeletal manifestations are numerous and are, perhaps, the most familiar components of the syndrome.[5] The length of the limbs is increased relative to the trunk (known as *dolichostenomelia*). This is quantified by measuring the lower segment length (top of the pubic ramus to the floor) divided into the upper segment length (height minus the lower segment length). In the Marfan patient, this ratio is greater than two standard deviations below the mean for age, race, and sex. The fingers of the patient with Marfan syndrome are long and thin (arachnodactyly); however, this feature is relatively subjective. The "thumb sign" is positive when the thumb, completely opposed within the clenched fist, protrudes outward beyond the ulnar border. The "wrist sign" is positive if the distal phalanges of the first and fifth fingers of one hand overlap when wrapped around the wrist of the opposite hand. Joint laxity is also characteristic but is of little diagnostic specificity. Pectus deformities are also common, including pectus excavatum, which is more common than pectus carinatum. Kyphosis, scoliosis, and a combination of both is also very common in this disorder.

The hallmark cardiovascular manifestations of Marfan syndrome include aortic root dilatation, expansion of the proximal ascending aorta, and mitral valve prolapse (MVP). Progressive dilatation of the aortic root and ascending limb of the aorta (also known as annulo-aortic ectasia) leads to aortic insufficiency and predisposes to aortic dissection and aortic rupture. Histologic examination of aortic specimens in Marfan syndrome reveal cystic medial necrosis, disruption of collagen fibers, and degeneration of the media which are probably the causes of decreased aortic tensile strength. Echocardiographic studies of aortic stiffness have demonstrated decreased aortic distensibility in patients with Marfan syndrome irrespective of aortic diameter.[7,8] The risk of aortic dissection and aortic insufficiency is greatest with severe aortic dilatation but dissection (particularly distal) may occur with even mild dilatation of the aorta.

De Paepe et al[4] recently suggested a revision of the diagnostic criteria that may more accurately diagnosis the condition. Their approach makes use of defined major and minor criteria from each of the above organ systems, as shown in Table 1. For an index case, in the absence of contributing family history the diagnosis is confirmed if major criteria are present in two systems with involvement of a third system. For the relative of an index case, the presence of one of the following criteria is necessary: (1) a first-degree relative who meets the diagnostic criteria; (2) presence of a mutation in the gene encoding fibrillin-1 (FBN1) known to cause the Marfan syndrome; or (3) presence of a haplotype around FBN1 known to be associated with confirmed Marfan syndrome in the family. In addition, a relative should display one major criterion in an organ system and involvement of a second organ system.[4]

Homocystcinuria should be considered in the differential diagnosis of patients presenting with features of Marfan syndrome. Patients with this disorder display ectopia lentis but are more likely to exhibit severe myopia and some degree of mental retardation. A positive cyanide-nitroprusside test confirms this diagnosis.[9]

Complications of Marfan syndrome can occur at any age. El Habbal[10] reviewed the serious cardiovascular sequelae (over a 10-year period) of 186 patients, 20 years of age or younger, who were diagnosed to have this disorder. Eight patients (4.3%) developed serious cardiovascular complications (see Table 2). Two patients died suddenly of rupture of the ascending aorta, 3 patients underwent aortic valve replacement for aortic insufficiency, 2 patients underwent emergency replacement of the ascending aorta, and 1 patient had symptomatic mitral regurgitation due to MVP. Paradoxically, in this study the finding of a negative family history was higher in patients who had serious complications than in those without. These authors also found that the incidence of seemingly unrelated cardiovascular abnormalities, ie, bicuspid aortic valve, atrial septal defect, and tetralogy of Fallot, was significantly higher than that seen in a normal population. Marsalese et al[11] reported on the follow-up of 81 patients with Marfan syndrome presenting primarily with aortic valve or root involvement. There were 31 deaths over a mean follow-up period of 99 months. Sixty-one percent were due to aortic dissection or rupture or sudden death. More recently, Silverman et al[12] examined survival and cause of death in a larger series of 417 patients with Marfan syndrome who were followed at referral centers; during this time 47 deaths were recorded. Approximately 21% were attributed to aortic rupture or dissection, whereas 6%

Table 1
Diagnostic Criteria for Marfan's Syndrome

	Skeletal System	Ocular System	Cardiovascular System
Major Criteria	1. pectus carinatum 2. pectus excavatum requiring surgery 3. dec. upper/lower segment ratio or arm span to height ratio to greater than 1.05 4. wrist and thumb signs 5. Scoliosis of >20° 6. Reduced elbow extension (<170°) 7. Medial displacement of medial malleolus causing pes planus 8. protusio acetabulae	1. ectopia lentis	1. dilatation of the ascending aorta with or without aortic regurgitation and involving at least the sinuses of Valsalva 2. Dissection of the ascending aorta
Minor Criteria	1. Moderate pectus excavatum 2. joint hypermobility 3. highly arched palate 4. characteristic facial appearance	1. abnormally flat cornea 2. increased axial length of globe 3. decreased miosis secondary to hypoplastic iris or ciliary muscle	1. Mitral valve prolapse with or without mitral regurgitation 2. dilatation of the main pulmonary artery without obvious cause below the age of 40 3. calcified mitral annulus below age 40 4. dilatation or dissection of the descending thoracic or abdominal aorta below age 50
	• At least two major criteria or one major criterion and two minor criteria	• At least two minor criteria	• One major or only one minor criteria.

Adapted from Reference 4.

Table 2
Ten-Year Follow-Up of Serious Cardiovascular Sequelae of Young Patients with Marfan Syndrome

Number of Patients	Serious Cardiovascular Manifestations	Age (yr)/Sex	Status
2	Rupture of ascending aorta	14/M, 19/M	Dead
1	Severe aortic regurgitation	18 1/2/M	Alive
2	Aneurysm of ascending aorta	7/F, 17/M	Alive
1	Dissection of ascending aorta	19/M	Alive
1	Repeated aortic valve surgery	19/M	Dead
1	Moderate mitral regurgitation with decreased exercise tolerance	8/F	Alive

M = male; F = female. Adapted from Reference 10.

were reported to be "sudden," with 15% of the deaths secondary to perioperative mortality and 8% related to congestive heart failure.

The actual incidence of ventricular arrhythmias in patients with Marfan syndrome is unknown. Chen et al[13] reported the case of a teenager with Marfan syndrome who presented with sudden death. They also published a series of 24 children, 8 of whom had evidence of ventricular dysrhythmias, including 3 with ventricular tachycardia. The incidence of ventricular arrhythmias was associated with a prolonged QT interval, especially when combined with MVP, in this small series.

The prevalence and natural history of MVP in Marfan syndrome appears distinct from MVP associated with other conditions in that serious mitral regurgitation develops in 1 of every 8 patients by the third decade.[14] Come et al[15] found MVP in 57% of 61 patients with Marfan syndrome. Pini et al[16] looked at mitral valve dimensions and motion in patients with Marfan syndrome and compared them to those in patients with primary MVP and normal subjects. These authors concluded that: (1) mitral valve billowing occurred more commonly in Marfan patients than in patients with primary MVP; (2) MVP in Marfan patients appeared to be due to mitral valve enlargement and abnormal chordae or abnormal mitral annular dispensability; (3) Marfan patients with MVP have low body weight and low systolic blood pressure; (4) Marfan patients with MVP more often have arachnodactyly than Marfan patients without MVP.

In the 1970s Marfan syndrome gained national attention when two Atlantic Coast Conference basketball players and an accomplished varsity swimmer with the disorder died suddenly within a 3-year period.[17] In 1986, Flo Hyman, an American volleyball star, died of aortic rupture while playing professionally in Japan.[18] Libertshon's review of the literature of 469 sudden deaths from cardiac causes in young persons from 1950 to 1993 revealed 6% of the deaths to be from dissecting aortic aneurysms and 9% of the deaths to be related to MVP.[19] In 1980, Maron et al[20] reported on sudden death in athletes younger than 35 years old. Seven percent were due to ruptured aorta, while a subsequent report based on a systemic tracking of US athletes from 1985 until 1995 reported that 5% of 158 deaths were due to aortic rupture.[21]

Come et al[15] reported physical exam findings of mitral valve disease and/or aortic regurgitation in 52% of patients with Marfan syndrome (MVP in 44% and aortic regurgitation in 23%). However, echocardiography was found to be more sensitive, revealing findings of mitral valve disease and/or aortic regurgitation in 82% of patients (MVP in 57% and aortic root enlargement in 69%). These authors found that the prevalence of MVP was equal in males and females, however aortic root enlargement was more prevalent in males (83% compared to 50%). It was also concluded that echocardiography was more sensitive than chest x-ray in detecting aortic root enlargement. Nuclear magnetic resonance has also shown promise in defining the extent of aortic root and proximal ascending aortic dilation.[22]

Recommendations for Athletic Participation

The 26th Bethesda Conference on Recommendations for Eligibility in Competition for Athletes with Cardiovascular Abnormalities recommends that athletes with Marfan syndrome that do not have a family history of premature sudden death and do not have evidence of aortic root dilatation or mitral regurgitation can participate in low and moderate static/low dynamic competitive sports classes IA and IIA.[23] The panel recommends measurement of aortic root dimension every 6 months for continued participation in sports. It is recommended that athletes with aortic root dilatation compete only in low-intensity competitive sports (class IA). Athletes with Marfan syndrome should not participate in sports that involve bodily collision.

Management

For over two decades it has been suggested that β-adrenergic blocking agents may reduce the risk of aortic root dissection in patients with Marfan syndrome. Based on theoretical considerations as well as experimental and clinical data on the management of patients with dissecting aortic aneurysms, β-blockers have long been considered the medical treatment of choice for patients with aortic aneurysms and Marfan syndrome. However, there are some experimental data that question the hemodynamic benefits of β-blockers in this disorder. Yin et al[24] performed cardiac catheterizations on nine patients with Marfan syndrome and concluded that although nitroprusside acutely increased aortic compliance, intravenous propranolol decreased aortic compliance. Nonetheless, clinical data seem to support the use of β-blockers in patients with this disorder. In 1994, Shores et al[25] published the results of an open-label randomized trial of propranolol in young patients with classic Marfan syndrome. Thirty-two patients were treated and 38 served as controls. The patients were monitored for an average of 9.3 years in the control group and 10.7 years in the treatment group. The average dose of propranolol was 212 ± 68 mg given in four divided daily doses. The rate of aortic root enlargement was significantly less in the propranolol-treated patients. Clinical endpoints such as aortic regurgitation, aortic dissection, cardiovascular surgery, congestive heart failure, and death were reached in five treatment patients and in nine patients in the control group. There was a significant survival benefit noted in the treatment group.

Surgery has proven to be clearly lifesaving for patients with Marfan syndrome. Silverman et al[12] recently reported a median probability of survival of 72 years among 417 patients followed at referral centers in the modern surgical era, compared to 48 years reported by Murdoch et al[26] in the classic natural history study published in 1972. Additionally, Finkbohner et al[27] reported on the long-term survival and complications of 103 patients with Marfan syndrome following aortic aneurysm repair. The median probability of survival in this population was 61 years; 53% of patients in this series had second operations. The factors that predicted the need for second aortic operations were hypertension, aortic dissection at the time of the first surgery, and a history of smoking. Marsalese et al[11] reported an increase in 5-year survival from 56% to 87.5% in Marfan patients operated in 1979 or later compared to an earlier surgical group.

Thus, although Marfan syndrome has become a treatable disorder, it is still an extremely serious medical problem that often leads to disqualification from competitive athletic activities. For physicians, patients, and families who need further information or support, the National Marfan Foundation is probably the best resource:

National Marfan Foundation (NMF)
382 Main Street
Port Washington, NY 11050
(516) 883–8712
(800) 8-MARFAN

References

1. Sun QB, Zhang KZ, Cheng TO, et al. Marfan syndrome in china: A collective review of 564 cases among 98 families. *Am Heart J* 1990;120(4): 934–948.
2. Schwartz H. Abraham Lincoln and the Marfan syndrome. *JAMA* 1964; 187:473–479.
3. Boucek RF, Noble NL, Gunja-Smith Z, Butler WT. The Marfan syndrome: A deficiency in chemically stable collagen cross links. *N Engl J Med* 1981; 305:988–991.
4. De Paepe A, Devereux RB, Dietz HC, et al. Revised diagnostic criteria for the Marfan syndrome. *Am J Med Genet* 1996;62:417–426.
5. Pyeritz RE, McKusick VA. The Marfan syndrome: Diagnosis and management. *N Engl J Med* 1979;300(14):772–777.
6. Child JS, Perloff JK, Kaplan S. The Heart of the matter: Cardiovascular involvement in Marfan's syndrome. (Editorial) *J Am Coll Cardiol* 1989; 14:429–431.
7. Hirata K, Triposkiadis F, Sparks E, et al. The Marfan syndrome: Abnormal aortic elastic properties. *J Am Coll Cardiol* 1991;18:57–63.
8. Jeremy RW, Huang H, Hwa J, et al. Relation between age, arterial distensability, and aortic dilatation in the Marfan syndrome. *Am J Cardiol* 1994;74:369–373.
9. Cruysberg JRM, Boers GHJ, Trijbels JMF, Deutman AF. Delay in diagnosis of homocysteinuria: Retrospective study of consecutive patients. *Br Med J* 1996;313:1037–1040.
10. El Habbal MH. Cardiovascular manifestations of Marfan's syndrome in the young. *Am Heart J* 1992;123:752–757.
11. Marsalese DL, Moodie DS, Vacante M, et al. Marfan's syndrome: Natural history and long-term follow-up of cardiovascular involvement. *J Am Coll Cardiol* 1989;14:422–428.
12. Silverman DI, Burton KJ, Gray J, et al. Life expectancy in the Marfan syndrome. *Am J Cardiol* 1995;75:157–160.
13. Chen S, Fagan LF, Nouri S, Donahoe JL. Ventricular dysrhythmias in children with Marfan's syndrome. *Am J Dis Child* 1985;139:273–276.
14. Pyeritz RE, Wappel MA. Mitral valve dysfunction in the Marfan syndrome. *Am J Med* 1983;74:797–807.
15. Come PC, Fortuin NJ, White RI Jr, et al. Echocardiographic assessment of cardiovascular abnormalities in the Marfan syndrome. *Am J Med* 1983; 74:465–474.
16. Pini R, Roman M, Kramer-Fox R, et al. Mitral valve dimensions and motion in Marfan patients with and without mitral valve prolapse. *Circulation* 1989;80:915–924.
17. McMillan RL. Sudden death in athletes and Marfan's syndrome. *Phys and Sports Med* 1978;June:105–109.
18. Demak R. Marfan syndrome: A silent killer. *Sports Illustrated* January, 1986.
19. Liberthson RR. Sudden death from cardiac causes in children and young adults. *New Engl J Med* 1996;334(16):1039–1044.
20. Maron BJ, Roberts WC, McAllister HA, et al. Sudden death in young athletes. *Circulation* 1980;62:218–229.
21. Maron BJ, Shirani J, Poliac LC, et al. Sudden death in competitive young athletes: Clinical, demographic, and pathologic profiles. *JAMA* 1996;276: 199–204.

22. Schaefer S, Peshock RM, Malloy CR, et al. Nuclear magnetic resonance imaging in Marfan's syndrome. *J Am Coll Cardiol* 1987;9:70–74.
23. Maron BJ, Mitchell JH. 26th Bethesda Conference: Recommendations for determining eligibility for competition in athletes with cardiovascular abnormalities. *J Am Coll Cardiol* 1994;24(4):846–897.
24. Yin FCP, Brin KP, Ting C-T, Pyeritz RE. Arterial hemodynamic indexes in Marfan's syndrome. *Circulation* 1989;79:854–862.
25. Shores J, Berger KR, Murphy EA, et al. Progression of aortic dilatation and the benefit of long-term β-adrenergic blockade in Marfan's syndrome. *N Engl J Med* 1994;330:1335–1341.
26. Murdoch JL, Walker BA, Halpern BL, et al. Life expectancy and causes of death in the Marfan syndrome. *N Engl J Med* 1972;286:804–808.
27. Finkbohner R, Johnston D, Crawford ES, et al. Marfan syndrome: Long term survival and complications after aortic aneurysm repair. *Circulation* 1995;91:28–33.

18

Dilated Cardiomyopathy and the Athlete

John J. Smith, MD, PhD

Cardiomyopathy is a general term for a family of diseases that affect systolic or diastolic function of the heart. In industrialized countries, coronary disease accounts for approximately 50% of cases of left ventricular systolic failure.[1] The balance of patients have nonischemic cardiomyopathies of which there are many etiologies. Often the proximate cause of myocardial failure is unknown and the cause defined as "idiopathic." The natural history of these diseases involves the progressive dilation of the left ventricle and, thus, the term *dilated cardiomyopathy* is often employed. In the following discussion the term *dilated cardiomyopathy* (DCM) refers to left ventricular systolic dysfunction due to nonischemic etiologies.

DCM is the cause of sudden death in athletes in approximately 3% of reported deaths.[2] The pathophysiology of DCM compromises cardiac reserve, thus limiting the ability of the athlete with DCM to effectively compete. Athletes affected by this condition may consult a physician if they experience exercise intolerance, but symptomatic arrhythmias and aborted sudden death may also bring these patients to medical attention. The more important question posed to the health practitioner is "when can the patient/athlete with DCM resume exercise?" This chapter reviews the history and pathophysiology of the condition, as well as the limited data base pertaining to exercise by this population, in order to assist in these decisions.

From Estes NAM, Salem DN, Wang PJ (eds). *Sudden Cardiac Death in the Athlete.* Armonk, NY: Futura Publishing Co., Inc.; ©1998.

Natural History of Dilated Cardiomyopathy

The natural history of patients with DCM is difficult to track for a number of reasons. First, the initiation of the cardiomyopathic process is usually unknown, often occurring during an asymptomatic period of the disease or with symptoms that may be confused with more common conditions such as influenza or upper respiratory tract infections. Second, there are a number of pathologic processes that follow a common pathway to DCM. The etiologic agent, which may be infectious, toxic, or proinflammatory, is absent at the time of diagnosis. Third, the clinical course is highly variable, with some patients remaining clinically stable for up to a decade or more.

Fuster and colleagues[3] reported the classic account of the course of patients with DCM who were referred to a tertiary care center. These authors reviewed the clinical course of 104 patients followed at the Mayo Clinic between 1960 and 1980.[3] Excluded from this cohort were patients with established coronary artery disease, hypertension, insulin-dependent diabetes mellitus, and systemic disease involving the heart. Suspected etiologies of the cardiomyopathy included excessive ethanol in 21% and antecedent viral infection in 20%. Patients in this "pre-vasodilator therapy era" series experienced a rapid downhill course to death with 50% surviving 2 years and 20% surviving 10 years. Of the patients who died, two thirds expired within 2 years of diagnosis. This classic study is not representative of the current era as suggested by Di Lenarda and coworkers.[4] Examining the mortality of patients presenting during one of three periods over the past two decades, these authors discovered that the 2- and 4-year survival rates of patients with DCM improved remarkably. The 4-year survival increased from 54% in the period ending in 1982 to 83% in the period ending in 1992. This improvement was observed following adjustment for severity of illness between the groups. Significant differences between the groups included greater use of angiotensin converting enzyme (ACE) inhibitors (35% versus 94%; early versus later cohort), greater use of β-adrenergic blockers (4% versus 86%), and less frequent use of any antiarrhythmic agent in the later group. During the period of these observations, there were no major changes in the detection of cardiomyopathy, indicating that the observed improvement in survival can be attributed to improvements in medical therapy.

Clinical observations allow for assessment of prognosis in patients with DCM. Redfield and coworkers[5] retrospectively tracked a cohort of patients with incidentally discovered nonischemic cardiomyopathy at the Mayo Clinic. Patients included in this series were asymptomatic at the time of discovery, although some had previously been symptomatic from heart failure (designated class I). All patients had a left ventricular ejection fraction (LVEF) of <0.5. The survival rate of the asymptomatic patients was not significantly different from that of the class I patients but both were considerably lower than expected for age- and gender-matched populations. The survival of asymptomatic patients was 100% at 2 years, but only 78% at 5 years, and 53% at 7 years. In comparison, the survival of placebo-treated patients in the Studies of Left Ventricular Dysfunction (SOLVD) Prevention Trial was even less optimistic, with a 4-year mortality rate of approximately 20% in a population that was asymptomatic at randomization. Only 20% of patients in SOLVD were classified as having nonischemic cardiomyopathy, but this study remains one of the few randomized trials to include relatively large numbers of asymptomatic patients with DCM. In summary, the clinical course of patients with DCM is variable, with evidence indicating an improvement in the survival over the past two decades.

Etiology of Dilated Cardiomyopathy

It is likely that the etiology of DCM plays an important role in the natural history. Dilation of the heart associated with systolic dysfunction is the final common path of a number of diseases, although the precise etiology is often difficult to establish. The common causes of DCM are grouped by familial, infectious, autoimmune, or toxic etiologies (Table 1), as well as "idiopathic" when no etiology is apparent after evaluation. Kasper and colleagues[14] carefully evaluated 673 patients with DCM and found no identifiable cause in nearly 50%. Other causes occurring with >1% frequency included myocarditis, coronary disease, peripartum cardiomyopathy, human immunodeficiency virus, ethanol abuse, drug-induced cardiomyopathies, connective tissue diseases, amyloidosis, hypertension, familial cardiomyopathies, metabolic diseases, and valvular heart disease. The contribution of inherited forms of DCM is probably underestimated. Many of the inherited defects leading to DCM are transmitted in an autosomal dominant or X-linked pattern.[6] Detection of members of these families requires a

Table 1
Causes of Dilated Cardiomyopathy

Familial	20% of patients will have a first-degree relative with similar condition.
Infectious	Probably the most common etiology, but difficult to establish.
Immune dysfunction	May occur with nonspecific activation of the immune response.
Toxic	Ethanol probably the most common etiologic agent.

high index of suspicion on part of the physician, the coach, or the athletic trainer.

The contribution of alcohol consumption to the development of DCM is probably underestimated. Because of ready accessibility of alcohol in all its forms, this form of cardiomyopathy may present when least expected. The most common mechanism of ethanol injury to the heart is the direct toxic effect, although deficiency of thiamine may further contribute to the left ventricular dysfunction (LVD). It is generally believed that there must be heavy consumption of ethanol for 10 years before alcohol cardiomyopathy becomes evident.[7] Suspicion, early detection, and total abstinence are the keys to therapy of this condition. Early in the clinical course, there is reversal of the acute toxic effects of ethanol on the heart and potential for recovery of ventricular function.[8]

Myocarditis is a common theme in discussions of the etiology of DCM and should be considered in patients who present with acute DCM. In an extensive clinicopathologic review of 673 patients presenting with DCM, biopsy evidence of myocarditis was found in 12%—approximately the same fraction in which unsuspected coronary disease was found (11%). An extensive discussion of this subject can be found in chapter 19, but a brief discussion of myocarditis, as it relates to DCM, is included here for completeness.

The reported incidence of myocarditis varies greatly in different reports. In a small series at the Massachusetts General Hospital, two thirds of patients presenting with symptoms of heart failure of less than 6 months in duration had biopsy evidence of myocarditis.[9] The shorter the interval between the onset of symptoms and the biopsy, the more likely that active myocarditis would be found on biopsy. Forty percent of these patients had a significant rise in left ventricular function and none of these patients died in the follow-up period. The role of endomyocardial biopsy in the evaluation of these patients is discussed later in this chapter.

Patients may present during an asymptomatic phase of their illness. Frequently many report a period of clinical deterioration that, after close questioning, can often be attributed to a viral illness or pneumonia. Patients may have a chest x-ray that reveals an enlarged heart, and the evaluation proceeds from there. Identification of patients with asymptomatic LVD is important because early therapy with ACE inhibitors can delay or prevent the onset of congestive heart failure (CHF).[10]

Evaluation of the Patient with Suspected Dilated Cardiomyopathy

The patient with unexplained heart failure or asymptomatic LVD should undergo a complete evaluation to exclude treatable causes of cardiomyopathy. The guidelines for evaluation of these patients were published by the Agency for Health Care Policy and Research (AHCPR).[11] The evaluation should include a careful history and physical examination to assess the clinical state of the patient and search for systemic diseases such as endocrine disorders, untreated systemic hypertension, and vasculitic processes. The laboratory evaluation should include measurement of renal function, electrolytes, thyroid function tests, and other specific labs suggested by the history and physical exam (such as iron studies in suspected iron-overload disease). There should be an assessment of left ventricular systolic function with echocardiography, radionuclide ventriculography, or contrast left ventriculography. The latter test is often performed in conjunction with coronary angiography when an ischemic etiology to the cardiomyopathy is being excluded. The clinical findings in DCM are summarized in Table 2.

The current AHCPR guidelines do not recommend serial assessment of left ventricular function. A fraction of patients presenting with severe heart failure will have significant clinical improvement accompanying an improvement in ventricular function. In the National Institutes of Health-sponsored Myocarditis study, there was a significant improvement in mean LVEF in both treatment and placebo groups apparent 28 weeks after randomization.[12] There was further but less significant improvement at 1 year in both groups. One can conclude that improvement in ventricular function can be expected and may have prognostic significance in the patients with myocarditis who don't die early. Steimle et al[13] reported that 49 of 297 consecutive patients with nonischemic DCM experienced an improvement of LVEF from an average of 0.22 to 0.49, with the entire group surviving with medical therapy alone an average 43 months. Also distinguishing this group were relatively normal hemodynamics, a short duration of symptoms, and higher serum sodium levels (an independent predictor of survival in many studies).[13] These patients often respond promptly to appropriate

Table 2
Clinical Features of Dilated Cardiomyopathy

History	Asymptomatic or symptoms of heart failure (exertional fatique or dyspnea).
Physical examination	Cardiomegaly, third and/or fourth heart sounds, evidence of valvular insufficiency.
Imaging (echocardiography or nuclear)	Cardiomegaly, depressed left ventricular (and commonly right ventricular) systolic function.
Electrocardiography	Sinus tachycardia, nonspecific ST segment changes, conduction delays, atrial and/or ventricular dysrhythmias.

medical therapy and therefore distinguish themselves as a low-risk group.

Considerable controversy remains regarding the role of endomyocardial biopsy in the evaluation of DCM. In the consecutive series of DCM patients reviewed by Kasper et al,[14] biopsy yielded a specific diagnosis in 115 patients (17%). Of these diagnoses, only 4 of the 673 patients in the study had a condition that could possibly respond to medical therapy (sarcoidosis), and one may argue that these particular patients could be diagnosed without a biopsy. Of the remaining 111 patients, 81 had myocarditis, 9 had Adriamycin cardiotoxicity, 14 had amyloidosis, and 4 had other rare conditions. Similar findings were reported by Chow et al,[15] with diagnostic findings of myocarditis seen in only 4.4% of 90 patients presenting with DCM and recent onset of symptoms. There is presently no rationale for routine endomyocardial biopsy in the evaluation of the patient with unexplained DCM, with possibly a single exception. When patients are being considered for urgent cardiac transplantation, endomyocardial biopsy may be needed to exclude active viral myocarditis, a contraindication to cardiac transplantation.[16]

Treatment of Dilated Cardiomyopathy

The therapy for DCM has undergone a revolution in the past decade. Treatment prior to the first Veterans Heart Failure Trial (V-HEFT-I) was limited to digoxin to improve performance of the failing heart and diuretics to alleviate the edematous state. Arnold Katz[17] was one of the first investigators to recognize that after the initial damage to the heart, progression of the condition is due to abnormal loading forces on the left ventricle. He proposed that the perpetuation of heart failure is due to abnormal loading forces placed on the heart rather than to a primary myocardial disease. It is now known that the abnormal load on the heart is due to activation of the plasma renin system, the sympathetic nervous system, and a number of other systemic and local organ neurohormonal systems.[18] Therapy directed against these upregulated systems has been shown to improve both symptoms and survival.

In the United States, the AHCPR has recommended treatment of individuals with asymptomatic and symptomatic LVD.[11] In addition to vasodilator therapy (ACE inhibitors recommended), therapy with digoxin and diuretics also have a role in treatment. The utility of each class of medications is discussed below.

Vasodilator Therapy

The rationale for vasodilator therapy as "firstline" treatment for the patient with LVD is now based on a wealth of clinical information.

It should be stated at the outset that many of the studies that have established vasodilator therapy were performed in populations with ischemic cardiomyopathy. Patients with DCM have also been included in a number of pivotal trials.[10,19–21] Any athlete detected to have asymptomatic LVD should be started on vasodilator therapy soon after the diagnosis is confirmed.

The SOLVD Prevention (asymptomatic) Trial[10] included patients with DCM or ischemic cardiomyopathy and remains one of the largest randomized trials of ACE inhibitor therapy to include DCM patients. In this trial there was an 8% reduction in total mortality and a 12% reduction in cardiovascular mortality, each not achieving statistical significance by predefined criteria. There was a 29% reduction in the combined endpoint of death or development of heart failure, which was highly statistically significant. Based on this trial, for 21 patients 5 years of treatment with enalapril would result in the prevention of one cardiovascular death or hospitalization for worsening heart failure. The importance of initiating ACE inhibitor therapy for patients found to have asymptomatic LVD cannot be overemphasized. By virtue of the cardiac reserve required for competitive athletics, patient/athletes with mild to moderate LVD may come to medical attention and offer an opportunity for the early initiation of this life-prolonging therapy.

There are several potential mechanisms by which inhibition of the renin-angiotensin system (RAS) mediates the clinical benefits described above. One obvious mechanism is the impact of these agents on neurohormones and particularly on plasma norepinephrine (PNE). The neurohormone substudy of the SOLVD Trial revealed that PNE levels are elevated in patients with symptomatic heart failure. In this trial, patients with asymptomatic LVD also had significantly higher levels of these neurohormones than did age-matched control subjects, but lower levels than patients with established heart failure.[18] The impact of enalapril therapy on PNE levels was greatest in the patients with symptomatic heart failure and only when PNE levels were elevated at baseline.[22] Despite these findings, ACE inhibitors have not been found to specifically reduce the incidence of sudden death in most studies and they have no impact on ventricular arrhythmias as assessed by ambulatory monitoring.

Enlargement of the heart, loss of contractile function, and the change to a globular shape are the structural hallmarks of DCM. Inhibition of tissue RAS results in favorable effects on ventricular and myocardial architecture. In the SOLVD Treatment Trial of symptomatic patients with cardiomyopathy, 1 year of ACE inhibition prevents progressive left ventricular dilatation.[23] Two weeks after withdrawal of enalapril in this trial, left ventricular end-diastolic volume (LVEDV) and left ventricular end-systolic volume (LVESV) returned to pretreatment values but not to the higher levels found in placebo-treated patients. Similar findings were observed in the patients with asymptomatic LVD, although these patients had a smaller LVEDV at randomization and proportionally smaller volume changes over the 2-year follow-up period.[24] These findings indicate that the favorable effects of enalapril were due to a combination of long-term effects on ventricular remodeling and a sustained impact on the stress (preload and afterload) placed on the ventricle. If ventricular function returns to "normal" with the administration of ACE inhibitors, these data would predict that ventricular function will somewhat deteriorate if ACE inhibitors are discontinued within the 2 years following diagnosis. The recovery of normal ventricular function has been proposed as one of the important prerequisites for athletes to return to competition.[25] Patient/athletes whose ventricular function improves with ACE inhibitor therapy to the point where they will return to competition should remain on these agents for at least 1 to 2 years and should be monitored carefully for deterioration in ventricular function if they are discontinued.

Reduction of ventricular arrhythmias has been proposed as one mechanism of mortality reduction. Pratt and coworkers[26] reviewed the SOLVD data base and reported that there was no significant differences in ventricular arrhythmias with enalapril therapy in either the Prevention or the Treatment Trials.[26]

Digoxin

One of the older herbal therapies still in routine clinical use, digoxin has been shown to improve the function of the failing heart with less impact on normal myocardium.[27] Improvement in functional capacity with addition of digoxin has been difficult to establish but withdrawal of the drug in a clinically stable patient has been associated with worsening symptoms.[28] The safety and efficacy of digoxin were unknown until recently.[29] The current recommendations for the use of digoxin include use in patients with activity intolerance despite clinically effective doses of ACE inhibitors and use in patients with LVD associated with atrial fibrillation. There is evidence that patients with LVD but without heart failure benefit,[30] but the risk-benefit ratio in these patients has not yet been assessed.

Diuretics

This class of medications is only useful for lowering the filling pressures of the left and right ventricles and relieving edematous states. These agents may cause intravascular volume and electrolyte depletion. Patients who require diuretic therapy for symptomatic heart failure associated with cardiomyopathy are unlikely to have sufficient cardiac reserve to engage in competitive athletics.

Other Therapy

A variety of other therapies for cardiomyopathy have been investigated and found to be associated with an adverse effect on survival despite a promising effect on exercise tolerance. All of these medications have failed to meet the approval of the Food and Drug Administration.

There are several drugs that remain in clinical trials. Amlodipine is a dihydropyridine calcium channel blocker with a long pharmacological half-life. It has been associated with favorable effects on exercise tolerance and survival. This has been particularly evident in the group of patients with nonischemic cardiomyopathy.[31] Promising results have also been reported with β-adrenergic blocking agents and particularly the class with α-adrenergic (vasodilating) properties.[32] Either or both of these classes of medications may be used routinely in the coming years in patients with DCM.

Arrhythmias and Sudden Death

There is little doubt that patients with DCM are at higher risk for sudden death. The predominant mechanism of sudden death in these patients is believed to be ventricular tachyarrhythmias.[33] Individuals with cardiomyopathy may be more susceptible to ventricular arrhythmias by virtue of higher baseline plasma norepinephrine, which increases further with physical exertion.[22] Other mechanisms of sudden death in this patient population include bradyarrhythmias and massive pulmonary emboli which may be difficult to distinguish clinically from ventricular arrhythmias. There are few data on the cardiac rhythm pres-ent at the time of cardiovascular collapse. Luu and coworkers[34] examined the cardiac rhythm of patients with cardiomyopathy at time of arrest and found that only 38% of the arrests were caused by ventricular tachycardia and fibrillation. The remaining patients in this series had severe bradycardia or pulseless electrical activity (electromechanical dissociation) at the time of cardiovascular collapse. The patients in this series were hospitalized at the time of arrest and are not likely representative of an ambulatory, less ill population.

Unfortunately there are no screening tests with acceptable sensitivity and specificity for predicting sudden death in patients with DCM. There is considerable controversy regarding the role of routine ambulatory rhythm monitoring in asymptomatic patients. Meinertz and coworkers[35] reported that the combination of a low LVEF and complex ventricular arrhythmias was predictive of sudden death. Unverferth and coworkers[36] found a similar association, but the number of patients with complex ventricular arrhythmias in this latter study was small.

Electrophysiology study (EPS) of DCM similarly is unreliable even when it comes to reproducing arrhythmias in patients with documented sustained ventricular arrhythmias. Screening asymptomatic patients with EPS has revealed inducibility ranging from 2.4% to 40%, depending on the stimulation technique used. Poor ventricular function is the most important predictor of inducibility and may serve as a surrogate predictor of survival.[37]

There are virtually no data on the predictive value of exercise testing for the endpoint of sudden death. Most series that examine exercise testing in patients are relatively small, short term, and not designed to correlate exercise arrhythmias with sudden death. The larger trials such as V-HeFT have only addressed the short-term safety of exercise testing patients with DCM.[38] In this study, only 1.6% of patients discontinued stress testing for arrhythmias (a predefined endpoint for stress testing). The low incidence of arrhythmias on stress testing unfortunately did not predict the relatively greater incidence of sudden death in these patients with mild to moderately symptomatic cardiomyopathy.

Implications of Dilated Cardiomyopathy for the Exercising Patient

LVD is a continuum, and labeling individuals "asymptomatic" is somewhat arbitrary. Many patients lead sedentary lives by choice and are therefore asymptomatic but may have significant exercise impairment when challenged. For example, 40 "asymptomatic" patients enrolled in the exercise substudy of the SOLVD Prevention Trial were found to have significant reductions in peak exercise time and oxygen consumption despite an absence of heart failure symptoms at baseline.[39] Therefore, exercise intolerance may occur in a patient who is otherwise asymptomatic. An athlete with DCM will likely seek medical attention earlier in the natural history of the illness than will a sedentary individual.

The adage "if it hurts, rest it" has been applied to the patient population with heart failure by generations of health care professionals. Until recently, the medical textbooks and literature recommended bed rest for the patient with cardiomyopathy. Clinical trials of enforced bed rest in a hospital, sometimes for up to 2 years, had demonstrated that heart size would return to normal or nearly normal in two thirds of patients.[40] During the period of hospitalization, those with alcoholic cardiomyopathies did not have access to ethanol, which may explain their improvement, and most of those with myocarditis were going to improve regardless of therapy. Unfortunately, two thirds of patients died during the study period and the 3.5 years of follow-up, suggesting that there was no impact of bed rest on the natural history of disease in the pre-ACE inhibitor era.

Most physicians would now consider enforced bed rest too restrictive a recommendation for patients with cardiomyopathy. Often cardiomyopathy patients are counseled to avoid all strenuous activities, including aerobic exercise. This recommendation is based more on tradition than scientific fact. The following discussion reviews the available data on efficacy and safety of exercise training by patients with cardiomyopathy.

One of the diagnostic criteria for the severity of cardiomyopathy is exercise intolerance. Before discussing exercise in heart failure patients, it is useful to review the response of the normal circulation to exercise. In order to meet the metabolic demands of the exercising muscle, there must be an increase in blood flow. Cardiac output must increase along with a reduction in tone of the resistance vessels in the cardiac and skeletal muscle beds. This is accomplished by activation of the sympathetic nervous system. In the local vascular beds, the release of metabolites from the exercising muscle (potassium ions, hyperosmolarity, and adenosine) further enhances blood flow.[41]

The heart augments cardiac output (the product of the heart rate and the stroke volume) by a number of mechanisms. With exercise, there is an increase in venous return to the heart, supported in part by the compression of veins coursing between the exercising muscles. The increase in stroke volume is due to contractile reserve (inotropic state) and recruitment of augmented preload (left ventricular diastolic distension). There is also an increase in cardiac output mediated by an increase in sympathetic tone and a withdrawal of vagal tone.[41]

As the ventricle fails, the contractile reserve also fails, due to a number of factors which include desensitization of β-adrenergic receptors. When contractile reserve fails, the ventricle may still recruit the augmented venous return by virtue of its diastolic distensibility, and thus augment stroke volume.[42] The preservation of preload reserve is one of the factors that distinguishes the asymptomatic from the symptomatic patients with cardiomyopathy.[42] In the normal heart, left ventricular relaxation is accelerated by adrenergic-mediated mechanisms that fail as the heart failure progresses. When the preload reserve mechanism fails, cardiac output may increase only by an increase in the heart rate, which may also be attenuated in patients with cardiomyopathy. The right ventricle may also contribute to exercise intolerance, either directly or due to its impact on the left ventricle. Dilation of the right ventricle and compression of the left ventricle due to restraint of the pericardium may also compromise left heart function.

There are a number of factors that contribute to the exercise limitation of patients with cardiomyopathy. Patients with cardiomyopathy report both dyspnea and fatigue in response to exercise, and either symptom may occur at a given percentage of the peak oxygen consumption.[43] There are no hemodynamic, ventilatory, or metabolic differences between patients who report dyspnea or fatigue as their "limiting" symptom.[44] Several studies have suggested that the major limiting factor to exercise for the patient with cardiomyopathy is delivery of oxygenated blood to the exercising muscle. Wilson and Mancini[43] reported that blood flow to the legs of exercising patients was significantly impaired in the group with cardiomyopathy.

Not all exercise intolerance in patients with cardiomyopathy is due to hemodynamic factors. Mancini and coworkers[45] demonstrated that 68% of patients with chronic symptomatic cardiomyopathy have reduced skeletal muscle mass. Conversely, fat stores as determined by triceps skinfold measurements are reduced in only 8% of patients. Using magnetic resonance spectroscopy, these investigators reported that the heart failure subjects had reduction of skeletal muscle phosphocreatine with a parallel increase in inorganic phosphorus compared with normal subjects. Furthermore, there was a delayed recovery of phosphocreatine stores after exercise. These data indicate a relative depletion of high energy stores in skeletal muscle, which may contribute to exercise intolerance.

If we accept the hypothesis that patients with cardiomyopathy may exercise, are there data that support a benefit from exercise training by these individuals? Few would question the utility of exercise training in patients following myocardial infarction but unfortunately there are limited data examining the benefit of training in nonischemic cardiomyopathies. Several studies have shown improvement in a number of cardiorespiratory parameters with exercise therapy in patients with left ventricular systolic dysfunction. Sullivan and coworkers[46] demonstrated that aerobic training of patients with cardiomyopathy for an average of 4 hours per week for 4 to 6 months resulted in a reduction of resting heart rate and a 23% increase in the peak oxygen consumption with exercise. While hemodynamics were not appreciably changed, there was a significant increase in exercising limb blood flow.[46] In a follow-up study, these investigators reported that exercise training resulted in a reduction in lactic acid production, a decrease in carbon dioxide production, and a longer exercise duration before anaerobic threshold was achieved.[47] This was not a randomized trial of exercise so this study cannot exclude the possibility that exercise tolerance would have increased with a less strenuous protocol.

Jette and coworkers[48] were among the first investigators to recognize the importance of a control group in the study of exercise in patients with cardiomyopathy. These investigators studied patients with ischemic cardiomyopathy, randomized to a 4-week exercise trial. They found, as did Sullivan et al,[46,47] that hemodynamics do not change appreciably with exercise training when compared to nonexercising control patients. The improvement in the exercising groups is likely due to correction of impaired vasodilation.[48] Coats and coworkers[49,50] designed a randomized, controlled crossover trial of aerobic exercise in patients with ischemic cardiomyopathy. These investigators reported a significant improvement in exercise capacity, an increase in cardiac output, and a shift in the balance of sympathetic-vagal tone in favor of enhanced vagal tone.[49] Restoration of autonomic control of the heart may play an important role in the response to emotional stress and exercise. This well-designed study was limited to patients with ischemic cardiomyopathy but the study's primary author proposed that *the benefits of exercise are not dependent on the etiology of heart failure*.[50] Further investigation of this problem should clarify if these observations can be extended to the patients with DCM.

The available trials of exercise therapy are inadequate to assess the impact of regular exercise on prognosis. The various controlled trials of exercise have found that improvement in exercise time is equivalent to that seen in the placebo-controlled trials of ACE inhibitor therapy. Exercise time is not a surrogate endpoint for mortality but there is a correlation between function status and survival. A properly designed and powered trial of exercise therapy is needed before a broad recommendation can be made.

Recommendations for the Patient/Athlete with Dilated Cardiomyopathy

Patient/athletes are likely to present for medical opinion in two manners. One group will be those patients with DCM who develop symptoms while training or during competition. These symptoms may include dyspnea or fatigue out of proportion to the conditioned state of the athlete. During the evaluation of these patients, it would be prudent to restrict the athlete from involvement in strenuous activity, particularly competition. At the time of initial detection, the practitioner will not know at what point in the natural history of the condition that the athlete resides. No assessment of the safety of competition can be made without further investigation and observation. The second group of patients will often come to the practitioner with a history of DCM in the past, now requesting clearance to resume training and competition. The evaluation and recommendations for exercise therapy in either group are similar.

Fully evaluate the new patients as described above. Exclude treatable causes of cardiomyopathy such as thyroid disease, valvular heart disease, and ethanol abuse. Indicators of a poor prognosis such as very poor left ventricular function, atrial fibrillation, evidence of right heart failure, a third heart sound on physical examination, or low serum sodium should dictate a conservative approach to physical activity (Table 3). These factors may not necessarily predispose an athlete to sudden death during competition or training, but unmonitored exercise in a patient with an adverse prognosis on clinical grounds cannot be considered prudent. Patient/athletes who have been fully evaluated and now present for clearance do not need a new evaluation, but it is prudent to consider the appropriateness of the original diagnosis.

Endomyocardial biopsy is not necessary to establish a diagnosis of myocarditis, but its presence may be suspected in a nonischemic cardiomyopathy of acute onset. The safety of exercise in a patient with proven or suspected myocarditis has not been established and should be discouraged. The Bethesda Conference on sudden death in the athlete has recommended that athletes with documented or suspected myocarditis not be allowed to exercise until heart size and function return to normal.[25] One should recall that patients recovering from documented myocarditis have the same prognosis as those with DCM (approximately 50% mortality at 5 years), which may assist the athlete in his/her decision making.

Medical therapy should be optimized and tailored to the severity of the condition. Patients with LVEF <0.4 should receive therapy with effective doses of an ACE inhibitor regardless of symptom status. Patients with persistent symptoms despite ACE inhibitor therapy should also receive digoxin. Edematous states may also require therapy with a loop diuretic. There may be a role for therapy with amlodipine and/or β-adrenergic blockers, although this role has yet to be defined.

Table 3
Factors Associated With an Adverse Prognosis in DCM

- Third heart sound
- Left bundle branch block
- Age >55 years
- Low serum sodium
- Advanced New York Heart Association functional class
- Atrial fibrillation
- Ventricular arrhythmias
- Large ventricular size
- Elevated plasma norepinepherine

DCM = dilated Cardiomyopathy.

There were insufficient data for participants in the Bethesda Conference on sudden death in the athlete to formulate a recommendation for participation of athletes with DCM.[25] Athletes who have been fully evaluated and observed for a minimum of 6 to 12 months may be considered for low-intermediate level, noncompetitive exercise. Such individuals should have stable or no symptoms on medication and none of the adverse prognostic factors listed in the table. They should also undergo symptom-limited exercise testing to assess functional capacity.[50] Peak oxygen consumption adds additional information about cardiopulmonary limitation versus deconditioning as the cause of activity limitation. There is no evidence that patients with advanced-class heart failure *symptoms* benefit from exercise training, but these patients benefit from low-level physical training to maintain their level of functioning. There is no lower limit of ventricular function, independent of symptoms, where exercise training is contraindicated. Patients with LVEF as low as 0.09 have been included in some of the trials described above.[49] Some authors have concluded that these patients have the most to gain from exercise training.[51] Patients with significant deconditioning or moderate heart failure may benefit from a structured rehabilitation program to improve their confidence.

In fully evaluated and treated patients, aerobic exercise training at 70% of peak oxygen consumption or greater (but below anaerobic threshold) is likely to achieve the optimal training benefit. Exercise is recommended for 20 to 60 minutes, 3 to 5 days per week. Coats et al[49] reported that compliance with an exercise regimen was directly correlated with the improvement in exercise time. There is no controlled study that supports an exercise prescription of isometric or weight training without aerobic exercise.

The best methods for arrhythmia screening are a careful history, measurement of ventricular function, and determination of atrial rhythm. Very poor ventricular function predicts an adverse prognosis, although it is not necessarily the mechanism of death. Similarly, patients with atrial fibrillation have a higher mortality rate and should be limited to low-level or monitored exercise.

Many of the studies of exercise training described in this chapter excluded patients with significant ventricular dysrhythmias on Holter monitoring. Unfortunately there is no test, invasive or noninvasive, that can reliably predict which patients are at risk for sudden death with exercise. Any patient experiencing symptoms suggestive of hemodynamically significant arrhythmias should not exercise until a full electrophysiologic evaluation is completed. If there is suspicion that the patient may be at risk for sudden death, exercise is not recommended until appropriate therapy has been instituted, and subsequent exercise should be limited to locations with rhythm monitoring and/or resuscitation apparatus.

References

1. Kannel W, Belanger A. Epidemiology of heart failure. *Am Heart J* 1991; 121:951–957.
2. Maron B, Shirani J, Poliac L, et al. Sudden death in young competitive athletes. *JAMA* 1996;276:199–204.
3. Fuster V, Gersh B, Giuliani E. The natural history of idiopathic dilated cardiomyopathy. *Am J Cardiol* 1981;47:525–531.
4. Di Lenarda A, Secoli G, Perkan A, et al. Changing mortality in dilated cardiomyopathy. *Br Heart J* 1994;72:S46–S51.
5. Redfield M, Gersh B, Bailey K, Rodeheffer R. Natural history of incidentally discovered, asymptomatic idiopathic dilated cardiomyopathy. *Am J Cardiol* 1994;74:737–739.
6. Michels V, Moll P, Miller D. The frequency of familial dilated cardiomyopathy in a series of patients with idiopathic dilated cardiomyopathy. *N Engl J Med* 1992;326:77–82.
7. Regan T. Alcohol and the cardiovascular system. *JAMA* 1990;264:377–384.
8. Nethala V, Brown E, Timson C, Patcha R. Reversal of alcoholic cardiomyopathy in a patient with severe coronary artery disease. *Chest* 1993;104: 626–629.
9. Dec G, Palacios I, Fallon J, et al. Active myocarditis in the spectrum of acute dilated cardiomyopathies. *N Engl J Med* 1985;312:885–890.
10. SOLVD Investigators. Effect of enalapril on mortality and the development of heart failure in asymptomatic patients with reduced left ventricular ejection fractions. *N Engl J Med* 1992;327:685–691.
11. Konstam M, Dracup K. *Heart Failure: Evaluation and Care of Patients with Left Ventricular Systolic Dysfunction. Clinical Practice Guideline, Volume 11.* Roskville, MD: US Department of Health and Human Services; 1994.
12. Mason J, O'Connell J, Herskowitz A, et al. A clinical trial of immunosuppressive therapy for myocarditis. *N Engl J Med* 1995;333:269–275.
13. Steimle A, Warner-Stevenson L, Fonarow G, et al. Prediction of improvement in recent onset cardiomyopathy after referral for heart transplantation. *J Am Coll Cardiol* 1994;23:553–559.
14. Kasper E, Agema W, Hutchins G, et al. The causes of dilated cardiomyopathy: A clinicopathological review of 673 consecutive patients. *J Am Coll Cardiol* 1994;23:586–590.
15. Chow L, Dittrich H, Shabetai R. Endomyocardial biopsy in patients with unexplained congestive heart failure. *Ann Intern Med* 1988;109: 535–539.
16. Mudge G, Goldstein S, Addonizio L, et al. 24th Bethesda Conference. Task force 3: Recipient guidelines/prioritization. *J Am Coll Cardiol* 1993;22: 21–31.
17. Katz A. Cardiomyopathy of overload. *N Engl J Med* 1990;322:100–110.
18. Francis G, Benedict C, Johnstone D, et al. Comparison of neurohormonal activation in patients with left ventricular dysfunction with or without congestive heart failure: A substudy of the Studies of Left Ventricular Dysfunction (SOLVD). *Circulation* 1990;82:1724–1729.
19. SOLVD Investigators. Effect of enalapril on survival in patients with reduced left ventricular ejection fraction and congestive heart failure. *N Engl J Med* 1991;325:293–302.

20. Cohn J, Archibauld D, Ziesche S, et al. Effect of vasodilator therapy on mortality in chronic congestive heart failure: Results of a Veterans Administration Cooperative Study. *N Engl J Med* 1986;314:1547–1552.
21. Cohn J, Johnson G, Ziesche S, et al. A comparison of enalapril with hydralazine-isosorbide dinitrate in the treatment of chronic congestive heart failure. *N Engl J Med* 1991;325:303–310.
22. Benedict C, Francis G, Shelton B, et al. Effect of long-term enalapril therapy on neurohormones in patients with left ventricular dysfunction. *Am J Cardiol* 1995;75:1151–1157.
23. Konstam M, Rousseau M, Kronenberg M, et al. Effects of the angiotensin converting enzyme inhibitor enalapril on the long term progression of left ventricular dysfunction in patients with heart failure. *Circulation* 1992; 86:431–438.
24. Konstam M, Kronenberg M, Rousseau M, et al. Effects of the angiotensin converting enzyme inhibitor enalapril on the long term progression of left ventricular dilatation in patients with asymptomatic systolic dysfunction. *Circulation* 1993;88(pt. 1):2277–2283.
25. Maron B, Isner J, McKenna W. Task force 3: Hypertrophic cardiomyopathy, myocarditis and other myopericardial diseases and mitral valve prolapse, 26th Bethesda Conference: Recommendations for determining eligibility for competition in athletes with cardiovascular abnormalities. *J Am Coll Cardiol* 1994;24:845–899.
26. Pratt C, Gardner M, Pepine C, et al. Lack of long-term ventricular arrhythmia reduction by enalapril in heart failure. *Am J Cardiol* 1995;75: 1244–1249.
27. Braunwald E, Bloodwell R, Goldberg L, Morrow A. Studies on digoxin. IV. Observations in man on the effects of digitalis preparations on the contractility of the non-failing heart and on total vascular resistance. *J Clin Invest* 1961;40:52.
28. Packer M, Gheorghiade M, Young D, et al. Withdrawal of digoxin from patients treated with angiotensin converting enzyme inhibitors. *N Engl J Med* 1993;329:1–7.
29. The Digitalis Investigators Group. The effect of digoxin on mortality and morbidity in patients with heart failure. *N Engl J Med* 1997;336:525–533.
30. Harvey R, Ferrer M, Cathcart R, Alexander J. Some effects of digoxin on the heart and circulation in man: Digoxin in enlarged hearts not in clinical heart failure. *Circulation* 1951;4:366.
31. Packer M, O'Connor C, Ghali J, et al. Effect of amlodipine on morbidity and mortality in severe chronic heart failure. *N Engl J Med* 1996;335: 1107–1114.
32. Packer M, Bristow M, Cohn J. Effect of Carvedilol on survival of patients with chronic heart failure. *Circulation* 1995;92(suppl 1):I–142.
33. Kjekshus J. Arrhythmias and mortality in congestive heart failure. *Am J Cardiol* 1990;65:42–48.
34. Luu M, Stevenson W, Stevenson L. Diverse mechanisms of unexpected cardiac arrest in advanced heart failure. *Circulation* 1989;80:1675–1680.
35. Meinertz T, Hofmann T, Kasper W, et al. Significance of ventricular arrhythmias in idiopathic dilated cardiomyopathy. *Am J Cardiol* 1984;53: 902–907.
36. Unverferth D, Magorien R, Moeschberger M, et al. Factors influencing the one year mortality of dilated cardiomyopathy. *Am J Cardiol* 1984;54: 147–152.

37. Meinertz T, Treese N, Kasper W, et al. Determinants of prognosis in idiopathic dilated cardiomyopathy as determined by programmed electrical stimulation. *Am J Cardiol* 1985;56:337–341.
38. Tristani F, Hughes C, Archibald D, et al. Safety of graded symptom-limited exercise testing in patients with congestive heart failure. *Circulation* 1987;76:VI54–VI58.
39. LeJemtel T, Liang C, Stewart D, et al. Reduced peak aerobic capacity in asymptomatic left ventricular dysfunction. A substudy of the Studies of Left Ventricular Dysfunction (SOLVD). *Circulation* 1994;90:2757–2760.
40. McDonald C, Burch G, Walsh J. Prolonged bed rest for the treatment of idiopathic cardiomyopathy. *Am J Med* 1972;52:41–50.
41. Shepherd J. Circulatory response to exercise in health. *Circulation* 1987; 76:1–10.
42. Konstam MA, Kronenberg M, Udelson J, et al. Effectiveness of preload reserve as a determinant of clinical status in patients with left ventricular dysfunction. *Am J Cardiol* 1992;69:1591–1595.
43. Wilson J, Mancini D. Factors contributing to the exercise limitation of heart failure. *J Am Coll Cardiol* 1993;22:93A–98A.
44. Sullivan M, Higgenbotham M, Cobb F. Increased exercise ventilation in patients with chronic heart failure: Intact ventilatory control despite hemodynamic and pulmonary abnormalities. *Circulation* 1987;77:552–559.
45. Mancini D, Walter G, Reichek N, et al. Contribution of skeletal muscle atrophy to exercise intolerance and altered muscle metabolism in heart failure. *Circulation* 1992;85:1364–1373.
46. Sullivan M, Higgenbotham M, Cobb F. Exercise training in patients with severe left ventricular dysfunction-Hemodynamic and metabolic effects. *Circulation* 1988;78:506–515.
47. Sullivan M, Higgenbotham M, Cobb F. Exercise training in patients with chronic heart failure delays ventilatory anaerobic threshold and improves submaximal exercise performance. *Circulation* 1989;79:324–329.
48. Jette M, Heller R, Landry F, Blumchen G. Randomized 4-week exercise program in patients with impaired left ventricular function. *Circulation* 1991;84:1561–1567.
49. Coats A, Adamopoulos S, Radaelli A, et al. Controlled trial of physical training in chronic heart failure. Exercise performance, hemodynamics, ventilation and autonomic function. *Circulation* 1992;85:2119–2131.
50. Coats A. Exercise rehabilitation in chronic heart failure. *J Am Coll Cardiol* 1993;22:172–177.
51. Conn E, Williams R, Wallace A. Exercise responses before and after physical conditioning in patients with severely depressed left ventricular function. *Am J Cardiol* 1982;49:296–300.

$$\boxed{19}$$

Myocarditis and the Athlete

David Portugal, MD and John J. Smith, MD, PhD

Introduction

The diagnosis and treatment of heart failure have undergone dramatic changes in recent years. In the Western world, coronary artery disease is the most common etiology. However, the nonischemic, nonvalvular dilated cardiomyopathies (DCMs) comprise a significant proportion of the world's cases of heart failure with approximately 700,000 to 800,000 patients in the US alone.[1,2] Although the exact incidence is unknown, many of these patients with idiopathic DCM are thought to have myocarditis early in the natural history of the illness.

According to the World Health Organization (WHO) Task Force, myocarditis or inflammatory cardiomyopathy is defined as an *inflammatory disease of the myocardium* diagnosed by *histological, immunological and immunohistochemical criteria.*[1] This rather broad definition exemplifies the historical ambiguity in diagnosing myocarditis. In his 1983 review, James[3] colorfully states that myocarditis is the *medical equivalent of a riddle wrapped in a mystery inside an enigma.*

The term *myocarditis* was introduced by Sobernheim in 1837,[4] although in 1812, Corvisart gave the first description of a clinical syndrome resembling myocarditis in his *Essai Sur les Maladies et les Lesions Organiques du Coeur.*[5] In the US, the term *pericarditis,* which was many times used interchangeably with *myocarditis,* appeared in the *Case Records of the Massachusetts General Hospital* as early as 1854.[6] However, it was not until the late 19th century and early 20th

From Estes NAM, Salem DN, Wang PJ (eds). *Sudden Cardiac Death in the Athlete.* Armonk, NY: Futura Publishing Co., Inc.; ©1998.

century that myocarditis could be linked to specific etiologies. Epidemics of mumps, influenza, and polio were associated with a high incidence of cardiac pathology, suggesting that the viral infection could result in cardiac dysfunction.[7] In the first half of the 20th century, some pathologists expressed uncertainty of the existence of myocarditis as a distinct entity. Then in 1942, Saphir[8] meticulously described his observations of the pathology. It is now known that there is a spectrum of etiologies leading to myocarditis. It is likely that enteroviruses account for the majority of human cases and serve as the etiologic agent in the murine model of myocarditis. The development of endomyocardial biopsy, serology, in situ hybridization, and polymerase chain reaction (PCR) have greatly enhanced our ability to define the disease. In the past decade, there have been significant advances in the management of complications related to myocarditis such as heart failure and arrhythmias. Due to several well-publicized cases involving athletes, there has also been a greater awareness of the potential for sudden death as a consequence of the disease. This chapter includes a review of myocarditis, including the current understanding of the etiology, pathophysiology, clinical presentation, diagnosis, and treatment of this condition. Also included are the current recommendations for the athlete/patient with proven or suspected myocarditis.

Pathophysiology/Mechanisms of Disease

Deciphering the mechanisms of the disease process is vital to understanding human pathology. The mouse has proven to be an excellent model for the study of the mechanisms likely to be operative in human myocarditis. In the 1960s investigators recognized that infecting mice with Coxsackie virus B (CVB) leads to sequences of events in the heart that bear striking resemblance to the human myocarditis.

In the mouse, the injury caused by viral infection follows three general pathways: direct myocardial cell destruction, secondary immunologic reaction, and finally, endothelial injury associated with microvascular spasm.[7] Myocyte destruction and immunologic injury occurs in two phases, acute and chronic.[9] Microscopically, the acute phase is marked by either patchy or diffuse areas of densely packed inflammatory cell infiltrate that surrounds necrotic myofibers.[10] During this time, viral invasion of the myocardium occurs, leading to a typical cytopathic effect characterized by myofibril destruction and vacuole formation. By the end of the first week of infection, neutralizing antibodies are produced and natural killer cells and macrophages begin the process of clearing the myocardium of virus. Thymus-derived (T) lymphocytes also begin to appear in the myocardium at this time; CD8+/cytotoxic lymphocytes (CTL) predominate early in the process, followed by CD4+/helper T-cells

(HTL), which soon exceed the number of CTLs present. Lymphocyte-mediated immunity plays a role in limiting the spread of the virus, but the activation of these immune cells appears to be responsible for the ongoing destruction of the myocardium.[7,10] In the chronic phase, which occurs over the next 6 months, the myocardium develops fibrosis, calcification, and hypertrophy in the remaining myocytes. The inflammatory process continues, but it occurs at a much lower intensity. Moreover, in contrast to the acute phase, it is no longer possible to culture the CVB virus during this period.

In addition to the direct cytopathic effect of viral infection and the immune-mediated myocardial destruction, there is injury caused by the alteration in the microvasculature. Silver and Kowalczyk[11] have noted the development of luminal narrowing and coronary obstruction from spasm and thrombus formation in acute murine myocarditis. The pathologic changes that result from the microvascular dysfunction have been noted and are similar to those changes seen in reperfusion injury. Verapamil and prazosin have been used in animal models to reverse the endothelial dysfunction and reduce the associated myocardial necrosis.[12] More recently, experiments of murine myocarditis have shown that nitric oxide, a potent endogenous vasodilator, plays a major role in the animals' defenses against viral infections.[13]

It is well established that myocarditis in humans is associated with many noninfectious etiologies. This fact has led some investigators to propose that myocarditis may be a predominantly immune-mediated disorder. The evidence to support this theory was found serendipitously when investigators noted that only certain strains of mice developed myocarditis to CVB-13.[14] Susceptible mouse strains exhibit high levels of viremia, partly due to late production of antibodies to the virus with subsequent delayed viral clearance. Furthermore, during the chronic phase of infection, when the virus can no longer be cultured from the tissue, the inflammatory process continues in the myocardium.

Immune sensitization to myosin heavy chains develops in both murine and human myocarditis.[15] Factor and coworkers[12] immunized mice with cardiac myosin alone, and found that these mice develop a disease that is histologically and immunologically identical to CVB-induced myocarditis.[14] Other investigators have detected the presence of cardiac-specific autoantibodies (eg, anti-α- and β-myosin heavy chain) in patients with DCM and in their symptom-free relatives.[16]

Despite these observations, it is clear that the theory of immune-mediated myocarditis does not explain the entire pathologic process. For example, athymic mice and mice with combined immunodeficiency are capable of developing viral myocarditis. In these mice, virus can no longer be cultured from the tissue, but remnants of viral RNA have been detected by in situ hybridization and PCR during the chronic phase of infection.[17] There is a direct correlation between the areas of the heart where viral RNA is detected and the areas with the most active inflammation histologically. Finally, if myocarditis is primarily an autoimmune disease, then immunosuppressive therapy would be expected to alter the course of the disease. To the contrary, immunosuppressive therapy with corticosteroids and cyclosporine has been shown to exacerbate infectious myocarditis in animals[18,19] and be ineffective in treatment of myocarditis in humans.[20]

Etiology

The reported causes of myocarditis are quite extensive, and can be classified by inciting agents: viral myocarditis, nonviral myocarditis, infectious myocarditis, drug-related myocarditis, and autoimmune myocarditis. A large number of cases remain where the etiologic agent cannot be established; they are thus classified as *idiopathic*. Giant-cell (GCM) and peripartum myocarditis are included in this latter group. The causes of myocarditis are listed in Table 1.

Infectious Myocarditis

Infectious agents are likely the most common etiology of myocarditis, with viral pathogens the most cited cause in industrialized nations. Surveillance of viral activity carried out by the WHO since the 1970s has demonstrated an association of enteroviruses, and specifically CVB, with myocardial disease.[21,22] Other common agents include the influenza viruses, Coxsackie A, cytomegalovirus, parainfluenza, and echovirus.

Cardiac involvement in infection with human immunodeficiency virus (HIV) is also quite common. The etiology of myocardial damage in HIV infection is often unclear, given the significant incidence of associated opportunistic infections, the toxicities of the drugs used to treat HIV, and the increase in autoimmune-related phenomena in these patients.[23] Nonetheless, cardiac disease is prevalent in this population, occurring in 25% to 50% of HIV-infected patients, although only approximately 10% of these patients have cardiac symptoms. Given the increasing prevalence of HIV infection in younger individuals, this is a particularly important etiology of myocarditis and is likely to contribute to cases of sudden cardiac death in young athletes. It is later in the course of the disease that patients may present with congestive heart failure (CHF) secondary to ventricular systolic dysfunction, pericardial effusion, and tamponade.[24]

Table 1
Causes of Myocarditis

I. Infectious

Viral
  Coxsackie B
  Influenza B
  Parainfluenza
  Echovirus
  Cytomegalovirus
  Poliovirus
  Adenovirus
  Influenza A
  Picornavirus
  Coxsackie A
  Human Immunodeficiency Virus

Bacterial
  Streptococcus
  Clostridia
  Pneumococcus
  Staphylococcus
  Diptheria
  Meningococcus
  Haemophilus
  Tularemia
  Brucellosis
  Mycoplasma
  Chlamydia

Fungal
  Aspergillosis
  Actinomycosis
  Blastomycosis
  Candidiasis
  Coccidiomyocosis
  Cryptococcosis
  Histoplasmosis

Spirochetal
  Lyme
  Leptospirosis
  Relapsing fever

Parasitic
  Cysticerosis
  Schistosomiasis
  Toxoplasmosis
  Trichinosis
  Trypanosomiasis

Rickettsial
  Rocky Mountain spotted fever
  Q fever
  Typhus

II. Drug-Related

Hypersensitivity
  Penicillin and derivatives
  Sulfonamides
  Phenytoin
  Carbamezepine
  Hydrochlorothizide
  Methyldopa
  Isoniazid
  Tetracycline

Toxic
  Cocaine
  Adriamycin
  Cobalt
  Chloroquine

III. Autoimmune

Systemic lupus erythematosis
Rheumatoid arthritis
Progressive systemic sclerosis (scleroderma)
Kawasaki's disease

Table 1 (continued)

IV. Idiopathic

Lymphocytic
Peripartum cardiomyopathy
Giant-cell

Other organisms have been implicated in the pathogenesis of myocarditis. *Chlamydia pneumoniae* (TWAR) myocarditis was implicated in the sudden deaths of several Swedish orienteers after ribosomal RNA from this organism was detected in the heart of one of the victims.[25] A subsequent report implicated this agent in the deaths of one third of the 15 Swedish orienteers who died unexpectedly between 1979 and 1992.[26] Awareness of the problem and modification of "training habits and attitudes" have been effective as there have been no further deaths in the past 5 years among Swedish orienteers.

Cardiac invasion of organisms is thought to account for most instances of acute bacterial myocarditis; however, toxins produced by certain organisms may be the cause of the myocardial injury in some infections. For example, *Corneybacterium diphtheriae* may produce myocarditis by elaboration of an exotoxin.[27] Similarly, the exotoxin produced in Clostridia infection also produces significant myocardial damage.[28]

Infectious myocarditis is most commonly characterized by ventricular dysfunction and chamber dilatation. This contrasts with Lyme carditis, a spirochetal infection caused by *Borrelia burgdorferi,* which is marked primarily by conduction abnormalities. Approximately 10% of patients with Lyme disease develop evidence of transient cardiac involvement. Most of these patients develop atrioventricular block, with the majority having complete heart block that commonly resolves but occasionally requires an electronic pacemaker.[29–31] The authors are not aware of any case report of sudden death in an athlete as a consequence of heart block from Lyme disease.

Outside the United States, Chagas' disease is the most common cause of inflammatory cardiac disease in certain regions of the world.[32] In Central and South America, approximately 20 million people are believed to be infected with *Trypanosoma cruzi,* the etiologic parasite in Chagas' disease, which is transmitted by the bite of a reduviid bug. The acute phase of the illness begins with fever, malaise, lymphadenopathy, hepatosplenomegaly, gastrointestinal symptoms, and meningeal irritation.[33] Some affected individuals develop acute infective myocarditis and may go on to manifest chronic Chagas' disease, which is characterized by cardiomegaly, CHF, ventricular arrhythmias, and sudden death.

The probability of developing infective myocarditis depends on a variety of factors, including the virulence of the organism as well as a number of host factors. Some individuals may develop a myopericarditis with fever, leukocytosis, pleuritic chest pain, and a pericardial rub on exam. Occasionally, a patient may present with chest pain, electrocardiogram abnormalities, and elevated creatine phosphokinase (CPK), suggestive of an acute myocardial infarction. More commonly, afflicted individuals will develop CHF symptoms with progressive dyspnea, orthopnea, signs of cardiomegaly with a ventricular gallop, and tachycardia out of proportion to the degree of heart failure.[2] With the onset of viral myocarditis, the patient may report a preceding flulike illness with upper respiratory or a gastrointestinal symptoms. Cardiac involvement usually develops 7 to 10 days later, although most individuals remain asymptomatic with only some nonspecific ST-T wave changes seen on ECG.

Autoimmune-Related Myocarditis

Cardiac involvement in the setting of autoimmune disease is commonly characterized by valvular, pericardial, or endocardial disease rather than myocarditis. Nonetheless, myocardial involvement has been described in association with these diseases. For example, the cardiac manifestations in systemic lupus erythematosus (SLE) include pericarditis and Libman-Sacks endocarditis. Clinical studies have described pericardial effusions occurring during the course of this disease in over half of patients studied.[34] Autopsy studies of patients with SLE have demonstrated histologic evidence of myocarditis in approximately 10% of individuals, often clinically inapparent during their lifetime.[35] Athletes with SLE should be screened with echocardiography before being allowed to participate in competitive athletic activities.

In rheumatoid arthritis, inflammatory rheumatoid nodules may rarely infiltrate the myocardium, compromising cardiac function, but frank myocarditis is very rare. Cardiac disease has also been described in progressive systemic sclerosis (PSS) or scleroderma and is part of the diffuse visceral involvement of many patients with these conditions. Pathologically, myocardial involvement in PSS is marked more by a patchy fibrosis, perhaps due to endothelial spasm, rather than by clear inflammatory injury.[36]

Since the initial description of the disease-syndrome years ago, Kawasaki's disease has become recognized as one of the leading causes of acquired heart disease in children.[37] The most dreaded complication of this disease is myocardial infarction due to coronary artery aneurysms, but ventricular dysfunction due to myocarditis occurs in a significant proportion of patients as well.[38] Fortunately, the process of myocardial inflammation resolves in most patients, with little clinical sequelae. Any patient/athlete with suspected Kawasaki's disease should not engage in strenuous activities during the acute and convalescent phase of the disease. Furthermore, the chronic changes in the coronary vessel may produce stenotic segments, which can lead to myocardial ischemia. Patients with healing Kawasaki's disease must be screened for coronary artery disease before being allowed to exercise.

Drug-Related Myocarditis

Myocardial inflammation due to pharmacological agents may either be due to a direct dose-related toxic effect or be secondary to a hypersensitivity reaction, which may occur anytime during the course of therapy.[39] The first description of this entity was in 1942 when French and Weller[40] described 126 patients with interstitial myocarditis with eosinophilic infiltration after sulfonamide administration. There is an extensive list of agents reported to cause hypersensitivity myocarditis, but a shorter list which includes sulfonamides, methyldopa, and penicillin and its derivatives likely accounts for 75% of all cases. Clinical diagnosis of hypersensitivity myocarditis is largely circumstantial and is usually proposed when signs of myocarditis are noted in the setting of a systemic drug reaction. Early recognition and removal of the offending agent may be lifesaving.

Cocaine use has became a significant cause of acquired heart disease, having been linked with acute myocardial infarctions, arrhythmias and sudden death, accelerated atherosclerosis, hypertension, cardiomyopathy, and myocarditis.[41,42] The effects of cocaine on the heart are largely due to its effect on the vasculature and its stimulation of catecholamine release. However, in autopsy studies of patients who died from cocaine intoxication, a mononuclear infiltrate with foci of necrosis has been noted as a prominent finding.[43] The extent of the inflammatory infiltrate appears to depend on the type of cocaine preparation, contaminants, route of drug delivery, and chronicity of drug abuse (see chapter 25).[44]

Physical Agents

The clinical spectrum of radiation-induced heart disease includes acute and chronic pericarditis, coronary artery disease, and rarely myocarditis, but manifestations are usually delayed and insidious in onset.[45] The pathologic findings usually include patchy fibrosis and reduction in capillary network with little evidence of acute inflammation.

Fortunately, in most case reports of radiation-induced myocarditis, patients received larger radiation doses than those used in practice today.[46]

Idiopathic Myocarditis

When the search for the etiology of myocarditis fails, the condition is often labeled *idiopathic*. Many of these cases are likely postviral but often the symptoms of left ventricular dysfunction that bring a patient to seek medical attention may occur late in the disease, far removed from the acute viral illness. The clinical presentation and natural history of idiopathic and viral myocarditis are largely indistinguishable. Moreover, given that both diseases have a similarly poor response to immunosuppressive therapy, the impetus to try to accurately distinguish one from the other is usually not necessary.

There are two forms of idiopathic myocarditis that are recognized as distinct entities: giant-cell myocarditis (GCM) and peripartum cardiomyopathy (PCM). In 1905 Saltikow described GCM in patients who demonstrated widespread degeneration of myocardial fibers and formation of multinucleated giant cells.[47] Most forms of myocarditis are characterized by a lymphocytic infiltrate. This is contrasted by the monocytic inflammatory cells in GCM. Some investigators have proposed that GCM is a separate pathologic process.[48] GCM may be idiopathic or it may be associated with other autoimmune or infectious illnesses including sarcoidosis, SLE, syphilis tuberculosis, and thyrotoxicoses. Compared to lymphocytic myocarditis, GCM has been reported to have a higher incidence of ventricular arrhythmias and a more rapidly fatal course. In a series by Davidoff et al,[49] only 20% of patients with GCM were alive and free from cardiac transplant at a follow-up of 2 years compared with 70% of patients with lymphocytic myocarditis. Given the unfavorable prognosis, patients diagnosed with GCM require close monitoring and possibly early listing for cardiac transplantation. Although there have been some case reports of patient recovery with immunosuppression, cardiac transplantation appears to be the only hope for survival in these patients.[50,51]

Another form of myocarditis whose cause remains unknown is PCM. This is a rare congestive cardiomyopathy that strikes women usually in the first 4 months of the postpartum period. The incidence ranges from 1 in 15,000 to 1 in 1300 live births.[52] Several investigators have noted a high incidence of lymphocytic infiltrates at the time of endomyocardial biopsy in these patients, suggesting inflammatory injury as the primary cause of the disease. Using more rigid pathologic criteria, Rizeq et al[53] found that only 3 out of 34 patients with PCM had evidence of myocarditis; the underlying cause of this condition remains unknown. Women with PCM should be treated in the same fashion as patients with DCM, with the same criteria applied for resumption of athletic activities.

Epidemiology of Myocarditis

The reported incidence of myocarditis has varied over the years. This variability is likely due to the diverse presentation of the disease, the difference in prevalence and virulence of etiologic agents, and the difficulty in making a clinical diagnosis. As recently as the early part of this century, at the time of autopsy pathologists would label a patient with any type of lesion in the myocardium as having had *chronic myocarditis*.[8] Autopsy series completed prior to the development of modern clinical and pathologic definition of myocarditis have estimated the incidence in the general population of myocarditis to be as high as 10%.[54] In contrast, more recent data suggest that the incidence may be much lower. In 12,747 consecutive autopsies performed at Malmo General Hospital in Sweden from 1975 to 1984, evidence of myocarditis was noted in only approximately 1% of patients.[5]

These series do not report the percentage of patients with histologic evidence of myocarditis who were symptomatic during their lifetime. Approximately 5% of individuals with viral infections will experience mild myocardial inflammation, but the impact of these subclinical infections on overall prognosis is impossible to determine.[55] Patients who present with symptomatic heart failure of unknown etiology are often considered to have myocarditis. Cohort studies have shown a 10% to 12% incidence of myocarditis in patients who either present with unexplained heart failure or are diagnosed with idiopathic DCM.[56,57]

Several investigators have proposed that myocarditis is direct precursor of DCM. Three lines of evidence support this hypothesis. First, mice surviving after infection with CVB-3 develop a DCM similar to that of humans.[58] The murine hearts have similar histologic findings to human DCM including myocardial scarring without inflammation, subendocardial thickening, and cardiac dilation. Second, higher titres of neutralizing antibodies to CVB have been found in patients with DCM than in control subjects.[59] In a retrospective study of 100 patients with cardiomyopathy, Cambridge and coworkers[60] reported elevated antiviral antibody titres in 30% of patients with "congestive cardiomyopathy," versus 2% of patients with noncardiomyopathic disease. Further evidence linking DCM and viral myocarditis comes from sophisticated molecular techniques that are capable of detecting viral RNA in biopsy specimens. Bowles and colleagues,[61] using the slot-blot technique and a radiolabeled probe complementary to enteroviral RNA in human endomyocardial biopsy specimens, found evidence of infection in 50% of biopsy samples in their patient cohort. In a prospective study that included 123 patients with new onset left ventricular dysfunction, Why and coworkers[62] reported that the presence of enteroviral RNA detected by hybridization was associated with a worse prognosis. The viral genome may contribute to the continuing pathophysiology of the disease, possibly by causing recurrent infection or inciting ongoing subclinical injury by the immune system. Alternatively, the viral genome may simply be a bystander in the myocardium, marking those patients with a poor outcome.[2]

Diagnosis

Laboratory Findings

The diagnosis of viral myocarditis can be established by the association of: (1) histologic evidence of myocarditis; (2) ventricular systolic dysfunction; and (3) evidence of viral infection. The evidence supporting a viral etiology includes a history of flulike illness combined with serology and/or positive viral culture. There must be a fourfold rise in neutralizing antibodies from paired acute- and convalescent-phase sera or the demonstration of a high titre of virus-specific serum immunoglobulin M (IgM) to have a "diagnostic" serology. Uncommonly, virus may be cultured from stool, pharyngeal secretions, or blood. Unfortunately, rarely these criteria are met in the patient presenting with new onset CHF, and the diagnosis of myocarditis must remain presumptive.

Other noninvasive testing used in myocarditis include ECG, nuclear imaging, and echocardiography. ECG abnormalities observed in myocarditis are varied and are listed in Table 2. Although the changes on ECG are nonspecific, particular findings may carry prognostic significance. In 45 patients with histologic evidence of myocarditis, Morgera et al[63] noted that the presence of left bundle branch block (LBBB) and abnormal QRS complexes predicted an adverse outcome. LBBB is commonly associated with extensive myocardial damage and may simply be a marker of severely impaired ventricular function.

Echocardiography (echo) or radionuclide ventriculography are commonly used to assess left ventricular function. In this setting, echo may be the superior imaging modality by virtue of its ability to show valve morphology, derive hemodynamic data, and identify ventricular thrombi. The presence of regional wall motion abnormalities was previously believed to be unlikely in myocarditis. Using echo, Italian investigators discovered that 64% of patients with biopsy-proven myocarditis exhibited heterogeneous ventricular wall motion including hypokinesis, akinesis, or dyskinesis adjacent to areas of preserved myocardial function.[64]

Table 2
ECG and ECHO Findings in Myocarditis

ECG:	LAE
	AV block
	RBBB
	LBBB
	ST abnormalities, usually ST depression, rarely ST elevation
	T wave inversions
	LVH criteria
	pathologic Q waves
	atrial and ventricular ectopy
	atrial and ventricular arrhythmias
ECHO:	LV dysfunction, global or regional
	LV cavity enlargement
	LVH
	ventricular aneurysms
	isolated or associated RV dysfunction
	pericardial effusions
	ventricular thrombi
	hemodynamic characteristics of diastolic dysfunction and restrictive heart disease

ECG = electrocardiogram; ECHO = echocardiogram; LAE = left atrial enlargement; AV = atrioventricular; RBBB = right bundle branch block; LBBB = left bundle branch block; LVH = left ventricular hypertrophy; LV = left ventricular; RV = right ventricular.

Radionuclide scanning has been applied to the diagnosis of myocarditis with variable results. Gallium-67, indium-111 antimyosin antibody, and technetium-99m pyrophosphate all have the ability to localize to sites of cardiac injury. These tests lack the ability to accurately distinguish inflammatory causes of ventricular dysfunction from other etiologies. O'Connell and coworkers[65] reported a sensitivity of 36% and a specificity of 98% for gallium cardiac imaging in the detection of myocarditis. Antimyosin antibodies are used to localize to areas of myocyte necrosis and, in one study, this technique possessed an 83% sensitivity and a 53% specificity for the diagnosis of myocarditis.[66] For calculating the sensitivity and specificity, endomyocardial biopsy was used as the "gold standard," yet cardiac biopsy has proven to be imperfect in the diagnosis of myocarditis.[67] Nuclear imaging may be helpful in determining prognosis. A normal scan predicts a lower likelihood of obtaining a "positive" endomyocardial biopsy, and also correlates with a lower probability that ventricular function will improve with time.[68]

Cardiac enzymes are often used to confirm myocyte death in myocarditis. The creatine phosphokinase MB fraction (CPK-MB) remains the standard test, but the accuracy of this test, as well as other biochemical markers of myocyte necrosis in the diagnosis of myocarditis, is unclear.[69] Newer markers of myocardial damage, such as troponin I, may offer more sensitive and specific evidence of the subtle and sustained injury that accompanies viral infection of the heart.[70]

Endomyocardial Biopsy

The technique of endomyocardial biopsy involves passage of a bioptome to the right ventricle via the right internal jugular vein or femoral vein to obtain samples of interventricular septal myocardium. Commonly, multiple samples are obtained to reduce the chances of missing the patchy areas of inflammation. Although this technique was first introduced in 1962, it was rarely used until the necessity to diagnose immunologic rejection in heart transplantation made the biopsy indispensable. The technique was also used to investigate unexplained heart failure in this early period. Etiologics of heart failure that may be detected by cardiac biopsy include: lymphocytic myocarditis, cardiac transplant rejection, amyloidosis, hemochromatosis, sarcoidosis, anthracycline cardiotoxicity, endocardial fibrosis, and hypereosinophilic syndrome.[71] Although histologic evidence of these diseases can be found in the biopsy specimens, many of these diseases can be diagnosed by other means. The remaining conditions, with the exception of cardiac transplant rejection, have no effective treatment and therefore do not require documentation of the diagnosis.

Physicians caring for patients with unexplained left ventricular dysfunction have used endomyocardial biopsy to establish a diagnosis. Pathologic criteria for myocarditis have been difficult to standardize, with the rates of "biopsy-proven" disease ranging from 3% to 63%.[72] To standardize the diagnostic histology of myocarditis, eight cardiac pathologists met in Dallas, Texas and established the "Dallas criteria."[73] These criteria were later used for the Multicenter Myocarditis Trial. Using these criteria, evidence of active or "borderline" myocarditis was diagnosed in only 10% of patients screened for inclusion in the study.[20] Thus, even in a selected population with recent onset heart failure symptoms, the diagnostic yield for this endomyocardial biopsy is quite low.

The histologic diagnoses established by the Dallas criteria are listed in Table 3, but unfortunately the different criteria neither suggest that a particular course of therapy is of benefit nor do they predict the prognosis once the diagnosis is established.[20,74] The low diagnostic yield and the lack of specific therapy and prognostic data for the diseases diagnosed by the procedure make endomyocardial biopsy unnecessary in the evaluation of the patient with suspected myocarditis. The

Table 3
Dallas Criteria

First Biopsy	
Active myocarditis	Inflammatory infiltrate, usually lymphocytes with adjacent myocyte damage
Borderline myocarditis	Sparse inflammatory infiltrate, myocyte damage not visualized on light microscopy
No evidence for myocarditis	No interstitial inflammatory infiltrate, no myocardial damage
Subsequent Biopsies	
Ongoing persistent myocarditis ± fibrosis	Degree of inflammatory infiltrate is same or worse compared to original biopsy specimen
Resolving/healing myocarditis ± fibrosis	Inflammatory infiltrate is decreased, fibroblasts and scar tissue are present
Resolved/healed myocarditis + fibrosis	No inflammatory infiltrate, no ongoing cellular necrosis, scar tissue may be present, adjacent compensatory hypertrophy may be present

sole exception to this recommendation is the patient with a rapid downhill course who may require urgent cardiac transplantation. In this group, active viral myocarditis should be excluded by biopsy. Animal studies have demonstrated exacerbation of viral myocarditis when immunosuppressive therapy, such as that used following transplantation, is initiated early in the course of the illness.[19]

Clinical Course and Prognosis

The clinical course of myocarditis remains unpredictable and therefore it is difficult to offer a general recommendation to the athlete/patient who presents for clearance to compete. The presence of inflammation on biopsy or nuclear imaging study appears to mark a group of patients, some of whom may experience improvement in ventricular function. This has not been the finding of all investigators who are attempting to correlate prognosis with biopsy findings.[75] Similarly, patients with an abnormal antimyosin antibody or gallium scan are more likely to have an improvement in ventricular function compared to patients with a "normal" scan[76]; however, this finding has not been validated in a large cohort of patients.

In the Myocarditis Treatment Trial, of the 111 patients enrolled in the study, 44 died or received a heart transplant after 5 years. The predictors of an adverse outcome in these patients included: (1) lower left ventricular ejection fraction (LVEF) at the time of enrollment; (2) use of a higher number of heart failure medicines; (3) longer duration of disease; and (4) lower serum levels of IgG antibodies.[20]

Serial assessment of ventricular function in the Multicenter Myocarditis Trial demonstrated that LVEF increases in the first year after diagnosis of lymphocytic myocarditis.[20] Unfortunately, the 5-year mortality is similar to that in other series of patients with heart failure (50% at 5 years; Figure 1), suggesting that myocarditis does not have a better prognosis than other causes of cardiomyopathy.

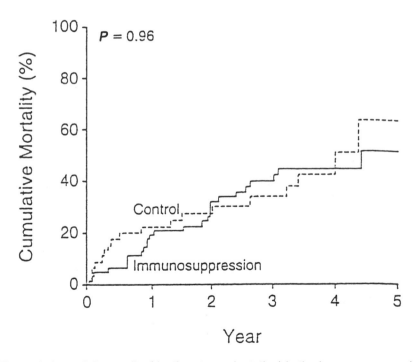

Figure 1. Actuarial mortality (death or transplantation) in the immunosuppression and control groups in patients with biopsy-proven myocarditis. There was no statistically significant difference between treatment groups. From Reference 20, with permission.

In addition to left ventricular dysfunction, the degree of right ventricular dysfunction may also be an independent predictor of worse outcome. In a retrospective analysis of 23 patients with histologic evidence of myocarditis, 10 of the 15 patients with impaired right ventricular function died or underwent heart transplantation at follow-up. In comparison, 1 of 8 patients with normal right ventricular function reached one of these endpoints.[77] Patients with worse right ventricular function were also more likely to have depressed left ventricular function, so it is unclear from this small patient series if assessment of right ventricular function adds prognostic information independent of left ventricular function.

Myocarditis and Sudden Death

Myocarditis is an infrequent cause of sudden death in the athlete. In two early patient series totaling approximately 50 patients, myocarditis or DCM was not considered the cause of death in any case.[78,79] In a broader series from the United States involving 158 athletes, 4 sudden deaths were attributed to myocarditis and another 4 to DCM.[80] A similar prevalence of myocarditis in athletic sudden death was reported by Roman and coworkers.[81] An explanation for the difference seen in these two eras may be simply that it took larger patient cohorts to detect a condition (sudden death from myocarditis) with a low incidence (<5%). Cyclic changes in the prevalence of the etiologic viruses or a rise in illicit drug use are alternative explanations for the observed differences.

The more common question to be addressed to the health care practitioner pertains to the risk of sudden death in the athlete with proven or presumed myocarditis, and to the issue of when athletic training can resume. It is clear that myocarditis is a cause of arrhythmias and minor electrocardiographic changes in athletes.[82] Supraventricular and ventricular arrhythmias can be seen in patients with active myocarditis as well as in those who are in the healing phase. These arrhythmias can produce a range of clinical problems from benign palpitations to sudden cardiac death.[83] Clinically silent myocarditis may result in ventricular arrhythmias in the population of patients with unexplained sudden death or medically refractory ventricular tachycardia. In an uncontrolled study, immunosuppressive therapy with corticosteroids resulted in improved control of arrhythmias.[84] The risk of ventricular arrhythmias does not completely abate with the resolution of inflammation in the heart.[85]

There are presently no clinical predictors of sudden death risk in patients with myocarditis. From the available clinical and investigational data, it would appear that early in the course of myocarditis, exercise may predispose to an adverse outcome, possibly from unfavorable loading forces placed on the heart by exercise, elevation of plasma norepinephrine, or a lack of therapy with angiotensin-converting enzyme (ACE) inhibitors during the preclinical, symptomatic phase of the illness. Even after resolution of acute inflammation and partial recovery of ventricular function, the patient remains at risk for dysrhythmias and therapy should be dictated by clinical symptoms and ventricular function. Beyond the acute and healing phase, the clinical behavior of patients with myocarditis parallels that of those with DCM. During this chronic phase, decisions regarding therapy and participation in athletics should be governed by the recommendations for patients with cardiomyopathy.[86]

Treatment

Despite significant strides in the classification and understanding of myocarditis, little progress has been made in the treatment of this condition. The Myocarditis Treatment Trial was a randomized, placebo-controlled study designed to evaluate the impact of immunosuppressive therapy on clinical outcome in patients with myocarditis. The trial randomized 111 patients with: (1) LVEF <45; (2) pathologic evidence of lymphocytic myocarditis; and (3) onset of heart failure within the previous 2 years. Patients were randomized into two treatment groups: prednisone plus cyclosporine, or azathioprine versus placebo. Twenty-eight weeks after randomization there was no significant difference in LVEF or survival between the two groups.[20] The actuarial mortality curve from this trial is shown in Figure 1.

Therapy is supportive for patients with a presumptive diagnosis of myocarditis. Patients may be critically ill during the acute phase of the illness but it is likely that the majority of patients are minimally symptomatic. Therapy for myocarditis then focuses on preventing the complications of the myocardial damage. The primary rule of therapy for this condition is the initiation of ACE inhibitor treatment when left ventricular systolic dysfunction is diagnosed, regardless of symptom status. In contrast to immunosuppressive therapy, ACE inhibitors have been shown to reduce mortality in patients with mild to severe heart failure associated with depressed left ventricular function.[87,88] In one study, patients with asymptomatic left ventricular dysfunction also had a trend toward reduction of mortality, but also experienced a reduction in the development of heart failure symptoms when treated with enalapril, the ACE inhibitor used in that trial.[89] There is evidence that ACE inhibitors prevent or slow the progressive left ventricular dilatation which follows myocardial injury. This benefit is partially lost if the therapy is withdrawn.[90] At present, there are no guidelines that dictate when ACE inhibitors may be discontinued in the patient recovering from myocarditis, but they clearly should be continued as long as left ventricular systolic function remains impaired.

Recommendations for the Athlete/Patient with Myocarditis

Athletes presenting with presumed myocarditis should discontinue training until evaluation is completed. Data from animal studies suggest that exercise during the acute phase of the disease leads to increased viral replication, more extensive myocyte necrosis, and a worse chance of survival.[91] The ventricular remodeling process of inflammation followed by fibrosis formation may create an arrhythmogenic milieu that could be unmasked with exercise.[82] The recent Bethesda Conference on athletes with cardiovascular disorders recognized the risk of sudden death in patients with myocarditis and recommended a convalescence period of 6 months after the onset of symptoms.[86] The practitioner or trainer who is supervising the athlete following recovery from myocarditis should remember that persistence of ventricular arrhythmia after the resolution of myocarditis has been noted in children and young adults.[85] At present, there are no validified clinical variables to stratify the risk of sudden death in these patients.

Patients with left ventricular dysfunction should be treated in a similar manner as patients with cardiomyopathy. This includes the use of ACE inhibitors and other medications as indicated. Patients with myocarditis secondary to other inflammatory conditions should receive specific therapy for those conditions, if indicated. Patients should be screened for treatable illness, such as HIV infection. Endomyocardial biopsy is not indicated except in severely ill patients who are being considered for urgent heart transplantation. In these patients with active viral infections, acute viral myocarditis must be ruled out in order to avoid exacerbating the infectious disease with immunosuppressive therapy. If nonviral infectious myocarditis is being considered, then biopsy may be indicated to determine appropriate therapy.

Myocarditis carries a prognosis similar to that of DCM. The 5-year mortality rate is roughly 50%, a fact which should be considered when the athlete/patient is making decisions that may impact on later life.

References

1. Richardson P, McKenna W, Bristow M, et al. Report of the 1995 World Health Organization/International Society and Federation of Cardiology Task Force on the definition and classification of cardiomyopathies. *Circulation* 1996;93:841–842.

2. Brown C, O'Connell J. Myocarditis and idiopathic dilated cardiomyopathy. *Am J Med* 1995;99:309–314.
3. James T. Myocarditis and cardiomyopathy. *N Engl J Med* 1983;308:39–41.
4. Olsen E. Myocarditis: A case of mistaken identity. *Br Heart J* 1983;50: 303–311.
5. Gravanis M, Sternby N. Incidence of myocarditis. *Arch Pathol Lab Med* 1991;115:390–392.
6. Christian H. Ten decades of interest in idiopathic pericarditis. *Am Heart J* 1951;42:645–651.
7. See D, Tilles J. Viral myocarditis. *Rev Inf Dis* 1991;13:951–956.
8. Saphir O. Myocarditis: A general review with and analysis of 240 cases. *Arch Pathol* 1942;33:88–137.
9. Sole N, Kuy O. Viral myocarditis: A paradigm for understanding the pathogenesis and treatment of dilated cardiomyopathy. *J Am Coll Cardiol* 1993;22:99A–105A.
10. Martino T, Lui P, Sole M. Viral infection and the pathogenesis of dilated cardiomyopathy. *Circ Res* 1994;74:182–188.
11. Silver M, Kowalczyk D. Coronary microvascular narrowing in acute murine Coxsackie B3 myocarditis. *Am Heart J* 1989;118:173–174.
12. Factor S, Minase T, Cho S, et al. Microvascular spasm in the cardiomyopathic syrian hamster: A preventable cause of focal myocardial necrosis. *Circulation* 1982;66:342–354.
13. Lowens C, Hill S, Lafond-Walker A, et al. Nitric oxide inhibits viral replication in murine myocarditis. *J Clin Invest* 1996;97:1837–1843.
14. Caforio A. Role of autoimmunity in dilated cardiomyopathy. *Br Heart J* 1994;72:30s–34s.
15. Lange L, Schreiner G. Immune mechanisms of cardiac disease. *N Engl J Med* 1994;330:1129–1135.
16. Caforio A, Keeling P, Zachar E, et al. Evidence from family studies for autoimmunity in dilated cardiomyopathy. *Lancet* 1994;344:773–777.
17. Klingel K, Hohenadi C, Canu A, et al. Ongoing enterovirus-induced myocarditis is associated with persistent heart muscle infection: Quantitative analysis of viral replication, tissue damage and inflammation. *Proc Natl Acad Sci U S A* 1992;89:314–318.
18. Tomioka N, Dishimoto C, Matsumori A, Kawai C. Effects of prednisolone on acute viral myocarditis in mice. *J Am Coll Cardiol* 1986;7:868–872.
19. O'Connell J, Reap E, Robinson J. The effects of cyclosporine on acute murine Coxsackie B3 myocarditis. *Circulation* 1986;73:353–359.
20. Mason J, O'Connell J, Herskowitz A, et al. A clinical trial of immunosuppressive therapy for myocarditis. *N Engl J Med* 1995;333:269–275.
21. Grist N, Reid D. Epidemiology of viral infections of the heart. In Banatvala J (ed): *Viral Infections of the Heart*. London: Edward Arnold; 1993:23–31.
22. Peters N, Polle-Wilson P. Myocarditis-continuing clinical and pathological confusion. *Am Heart J* 1991;121:942–947.
23. Hershowitz A, Wu T, Willoughby S, et al. Myocarditis and cardiotropic viral infection associated with severe left ventricular dysfunction in late stage infection with Human Immunodeficiency Virus. *J Am Coll Cardiol* 1994;24:1025–1032.
24. Beschorner W, Baughman K, Turnicky R, et al. HIV-associated myocarditis, pathology and immunopathology. *Am J Pathol* 1990;137:1365–1371.
25. Wesslen L, Pahlson C, Friman G. Myocarditis caused by Chlamydia pneumoniae (TWAR) and sudden unexpected death in a Swedish elite orienteerer. *Lancet* 1992;240:427–428.

26. Wesslen L, Pahlson C, Lindquist O, et al. An increase in sudden unexpected cardiac deaths among young Swedish orienteers during 1979–1992. *Eur Heart J* 1996;17:902–910.
27. Stockins B, Lanas F, Saavedra J, Opazo J. Prognosis in patients with diphtheria myocarditis and bradyarrhythmias. Assessment of results of ventricular pacing. *Br Heart J* 1994;72:190–191.
28. Stevens D, Troyer B, Merrick D, et al. Lethals effects and cardiovascular effects of purified alpha and theta toxins from clostridium perfringens. *J Infect Dis* 1988;157:272–279.
29. Linde MVD. Lyme carditis: Clinical characteristics of 105 cases. *Scand J Infect Dis* 1991;77(suppl):81–84.
30. Habib G, Mann D, Zoghbi W. Normalization of cardiac structure and function after regression of cardiac hypertrophy. *Am Heart J* 1994;128: 333–343.
31. Haywood G, O'Connell S, Gray H. Lyme carditis: A United Kingdom perspective. *Br Heart J* 1993;70:15–16.
32. Hagar J, Rahimtoola S. Chagas disease in the United States. *N Engl J Med* 1991; 325:763–769.
33. Morris S, Tanowitz H, Wittner M, Bilezikian J. Pathophysiological insights into the cardiomyopathy of Chagas disease. *Circulation* 1990;82: 1900–1909.
34. Doherty N, Siegel R. Cardiovascular manifestations of systemic lupus erythematosis. *Am Heart J* 1985;110:1257–1265.
35. Hejtmancik M, Wright J, Quint R, Jennings F. The cardiovascular manifestations of systemic lupus erythematosis. *Am Heart J* 1964;119:119–130.
36. Bulkley B, Ridolfi R, Salyer W, Hutchins G. Myocardial lesions of progressive systemic sclerosis: A cause of cardiac dysfunction. *Circulation* 1976;53:483–490.
37. Hiraishi S, Yashiro K, Oguchi K, et al. Clinical course of cardiovascular involvement in the mucocutaneous lymph node syndrome: Relation between clinical signs, carditis and development of coronary arterial aneurysms. *Am J Cardiol* 1981;47:323–329.
38. Fujiwara H, Hamashima Y. Pathology of the heart in Kawasaki's disease. *Pediatrics* 1978;61:100–107.
39. Kounis N, Zavras G, Soufras G, Kitrou M. Hypersensitivity myocarditis. *Ann Allergy* 1989;62:71–73.
40. French A, Weller C. Interstitial myocarditis following the clinical and experimental use of sulfonamide drugs. *Am J Pathol* 1942;18:122–130.
41. Taselaar H, Karch S, Stevens B, Billingham M. Cocaine and the heart. *Hum Pathol* 1987;18:195–199.
42. Isner J, Chokshi S. Cardiovascular complications of cocaine. *Curr Prob Cardiol* 1991;64:94–123.
43. Virmani R, Robinowitz M, Smialek J, Smyth D. Cardiovascular effect of cocaine: An autopsy study of 40 patients. *Am Heart J* 1988;115:1068–1075.
44. Kloner R, Hale S, Alker K, Rezkalla S. The effects of acute and chronic cocaine use on the heart. *Circulation* 1992;85:407–418.
45. Loyer E, Delpassand E. Radiation induced heart disease—imaging features. *Semin Roentgenol* 1993;28:321–332.
46. Stewart J, Fajardo L. Radiation induced heart disease—an update. *Prog Cardiovasc Dis* 1984;27:173–194.
47. McFalls E, Hosenpud J, McAnulty J, et al. Granulomatous myocarditis: Diagnosis by endomyocardial biopsy and response to corticosteroids in two patients. *Chest* 1986;89:509–511.

48. Mason J. Distinct forms of myocarditis. *Circulation* 1991;83:1110–1111.
49. Davidoff R, Palacios I, Souther J, et al. Giant cell versus lymphocytic myocarditis: A comparison of their clinical features and long-term outcomes. *Circulation* 1991;83:953–961.
50. Nieminen M, Salminen U, Taskinen E, et al. Treatment of serious heart failure by transplantation in giant cell myocarditis diagnosed by endomyocardial biopsy. *J Heart Lung Transplant* 1994;13:543–547.
51. Desjardins V, Pelletier G, Leung T, Waters D. Successful treatment of severe heart failure caused by idiopathic giant cell myocarditis. *Can J Cardiol* 1992;8:788–791.
52. Lampert M, Lang R. Peripartum cardiomyopathy. *Am Heart J* 1995;130: 860–870.
53. Rizeq M, Rickenbacher P, Fowler M, Billingham M. Incidence of myocarditis in peripartum cardiomyopathy. *Am J Cardiol* 1994;74:474–477.
54. Kline L, Kline T, Saphir O. Myocarditis in senescence. *Am Heart J* 1963;65:446–457.
55. Richardson P, Why H. Clinical spectrum of viral heart disease. In Banatvala J (ed): *Viral Infections of the Heart.* London: Edward Arnold; 1993:59–81.
56. Chow L, Dittrich H, Shabetai R. Endomyocardial biopsy in patients with unexplained congestive heart failure. *Ann Intern Med* 1988;109:535–539.
57. Kasper E, Agema W, Hutchins G, et al. The causes of dilated cardiomyopathy: A clinicopathological review of 673 consecutive patients. *J Am Coll Cardiol* 1994;23:586–590.
58. Reyes M, Ho K, Smith F, Lerner A. A mouse model of dilated type cardiomyopathy due to Coxsackie virus B3. *J Infect Dis* 1981;144:232–236.
59. Keeling P, Lukaszyk A, Poloniecki J, et al. Prospective case control study of antibodies to Coxsackie B virus in idiopathic dilated cardiomyopathy. *J Am Coll Cardiol* 1994;23:593–598.
60. Cambridge G, MacArthur C, Waterson A, et al. Antibodies to Coxsackie B viruses in congestive cardiomyopathy. *Br Heart J* 1979;41:692–696.
61. Bowles N, Olsen E, Richardson P, Archard L. Detection of Coxsackie B virus specific RNA sequences in myocardial biopsy samples from patients with myocarditis and dilated cardiomyopathy. *Lancet* 1986;1:1120–1123.
62. Why H, Meany B, Richardson P, et al. Clinical and prognostic significance of detection of enteroviral RNA in the myocardium of patients with myocarditis or dilated cardiomyopathy. *Circulation* 1994;89:2582–2589.
63. Morgera T, Dilenarda A, Dreas L, et al. Electrocardiography of myocarditis revisited: Clinical and prognostic significance of electrocardiographic changes. *Am Heart J* 1992;124:455–466.
64. Pianamonit B, Albed E, Cigalotto A, et al. Echocardiographic findings in myocarditis. *Am J Cardiol* 1988;62:2285–2291.
65. O'Connell J, Henkinn R, Subramanian R, et al. Gallium 67 imaging in patients with dilated cardiomyopathy and biopsy-proven myocarditis. *Circulation* 1984;70:58–62.
66. Dec G, Palacios I, Yasuda T, et al. Antimyosin antibody cardiac imaging: Its role in diagnosis of myocarditis. *J Am Coll Cardiol* 1990;16:97–104.
67. Jain D, Zaret B. Antimyosin cardiac imaging in acute myocarditis. *J Am Coll Cardiol* 1990;16:105–107.
68. Narula J, Khaw B, Dec G, et al. Diagnostic accuracy of antimyosin scintigraphy in suspected myocarditis. *J Nucl Cardiol* 1996;3:371–381.
69. Adams J, Abendscein D, Jaffe A. Biochemical markers of myocardial injury: Is MB creatine kinase the choice for the 1990's. *Circulation* 1993;88: 750–762.

70. Smith S, Ladenson J, Mason J, Jaffe A. Elevations of cardiac troponin I associated with myocarditis, experimental and clinical correlates. *Circulation* 1993;88:163–167.
71. Mason J, O'Connell J. Clinical merit of endomyocardial biopsy. *Circulation* 1989;79:971–979.
72. Baandrup U, Olsen E. Critical analysis of endomyocardial biopsies from patients suspected of having myocarditis. *Br Heart J* 1981;45:475–486.
73. Aretz H. Myocarditis: The Dallas criteria. *Hum Pathol* 1987;18:619–624.
74. Lieberman E, Hutchins G, Herskowitz A, et al. Clinicopathological description of myocarditis. *J Am Coll Cardiol* 1991;18:1617–1626.
75. Dec G, Fallon J, Southern J, Palacios I. Relation between histologic findings on early repeat right ventricular biopsy and ventricular function in patients with myocarditis. *Br Heart J* 1988;60:332–337.
76. Jarula J, Khaw B, Dec G. Diagnostic accuracy of antimyosin scintigraphy in suspected myocarditis. *J Nucl Cardiol* 1996;3:371–381.
77. Mendes L, Dec G, Picard M, et al. Right ventricular dysfunction: An independent predictor of adverse outcome in patients with myocarditis. *Am Heart J* 1994;128:301–307.
78. Corrado D, Theine G, Nava A, et al. Sudden death in young competitive athletes: Clinicopathological correlations in 22 cases. *Am J Med* 1990; 89:588–596.
79. Maron B, Roberts W, McAllister H, et al. Sudden death in young athletes. *Circulation* 1980;62:218–229.
80. Maron B, Shirani J, Poliac L, et al. Sudden death in young competitive athletes. *JAMA* 1996;276:199–204.
81. Roman G, Wessien L, Karajalainen J, Rolf C. Infectious and lymphocytic myocarditis: Epidemiology and factors relevant to sports medicine. *Scand J Med Sci Sports* 1995;5:269–278.
82. Zeppilli P, Santini C, Palieri V, et al. Role of myocarditis in athletes with minor arrhythmias and/or echocardiographic abnormalities. *Chest* 1994; 106:373–380.
83. Woodruff J. Viral myocarditis: A review. *Am J Pathol* 1980;101:427–484.
84. Vignola P, Aonuma K, Swaye P, et al. Lymphocytic myocarditis presenting as unexplained ventricular arrhythmias: Diagnosis with endomyocardial biopsy and response to immunosuppression. *J Am Coll Cardiol* 1984;4: 812–819.
85. Friedman R, Kearney D, Moak J, et al. Persistence of ventricular arrhythmia after resolution of occult myocarditis in children and young adults. *J Am Coll Cardiol* 1994;24:780–783.
86. Maron B, Isner J, McKenna W. Task force 3: Hypertrophic cardiomyopathy, myocarditis and other myopericardial diseases and mitral valve prolapse, 26th Bethesda Conference: Recommendations for determining eligibility for competition in athletes with cardiovascular abnormalities. *J Am Coll Cardiol* 1994;24:845–899.
87. CONSENSUS Study Group. Effects of enalapril on mortality in severe congestive heart failure. *N Engl J Med* 1987;316:1429–1435.
88. SOLVD Investigators. Effect of enalapril on survival in patients with reduced left ventricular ejection fraction and congestive heart failure. *N Engl J Med* 1991;325:293–302.
89. SOLVD Investigators. Effect of enalapril on mortality and the development of heart failure in asymptomatic patients with reduced left ventricular ejection fractions. *N Engl J Med* 1992;327:685–691.

90. Konstam M, Rousseau M, Kronenberg M, et al. Effects of the angiotensin converting enzyme inhibitor enalapril on the long term progression of left ventricular dysfunction in patients with heart failure. *Circulation* 1992; 86:431–438.
91. Gaimaitian B, Chason J, Lerner A. Augmentation of the virulence of murine Coxsackie B3 myocardiopathy by exercise. *J Exp Med* 1970;131: 1121–1136.

20

Sudden Cardiac Death in Athletes with Congenital Heart Disease

Paul C. Gillette, MD

Young patients with congenital heart disease often want to participate in organized athletics. In the United States, this is almost a rite of passage for the teenage years. In previous decades, young patients with congenital heart disease received no definitive treatment. Currently many such patients have had their definitive treatment prior to reaching an age where organized athletics are an issue. Modern surgical techniques can repair most defects early in life with little residua or sequela. Not every case, however, has a perfect repair, and some patients still suffer myocardial or conduction system damage before or during the repair.[1] In addition, as more and more extremely severe defects are effectively palliated, a number of children will grow into adolescence with major structural or physiologic abnormalities that cannot be repaired by current techniques. Obviously, cardiac transplantation is not a cure for their problems; it only trades one disease and one set of physiologic abnormalities for another.

For the purpose of this chapter, some important forms of congenital heart disease that are covered in other chapters are excluded.[2] These include the Marfan syndrome, Wolff-Parkinson-White syndrome, the long QT syndrome, coronary artery anomalies, and hypertrophic cardiomyopathy. Arrhythmogenic right ventricular dysplasia is also

From Estes NAM, Salem DN, Wang PJ (eds). *Sudden Cardiac Death in the Athlete.* Armonk, NY: Futura Publishing Co., Inc.; ©1998.

probably a congenital defect, and, is also covered elsewhere in this volume.[3]

It is critical to remember that each condition discussed has a peak of risk in the teenage and preteenage years. The natural history of these disorders after the patient reaches adulthood (>21 years) is the same as that of the younger survivors. The exact reason for the increased risk of sudden death in the 10- to 18-year age group is unknown. Developmental, physical, and physiologic changes probably account for part of the change, but extrinsic factors such as increased participation in organized activity are also likely to play a role. Mental stress, legal pharmacological stresses (such as caffeine), and illegal drugs,[4] probably also play an inciting role.

The preparticipation history and physical should begin early in organized sports.[5] Society dictates an ever-increasing stress on younger and younger athletes. Physicians can have little affect on societal stresses, but we can try to select specific athletics that are safe for each individual patient. The preparticipation history and physical should ideally be performed by the patient's personal physician, who has a knowledge of historical events that might be of importance. Unfortunately, many patients of this age do not have a personal physician either because of financial considerations or because children of this age are "healthy." Regardless of which physician performs this examination, it must be taken seriously and not seen as "paperwork to fill out." The patient's personal history and family history are extremely important and should be obtained from a responsible adult if possible (see chapter 4). It is the author's opinion that an electrocardiogram (ECG) should be obtained one or several times during an athlete's career.

The decision as to whether a patient with known congenital heart disease can participate and at what level is a difficult one. Guidelines have been prepared by the American College of Cardiology through several Bethesda conferences.[6-8] Certain defects have historically been known to carry a higher risk of sudden death.

One of the most common of these defects is congenital valvular aortic stenosis.[2,5,9] This is a defect that cannot be cured with present-day techniques. Patients with moderate or severe cases should be prohibited from participation in competitive sports, even after surgical or catheter palliation. Palliation is always only partial and often leads to aortic insufficiency. Usually in the late teenage years or early adulthood, valve replacement is necessary. It is possible that longer follow-up of early Ross repairs (using the patient's pulmonary valve in the aortic position) will allow some participation. It is equally likely that before a patient is considered a candidate for a Ross procedure, significant myocardial damage has occurred and that the pulmonary valve will develop physiologic abnormalities in the aortic position. It is unlikely that any patient with significant valvular aortic stenosis should be allowed to participate in competitive, organized athletics. Patients with a gradient of <50 mm Hg by catheter or a mean gradient of <50 mm Hg by echocardiogram pose a difficult clinical problem. Most will progress and should be excluded from participation at an early age. Those with gradients <20 mm Hg at rest, normal ECGs, and normal wall thickness by echocardiogram, who have a normal treadmill stress test, may be considered to be at low risk for sudden death.

Patients with membranous subaortic stenosis who had surgical repair before any evidence of myocardial damage or aortic valve damage occurred and who have no surgical sequelae may be considered in the same group as those with mild valvular aortic stenosis. Patients with mild pulmonary valve stenosis and no other abnormalities may be allowed full participation.[6] Patients with severe valvular pulmonary stenosis who are treated by surgery or catheter may have significant myocardial fibrosis and may be at risk for arrhythmia. Patients who have had successful catheter treatment in infancy may escape myocardial damage or spontaneously repair it and may be considered individually by noninvasive testing.

Patients who have no sequelae 6 months after having undergone successful atrial septal defect repair (particularly if performed early in life) are probably at low risk and should be allowed participation.[6] The same would hold true for patients with excellent results from an early ventricular septal defect repair, particularly those done without a ventriculotomy; however, careful evaluation for residual problems or sequelae is important.

Individuals with very small atrial or ventricular septal defects that do not require surgery may be considered for participation. These patients usually have a left to right shunt of ≤1.25:1 and normal intracardiac pressures.

Children who have coarctation of the aorta often have diffuse vascular and aortic valve disease. Although modern surgical and catheter therapy can virtually eliminate a transaortic pressure gradient at the site of the coarctation, important anatomic and physiologic abnormalities usually remain. The most serious is a propensity to develop hypertension despite the absence of a coarctation. The possibility of aneurysms, either of the thoracic aorta or the cerebral circulation, are also troubling, as is the early development of coronary disease if surgery was performed relatively late. The bicuspid aortic valve often present is an additional problem, as it may progress to aortic stenosis. The flow abnormalities associated with the bicuspid aortic valve also sometimes cause aneurysmal dilation of the ascending aorta. For all of these reasons, it is an unusual patient with coarctation of the aorta who can participate safely in organized athletics.[2]

Patent ductus arteriosus is usually cured by device or surgical closure at an early age. The left ventricular dilation usually regresses and after several years participation may be possible. A very small patent ductus presents no physiologic abnormality and allows full participation.

Very complex congenital heart defects usually cannot be completely repaired. Tetralogy of Fallot, except for the most mild forms, fits in this category.[6] Even the best repairs often leave the patient with some pulmonary stenosis and create pulmonary insufficiency. It is unclear if the right ventricular myocardium ever fully recovers. The best hope lies in early repair. Midterm results of this approach, pioneered by the group at Boston Children's Hospital, are encouraging, but at least another decade will be required to fully settle this issue. In general, patients postoperative for tetralogy of Fallot cannot safely be allowed to participate in organized athletics.

The management of patients with d-transposition of the great arteries has undergone dramatic change in the last decade. The venous repair (Mustard/Senning) has been replaced by the arterial repair. Patients who have undergone venous repair have important physiologic and electrical abnormalities and cannot be allowed to participate in organized athletics. Some patients who undergo neonatal arterial switch repair may reach adolescence with nearly normal hearts and may be fit to participate fully, although supportive research is yet to be seen. A thorough evaluation for coronary artery insufficiencies, aortic insufficiency, and supravalvular pulmonary stenosis is required.

Patients with a single ventricle who have had a Fontan repair, although well palliated, will never have normal enough physiology to participate in organized athletics.[6] Patients with single ventricle who have not had a Fontan are also unfit for full participation. As a general rule, any patient with cyanosis at rest should not be allowed to participate in competitive sports because of myocardial hypertrophy and fibrosis.[10]

Some congenital cardiac defects have great variability in severity, which directly influences the ability of affected patients to participate in athletics. Ebstein's anomaly and congenitally corrected "L" transposition are in this category.[11] In their mildest forms, there is no physiologic abnormality and full participation is possible. At the other end of the spectrum severe physiologic abnormalities are present and participation is not possible.

Patients with congenital complete atrioventricular block may participate, either with or without a pacemaker, if there are no other abnormalities. Having a pacemaker prohibits participation in contact sports such as football and hockey. In this regard, competitive organized athletics must be differentiated from contact athletics.[7]

There is a trend to try to orient young people toward athletic endeavors in which they might participate throughout their lives. Golf, tennis, and aerobics are in this category. This is almost surely a positive trend, but it is pushing us to new grounds where less information is available. These sports probably are less likely to precipitate arrhythmias and sudden death and may even condition the cardiovascular system and decrease the occurrence of arrhythmias and sudden death. Heavily competitive singles tennis may, in some cases, overstress the congenitally abnormal heart. Some levels of aerobics may also be too much, whereas lower levels may be positive.

Thus, although the numbers may be small for patients with congenital heart disease, and although there are now guidelines, the physician must still make individual decisions about individual patients.[8]

References

1. Denfield SW, Garson A Jr. Sudden death in children and young adults. *Pediatr Clin North Am* 1990;37(1):215–231.
2. Basso C, Frescura C, Corrado D, et al. Congential heart disease and sudden death in the young. *Hum Pathol* 1995;26(10):1065–1072.
3. Corrado D, Thiene G, Nava A, et al. Sudden death in young competitive athletes: Clinicopathologic correlations in 22 cases. *Am J Med* 1990;89: 558–596.
4. Win-Kuang S, Edwards WD, Hammill SC, et al. Sudden unexpected nontraumatic death in 54 young adults: A 30-year population-based study. *Am J Cardiol* 1995;76:148–152.
5. Maron BJ, Thompson PD, Puffer JC, et al. Cardiovascular pre-participation screening of competitive athletes. A statement for health professionals from the Sudden Death Committee (Clinical Cardiology) and Congenital Cardiac Defects Committee (Cardiovascular Disease in the Young), American Heart Association. *Circulation* 1996;94(4):850–855.
6. Graham TP, Bricker JT, James FW, et al. Task force 1: Congenital heart disease 26th Bethesda Conference. *J Am Coll Cardiol* 1994;24(4):867–873.
7. Mitchell JH, Haskell WL, Raven PB. Classification of sports. 26th Bethesda Conference. *J Am Coll Cardiol* 1994;24(4):864–866.
8. Recommendations for determining eligibility for competition in athletes with cardiovascular abnormalities. 26th Bethesda Conference. *J Am Coll Cardiol* 1994;24(4):845–899.
9. Lambert EC, Menon VA, Wagner HR, et al. Sudden unexpected death from cardiovascular disease in children. *Am J Cardiol* 1974;34:89.
10. Hegerty A, Anderson RH, Deanfield JE. Myocardial fibrosis in tetralogy of Fallot: Effect of surgery or part of the natural history? *Br Heart J* 1988;59:123. Abstract.
11. Rossi L, Thiene G. Mild Ebstein's anomaly associated with supraventricular tachycardia and sudden death: Clinicomorphologic features in 3 patients. *Am J Cardiol* 1984;53:332–334.

21

Coronary Anomalies as a Cause of Sudden Death in the Athlete

Melvin D. Cheitlin, MD

Sudden death at any age is always shocking and unexpected. Most often it occurs in elderly patients with known heart disease. Sudden death on the athletic field is more than shocking. It happens to young, active people, negating the preconceived idea that exercise protects against heart disease. It happens to the people who are least likely to have a cardiac event—active, even hyperactive, young people. When sudden death occurs, it generates intense interest from the press, and it regenerates interest in screening athletes with use of various tests other than the history and physical examination before allowing them to participate in athletics; even though the studies that have been done have shown this to be futile.[1–5]

Sudden death occurring during sports is, fortunately, a rare event. Various estimates of the prevalence of sudden death during athletics or vigorous exercise have been published. Ades[6] reported four cases of sudden death occurring per million athletes per year. Van Camp,[7] using statistics from the National Federation of State High School Associations (NFSHA), estimated 10 to 25 sudden cardiac deaths per year in the group younger than 30 years old. Excluding joggers with known coronary disease, the prevalence of sudden cardiac death is 1 for every 15,240 joggers per year.[8] Phillips and colleagues[9] reported 1 death annually for

From Estes NAM, Salem DN, Wang PJ (eds). *Sudden Cardiac Death in the Athlete.* Armonk, NY: Futura Publishing Co., Inc.; ©1998.

every 735,000 exercising Air Force recruits. This population is screened before induction into the Air Force, and therefore is not comparable to the general population. In the general population of men younger than age 30, in a report from Rhode Island, there was 1 death during recreational exercise for every 280,000 people.[10] Van Camp and colleagues,[11] over a 10-year period, reported nontraumatic sports deaths in 126 high school athletes and in 34 college athletes. The estimated death rate in male athletes was five times as high as in female athletes: 7.47 versus 1.33 per million athletes per year.[11]

Although sudden death on the athletic field is a rare occurrence, when it does occur, cardiac disease is the major nontraumatic cause.[11–16]

The causative cardiac disease seen in these athletes older than age 35 is, overwhelmingly, coronary artery disease. Waller[17] reported that in this age group, 90% of the deaths occurred due to coronary disease. In the series by Ragosta and colleagues,[10] of 75 recreational joggers older than 30 years of age who died, 95% had coronary artery disease. In most series, the most common etiology in patients younger than 35 years old is hypertrophic cardiomyopathy.[12,13,18,19] Often, the second most frequent cause is coronary anomalies.[12,18] McCaffrey and colleagues[12] reviewed seven studies with literature of sudden death in athletes 30 years of age or younger. Of 84 such deaths, 20 (24%) were associated with hypertrophic cardiomyopathy and 15 (18%) with coronary artery anomalies.[12] Congenital coronary anomalies have been reported as a cause of sudden death in 12% to 14% of athletes younger than age 35.[20,21] Although some series suffer from referral bias, coronary anomalies do occur in most reports of sports-related sudden death in young people.

Types of Coronary Anomalies Seen (Figure 1)

. Classification of coronary anomalies has been proposed by Roberts[22]:

1. Anomalous origin of one or both coronary arteries from the pulmonary artery
2. Anomalous origin of one or both coronary arteries from the aorta:
   (a) Left coronary artery from the right sinus of Valsalva
   (b) Right coronary artery from the left posterior sinus of Valsalva
   (c) Left circumflex coronary artery from the right sinus of Valsalva
   (d) Anomalous origin of a coronary artery from the right posterior sinus of Valsalva
   (e) Right coronary artery and left anterior descending coronary artery from the right sinus of Valsalva

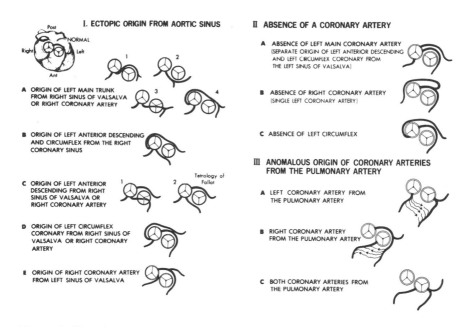

Figure 1. Classification of anomalies of the coronary arteries. From Reference 41, with permission.

3. A single coronary ostium from the aorta:
   (a) A single right coronary ostium
   (b) A single left coronary ostium
4. Coronary arteriovenous, coronary cameral, or coronary pulmonary artery fistulae
5. Congenital/hypoplastic coronary artery

Some of these coronary anomalies create serious compromise of coronary blood flow and myocardial ischemia and, therefore, without correction, are incompatible with athletics or even survival for any period of time. Such is the case with anomalous origin of the left coronary artery from the pulmonary artery or anomalous origin of both coronary arteries from the pulmonary artery; therefore, with the exception of unique case reports, these disorders are not seen in athletics. Other coronary anomalies almost never produce ischemia. Such is the case with a single coronary artery or high-origin arteries of a coronary artery from the aorta, or anomalous coronary artery to pulmonary artery fistula, which is almost always small and asymptomatic.[23]

The most common coronary anomaly found in young people who have died suddenly on the athletic field, whether during or immediately after exercise, is that of the left coronary artery from the anterior sinus of Valsalva.[12,18,21,24] Of the two anomalies of origin, the right coronary from the left sinus of Valsalva is the slightly more common coronary anomaly.[25] Jokl and colleagues[26] first reported isolated case reports of children and adolescents dying suddenly with the only abnormality being the left coronary artery arising from the right sinus of Valsalva. In 1974, Cheitlin and colleagues[24] reported an autopsy series from the Armed Forces Institute of Pathology (AFIP). There were 51 cases: 33 with the left coronary artery from the right sinus of Valsalva, and 18 with the right coronary artery from the left sinus of Valsalva. Nine patients died suddenly, seven during or immediately after exercise, all with the left coronary artery coming from the right sinus of Valsalva. There were no sudden deaths in the patients with the right coronary artery coming from the left posterior sinus of Valsalva. The major difference between those who died suddenly and the others was that the mean age in the sudden death group was 20 years (range 13 to 36), versus 57.3 years (range 24 to 87). Although in this series, there were no sudden deaths in the group with the right coronary artery coming from the left posterior sinus of Valsalva, Roberts and colleagues[27] reported a series with five sudden deaths in patients with this anomaly.

Most sudden deaths associated with anomalous origin of a coronary artery from the aorta have been in the anomalies where the left coronary artery arises from the anterior sinus of Valsalva.[24,25,28] Liberthson and colleagues[28] reported their own nine autopsied cases and 18 previously reported cases. No patients with the right coronary artery arising from the left posterior sinus of Valsalva were known to have related ventricular tachycardia, syncope, or sudden death. The mean age of these patients was 54 years. Of the 20 autopsied patients with the left coronary arising from the anterior sinus of Valsalva, all died suddenly after physical exertion. The mean age of these patients was 16 years (range 1 to 36).

In a later series for the AFIP, Taylor and colleagues[25] reported 49 cases where the left main coronary arose from the anterior sinus of Valsalva or as a first branch of the right coronary artery. Of these 49 patients, 28 (57%) died suddenly and 18 of those 28 (64%) died during or soon after exercise. Of the 28 patients where the left coronary passed posteriorly between the right ventricular outflow tract and the aorta, 23 (82%) died suddenly. There were 52 cases of the right coronary artery arising from the left posterior sinus of Valsalva. In this group, 13 (25%) died suddenly.[25]

As it arises from the aorta, the coronary artery usually takes an oblique course, resulting in an oval, or even slitlike, ostium. The left main coronary artery, after arising from the anterior sinus of Valsalva or as a first branch from the right coronary artery, can take four possible courses (Figure 1)[25]:

1. Anterior to the right ventricular outflow tract, bifurcating into the left anterior descending and left circumflex as it reaches the anterior interventricular groove;

2. left posterior, between the right ventricular outflow tract and the aorta, passing to its usual position under the left atrial appendage before bifurcating;
3. The left coronary artery can dive into the myocardium, ride along the subendocardium of the crista supraventricularis, and rise to the epicardium at the proximal portion of the anterior interventricular groove before bifurcating;
4. The left coronary artery can pass posteriorly to the right and posterior to the aorta, to its usual position before bifurcating

The right coronary artery from the left posterior sinus of Valsalva can take two courses: (1) anteriorly, between the right ventricular outflow tract and aorta to the right atrioventricular (AV) groove; (2) Posterior to the aorta, to the right AV groove.

The vast majority of young patients who have died during or immediately after an athletic activity have had the left coronary artery arise from the anterior sinus of Valsalva, where the left main coronary artery passes between the right ventricular outflow tract and the aorta (Figure 2). Fewer patients with the right coronary artery arising from the left posterior sinus of Valsalva and passing anteriorly between the

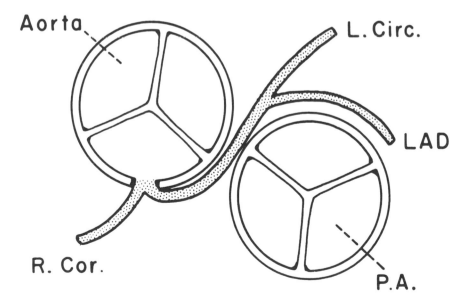

Figure 2. Diagram of the anomalous origin of the left coronary artery from the anterior sinus of Valsalva. R. Cor. = right coronary artery; L. Circ. = left circumflex; LAD = left anterior descending; P.A. = pulmonary artery. From Reference 24, with permission.

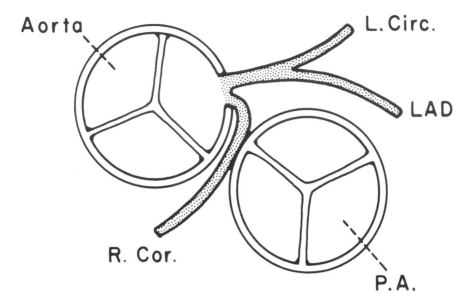

Figure 3. Diagram of the anomalous origin of the right coronary artery from the left sinus of Valsalva. R. Cor. = right coronary artery; L. Circ. = left circumflex; LAD = left anterior descending; P.A. = pulmonary artery. From Reference 24, with permission.

right ventricular outflow tract and the aorta die suddenly during athletic activity (Figure 3). There are occasional deaths reported in athletes with a single coronary artery; it occurs more often when the single coronary artery arises from the anterior sinus of Valsalva than when it arises from the left posterior sinus of Valsalva.[25] Pete Maravich, a professional basketball player who died in 1980 at age 40 while playing a "pick-up" basketball game, is the most famous example of the association of this anomaly with sudden death. Occasional sudden deaths have been reported in patients with a hypoplastic left coronary artery.[25]

The mechanism of sudden death in such circumstances is almost certainly acute ischemia, involving a large portion of the left ventricular myocardium and producing ventricular tachycardia and ventricular fibrillation. The myocardial ischemia results from sudden obstruction occurring at the origin of the anomalous coronary artery. There is little direct evidence for this, except for the finding in some patients of myocardial fibrosis, and even myocardial infarct, in the area supplied by an anomalous coronary artery.[24,25,28] In some patients who died suddenly, severe chest pain was reported days or weeks before death.[29,30] In those patients who were being monitored by electrocardiogram (ECG) at the time of their acute event, the mechanism of sudden death was ventricular fibrillation.[24,29]

There are patients seen with anomalous coronary arteries and obstructive atherosclerosis within the anomalous coronary artery or involving other coronary arteries. These patients are older, usually over age 40. In these patients, symptoms and signs of myocardial ischemia most likely relate to the obstructive disease and not the anomalous origin of the coronary artery.

The mechanism for ischemia with a large arteriovenous or coronary-cameral fistula, where coronary blood flow through the anomalous connection can be very large, is probably a coronary steal, with low perfusion pressure in the artery to the distal dependent myocardium.[31]

The mechanism of the sudden obstruction of the proximal anomalous coronary artery is still unknown. Whatever the mechanism, it must account for the fact that the patient who may have died suddenly during exercise had done the same or more exercise multiple times in the past, without any symptomatology or impairment. There are reports of patients who had maximal stress tests after their first episode of syncope, where the stress tests were totally normal; this suggests that the myocardial ischemia is not necessarily reproducible by stress test or possibly by any noninvasive procedure.[24] The second fact that must be considered is that almost all patients with this anomaly who have had exercise-related sudden death have been young, most younger than 35 years old.[24,25,28] Older patients with the same coronary anomaly do not seem to be at risk of sudden death. It is probable that once the vulnerable period has passed, those patients with the coronary anomaly at risk of sudden death have been triaged out and the older patients remain where the mechanism for sudden coronary obstruction and death does not exist.

The following mechanisms have been proposed for the sudden onset of myocardial ischemia and arrhythmic death[24,25]:

1. Compression of the left main coronary between the right ventricular outflow tract and the aorta (this was first proposed by Jokl et al[26]; it is difficult to see how a normal pulmonary artery pressure, with exercise, can compress a coronary artery with normal or elevated systemic arterial pressure);
2. Kinking of the coronary artery as it arises from the aorta;
3. Sudden compression of the slitlike ostium of the anomalous artery by expansion of the aorta and pulmonary artery[24,32] during exercise (this was first proposed by Cheitlin and colleagues,[24] and remains the favored explanation);
4. Spasm of the left coronary artery in the passage between the pulmonary artery-right ventricular outflow tract and the aorta.

In a recent study, Taylor and colleagues[33] examined hearts of 13 patients with anomalous origin of the right coronary artery from the left posterior sinus of Valsalva, and nine patients with the left coronary artery from the right sinus of Valsalva. There were 13 patients who died suddenly (group I) and nine who died of causes unrelated to the anomalous coronary artery (group II). The ostium and initial course of the anomalous coronary artery were examined and the angle of origin, the geometry and size of the coronary ostium, the position of the ostium in the coronary sinus, and the length of the coronary within the aortic wall were all measured. There were no significant differences in any of these measurements between groups I and II. Age ≥ 30 years was the only variable associated with a decreased risk for sudden death. There is, therefore, no simple anatomic relationship of the ostium or initial course of the anomalous coronary artery that predicts the possibility of sudden death.

It has recently been proposed that spasm of the anomalous left coronary artery could occur if endothelial injury occurred, possibly related to the position of the artery between the right ventricular outflow tract and the aorta.[33] With exercise, the systolic expansion of the aorta and pulmonary artery could injure the coronary endothelium and the increased sympathetic tone and outpouring of catecholamines could precipitate coronary spasm. Such endothelial injury would be sporadic and might account for the unpredictable episodes of sudden coronary obstruction.

Symptoms and Signs in Patients with Anomalous Coronary Arteries

Most patients who have both coronary arteries arising from a single sinus of Valsalva are asymptomatic; this condition usually is found by coronary arteriography that is done when the patient has atypical chest pain or for other unrelated reasons. Presently, some patients are found incidentally by echocardiography[34,35] or NMR[36,37] done for reasons unrelated to the anomalous coronary artery.

In some series, chest discomfort has been reported; and in many, a history of previous syncope has been obtained, usually associated with exercise.[24,28] An evaluation of cases from the literature reports exertional syncope or exertional chest pain in nearly one third of patients.[28] Given the secondary gain from not reporting transient symptoms in a person aspiring to competitive athletics or already engaged in collegiate or professional sports, it is possible, even likely, that such patients will not report their symptoms, even if asked. In many patients who died suddenly with these anomalies, careful questioning of friends and family and review of records have failed to reveal any evidence of previous symptomatology or abnormal physical findings; this is in spite of the rare individual with a coronary-cameral or coronary arteriovenous fistula who might have been expected to have a murmur, usually a continuous murmur.

In patients who are suspected to have a possible coronary anomaly (usually young patients who have angina-like pain on activity) or patients with a history of syncope with or immediately after activity, a stress exercise ECG, with or without radionuclide myocardial perfusion scan, is frequently performed. In two patients who had been resuscitated and were found to have an anomalous coronary artery, Cheitlin et al did maximal stress tests, and both times they were entirely normal.[24] In a third case, a young woman referred to Cheitlin after she had died suddenly after a physical proficiency run, there was a history of chest pain and a negative maximal stress test. Since, as previously mentioned, these patients had performed the same or more exercise many times before the exercise that preceded sudden death, it is probable that coronary obstruction is not always present, but occurs episodically for reasons not yet known. It is possible that stress tests using dobutamine, ECG, or echo might reproduce the occlusion, but this could be dangerous.

It is important, especially in the older patient, to perform a stress test with radionuclide myocardial perfusion imaging. If the myocardial perfusion defect is not in the area subserved by the anomalous coronary artery, it is likely that the observed ischemia is due to lesions in other normally arising vessels and not to obstruction of the anomalous coronary artery.

Identification of Suspected Coronary Anomaly

Anomalous coronary arterial origin should be suspected in young patients who have chest pain or syncope associated with or immediately following activity. As stated, exercise stress tests with or without thallium or sestamibi perfusion scanning may be performed, and if positive, a coronary arteriogram should be done. Unfortunately, a negative exercise study does not rule out a potentially dangerous coronary anomaly, and so further noninvasive imaging should be performed when suspicion is high. Although it is possible to identify the origin of the left and right coronary artery using transthoracic two-dimensional (2-D) Doppler imaging, most often the origin of one or both coronary arteries cannot be identified.[34] With transesophageal echocardiography, it is much more likely that the origin of both vessels will be seen.[37,38] If they are in the appropriate position and the vessel size is normal, consistent with a normal coronary blood flow, a serious coronary anomaly can be ruled out. With manipulation, it is possible to identify the proximal course of the coronary artery, and to identify those vessels passing between the right ventricular outflow tract and the aorta.

Both magnetic resonance imaging (MRI)[37–39] and computed tomography (CT) scanning[40] have been useful in identifying the origin and proximal course of the coronary anomaly, and if the vessels cannot be identified by 2-D Doppler echocardiography, then these are good noninvasive studies that can rule out anomalous origin of one or both coronary arteries and significant coronary AV fistulae.

If an anomalous coronary vessel is seen or if the origin of the coronary arteries cannot be visualized, then coronary arteriography is the only way to identify and fully evaluate these anomalies.

Treatment

In older patients with no symptoms of exertional chest discomfort, presyncope, or syncope, finding the coronary anomaly usually studied for some unrelated reason probably has no significance and needs no therapy, since most patients with anomalous origin of the coronary arteries who die suddenly are younger than 35 years of age. If the patient has coronary atherosclerotic fixed obstruction in other coronary arteries or in the anomalous coronary artery, the patient should be treated in the same manner as other patients with coronary artery disease. Unfortunately, most patients at risk with this coronary anomaly of origin have no premonitory symptoms or signs, and present for the first time with unexpected, shocking sudden death.

In the young patient with evidence of ischemia such as angina or myocardial ischemia by stress or perfusion testing, or a history of presyncope or syncope that is not clearly vagal, if an anomalous coronary artery is found, bypass surgery or enlargement of the ostium by removing the common wall of the coronary artery and aorta and making a funnel-like ostium into the coronary artery should be done.[24,28]

Since this anomaly is so rare, and noninvasive methods to identify it so expensive, it is clear that there is no screening possible for this lesion.

Conclusions

Next to trauma, cardiac disease is the most common cause of sudden death on the athletic field. In most studies, coronary anomalies are a common cardiovascular cause of death, second only to hypertrophic cardiomyopathy. Anomalous origin of both coronaries from the same sinus of Valsalva, especially origin of the left coronary from the anterior sinus of Valsalva, is the most frequent of the coronary anomalies associated with sudden death in athletes. Most often, sudden death occurs with or after exercise and many patients have had a history of exertional syncope or chest pain prior to the fatal episode. In all studies, patients who have experienced sudden death with this anomaly have been younger than 30 to 35 years old. Older patients with the anomaly have, therefore, shown that they are not susceptible to this tragic accident.

It is clear that not all people with such anomalies are at risk of sudden death, since many have lived a full life and die of unrelated problems. It is also clear that even athletes who die suddenly with this anomaly have done similar or more exercise many times before without problems. Apparently, sudden occlusion of the coronary artery, presumably collapse of the ostium, is episodic and, at present, not reliably reproducible by stress tests. There are many theories regarding the mechanism of the sudden occlusion, but none have been proved.

Since both sudden death among athletes and coronary anomalies are rare, it is not possible to screen all athletes for this potential problem. However, any athlete with exertional syncope or presyncope that is not clearly vagal, or exertional chest discomfort, should be studied. Usually an exercise test with or without radioisotope myocardial perfusion is the first approach. If there is ischemia, or even with a negative test if suspicion is high, a 2-D echo Doppler looking for the origin of both coronary arteries can be performed. If the coronary origins are normal, no further evaluation is necessary. If the origins of both coronary arteries cannot be identified, transesophageal echocardiography may be definitive. If suspicion remains high, an MRI or CT scan can frequently demonstrate the origin and initial course of both arteries. If none of these techniques are successful and suspicion is still high, then coronary arteriography is definitive.

If such an anomaly is found in a symptomatic patient younger than age 30, or an asymptomatic patient with demonstrable ischemia in the appropriate myocardial segment, bypass surgery or surgery to enlarge the ostium is indicated. Less clear is what should be done in the asymptomatic young patient where this anomaly is found incidentally. At the present time, most would recommend surgery. When this anomaly is found in a patient older than 30 to 35 years old, if there are symptoms of exertional syncope or if ischemia can be demonstrated in the appropriate myocardial region, then surgery is indicated. However, if the patient has another explanation for the symptoms, such as coronary atherosclerosis, or if no ischemia can be shown in the appropriate myocardial segment, then the symptoms are probably unrelated to the coronary anomaly and no surgery for the coronary anomaly is indicated.

References

1. Maron BJ, Bodison SA, Wesley YE, et al. Results of screening a large group of intercollegiate competitive athletes for cardiovascular disease. *J Am Coll Cardiol* 1987;10:1214–1221.

2. Lewis JF, Maron BJ, Diggs JA, et al. Preparticipation echocardiographic screening for cardiovascular disease in a large, predominantly black population of collegiate athletes. *Am J Cardiol* 1989;64:1029–1033.
3. Epstein SE, Maron BJ. Sudden death and the competitive athlete: Perspectives on preparticipation screening studies. *J Am Coll Cardiol* 1986; 7:220–230.
4. LaCorte MA, Boxer RA, Gottesfeld IB, et al. EKG screening program for school athletes. *Clin Cardiol* 1989;12:42–44.
5. Rich BSE. Sudden death screening. *Med Clin North Am* 1994;78:267–288.
6. Ades PA. Preventing sudden death. Cardiovascular screening of young athletes. *Phys Sportsmed* 1992;20(9):75–76,79–82,85,89.
7. Van Camp SP. Sudden death. *Clin Sports Med* 1992;11:273–289.
8. Fahrenbach MC, Thompson PD. The preparticipation sports examination. Cardiovascular considerations for screening. *Cardiol Clin* 1992;10: 319–328.
9. Phillips M, Robinowitz M, Higgins JR, et al. Sudden cardiac death in Air Force recruits. A 20-year review. *JAMA* 1986;256:2696–2699.
10. Ragosta M, Crabtree J, Sturner WQ, et al. Death during recreational exercise in the state of Rhode Island. *Med Sci Sports Exerc* 1984;16:339–342.
11. Van Camp SP, Bloor CM, Mueller FO, et al. Nontraumatic sports death in high school and college athletes. *Med Sci Sports Exerc* 1995;27:641–647.
12. McCaffrey FM, Braden DS, Strong WB. Sudden cardiac death in young athletes: A review. *Am J Dis Child* 1991;145:177–183.
13. Maron BJ, Roberts WC, McAllister HA, et al. Sudden death in young athletes. *Circulation* 1980;62:218–229.
14. Thomas RJ, Cantwell JD. Sudden death during basketball games. *Phys Sportsmed* 1990;18(5):75–78.
15. Topaz O, Edwards JE. Pathologic features of sudden death in children, adolescents, and young adults. *Chest* 1985;87:476–482.
16. Jensen-Urstad M. Sudden death and physical activity in athletes and nonathletes. *Scand J Med Sci Sports* 1995;5:279–284.
17. Waller BF. Sudden death in middle-aged conditioned subjects: Coronary atherosclerosis is the culprit. *Mayo Clin Proc* 1987;62:634–636.
18. Maron BJ, Epstein SE, Roberts WC. Causes of sudden death in competitive athletes. *J Am Coll Cardiol* 1986;7:204–214.
19. Wight JN Jr, Salem D. Sudden cardiac death and the "athlete's heart." *Arch Intern Med* 1995;155:1473–1480.
20. Burke AP, Farb A, Virmani R, et al. Sports-related and non-sports-related sudden cardiac death in young adults. *Am Heart J* 1991;121:568–575.
21. Burke AP, Farb A, Virmani R. Causes of sudden death in athletes. *Cardiol Clin* 1992;10:303–317.
22. Roberts WC. Major anomalies of coronary arterial origin seen in adulthood. *Am Heart J* 1986;111:941–963.
23. Chu E, Cheitlin MD. Diagnostic considerations in patients with suspected coronary artery anomalies. *Am Heart J* 1993;126:1427–1438.
24. Cheitlin MD, De Castro CM, McAllister HA. Sudden death as a complication of anomalous left coronary origin from the anterior sinus of Valsalva. A not-so-minor congenital anomaly. *Circulation* 1974;50:780–787.
25. Taylor AJ, Rogan KM, Virmani R. Sudden cardiac death associated with isolated congenital coronary artery anomalies. *J Am Coll Cardiol* 1992;20: 640–647.
26. Jokl E, McClellan JT, Williams WC, et al. Congenital anomaly of the left coronary artery in young athletes. *Cardiologia (Basel)* 1966;49:253–258.

27. Roberts WC, Siegel RJ, Zipes DP. Origin of the right coronary artery from the left sinus of Valsalva and its functional consequences: Analysis of 10 necropsy patients. *Am J Cardiol* 1982;49:863–868.

28. Liberthson RR, Dinsmore RE, Fallon JT. Aberrant coronary artery origin from the aorta. Report of 18 patients, review of the literature and delineation of natural history and management. *Circulation* 1979;59:748–754.

29. Leberthson RR, Dinsmore RE, Bharati S, et al. Aberrant coronary artery origin from the aorta. Diagnosis and clinical significance. *Circulation* 1974;50:774–779.

30. Cohen LS, Shaw LD. Fatal myocardial infarction in an 11 year old boy associated with a unique coronary artery anomaly. *Am J Cardiol* 1967;19: 420–423.

31. Wilde P, Watt I. Congenital coronary artery fistulae: Six new cases with a collective review. *Clin Radiol* 1980;31:301–311.

32. Barth CW 3d, Roberts WC. Left main coronary artery originating from the right sinus of Valsalva and coursing between the aorta and pulmonary trunk. *J Am Coll Cardiol* 1986;7:366–373.

33. Taylor AJ, Byers JP, Cheitlin MD, et al. Anomalous right or left coronary artery from the contralateral coronary sinus: "High-risk" abnormalities in the initial coronary artery course and heterogenous clinical outcomes. *Am Heart J* 1997;133:428–435.

34. Daliento L, Fasoli G, Mazzucco A. Anomalous origin of the left coronary artery from the anterior aortic sinus: Role of echocardiography. *Int J Cardiol* 1993;38:89–91.

35. Fernandes F, Alam M, Smith S, et al. The role of transesophageal echocardiography in identifying anomalous coronary arteries. *Circulation* 1993; 88:2532–2540.

36. Post JC, van Rossum AC, Bronzwaer JG, et al. Magnetic resonance angiography of anomalous coronary arteries. A new gold standard for delineating the proximal course? *Circulation* 1995;92:3163–3171.

37. Alam M, Brymer J, Smith S. Transesophageal echocardiographic diagnosis of anomalous left coronary artery from the right aortic sinus. *Chest* 1993;103:1617–1618.

38. Smolin MR, Gorman PD, Gaither NS, et al. Origin of the right coronary artery from the left main coronary artery identified by transesophageal echocardiography. *Am Heart J* 1992;123:1062–1065.

39. Doorey AJ, Wills JS, Blasetto J, et al. Usefulness of magnetic resonance imaging for diagnosing an anomalous coronary artery coursing between aorta and pulmonary trunk. *Am J Cardiol* 1994;74:198–199.

40. Mousseaux E, Hernigou A, Sapoval M, et al. Coronary arteries arising from the contralateral aortic sinus: Electron beam computed tomographic demonstration of the initial course of the artery with respect to the aorta and the right ventricular outflow tract. *J Thorac Cardiovasc Surg* 1996; 112:836–840.

41. Cheitlin MD. Coronary arterial anomalies. In Parmley WW, Chatterjee K (eds): *Cardiology, Volume 2.* Chapter 55;1–14.

22

Sudden Death in the Athlete:

Atherosclerotic Coronary Artery Disease

Paul D. Thompson, MD

Introduction

Atherosclerotic coronary artery disease (CAD) is the predominant cause of exercise-related deaths in adults variously defined as individuals over age 30, 35, or 40 years. Ragosta et al[1] examined the cause of death in 81 individuals who died during recreational exercise in the state of Rhode Island between January 1, 1975 and May 1, 1982. CAD was deemed responsible for 71 (87%) of the deaths in individuals over age 30 years. "Hypertensive cardiovascular disease" (2 cases), a dissecting aortic aneurysm (1 case), and a cerebrovascular accident (1 case) accounted for the remaining deaths. Consequently, all of the deaths in subjects older than age 30 were attributed to atherosclerotic vascular disease and 90% were probably due to coronary atherosclerosis. In contrast, CAD is a rare cause of exercise-related death in younger subjects. Only 3 of 100 cardiovascular deaths occurring within 1 hour of vigorous exercise in high school and college athletes were caused by CAD.[2] Such deaths in young athletes are often associated with marked hypercholesterolemia,[3] suggestive of low-density lipoprotein receptor deficiency or defect.

From Estes NAM, Salem DN, Wang PJ (eds). *Sudden Cardiac Death in the Athlete.* Armonk, NY: Futura Publishing Co., Inc.; ©1998.

The Incidence and Risk of Exercise–Related Coronary Artery Disease Events

The risk of cardiac events during exercise has not been defined for an athletic population, but several studies have examined the risk of sudden death during exercise in the general population. These studies suffer from the low incidence of exercise-related deaths so that small changes in the number of deaths would greatly affect the incidence estimates. Nevertheless, such studies leave little doubt that vigorous exercise can provoke sudden death in individuals with occult CAD.

Thompson et al[4] estimated the risk of sudden death during jogging among men aged 30 through 65 years in Rhode Island from 1975 through 1980. There were only 10 deaths in this age group: all were in men, and all were due to CAD. The absolute incidence of exercise-related deaths was low at only 1 death per year for every 7620 joggers. Nevertheless, the incidence of jogging-related sudden death for the Rhode Island population was sevenfold greater than the death rate during sedentary activities. Half of the victims had known CAD by history or electrocardiogram (ECG) criteria. If these men are eliminated and it is assumed that no other joggers had known CAD, the annual incidence of sudden death can be estimated as 1 per every 15,240 previously healthy joggers.

Similarly, Siscovick et al[5] calculated the risk of exertion-related cardiac arrest during vigorous exercise among previously healthy subjects in Seattle. The absolute incidence of cardiac arrest, based on nine events, was only 1 per 18,000 men, but again the relative rate of sudden death was higher during exercise than during sedentary activities. In men who expended ≤ 112 kcal per week in activities requiring ≥ 6 kcal per minute, the relative risk was increased 56 times over rest, whereas the relative risk was increased only fivefold in men who spent ≥ 144 minutes per week in such activities. This study demonstrates that regular exercise reduces the chance of sudden death during exercise, but that exercise transiently increases the risk of cardiac arrest even among habitually active individuals.

These results were obtained in the general population and not in a defined population of middle-aged athletes. Maron et al[6] calculated the frequency of cardiac arrest among 215,413 participants in the Marine Corps and Twin Cities Marathons from 1976 to 1994. There were four deaths, or 1 death per 50,000 participants, over this time span. If a marathon time of 4 hours was used, the death rate was 1 per every 215,000 hours of competition. This number greatly exceeds the incidence of cardiac arrest of 1 death per every 4.8×10^6 hours among the most active group in Seattle and is consistent with the concept that prolonged competitive tasks increase the exercise risk.[5] Again, however, these calculations are based on too few events to support firm conclusions.

In the Rhode Island and the Seattle studies,[4,5] the increased risk of exercise-related sudden death compared to other activities was greatest among the youngest adults. In Rhode Island the relative risk of jogging versus more sedentary activities was 99, 13, and 5 times greater than at rest in men aged 30 to 39, 40 to 49, and 50 to 59 years, respectively. The number of deaths per hour of jogging varied from 1 per 482,600 hours to 1 per 309,400 hours for the youngest and oldest groups, suggesting approximately equivalent hourly event rates. In Seattle, 6 of the 9 cases of cardiac arrest occurred in men younger than age 45. The younger men spent more time exercising, however, so that the cardiac arrest incidence figures were actually similar in the older and younger men.[5,7] Consequently, it appears that in young men, the higher relative risk of death during vigorous exercise is due in part to the much lower risk of sudden death in this age group during sedentary activities. This interesting observation supports the concept that vigorous exercise does indeed transiently increase the risk of sudden death from CAD, especially among young subjects.

Sudden cardiac death (SCD) is not the only CAD exercise-related complication. Exercise also increases the risk of acute myocardial infarction (MI).[8,9] Mittleman et al[8] examined the relative risk of suffering a MI during or within 1 hour of exercise requiring 6 metabolic equivalents (METS) (an estimated 21 mL of O_2/kg/min for a 70 kg person). The study population was derived from 22 community and 23 tertiary care hospitals in the United States. Of 1228 MI patients qualifying for inclusion, only 54 (4.4%) patients experienced initial symptoms of their MI during or within 1 hour of exercise. Three comparisons were performed: within the MI patients between their habitual level of activity and their activity within an hour of their MI; within the patients between the day of their MI and the same time period a day earlier; and between patients and community controls. In each of these three comparisons, the relative risk of an MI during or soon after exercise was at least 5.6-fold greater than the risk during less vigorous activity. Common activities associated with MI included lifting or pushing (18%), isotonic activities such as jogging (30%), and yard work such as gardening and chopping wood (52%). In patients who were usually sedentary, the relative risk was 107-fold higher during exercise than at rest, whereas in those who habitually exercised at least five times weekly, the relative risk was only 2.7-fold higher. Diabetics had a relative risk of an exercise-related MI that was 18.9 times higher than their risk while at rest.

Willich et al[9] compared the frequency of MIs during or within 1 hour of exercise requiring 6 or more METS with the frequency of MIs during less vigorous activity in Berlin and Augsburg, Germany. Two comparisons were performed: a within-patient comparison, using the patient's usual frequency of exertion to calculate the expected chance of an MI occurring with exertion compared to the actual frequency, and a comparison between patients and a telephone control group. The control group was asked to describe their activity at the time those MI victims suffered their event. Over a 2-year period there were 1194 patients who agreed to participate. Of these, 69 patients (5.8%) had an exercise-associated MI. The patient group was not restricted to patients with first MI and consequently had more prior MIs, more cardiac risk factors, and used more cardiac medications than the telephone controls. Nevertheless, after adjusting for these differences, the relative risk of an MI during exercise was 2.1 higher than at rest. The same increase in relative risk was also found for the within-subject comparison.

These studies support the conclusion that exercise also transiently increases the risk of acute MI. Both studies suffered in that there were relatively few exercise-related events. In addition, these studies are not readily applicable to either athletes or the healthy population because both studies included patients with known heart disease.

The present author know of no studies that provide an absolute incidence of MI during vigorous exercise in previously healthy individuals. The incidence of exercise-related MI can be estimated from other data.[10] Among previously healthy hypercholesterolemic men in the Lipid Clinics Primary Prevention Trial, there were seven times as many MIs during exercise as there were SCDs.[11] If we assume an absolute risk of sudden death during exercise as 1 death per 15,000[4] to 1 death per 18,000[5] healthy men, and if the risk of MI is assumed to be seven times more frequent, there is an absolute annual incidence of 1 MI during exertion for every 2142 to 2571 exercising men. This estimated risk is not trivial, but has not been validated in population-based studies. The annual rate of exercise MIs could range from 1 per 571 to 1 per 3714 men per year if 95% confidence limits for sudden death during exercise from the Rhode Island study (l death per 4000 to 26,000 men per year)[4] are used to calculate the incidence. It must be emphasized, however, that these MI incidence figures are estimated from sudden deaths in the general population and are unlikely to be representative of the risk in athletes. It is suspected that the MI risk is reduced in athletes, since frequent physical exertion appears to protect against exercise-related events.[5,8]

The Pathology of Exercise–Related Coronary Artery Disease Events

The coronary artery pathologic findings among previously asymptomatic subjects who die during exertion are consistent with those for atherosclerotic plaque rupture and acute coronary artery occlusion.[12,13]

In 1975, Black et al[12] reported clinical, autopsy, or angiographic evidence of acute plaque rupture in 13 patients who developed coronary syndromes during vigorous exertion. More recently, Ciampricotti et al[14] performed acute coronary angiography on 13 athletes who sustained a CAD event within 1 hour of sports participation. Seven had suffered an exercise-related MI and six had survived an exercise-related cardiac arrest. All were considered physically well trained and all spent an average of ≥5 hours per week in exercise activities. Coronary angiography demonstrated coronary thrombosis in all sudden death survivors and in three of those with acute MI. After reperfusion, an eccentric atherosclerotic plaque consistent with prior plaque rupture was demonstrated in eight cases. These pathologic and clinical findings are identical to those reported for SCD and acute MI not related to exertion in previously asymptomatic adults in the general population.[15]

In contrast, patients with known coronary heart disease who die during exertion often do not demonstrate evidence of an acute coronary lesion or myocardial injury,[16] suggesting that ventricular fibrillation from myocardial scarring is the proximate cause of death.

The Mechanism for Exercise-Related Acute Cardiac Events

Several hypotheses have been advanced to explain how physical exertion could provoke plaque rupture and coronary thrombosis.[17] No less an expert than Master,[18] originator of the Master step test, suggested that exercise does not provoke cardiac events, but that the increased myocardial oxygen demand associated with exercise amplifies symptoms of a preexisting infarct. Alternatively, exercise might have a more direct role in injuring coronary arteries.

In what now reads as a very clairvoyant discussion, Black et al[12] suggested that the increased "twisting and bending" of coronary arteries during vigorous exertion increases the frequency of plaque rupture and that "Black's Crack in the Plaque" is responsible for most exertion-related acute coronary events. They emphasized that the coronary arteries are subjected to five "stress motions," including a ballooning action from the pulsation of blood, an accordion motion associated with lengthening and contracting during the cardiac cycle, a twisting motion, acute bending during contraction, and flow currents. All of these motions are exacerbated by the increase in heart rate and contractility produced by exercise as well as by exaggerated changes in cardiac systolic and diastolic dimensions. Furthermore, exercise dilates normal coronary arteries but can induce coronary artery spasm in diseased artery segments.[19] Such spasm on a noncompliant atherosclerotic plaque can induce plaque rupture.

Alternatively, exercise can increase thrombosis by augmenting catecholamine-induced platelet aggregation or by deepening existing coronary fissures. Such exercise-induced platelet aggregation has been documented and appears to be greater in sedentary subjects.[20] Physical exertion also increases systolic blood pressure, thereby increasing shear forces in the coronaries and possibly increasing coronary fissuring. Plaque rupture without coronary thrombosis is common. Coronary plaque fissures without thrombosis were found in 17% of people who died of noncoronary atherosclerosis and in 9% of subjects who died in motor vehicle accidents and suicides.[21] Consequently, it may be that vigorous exercise induces coronary thrombosis on mildly fissured coronary plaques that would have otherwise remained asymptomatic.

The latter hypothesis implies that such affected individuals would have escaped their acute coronary event if they had not exercised. This issue is difficult to address directly, but a study from the 1978 Rhode Island blizzard suggests that victims of exertion-related cardiac events would have suffered a similar fate in the near future.[22] In February of 1978 a blizzard dumped 50 inches of snow on the state in 24 hours. The CAD death rate increased from the usual February average of 27 deaths per day to 48 deaths per day on the day of the storm and for 3 of the next 5 days. The death rate subsequently decreased for the remainder of the month so that the average daily death rate for February 1978 appears unchanged from the prior five Februarys. Such results suggest that the physical and emotional burden of the storm affected people who would have succumbed to CAD in the near future.

Preventing Exercise–Related Coronary Artery Disease Events in Athletes

Efforts to prevent exercise-related CAD events in athletes require identification of potential victims before an event. Unfortunately, the profile of athletes who develop CAD events may be different from the profile of individuals in the general population who experience an exercise-related SCD or MI. For example, Thompson et al[13] reported 18 individuals who died during or immediately after exercise, 13 of whom died of CAD. Six of these 13 experienced prodromal symptoms of CAD. Similarly, Noakes[23] summarized 36 cases of SCD or MI in marathon runners and found prodromal symptoms in 71% of the 28 cases where information was available. In contrast, Ciampricotti et al[24] compared the clinical characteristics of 36 well-conditioned athletes who suffered SCD, MI, or unstable angina within 1 hour of exertion with those of 36 other men. Prodromal symptoms were experienced by 47% of the sedentary men but by only 8% of the athletes. Risk factors for heart disease, including hypertension (19% versus 33%), hypercholesterolemia (14% versus 56%), and cigarette smoking (58% versus 94%), were less frequent in the athletes. Ages for the two groups were similar, but the athletes had less multiple vessel disease, fewer coronary stenoses, and less severe stenoses in the culprit and nonculprit vessels. The authors interpret these data as an indication that exercise prevents severe CAD; but an alternative interpretation is that vigorous exercise provokes CAD events in individuals with less severe disease and before their disease would otherwise become manifest. This issue is unresolved but it does appear that athletes who suffer exercise-related CAD events have fewer risk factors than individuals in the general population with CAD, and it is unlikely that potential victims of exercise-related CAD can be identified by risk factors alone.

It is also not clear that exercise testing can reliably identify athletes who are at risk for CAD events. The American College of Sports Medicine recommends that high-risk individuals undergo exercise stress testing prior to vigorous exercise.[25] The "high risk" classification includes men older than 40 and women older than 50 years of age, individuals with more than one coronary disease risk factor, and those with known coronary disease. The American Heart Association, however, considers exercise testing prior to exercise programs "controversial."[26]

Exercise testing in asymptomatic adults is a poor predictor of the major cardiac complications during exercise, acute MI, and SCD. A true positive exercise test requires a hemodynamically significant coronary obstruction, whereas acute coronary events often involve plaque rupture and thrombosis at the site of previously nonobstructive atherosclerotic plaque.[27]

Studies that evaluate the utility of exercise testing in ostensibly healthy populations support this hypothesis. McHenry et al[28] reported a study of 916 Indiana state troopers who underwent maximal exercise tests, had repeat testing at intervals of 1 to 5 years, and were followed for a mean of 12.7 years. Only 61 men (6.6%) ever demonstrated a positive ECG response to exercise. Of these, 21 (32%) developed clinical signs of coronary disease including angina pectoris in 18, an acute MI in 1, and sudden death in 1. An additional asymptomatic man underwent coronary bypass surgery. Among the 833 men with normal ECG responses, only 44 (5%) subsequently developed clinical coronary disease: 25 developed an infarct, 7 died suddenly, and 12 developed angina. These data suggest that a positive exercise test identifies individuals with hemodynamically significant coronary lesions, but that these lesions are often tolerated until the appearance of angina.

Screening only individuals at high risk produces similar results. Exercise testing was used to screen for heart disease in 3617 men participating in the Lipid Research Clinics Primary Prevention Trial.[11]

All men had prerandomization low-density lipoprotein cholesterol values >4.91 (190) mMol/L (mg/dL). Exercise tests to 90% of age-predicted maximal heart rate were performed at baseline and annually thereafter. Sixty-two men developed an exercise-related event: 54 acute MIs and 8 sudden deaths. Only 11 of the 62 events occurred in men with a positive exercise test. The predictive value of a positive exercise test for an acute exercise event was only 4%, in part because such events are rare. The authors concluded that routine exercise testing is not effective in preventing acute cardiac events even in high-risk populations.

Recommendations

The present author maintain that prevention of exercise-related CAD events in athletes will be extremely difficult because of the rarity of such events and the poor predictive value of exercise testing for the major CAD events provoked by exercise. They do recommend that middle-aged athletes follow the standard approach to CAD prevention. Smoking cessation may be especially important in athletes because several European authors have noted a high rate of cigarette use among athletes who suffer exercise-related CAD events.[29] Athletes should also understand that cocaine use might accelerate the development of atherosclerotic CAD[30] as well as provoke coronary spasm.

Physicians should inform exercising adults of the nature of prodromal cardiac symptoms, especially the fact that cardiac discomfort is often not perceived as "pain" but as discomfort, tightness, or heartburn. New symptoms of exercise intolerance, such as exercise syncope, unusual dyspnea, and chest discomfort, should be carefully evaluated in athletes of all ages since at least some victims of exercise-related events had complained of such symptoms which they or their physicians ignored.[13] The present author also suggest that individuals who officiate at events involving middle-aged athletes learn and update yearly their cardiopulmonary resuscitation skills. Such individuals may be present when athletes suffer an exercise-related CAD event and may be able to prevent some of these exercise-related tragedies. Finally, athletes with known CAD should be encouraged to follow the recommendations of 26th Bethesda Conference on Recommendations for Determining Eligibility for Competition in Athletes with Cardiovascular Abnormalities. These guidelines restrict patients with known CAD from competing in sports that place a moderate or high aerobic demand on the cardiovascular system as defined by that conference.[31] Such patients are, however, encouraged to participate in an exercise training program for its cardiovascular benefits.

References

1. Ragosta M, Crabtree J, Sturner WQ, et al. Death during recreational exercise in the state of Rhode Island. *Med Sci Sports Exerc* 1984;16:339–342.
2. Van Camp SP, Bloor CM, Mueller FO, et al. Nontraumatic sports death in high school and college athletes. *Med Sci Sports Exerc* 1995;27:641–647.
3. Maron BJ, Roberts WC, McAllister HA, et al. Sudden death in young athletes. *Circulation* 1980;62:218–229.
4. Thompson PD, Funk EJ, Carleton RA, et al. Incidence of death during jogging in Rhode Island from 1975 through 1980. *JAMA* 1982;247: 2535–2538.
5. Siscovick DS, Weiss NS, Fletcher RH, et al. The incidence of primary cardiac arrest during vigorous exercise. *N Engl J Med* 1984;311:874–877.
6. Maron BJ, Poliac LC, Roberts WO. Risk for sudden cardiac death associated with marathon running. *J Am Coll Cardiol* 1996;28:428–431.
7. Siscovick DS. Risks of exercising: Sudden cardiac death and injuries. In Bouchard C, Shephard RJ, Stephens T, et al. (eds): *Exercise, Fitness, and Health: A Consensus of Current Knowledge*. Champaign: Human Kinetics Books; 1990:707–713.
8. Mittleman MA, Maclure M, Tofler GH, et al. Triggering of acute myocardial infarction by heavy exertion: Protection against triggering by regular exercise. *N Engl J Med* 1993;329:1677–1683.
9. Willich SN, Lewis M, Lowell H, et al. Physical exertion as a trigger of acute myocardial infarction. *N Engl J Med* 1993;329:1684–1690.
10. Thompson PD, Fahrenbach MC. Risks of exercising: Cardiovascular including sudden cardiac death. In Bouchard C, Shephard RJ, Stephens T, et al. (eds): *Exercise, Fitness, and Health: A Consensus of Current Knowledge*. Champaign: Human Kinetics Books; 1990:707–713.
11. Siscovick DS, Ekelund LG, Johnson JL, et al. Sensitivity of exercise electrocardiography for acute cardiac events during moderate and strenuous physical activity: The lipid research clinics coronary primary prevention trial. *Arch Intern Med* 1991;151:325–330.
12. Black A, Black MM, Gensini G. Exertion and acute coronary artery injury. *Angiology* 1975;26:759–783.
13. Thompson PD, Stern MP, Williams P, et al. Death during jogging or running: A study of 18 cases. *JAMA* 1979;242:1265–1267.
14. Ciampricotti R, Gamal MIH, Bonnier JJ, et al. Myocardial infarction and sudden death after sport: Acute coronary angiographic findings. *Cathet Cardiovasc Diagn* 1989;17:193–197.
15. Davies MJ, Thomas AC. Plaque fissuring—the cause of acute myocardial infarction, sudden ischaemic death, and crescendo angina. *Br Heart J* 1985;53:363–373.
16. Cobb LA, Weaver WD. Exercise: A risk for sudden death in patients with coronary heart disease. *J Am Coll Cardiol* 1986;7(1):215–219.
17. Thompson PD. The relative risk of myocardial infarction during exercise. In Fletcher GF (ed): *Cardiovascular Response to Exercise*. Mount Kisco: Futura Publishing Company; 1994:291–300.
18. Master A. Activities associated with the onset of acute coronary artery occlusion. *Am Heart J* 1939;18:434–443.
19. Gordon JB, Ganz J, Nabel EG, et al. Atherosclerosis influences the vasomotor response of epicardial coronary arteries to exercise. *J Clin Invest* 1989;83:1946–1952.

20. Kestin AS, Ellis PA, Barnard MR, et al. Effect of strenuous exercise on platelet activation state and reactivity. *Circulation* 1993;88:1502–1511.
21. Davies MJ, Bland JM, Hangartner JRW, et al. Factors influencing the presence or absence of acute coronary artery thrombi in sudden ischaemic death. *Eur Heart J* 1989;10:203–208.
22. Faich G, Rose R. Blizzard morbidity and mortality: Rhode Island, 1978. *Am J Public Health* 1979;69(10):1050–1052.
23. Noakes TD. Heart disease in marathon runners: A review. *Med Sci Sports Exerc* 1987;19:187–194.
24. Ciampricotti R, Deckers JW, Taverne R, et al. Characteristics of conditioned and sedentary men with acute coronary syndromes. *Am J Cardiol* 1994;73:219–222.
25. Mahler DA, Froelicher VF, Miller NH, York TD. Health screening in risk stratification. In *ACSM's Guidelines for Exercise Testing and Prescription, 5th Edition.* Baltimore, MD: Williams and Wilkins; 1995:25. (Kenney WL, Humphrey RH, Bryant CX, eds.)
26. Schlant RC, Blomqvist CG, Brandenburg RO, et al. Guidelines for exercise testing: A report of the Joint American College of Cardiology/American Heart Association Task Force on Assessment of Cardiovascular Procedures (subcommittee on exercise testing). *Circulation* 1986;74:653A–667A.
27. Little WC, Constantinescu M, Applegate RJ, et al. Can coronary angiography predict the site of a subsequent myocardial infarction in patients with mild-to-moderate coronary artery disease? *Circulation* 1988;78:1157–1166.
28. McHenry PL, O'Donnell J, Morris SN, et al. The abnormal exercise electrocardiogram in apparently healthy men: A predictor of angina pectoris as an initial coronary event during long-term follow-up. *Circulation* 1984;70:547–551.
29. Pic A, Broustet JP, Saliou B, et al. Coexistence of vigorous exercise and heavy smoking in triggering acute myocardial infarction in men under 35 years—fact or fiction? In Roskamm H (ed): *Myocardial Infarction at Young Age.* Berlin, New York: Springer-Verlag; 1981:108–114.
30. Kolodgie FD, Virmani R, Cornhill JF, et al. Increase in atherosclerosis and adventitial mast cells in cocaine abusers: An alternative mechanism of cocaine-associated coronary vasospasm and thrombosis. *J Am Coll Cardiol* 1991;17:1553–1160.
31. Maron BJ, Mitchell JH. 26th Bethesda Conference: Recommendations for determining eligibility for competition in athletes with cardiovascular abnormalities. *J Am Coll Cardiol* 1994;24:845–899.

23

Sudden Cardiac Death in Athletes:

Valvular Heart Disease

Carey D. Kimmelstiel, MD, Gregory D. Russell, MD, and Deeb N. Salem, MD

Competitive athletes represent what is typically thought to be the healthiest, most conditioned segment of our society. Despite this perception, sudden death in competitive athletes has gained public interest in large part due to recent deaths of high-profile athletes.

Cited statistics estimate that 5 of 100,000 young athletes have a condition that predisposes them to sudden death; the annual incidence of sudden cardiac death is 0.0005% per year.[1] Some activities, such as jogging, are associated with higher rates of sudden death among previously asymptomatic individuals.[2,3]

This chapter specifically reviews valvular heart disease as a cause of sudden death in athletes. It highlights the two valvular lesions reported to cause death in this population, examines available data from published series, and describes putative pathophysiologic mechanisms. Aortic stenosis (AS) and mitral valve prolapse (MVP) are the two lesions that account for most valvular precipitants of sudden cardiac death in athletes. This chapter summarizes exercise limitations in patients with these and other types of valvular heart disease.

From Estes NAM, Salem DN, Wang PJ (eds). *Sudden Cardiac Death in the Athlete.* Armonk, NY: Futura Publishing Co., Inc.; ©1998.

Causes of exercise-related sudden cardiac death are age-dependent. Younger athletes are more likely to succumb due to hypertrophic cardiomyopathy or coronary anomalies, while older athletic participants often harbor atherosclerotic coronary artery disease.[3-9] Valvular heart disease has been reported as a cause of sudden cardiac death in the general populace. In multiple series of younger populations who die suddenly, valvular heart disease is cited as the etiology in 0% to 28% of patients reported.[10,11] In younger patients with known heart disease, early series reported valvular disease as the inciting cause of death in up to 17%.[11] When athletic participants die suddenly, a structural abnormality is most often found.[1,6] However, valvular disease represents the etiology of a far smaller percentage of sudden deaths compared with the general populace. In published series and reviews of sudden death in athletes, valvular disease is cited as the etiologic factor on average, approximately 4% of the time, with a frequency of 0% to 10%.[1,2,6,12-20]

Mitral Valve Prolapse

MVP is a common and usually benign condition when it is not associated with Marfan syndrome or other connective tissue disorders. However, in a review of 74 sudden deaths associated with strenuous exertion or sports in individuals ranging from 11 to 35 years of age, 5% were attributed to MVP.[11]

MVP has been reported to occur in 4% to 7% of the general population.[21] The diagnosis of MVP is made by cardiac auscultation and/or echocardiographic examination. Common symptoms include dyspnea, lightheadedness, chest pain, palpitations, and syncope, although many patients are asymptomatic. Electrocardiographic abnormalities include ST segment and T wave changes that may appear at rest or during electrocardiogram (ECG) stress testing. The physical examination is associated with a midsystolic click with or without a systolic murmur. Dissolution of collagen or dysgenesis of the chordae and pars fibrosa appear to be the primary pathologic disorders that lead to valvular prolapse or billowing.[21]

Sudden death is estimated to occur in 0.02% of MVP patients without significant mitral regurgitation, and perhaps in as many as 1% of those patients with severe mitral regurgitation.[22] The mechanism for MVP-associated sudden death is postulated to be ventricular arrhythmia[22] or bradycardia (Table 1). In reviewing the literature, Khandheria and Segal[23] noted ventricular arrhythmias, sinus bradycardia, and sinus arrest in the absence of ventricular escape as possible causes but concluded that there were not enough data available to recognize a

Table 1
Possible Mechanisms for SCD in MVP

Ventricular arrhythmias
Sinus bradycardia and sinus arrest without escape rhythm
Long QT interval
Significant mitral regurgitation

SCD = sudden cardiac death; MVP = mitral valve prolapse.

high-risk group. Marks et al[24] studied 459 patients with MVP and concluded that patients with mitral valve leaflet thickening and redundancy had a significantly higher risk of infective endocarditis, moderate to severe mitral regurgitation, and the need for valve replacement
than those that did not have these echocardiographic abnormalities.
These findings, however, did not help to identify patients at risk of sudden death.[24] There does seem to be some evidence that patients with
MVP and significant mitral regurgitation may be at higher risk of complex ventricular arrhythmias and sudden death.[25]

Although QT interval prolongation has been related to arrhythmias and sudden death in MVP, this association has not always been
consistent and has been challenged by some investigators.[26,27] In a review of 589 cases of arrhythmias associated with MVP, Swartz et al[28]
noted ventricular tachycardia in 6.3% of patients, paroxysmal
supraventricular tachycardia in 6.1% of patients, and sudden death in
1.4% of patients. However, sudden death is likely to be due to ventricular arrhythmias in the setting of left ventricular dysfunction resulting from mitral regurgitation.

Wooley[21] has suggested that the MVP syndrome is due to an inherited disorder of centrally mediated autonomic and adrenergic function. He cites data that document increased frequency of ventricular
extrasystoles which parallel rises in urinary excretion of epinephrine
and norepinephrine.[29] In a recent study, Babuty et al[30] found a high
prevalence of ventricular arrhythmias and late potentials in 58 consecutive MVP patients evaluated by noninvasive studies. The prognostic implication of these findings is uncertain, as clinical follow-up of
this population was not reported. Increased patient age and mitral regurgitation seem to be the factors that predisposed to complex ventricular arrhythmias. Electrophysiologic testing did not appear to identify the MVP group with a higher risk of ventricular arrhythmias.[30]
While several studies relate the incidence of dysrhythmias to the occurrence of sudden death, a number of studies dispute this relationship.[4] Additionally, some investigators have noted low sensitivity,
specificity, and predictive value for sudden death in MVP patients in

whom complex ventricular ectopy has been recorded during ambulatory electrocardiographic monitoring.[26] This poses obvious problems in prediction of risk for athletes discovered to have MVP and ventricular ectopy.

Although MVP is cited with a definable frequency as a cause of sudden death in athletes, there is in fact little evidence that malignant arrhythmias or sudden death are exercise related in MVP.[7,9] The majority of sudden deaths attributed to MVP do not occur with exercise, and death in the setting of MVP almost never occurs in trained athletes.[6,9,31] In addition, complex ventricular arrhythmias, when detected in the clinical setting of MVP, are associated with low sensitivity, low specificity, and poor predictive value for subsequent sudden death.[25]

Further difficulties in ascribing a precise link between sudden death and MVP in athletes (Table 2) relate to the fact that when studied at necropsy, subjects whose death has been attributed to MVP have been found to harbor other cardiac disorders that might have directly or indirectly caused demise. Such associated anomalies include marked increases in left ventricular mass,[5,20] right ventricular dilation and hypertrophy,[3,32] conduction system disease including the presence of accessory pathways,[3,14,32] coronary artery hypoplasia,[5] and right and left ventricular myocardial abnormalities.[14] In addition, selected cases of sudden death ascribed to MVP in younger patients may have been caused by inherited defects unrelated to MVP.[4] Finally, the fraction of sudden deaths in athletes attributed to MVP is similar to the prevalence of MVP in the general population, raising the possibility that the presence of MVP in the hearts of dying athletes represents an epiphenomenon.

Athletes with asymptomatic MVP, no evidence of coexisting connective tissue disorder (eg, Marfan syndrome), and no evidence of mitral regurgitation should be reassured that their condition is generally benign and should have no limits placed on their activities. Athletes with MVP and a history of syncope should be evaluated by Holter mon-

Table 2
Problems Linking MVP to SCD in Athletes

- Poor sensitivity, specificity, and predictive value of arrhythmias for SCD

- Little evidence that malignant arrhythmias or sudden death are exercise related

- MVP hearts frequently harbor significant other pathology

- Similar incidence of MVP in SCD and general populations

MVP = mitral valve prolapse; SCD = sudden cardiac death.

itoring and stress testing. Athletes with MVP and arrhythmogenic syncope, disabling chest pain, significant mitral regurgitation and cardiomegaly, Marfan syndrome, a family history of sudden death from MVP, or repetitive forms of sustained ventricular arrhythmias (particularly if symptomatic) should be disqualified from performing strenuous physical activities.[31]

Aortic Stenosis

Syncope and sudden death have been associated with AS for nearly 300 years.[33] Syncope is a frequent symptom of AS, reported to occur in 15% to 30% of symptomatic patients regardless of its etiology.[33] Exertional syncope has been recognized as a risk inherent to AS since initial case reports were noted in the early part of the 20th century.[33] Sudden death has long been known to be related to syncopal attacks,[34] and in older literature is documented as the presenting symptom in up to 5% of cases.[33] Its current frequency in the surgical era is difficult if not impossible to define.

Several mechanisms have been postulated to account for exertional syncope in AS (Table 3). Carotid sinus hypersensitivity or cerebral ischemia have previously been suggested as important mechanisms. Confirmatory data for both of these postulated mechanisms are generally lacking.[34] Arrhythmias have previously been thought to account for syncope in AS, and indeed they have been documented to occur in this disorder. Some authors have reported ventricular arrhythmias in AS that improve after aortic valve replacement,[35] while others have found no relationship between severity of valvular disease and the grade of ventricular ectopic activity.[36] Most importantly, Schwartz et al[37] reported the results of 72 hours of continuous monitoring in nine patients with AS, during which time they observed 14 syncopal episodes.[37] The initial manifestation in these patients was hypotension. Ventricular tachyarrhythmias, when present, occurred at least 20 seconds after the onset of syncope, suggesting a secondary role for arrhythmias instead of a causative one.[37]

Table 3
Postulated Mechanisms of Syncope in AS

Carotid sinus hypersensitivity
Cerebral ischemia
Arrhythmias
Sudden LV dysfunction
Malfunction LV baroreceptors

AS = aortic stenosis; LV = left ventricular.

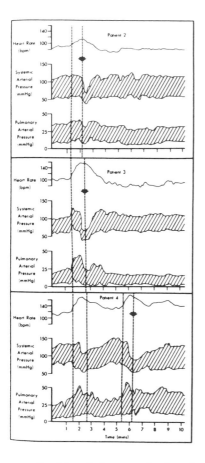

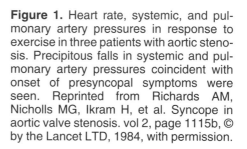

Figure 1. Heart rate, systemic, and pulmonary artery pressures in response to exercise in three patients with aortic stenosis. Precipitous falls in systemic and pulmonary artery pressures coincident with onset of presyncopal symptoms were seen. Reprinted from Richards AM, Nicholls MG, Ikram H, et al. Syncope in aortic valve stenosis. vol 2, page 1115b, © by the Lancet LTD, 1984, with permission.

Sudden left ventricular dysfunction has been cited as a cause of syncope in AS[38]; however, there are no confirmatory data. Furthermore, left ventricular dysfunction seems unlikely since syncope in this disorder occurs most commonly in the setting or normal left ventricular systolic function.[39]

The preponderance of evidence suggests that the mechanism of exertional syncope (which may eventuate in sudden death) in AS involves malfunction of left ventricular baroreceptors. This phenomenon, initially hypothesized in 1971[34] postulates that exercise induces an abrupt rise in left ventricular pressure that is unaccompanied by a similar increase in aortic pressure, leading to excessive activation of left ventricular baroreceptors. Vagal afferents transmit inhibitory impulses to the brain stem, leading to vagally mediated arterial and venous vasodilation, consequent hypotension, and reduced cardiac output.[40]

Experimental and clinical data support this mechanism as being responsible for exercise-induced syncope in AS. Ventricular stretch receptors were histologically identified in 1939.[33] Aviado and colleagues[41] documented that experimentally induced rises in left ventricular pressure caused reflex vasodilation in vascularly isolated lower extremities. Mark et al[42] documented upper-extremity vasodilation during leg exercise in AS patients, while control subjects vasoconstricted during leg exercise; AS patients were seen to vasoconstrict normally following aortic valve replacement.

Richards and coauthors[43] noted presyncope associated with systemic and pulmonary arterial hypotension in response to exercise in AS patients. Hypotension and presyncope were seen in response to abrupt symptom-limited exercise; submaximal exercise led to blunted rise in blood pressure (Figure 1), lending further support to the concept of baroreceptor involvement.[43] Finally, Lombard and Selzer,[39] reporting on a large series of AS patients, have noted higher left ventricular systolic pressures in those with syncope compared to those without.

Exercise Recommendations and Limitations for Patients with Acquired or Congenital Valvular Heart Disease

In order to make recommendations as specific as possible, it is necessary to attempt to classify exercise or sports according to type and intensity, as well as risk, with respect to physical impact and consequences of syncope. Exercise and sports can be broadly divided into two categories, static and dynamic.[44,45] These represent the two extremes of a continuum between exercise in which muscles apply force with little motion, static or isometric, and exercise in which muscles apply force with a large degree of resultant motion, dynamic or isotonic. An example of the former is weight lifting, of the latter, long-distance running.

The main difference between these types of exercise is that as the degree of motion increases, more work is done. During dynamic exercise there is a larger increase in heart rate, stroke volume, cardiac output, and oxygen consumption when compared to static exercise. There is also a reduction in systemic vascular resistance and in diastolic blood pressure seen in dynamic exercise but not in static exercise. In general, the effect of dynamic exercise on the vascular system is more of a volume load, verses a pressure load in static exercise. As a result, increased ventricular mass is seen in athletes participating in both static and dynamic exercise. Dynamic exercise tends to also increase chamber size, whereas static does not.[46]

A classification scheme for sports and exercise has been described[44] and uses a division of three increasing levels of intensity for both static and dynamic effort: I, II, III, and A, B, C, respectively. The spectrum ranges from sports with both low static and low dynamic components (IA) (eg, golf) to high static and high dynamic effort such as cycling (IIIC). Additional notation is made for those sports that carry a higher potential risk of collision or risk resulting from syncope. This scheme is used to outline general guidelines for allowable exercise for patients with valvular disorders. One must also be cognizant of the potential cardiovascular effects of emotional stress and increased sympathetic tone often seen at any level of exercise.

What follows is a synopsis of descriptions of gradations of severity of various valvular lesions, followed by general recommendations of exercise prescription for patients with specific valvular anomalies. The interested reader is referred to more comprehensive reviews of this topic.[47]

Congenital Valvular Heart Disease

Although there are a wide variety of congenital heart defects which require special attention when considering exercise recommendations, only those associated with valvular disease are considered here.[48] These include congenital AS, pulmonic stenosis, and Ebstein's anomaly.

Aortic Valve Stenosis

AS that appears in childhood is often quantified by physical examination, ECG, Doppler echocardiography, and cardiac catheterization. The peak instantaneous transvalvular gradient is used to characterize severity: ≤20 mm Hg, mild; 21 to 49 mm Hg, moderate; and ≥50 mm Hg, severe. Since this disease carries a small but measurable risk of sudden death, a thorough evaluation is indicated for those with a history of fatigue, dizziness, chest pain, or syncope. Severe AS carries a higher risk of sudden death; 20% to 40% of such events occur during exercise.[10,49,50]

Patients with mild AS can participate at all levels of intensity provided they have normal exercise tolerance and ECG and no history of exertional chest pain, syncope, or symptomatic arrhythmia. Those with moderate AS can participate in exercise with low static and low to moderate dynamic intensity, or moderate static and low dynamic intensity (classes IA, IB, and IIA), as long as there is mild or no left ventricular hypertrophy (LVH) by echocardiography or LVH strain by ECG, normal exercise tolerance test, and none of the above-described symptoms. Individuals with severe AS should not participate in competitive sports or exercise.[48] AS treated by surgical or interventional techniques should be guided by the resultant degree of stenosis, the need for anticoagulation, as well as any potential aortic valve regurgitation as discussed below.

Pulmonic Valve Stenosis

This lesion is usually diagnosed by physical exam and further characterized by evidence of right ventricular hypertrophy on exam or ECG, and transvalvular gradient measured by Doppler. The stenosis is considered mild if the peak gradient is <40 mm Hg, moderate if 40 to 70 mm Hg, and severe if >70 mm Hg.

Individuals with a peak gradient <50 mm Hg with normal RV function and no adverse symptoms are not limited with respect to exercise. For patients with a peak gradient >50 mm Hg, only low-intensity exercise is recommended.[48] Most of these patients undergo balloon valvuloplasty or surgical valvulotomy and are then guided by the residual gradient.[48]

Ebstein's Anomaly

There is a wide range of severity with this malformation in which the tricuspid valve is displaced downward leading to "atrialization" of the right ventricle. Ebstein's anomaly is associated with mild to severe tricuspid valve regurgitation, as well as a range of arrhythmias and associated cardiac anomalies such as the Wolff-Parkinson-White syndrome.

Those patients with mild disease—nearly normal heart size, without evidence of cyanosis or arrhythmia—are not limited with respect to exercise. For those with tricuspid regurgitation of at least moderate severity but with no arrhythmia, low-intensity exercise is allowed. Patients with severe disease should not participate in competitive sports or exercise.[48] If surgical correction is performed, then low-intensity exercise is permitted as long as the above criteria are met.

Acquired Valvular Heart Disease

As with congenital valvular heart disease, diagnosis of acquired valvular disease is usually accomplished by use of a complete history and physical exam. Characterization of the severity of the lesion is often aided by the use of echocardiography, cardiac catheterization, and occasionally radionuclide studies for estimating regurgitant volumes in severe valvular dysfunction. Mild or trivial regurgitant jets are a common incidental finding on echocardiography and are seen on at least one valve in athletes in up to 90% of cases.[51] When valvular abnormalities coexist with other cardiac diseases such as ischemic or idiopathic cardiomyopathies, the most restrictive lesion should be used to guide exercise prescription, with potential additive effects of other lesions. The recommendations that follow are presented as general guidelines and will often need to be tailored to individual patients.[47]

Mitral Stenosis

This lesion is usually a result of rheumatic disease; it is occasionally due to mitral annular calcification. Patients with severe mitral stenosis are usually symptomatically limited with exercise, owing to the consequent increases in left atrial and pulmonary capillary pressures. Patients who are asymptomatic during exercise are still subject to potential long-term deleterious effects of repeated increases in pulmonary capillary pressure. The long-term effect on the lungs and right ventricle are not well understood, but must be considered when counseling a patient. The severity of mitral stenosis as well as the degree of pulmonary hypertension can usually be estimated using Doppler echocardiography. The severity is considered mild for valve areas >1.5 cm^2, exercise pulmonary artery wedge pressure (EPAWP) ≤20 mm Hg, or resting pulmonary artery systolic pressure (RPASP) <35 mm Hg; moderate for valve areas 1.1 to 1.4 cm^2, EPAWP ≤25 mm Hg, or RPASP ≤50 mm Hg; and severe for valve areas <1.1 cm^2, EPAWP >25 mm Hg, or RPASP >50 mm Hg.

For patients in atrial fibrillation on anticoagulation, the risk of bleeding should be considered in activities with risk of trauma. Patients in sinus rhythm with mild mitral stenosis should not be limited. Those with atrial fibrillation with mild stenosis, atrial fibrillation or sinus rhythm with moderate stenosis, or those with EPASP <50 mm Hg can participate in low to moderate static and dynamic exercise.[47] Individuals with mild stenosis but EPASP between 50 and 80 mm Hg should be limited to low to moderate static and low dynamic exercise and those with severe stenosis or EPASP >80 mm Hg should not participate in competitive sports or exercise.[47]

Mitral Regurgitation

There are many etiologies for mitral regurgitation, but in this chapter only primary valvular disease is considered. Mitral regurgitation can usually be diagnosed by physical exam, although its severity is often difficult to quantitate. The primary hemodynamic consequence is increased diastolic left ventricular volume and increased left atrial pressure. Global left ventricular function may appear normal in spite of underlying depressed myocardial performance due to the low-resistance regurgitant flow and subsequent decrease in apparent afterload. Several echocardiographic parameters are used to estimate severity, such as systolic reversal of pulmonary vein flow or flow visualized into the left atrial appendage or pulmonary veins by color Doppler, as well as the cross-sectional area of the jet.[52] Similar visual criteria are used when judging severity by contrast left ventriculography. Over time, significant mitral regurgitation will lead to increasing left ventricular volume and decreasing systolic function. Patients should therefore be followed with serial echocardiograms for these measurements. One must consider that in the trained athlete, the upper limit of normal left ventricular volume is increased.

Patients in normal sinus rhythm with normal left ventricular size and function are not limited. Those with normal left ventricular function with mild enlargement should be limited to low and moderate static and dynamic sports and exercise.[47] If atrial fibrillation is present, exercise testing should be done to ensure that the rate response is not excessive. High dynamic exercise can be considered in selected athletes.[47] Those with significant left ventricular enlargement or any degree of decreased function should not participate in competitive sports or exercise.[47]

Aortic Stenosis

There are three common etiologies of AS: rheumatic, degenerative-calcific, and congenital. Diagnosis, as well as estimation of severity, is usually easily made by physical exam. Quantification of severity can usually be done reliably with use of Doppler echocardiography, especially in the setting of normal left ventricular function. The symptom triad of left ventricular failure, angina, and syncope usually occurs late in the course of disease and correlates with the incidence of sudden death.[53] In patients with acquired AS and normal left ventricular systolic function, severity is classified by the mean transvalvular gradient. Stenosis is considered mild for gradients ≤20 mm Hg, moderate if 21 to 39 mm Hg, and severe for ≥40 mm Hg. Serial evaluations are recommended to document disease progression.

A history of syncope with any degree of stenosis should be regarded as potentially life-threatening and warrants thorough investigation. Patients without a history of syncope, with mild or mild to moderate stenosis, can engage in low-intensity exercise or sports.[47] Selected patients may increase intensity to moderate static and dynamic, provided exercise testing reveals no significant arrhythmia, ST segment depression, or abnormal blood pressure response.[47] Patients with severe AS should not participate in competitive sports or exercise.

Aortic Regurgitation

The most common causes of aortic regurgitation are congenital bicuspid aortic valve, rheumatic heart disease, diseases involving the valve or annulus such as infective endocarditis, or aortic root disorders such as Marfan syndrome. Significant aortic regurgitation eventually leads to left ventricular volume overload and congestive heart failure. Severity of aortic regurgitation can be assessed by physical exam, aortic root angiography, and Doppler echocardiography. Hemodynamic severity is considered mild if there are minimal or absent peripheral signs with normal left ventricular size, moderate if there are peripheral signs and mild to moderately increased ventricular size with normal function, and severe if there are peripheral signs with severe ventricular enlargement or if there is left ventricular dysfunction with any degree of ventricular enlargement.

Patients with mild to moderate aortic regurgitation and normal or mildly increased left ventricular size are not limited in athletic participation. Those with mild to moderate aortic regurgitation and moderate left ventricular enlargement can, in selected cases, participate in low to moderate static and up to high dynamic exercise. Patients with severe regurgitation or with symptoms of congestive heart failure should not participate in competitive sports or exercise. Any individual with aortic regurgitation and markedly dilated ascending aorta should refrain from competitive sports or exercise.

Tricuspid Valve Disease

Primary tricuspid valve disease is seldom significant. The long-term effects of tricuspid regurgitation in the absence of preceding right ventricular failure or pulmonary hypertension are unknown. The severity of tricuspid regurgitation can be estimated with Doppler echocardiography. In patients with primary tricuspid regurgitation and right atrial pressure ≤20 mm Hg, there is no limitation to athletic participation. Acquired tricuspid stenosis is almost always a result of rheumatic heart disease and most frequently coexists with mitral stenosis. Activity guidelines are based on the limitations presented by mitral stenosis.[47]

Multivalvular Disease

In general, patients with significant multivalvular disease should not participate in competitive sports or exercise. Further recommendations may be based primarily on the most significant lesion, with consideration of the potential additive hemodynamic effects of multiple mild to moderately diseased valves.[47]

Prosthetic Valves

Even in optimal cases of valve replacement there is usually some residual transvalvular gradient.[54] The long-term hemodynamic effect of repetitive exercise in these cases is unknown. Hemolysis is less of a concern with the newer generation mechanical valves, but mechanical valves still are inherently less efficient compared to native valves, with more mass and resultant inertia. For this reason, one might expect higher gradients and lower generated cardiac outputs with increased heart rates in response to exercise, but there are very little data available that address this issue.[47] Exercise testing may be used to estimate an individual patient's response to hemodynamic stress.[47]

All patients receiving anticoagulation should avoid activity with risk of trauma. Those patients not taking anticoagulation, who have a prosthetic or bioprosthetic mitral valve and normal valvular function and normal or near normal left ventricular function, can participate in low to moderate static and dynamic exercise or sports.[47] Patients as above with a prosthetic or bioprosthetic aortic valve can participate in low-intensity exercise, with some exceptions able to engage in low to moderate activity.

The preceding discussion has reviewed valvular causes of sudden death in athletes. Valvular disease appears to be an uncommon etiology of sudden death in this population. Early studies that reported on this syndrome may have overestimated the frequency with which valvular disease led to sudden death, due to an overestimation of deaths due to MVP. Clearly, improved diagnostic methods have aided in the early diagnosis of valvular disease and have mitigated the incidence of sudden death in afflicted athletes. As detailed previously, sudden death in AS is most often related to exertion and is probably due to a baroreceptor-mediated mechanism. Sudden cardiac death in athletes with MVP may be related to coexisting abnormalities; its pathogenesis is unclear, but may be arrhythmogenic.

Classification of sports by the intensity of static and dynamic components allows for a more rational prescription of exercise in patients with specific valvular abnormalities. Adherence to published guidelines should reduce risk in affected individuals.

References

1. Epstein SE , Maron BJ. Sudden death and the competitive athlete: Perspectives on preparticipation screening studies. *J Am Coll Cardiol* 1986;7:220–230.
2. Thompson PD. The cardiovascular complications of vigorous physical activity. *Arch Intern Med* 1996;156:2297–2302.
3. Rich BSE. Sudden death screening. *Med Clin North Am* 1994;78:267–287.
4. McCaffrey FM, Braden DS, Strong WB. Sudden cardiac death in young athletes. *Am J Dis Child* 1991;145:177–183.

5. Maron BJ, Shirani J, Poliac LC, et al. Sudden death in young competitive athletes. *JAMA* 1996;276:199–204.
6. Maron BJ, Epstein SE, Roberts WC. Causes of sudden death in competitive athletes. *J Am Coll Cardiol* 1986;7:204–214.
7. Wight JN, Salem D. Sudden death and the 'athlete's heart.' *Arch Intern Med* 1995;155:1473–1480.
8. Steinberger J, Lucas RV, Edwards JE, et al. Causes of sudden unexpected cardiac death in the first two decades of life. *Am J Cardiol* 1996;77:992–995.
9. Burke AP, Farb A, Virmani R. Causes of sudden cardiac death in athletes. *Cardiol Clin* 1992;10:303–317.
10. Driscoll DJ, Edwards WD. Sudden unexpected death in children and adolescents. *J Am Coll Cardiol* 1985;5:118B–121B.
11. Liberthson RR. Sudden death from cardiac causes in children and young aduits. *N Engl J Med* 1996;334:1039–1044.
12. Phillips MM, Robinowitz M, Higgins JR, et al. Sudden cardiac death in air force recruits. *JAMA* 1986;256:2696–2699.
13. Maron BJ, Poliac LC, Roberts WO. Risk for sudden death associated with marathon running. *J Am Coll Cardiol* 1996;28:428–431.
14. Corrado D, Thiene G, Nava A, et al. Sudden death in young competitive athletes: Clinicopathologic correlations in 22 cases. *Am J Med* 1990;89:188–196.
15. Burke AP, Farb A, Virmani R, et al. Sports-related and non-sports-related sudden death in young adults. *Am Heart J* 1991;121:568–575.
16. Chillag SA. Is exercise-related sudden death preventable? *Your Patient and Fitness* 1991;5:6–10.
17. Thompson PD, Stern MP, Williams P, et al. Death during jogging or running. *JAMA* 1979;242:1265–1267.
18. Virmani R, Robinowitz M, McAllister HA. Nontraumatic death in joggers. *Am J Med* 1982;72:874–882.
19. Northcote RJ, Evans AD, Ballantyne D. Sudden death in squash players. *Lancet* 1984;148–150.
20. Maron BJ, Roberts WC, McAllister HA, et al. Sudden death in young athletes. *Circulation* 1980;62:218–229.
21. Wooley CF. The mitral valve prolapse syndrome. *Hosp Pract* 1983;163–174.
22. Singh RG, Devereux RB. Mitral valve prolapse: A review of current management. *Cardiology* 1993;Nov:77–80.
23. Khandheria B, Segal B. Sudden death and mitral valve prolapse. *Prac Cardiol* 1984;10:160–165.
24. Marks AR, Choong CY, Sanfilippo AJ, et al. Identification of high-risk and low-risk subgroups of patients with mitral valve prolapse. *N Engl J Med* 1989;320:1031–1036.
25. Kligfield P, Hochfeiter C, Kramer H, et al. Complex arrhythmias in mitral regurgitation with and without mitral valve prolapse: Contrast to arrhythmias in mitral valve prolapse without mitral regurgitation. *Am J Cardiol* 1985;55:1545–1549.
26. Kligfield P, Levy D, Devereux RB, Savage DD. Arrhythmias and sudden death in mitral valve prolapse. *Am Heart J* 1987;113:1298–1307.
27. Cowan MD, Fye WB. Prevalence of QTc prolongation in women with mitral valve prolapse. *Am J Cardiol* 1989;63:133–134.
28. Swartz MH, Teichholz LE, Donoso E. Mitral valve prolapse: A review of associated arrhythmias. *Am J Med* 1977;62:377–389.
29. Boudoulas H, Reynolds JC, Mazzaferri E, et al. Metabolic studies in mitral valve prolapse syndrome. *Circulation* 1980;61:1200–1205.

30. Babuty D, Cosnay P, Breuillac JC, et al. Ventricular arrhythmia factors in mitral valve prolapse. *PACE* 1994;17:1090–1099.
31. Jeresaty RM. Mitral valve prolapse: Definition and implications in athletes. *J Am Coll Cardiol* 1986;7:231–236.
32. Bharati S, Bauernfeind R, Miller LB, et al. Sudden death in three teenagers: Conduction system studies. *J Am Coll Cardiol* 1983;1:879–886.
33. Bump TE. Sudden death and syncope in aortic stenosis. *Cardiology* 1989;121–124.
34. Selzer A. Changing aspects of the natural history of valvular aortic stenosis. *N Engl J Med* 1987;317:91–98.
35. Olshausen KV, Amann E, Hofmann M, et al. Ventricular arrhythmias before and late after aortic valve replacement. *Am J Cardiol* 1984;53:143–146.
36. Klein RC. Ventricular arrhythmias in aortic valve disease: Analysis of 102 patients. *Am J Cardiol* 1984;53:1079–1083.
37. Schwartz LS, Goldfischer J, Sprague GJ, et al. Syncope and sudden death in aortic stenosis. *Am J Cardiol* 1969;23:647–658.
38. Flamm MD, Braniff BA, Kimball R, et al. Mechanism of effort syncope in aortic stenosis. *Circulation* 1967;36:II–109.
39. Lombard JT, Selzer A. Valvular aortic stenosis. *Ann Intern Med* 1987; 106:292–298.
40. Grech ED, Ramsdale DR. Exertional syncope in aortic stenosis: Evidence to support inappropriate left ventricular baroreceptor response. *Am Heart J* 1991;121:603–606.
41. Aviado DM, Li TH, Calesnick B, et al. Cardiovascular adjustments to pressure changes in left ventricle and peripheral arteries. *Fed Proc* 1951;10:7.
42. Mark LA, Kioschos M, Abboud FM, et al. Abnormal vascular response to exercise in patients with aortic stenosis. *J Clin Invest* 1973;52:1138–1146.
43. Richards AM, Nicholls MG, Ikram H, et al. Syncope in aortic valvular stenosis. *Lancet* 1984;2:1113–1116.
44. Mitchell JH, Haskell WL, Raven PB. 26th Bethesda Conference: Classification of sports. *J Am Coll Cardiol* 1994;24:864–866.
45. Asmussen E. Similarities and dissimilarities between static and dynamic exercise. *Circ Res* 1981;48:I3–I10.
46. Pelliccia A, Maron BJ, Spataro A, et al. The upper limit of physiologic cardiac hypertrophy in highly trained elite athletes. *N Engl J Med* 1991;324:295–301.
47. Cheitlin MD, Douglas PS, Parmley WW. 26th Bethesda Conference: Acquired valvular heart disease. Task Force 2. *J Am Coll Cardiol* 1994;24:874–879.
48. Graham TP, Bricker JT, James FW, et al. 26th Bethesda Conference: Congenital heart disease. Task Force 1. *J Am Coll Cardiol* 1994;24:867–873.
49. Lambert EC, Menon VA, Wagner HR, et al. Sudden unexpected death from cardiovascular disease in children. *Am J Cardiol* 1974;34:89–96.
50. Doyle EF, Arumugham P, Lara E, et al. Sudden death in young patients with congenital aortic stenosis. *Pediatrics* 1974;53:481–489.
51. Douglas PS, Berman GO, O'Toole ML, et al. Prevalence of multivalvular regurgitation in athletes. *Am J Cardiol* 1989;64:209–212.
52. Spain MG, Smith MD, Grayburn PA, et al. Quantative assessment of mitral regurgitation by Doppler color flow imaging: Angiographic and hemodynamic correlations. *J Am Coll Cardiol* 1989;13:585–590.
53. Frank S, Johnson A, Ross JJ. Natural history of valvular aortic stenosis. *Br Heart J* 1973;35:41–46.
54. McClung JA, Stein JH, Ambrose JA, et al. Prosthetic heart valves: A review. *Prog Cardiovasc Dis* 1983;26:237–270.

24

Syncope in the Athlete

Gregory F. Michaud, MD, Paul J. Wang, MD, and
N.A. Mark Estes III, MD

Introduction

Syncope is the sudden loss of consciousness and postural tone, with spontaneous and complete recovery after a brief duration. Aborted sudden death, although it may initially appear similar to a syncopal spell, requires intervention such as defibrillation or cardiopulmonary resuscitation. The distinction between syncope and aborted sudden death is crucial because the prognosis for sudden death survivors is poor. Syncope is associated with a favorable prognosis in the majority of patients who do not have structural heart disease. However, it may herald sudden death in a particular subset of patients with structural heart disease or certain electrophysiologic abnormalities such as ventricular preexcitation or long QT syndrome (LQTS). It is incumbent upon the physician to determine, through an evaluation that includes history, physical examination, electrocardiogram (ECG), and selective use of other tests, which patients are at high risk of cardiovascular death.

Athletes with syncope provide a unique challenge in that apparently abnormal cardiovascular findings are present in many athletes who do not have organic heart disease. Benign arrhythmias, mild to modest myocardial hypertrophy, and electrocardiographic changes

From Estes NAM, Salem DN, Wang PJ (eds). *Sudden Cardiac Death in the Athlete.*
Armonk, NY: Futura Publishing Co., Inc.; ©1998.

that mimic ischemia frequently result from intense cardiovascular training. Additionally, although the incidence of sudden death in athletes is low, the loss of an athlete typically sends shock waves through a community and garners intense local publicity. This chapter concentrates on the etiologies and diagnosis of syncope in the athlete.

Epidemiology

Syncope is common in apparently healthy populations, but there are no data on the precise incidence and prevalence of syncope in athletes. In the Framingham Study, 5209 subjects 30 to 62 years old were followed for a period of 26 years, during which 3% of men and 3.5% of women had syncope. The majority of episodes (79% in males, 88% in females) were in the absence of a concurrent cardiovascular or neurological disease. The prevalence increased from 0.7% in the youngest subjects to 5.6% in the elderly.[1] Up to 40% of healthy persons in selected populations are reported to have at least one syncopal episode over a lifetime, although many episodes are related to alcohol ingestion and trauma.[2] Syncope accounted for 3% of emergency room visits at a large teaching hospital in Boston (1978 to 1979); 36% of these patients were admitted for further evaluation.[3]

Pathophysiology

Syncope generally results from a sudden decrease in cerebral blood flow to the brain stem reticular activating system. It is possible for patients with seizures, hypoglycemia, or hypoxemia to have syncope with normal cerebral blood flow.[4] Hypoglycemia as an etiology of syncope is rare, particularly in the absence of diabetes.[5–7] Seizures can usually be differentiated from syncope by a careful history and possibly by an electroencephalogram (EEG) or cerebral imaging study, although tonic-clonic activity is noted, at times, with syncopal episodes.[4] Patients with syncope in the absence of underlying cerebrovascular disease generally do not have prolonged periods of impaired consciousness as do patients with seizures who may have a postictal state. Syncope from hypoxemia occurs most frequently in patients with obvious underlying cardiopulmonary disease.

Cerebral blood flow is maintained over a wide range of perfusion pressures via an autoregulatory mechanism that maintains oxygen delivery within 50- to 60-mL O_2/min/100 gram brain tissue. It is estimated that loss of consciousness ensues when oxygen delivery falls below 3.5 mL/min/100 gram for more than 8 to 10 seconds, although

Table 1
Mechanisms of Syncope and Underlying Structural Heart Disease

Mechanisms	Associated Cardiovascular Conditions
Neurally mediated syncope	Generally no structural heart disease
Ventricular arrhythmias	Hypertrophic cardiomyopathy Arrhythmogenic right ventricular cardiomyopathy Long QT syndrome Dilated cardiomyopathy Myocarditis Valvular heart disease Congenital malformations Drug abuse No structural heart disease
Supraventricular arrhythmias (including atrial flutter and fibrillation)	Wolff-Parkinson-White syndrome Hypertrophic cardiomyopathy Aortic stenosis Pulmonary hypertension Congenital malformations No structural heart disease
Bradycardia	Physiologic response to training Congenital complete heart block Congenital malformations Long QT syndrome Conduction system disease
Reduced cardiac output	Aortic stenosis Hypertrophic cardiomyopathy Left atrial myxoma Pulmonary hypertension Severe volume and salt depletion

sudden drops require less of a reduction.[8] Sudden decreases in cerebral blood flow may occur secondary to decreases in cardiac output or systemic vascular resistance. Decreases in cardiac output may be due to obstruction of left or right ventricular outflow, myocardial pump failure, or arrhythmias. A decrease in systemic vascular resistance or venous return may result from neurally mediated cardiovascular reflexes, orthostasis from drugs, poor oral intake, or dysautonomia. Focal decreases in cerebral blood flow may also result in syncope, such as in transient ischemic attacks of the posterior cerebral circulation and subclavian steal syndrome.

Causes of Syncope

The etiologies of syncope in a general population span a broad range, from relatively benign conditions to life-threatening illnesses. Excellent reviews of syncope with a broader scope are available.[9–12] In studies that evaluate sudden death in the athlete, it is apparent, retrospectively, that a number of athletes with organic heart disease had syncopal episodes prior to sudden death.[13,14] In athletes younger than 35 years, the organic cardiovascular cause most frequently associated with sudden death is hypertrophic cardiomyopathy (HCM).[15–20] Less commonly reported are anomalous coronary arteries, Marfan syndrome, myocarditis, and dilated cardiomyopathy.[21] Arrhythmogenic right ventricular dysplasia (ARVD) has a high incidence in the Veneto region of Italy.[13,21,22] Valvular heart disease, conduction abnormalities, and sarcoid are rarely associated with sudden cardiac death in the young athlete. LQTS and the Wolff-Parkinson-White syndrome (WPW) are associated with an increased risk of sudden death, but may be under-reported in athletes because autopsy findings are absent or easily overlooked. In more than 80% of athletes aged greater than 35 years, coronary artery atherosclerosis is the predominate cause of sudden death.[23]

The list of causes of syncope is generally the same in athletes as in the general population. Neurally mediated hypotension and bradycardia are the leading causes in athletes without structural heart disease. Although ventricular and supraventricular arrhythmias, bradyarrhythmias, and reduced cardiac output states are more often seen to cause syncope in patients with structural heart disease, they may also contribute to episodes in athletes free of organic heart disease. Table 1 relates these mechanisms of syncope to underlying structural heart disease, if present.

Diagnosis (Figure 1)

A particular concern of athletes with syncope and their families is that an important cardiac diagnosis will be missed; especially after the high-profile case of Reggie Lewis in 1993. Mr. Lewis was a Boston Celtics professional basketball star who underwent a series of diagnostic tests after experiencing syncope in the midst of a game. The diagnosis, made public through a press conference with his physician, was neurocardiogenic syncope. Shortly thereafter, he suffered a cardiac arrest from ventricular fibrillation. An autopsy revealed focal cardiomyopathy, a structural abnormality of the myocardium that is a substrate for ventricular arrhythmias. The appropriate diagnostic evaluation of athletes with syncope, including those who experience

Athlete with Syncope

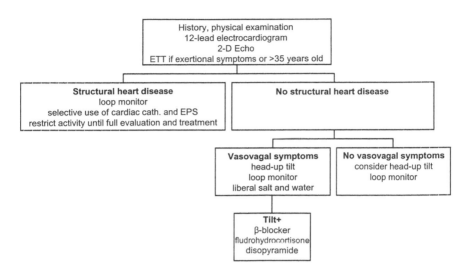

Figure 1. An algorithm for the evaluation and treatment of the athlete with syncope.

symptoms during exercise, is of crucial importance in assessing the stricken athlete's risk of sudden death.

The personal history is a cornerstone in the evaluation of an athlete with syncope. Premonitory symptoms such as yawning, nausea, diaphoresis, epigastric discomfort, and pallor often precede the common faint or vasovagal syncope, which may occur in response to pain, sight of blood, hunger, fatigue, crowding, exhaustion, stress, and other precipitors. Syncope may occur repetitively in certain situations such as postprandially, after alcohol or drug use, or with coughing, deglutition, micturition, or defecation. Syncope without premonition, associated with significant physical injury, accompanied by palpitations, and occurring at or near the peak of exercise mandates the physician to exclude organic heart disease and a possible primary arrhythmic etiology. A detailed personal medical and drug history (prescription, nonprescription, recreational) is essential. The number of syncopal episodes and the duration since the first episode are important facts. Recurrent syncope over many years is generally associated with a benign cause. Recurrent syncope over a short duration increases the likelihood of organic heart disease.[24] The hydration and nutritional status of the athlete should also be assessed. A history of sudden death or cardiac disease in a young family member should warrant further investigation, since many of the organic causes of sudden death in athletes, including HCM, LQTS, and, in some cases, ARVD, have strong genetic predispositions.

Physical examination may yield clues to underlying heart disease. Aortic stenosis, atrial myxoma, pulmonary hypertension, and HCM with left ventricular (LV) outflow obstruction should be readily apparent by auscultation if maneuvers are performed that will unmask an obstructive murmur, such as listening to the heart while the patient squats and stands or during the Valsalva maneuver. A thorough neurological examination should be performed, but is often not helpful in the exclusion of seizures as an alternative diagnosis. The results of history and physical examination determine the underlying cause in 56% to 85% of patients with syncope,[3,6,25] although these data have not been confirmed in athletes.

Noninvasive testing should include an ECG, which adds an additional 2% to 11% diagnostic yield.[3,6,25] The ECG will be abnormal in the overwhelming majority of athletes with organic heart diseases such as HCM, LQTS, ARVD, aortic stenosis, myocarditis, and dilated cardiomyopathy. Unfortunately, 13% to 30% of athletes with structurally normal hearts will have ST segment and T wave abnormalities that mimic organic heart disease. For patients with frequent recurrent syncope, an ambulatory electrocardiographic loop recorder should be provided if an arrhythmic etiology is suspected. A loop monitor continuously records and erases the ECG, usually in two leads, so that several minutes are saved before and after the patient triggers an event by pushing a button on the recording box. The echocardiogram is an essential tool for excluding structural heart disease, particularly HCM, valvular disease, and ARVD, in the athlete with syncope. A standard exercise test will reproduce symptoms in relatively few patients with exercise-induced syncope, but should be performed in most patients, particularly athletes older than 30 years, for whom the prevalence of symptomatic coronary artery disease rises dramatically. Tilt table testing has been advocated as a sensitive and specific tool for determining the predisposition to neurocardiogenic syncope; but the lack of specificity for endurance athletes requires cautious interpretation of the results.[26]

Invasive testing should be reserved for select patients. Cardiac angiography may be used in patients with known or suspected coronary artery disease or anomalous coronary arteries. Anomalous coronary arteries may also be diagnosed with magnetic resonance imaging and transesophageal echocardiography. Electrophysiologic studies (EPS) are associated with a risk of myocardial infarction and death in less than 0.1% of patients undergoing the procedure, and deep vein thrombosis, cardiac perforation, pulmonary embolus, and arteriovenous fistulae are associated with a risk of myocardial infarction and death in less than 1%.[27] Although EPS are safe, the sensitivity, specificity, and predictive value depend on the clinical presentation, findings on EPS, and the underlying cardiac structural abnormality. In general, EPS may be useful in patients with WPW, ARVD, dilated cardiomyopathy, or suspected supraventricular or ventricular tachycardia. The diagnostic utility in patients with HCM is debated. EPS generally are not useful in patients with LQTS.

The mechanisms of syncope, as outlined in Table 1, and the associated disease states are discussed below.

Neurally Mediated Syncope

There are few studies or case series that look exclusively at the etiology of syncope in athletes without organic heart disease.[28–35] It was previously believed that syncope in association with exercise was the initial presentation of a serious underlying cardiovascular disorder. Reports of exercised-induced syncope in patients without organic heart disease have made it clear that neurocardiogenic syncope may occur occasionally at peak exercise, but usually occurs 1 to 10 minutes after abrupt cessation of exercise.[36–40] Still, neurocardiogenic syncope, when it occurs at peak exercise or within seconds of termination, is a diagnosis of exclusion.

Numerous receptors and factors may play a role in triggering neurally mediated bradycardia and hypotension.[41] Arterial baroreceptors are primarily located on the aortic arch and the carotid sinus. The baroreceptors respond to changes in blood pressure via afferent neural fibers connecting to the brain stem. A fall in blood pressure causes a decrease in the firing rate of these receptors, an efferent increase in sympathetic tone, and withdrawal of parasympathetic output. A rise in blood pressure has the opposite effect on baroreceptors. Ventricular mechanoreceptors located in the inferior myocardium respond to increased contractility by increasing vagal tone and withdrawing sympathetic output. Chemoreceptors located in the aortic and carotid bodies respond to decreases in PO_2 and increases in PCO_2 by increasing minute ventilation and promoting musculoskeletal vasoconstriction and bradycardia. The complex interaction of the receptors described above and modulation of the afferent signals from these receptors by the brain to maintain blood pressure and heart rate homeostasis, however, is poorly understood.

An abnormal response to tilt table testing is thought to be a marker for predisposition to neurally mediated syncope. Upright posture results in pooling of venous blood in the lower extremities, which is compensated for by sympathetically mediated peripheral vasoconstriction, elevated heart rate and, increased inotropy. A normal individual maintains a slightly lower systolic pressure and an increased diastolic pressure and heart rate in the erect posture. Patients with neurally mediated syncope are thought to have abnormal activation of cardiac mechanoreceptors in response to increased inotropy. The afferent limb of the reflex, via the so-called C-fibers to the brain stem, causes an efferent withdrawal of sympathetic output and an increase in parasympathetic tone, resulting in hypotension and bradycardia. The cerebral vasculature also responds abnormally in patients with tilt-induced syncope, ie, vasoconstriction instead of dilation in the face of hypotension.

Recurrent syncope may be seen in the well-trained athlete who does not have organic heart disease.[42] There are numerous cases of exercise-associated asystole reported in the medical literature.[28,29,31,32,40,43] These patients were shown to have no coronary artery disease or structural abnormalities, and ranged in age from 22 to 53 years old. Asystolic periods ranged from 10 to 60 seconds and occurred from 15 seconds to 10 minutes after cessation of exercise. In one patient, syncope occurred briefly after starting exercise. Reported follow-up was too limited and treatment too inconsistent to draw any conclusions. All episodes were presumed to be of neurocardiogenic origin, although tilt tests were available in only 3 of 7 patients.

The first report of tilt table testing used to guide therapy in a well-conditioned athlete was published in 1989.[44] It is not clear whether any of the patient's syncopal spells were related directly to exercise. Since then there have been several small series that looked at tilt table testing in the evaluation of athletes with recurrent syncope.[26,36–38] In the first series of 24 young athletes, inclusion criteria were two or more episodes of witnessed syncope related to exercise in the preceding 6 months, and no etiology despite careful history, physical examination, ECG, echocardiogram, exercise test, fasting glucose, EEG, and brain magnetic resonance imaging.[26] All patients had complete loss of consciousness during or shortly after exercise. Seven patients suffered injuries, even bone fractures. All patients underwent tilt testing to 80° for 30 minutes and, if syncope was not induced, an additional 30 minutes with isoproterenol infusion at 1 μg/min[-1] after a 5-minute respite in the supine position. This was repeated to a maximum dose of 3 μg/min[-1]. Nineteen of 24 patients had syncope induced by tilt testing; 10, without isoproterenol infusion. None of the 10 athletic controls had syncope. During a follow-up period of 23 ± 7 months, many of the tilt-positive patients who were treated with fludrohydrocortisone, β-blockers, scopolamine patches, disopyramide, and combinations thereof were asymptomatic. Of the tilt-negative patients, 2 of 5 had recurrent syncopal spells.

A second series of five patients with exercise-induced syncope and a wide age range were evaluated by exercise test and tilt table after organic heart disease was excluded.[36] All had syncope or presyncope induced on the treadmill in the midst of exercise. This group is distinct from the first group, who also had syncope during or shortly after exertion, but in whom symptoms could not be reproduced on the treadmill. All five of these patients had an abnormal tilt test. Four patients responded to β-blockers or disopyramide and the fifth elected to receive no drug therapy.

The next series was a group of 42 young patients with exercise-induced syncope and no organic heart disease, although three received cardiopulmonary resuscitation and therefore might be better classified as sudden death survivors. Ten control patients had syncope unrelated to exercise.[37] A positive tilt test was seen with equal preponderance between the groups, suggesting that neurally mediated syncope may occur frequently in young patients without organic heart disease and frequent recurrent syncope. All of the patients with exercise-induced syncope were alive at up to 7 years of follow-up. Six of 10 were taking β-blockers and 6 of 10 had resumed exercise.

The longest follow-up period was 35 ± 9 months in a group of 17 young patients without organic heart disease and presumed neurocardiogenic syncope associated with exercise.[38] All patients had abnormal responses to tilt table testing, but 65% required isoproterenol infusion. Therapy was individualized and tailored in some patients by assessment of tilt table response. Only 2 of the 17 patients did not resume athletics after treatment.

Presently, it is apparent that in small series of athletic patients with exercise-induced syncope and no organic heart disease, neurally mediated hypotension and bradycardia predominate as the cause of syncope. The follow-up time is too short to make any general recommendations concerning long-term prognosis. Treatment aimed at neurally mediated syncope seems most appropriate, but no studies that methodically evaluate drug, dietary, or behavioral therapy are available in patients with exercise-induced syncope and a positive tilt table test. From the limited data available, it appears to be safe for those patients treated successfully with drugs to resume exercise.

Ventricular Arrhythmias

Symptomatic ventricular arrhythmias associated with organic heart disease carry a poor prognosis in athletes with syncope. Frequently associated disease states include HCM, ARVD, LQTS, dilated cardiomyopathy, myocarditis, congenital and valvular disease, and drug abuse.

Idiopathic ventricular tachycardias may occur in the right or left ventricle in individuals without structural heart disease and the diagnosis carries an excellent prognosis with medical or ablative therapy. In the right ventricle, the site of origin usually lies in the outflow tract and gives a left bundle branch block (LBBB) pattern with an inferior axis on the 12-lead ECG. This entity, also known as repetitive monomorphic ventricular tachycardia, occurs frequently with exertion and often is not inducible with ventricular extrastimuli. The idiopathic left ventricular tachycardia is frequently inducible and verapamil sensitive. A right bundle branch block (RBBB) pattern is usually seen. Idiopathic left or right ventricular tachycardias seldom cause syncope. Organic heart disease, such as ARVD, LQTS, and HCM, must be carefully excluded. Both forms are quite amenable to radiofrequency ablation, with a cure rate in excess of 90%. Athletes with idiopathic ventricular tachycardia may safely resume competition with ablative or drug therapy.

Hypertrophic Cardiomyopathy

HCM is a common genetic malformation of the heart that occurs, with a diversity of pathologic and clinical features, in 1 out of 500 young adults in the general population. Patients with HCM may be asymptomatic or may suffer from severe heart failure symptoms. Some die suddenly, often without prior warning.[15,45,46] Annual mortality figures range from 3% to 4% per year at tertiary referral centers to 1% per year in the general population.[47]

Syncope may occur from a number of mechanisms in athletes with HCM. Ventricular arrhythmias are probably the most common cause of sudden death and, possibly, syncopal episodes. The dynamic interplay of poor diastolic filling and coronary perfusion, and LV outflow obstruction associated with exercise in athletes with HCM, make supraventricular arrhythmias, sinus tachycardia, orthostasis, and low systemic vascular resistance poorly tolerated. Patients with HCM have a high prevalence of abnormal tilt table responses, possibly related to increased LV wall tension and contractility, which may trigger mechanoreceptors in the inferior LV myocardium.[48] Bradyarrhythmias from sinus node dysfunction or atrioventricular (AV) block may also contribute to syncope and sudden death.[49,50]

Isolated and remote episodes of syncope are reported in patients with HCM.[47] It is not common, however, for patients to have reported a syncopal episode prior to sudden death.[15,46] Since it is not clear that patients with a single episode of syncope are at high risk of sudden death, further risk stratification is warranted prior to treatment recommendations. The absence of symptom onset at a young age, marked hypertrophy (>20 mm Hg), nonsustained ventricular tachycardia, family history of premature death from HCM, and an abnormal blood pressure response with exercise place the patient at low risk for sudden death.[47] These patients should be evaluated with a 24-hour Holter monitor and exercise test.[51] The role of EP testing in patients with HCM and syncope is debatable. Even sudden cardiac death survivors with HCM are rarely inducible to sustained ventricular arrhythmias with up to two ventricular extrastimuli. Asymptomatic patients are often inducible to polymorphic ventricular tachycardia or ventricular fibrillation with tight coupling intervals and three ventricular extrastimuli. The poor sensitivity and specificity of EP testing in patients with HCM and syncope make the results difficult to interpret.

Patients with recurrent syncopal spells are probably at higher risk for sudden death. Treatable entities such as supraventricular or ventricular tachycardias, bradyarrhythmias, and marked outflow obstruction should be investigated. In addition to Holter monitoring and an exercise test, electrophysiologic evaluation or loop monitors to uncover unexpected supraventricular tachycardia or bradyarrhythmias may be useful. Tilt table testing may be considered, but its poor specificity makes the test less useful. Athletes with HCM, an isolated syncopal episode, and no risk markers for sudden death should be allowed to participate in competitive sports. Patients with multiple syncopal episodes or other risk markers for sudden death should refrain from competitive athletics.

Arrhythmogenic Right Ventricular Dysplasia

ARVD involves fatty replacement of the free wall of the right ventricle. The condition predominates in men and is discovered in 80% of individuals before they reach age 40. The highest reported incidence of ARVD associated with sudden death is 20%, in the Veneto region of Italy.[22] The incidence in other series ranges from <1% in Maryland[52] to 5% in Lyon, France.[53] These regional variations are probably due to a number of influences. Genetic inheritance is autosomal dominant. Additionally, the heightened awareness and skill of the physicians performing autopsies is most likely a factor, since the diagnosis may be difficult to make on gross inspection of the heart. Finally, Italian physicians are mandated to screen all athletic participants, and athletes with HCM are likely to be excluded from competition.

A history of syncope or palpitations is seen in a majority of patients with ARVD.[21,22] Most of the sudden deaths in the Italian series[22] were related to exercise. Treadmill exercise protocols or isoproterenol infusions may precipitate ventricular ectopy or salvos of ventricular tachycardia.[54] Up to 80% of patients with ARVD presenting with a ventricular arrhythmia will have sustained monomorphic ventricular tachycardia inducible with ventricular extrastimuli.[55] Since the ectopy arises from the right ventricular free wall, it has an LBBB morphology and usually an axis between -90° and +100°. Patients with a history of syncope and ARVD should be excluded from competitive athletics. An implantable defibrillator, together with either β-blocker or sotalol drug therapy, may allow the individual to safely enjoy limited physical activity, although this has not been proven in a clinical trial.

The Long QT Syndrome

LQTS is a genetically inherited disorder of repolarization, characterized by prolonged QT intervals, QT interval heterogeneity and lability, and polymorphic ventricular tachycardia, known as torsades de pointes. Three gene mutations have been identified with LQTS, each encoding a different ion channel.[56] The SCN5A gene encodes the sodium channel and is linked to chromosome 3. The HERG gene is linked to chromosome 7 and gives rise to a delayed rectifier potassium channel. The KVLQT1 gene appears to encode a potassium channel and is linked to chromosome 11. The incidence of sudden death varies greatly from one affected family to another and from one gene mutation to another.

Syncope in an individual with long QT syndrome is almost always attributable to torsades de pointes ventricular arrhythmia, which may occasionally degenerate into ventricular fibrillation and cause sudden death. These bouts of polymorphic ventricular tachycardia are often driven by adrenergic or pause-dependent (short-long-short RR intervals) mechanisms. Syncope is associated with intense emotions in 47% of patients, 20% upon awakening, 41% with exertion, and 8% by unexpected, loud auditory stimuli such as the ringing of an alarm clock.[57] Patients with LQTS and syncope are at high risk for recurrent syncope and sudden death without appropriate therapy, such as β-blockers, pacemaker, or left cervicothoracic sympathetic ganglionectomy. Patients with adequate therapy may resume ordinary activity but must be considered ineligible for competitive athletics and should be warned against strenuous physical exertion.

Dilated Cardiomyopathy

Despite the associated high mortality and sudden death rate, dilated cardiomyopathy is a rare cause of sudden death in young athletes, probably because athletes are more likely to present with heart failure symptoms that significantly impair performance. Nonetheless, patients with dilated cardiomyopathy and syncope are reported to have an increased risk of sudden death.[58] Further tools for risk stratification and diagnosis are limited. Patients with nonsustained ventricular tachycardia, severely reduced LV function, and ventricular arrhythmias induced with programmed electrical stimulation are at high risk of sudden death.[59] The negative predictive value of programmed stimulation for sudden death, however, is poor.[60-63] This may be explained partly by the observation that sudden death from ventricular tachycardia or ventricular fibrillation in the heart failure population occurs less often than previously imagined. In a study of hospitalized patients with advanced heart failure, the continuous ECG monitor showed a ventricular arrhythmia in only 40% of patients with cardiac arrest. The remaining patients had severe bradycardia or pulseless electrical activity documented.[64] Likewise, the etiologies of syncope are diverse in patients with dilated cardiomyopathy and poor LV function. Definitive therapies for known or suspected ventricular arrhythmias include amiodarone and the implantable defibrillator. Dual-chamber pacing is indicated in patients with known or suspected sinus bradycardia or AV block, if sinus rhythm can be maintained. Although patients may benefit from monitored exercise programs,[65] there are no data available concerning competitive and strenuous athletics.

Congenital Heart Disease

Ventricular arrhythmias are common following repair of the ventricles in congenital heart disease (CHD). Most related studies are in patients with repair of tetralogy of Fallot, of whom 1% to 7% will experience late ventricular arrhythmias or sudden death.[66] Late sudden death in other forms of repaired CHD occur in 18% of patients with double-outlet right ventricle, 4% with ventricular septal defect (VSD), and 18% with truncus arteriosus with single pulmonary artery. Conduction disturbances are also common following repair of CHD. For instance, more than 80% of patients will have complete RBBB following repair of tetralogy of Fallot and 10% to 15% of that subset will have left anterior fascicular block.[67] A small percentage will have first-degree AV block as well. It can be a challenge to discriminate bradycardic syncope from tachycardic syncope, since many patients with repaired CHD will have conduction abnormalities on the surface ECG.

There are little data on the use of EPS in postoperative CHD patients with syncope. Most of these patients have evidence of sinus node or conduction disease. The significance of inducible arrhythmias is unclear. In a study of 27 postoperative tetralogy of Fallot patients, 4 had a history of syncope, 2 had inducible sustained ventricular tachycardia, and 2 had inducible nonsustained ventricular tachycardia. Five additional patients with poor right ventricular hemodynamics and complex ambient ventricular ectopy had inducible ventricular arrhythmias.[68] In a large multicenter study of 359 postoperative tetralogy of Fallot patients, 17% had inducible ventricular arrhythmias. Inducibility correlated with a history of syncope or presyncope.[69] It appears that a substantial number of postoperative CHD patients have syncope from ventricular arrhythmias. Treatment options include antiarrhythmic agents, radiofrequency ablation, or the implantable cardioverter defibrillator.

Myocarditis

Myocarditis is a rare inflammatory disease of the myocardium, in which immune-mediated destruction of myocardial cells and the microvasculature cause acute and chronic ventricular dysfunction. In the acute phase, the patient may experience chest pain, dyspnea, and ventricular or supraventricular arrhythmias following or concurrent with a flulike illness. The clinical course of acute myocarditis varies tremendously and some patients with impaired myocardial function may recover significantly. The chronic phase of myocarditis parallels that of dilated cardiomyopathy, which is considered elsewhere.

Acute myocarditis is an uncommon clinical entity, therefore natural history and management experience is limited. Myocarditis accounts for sudden death in less than 5% of individuals aged less than 35 years.[15,16,18,20,21,70–73] The mortality associated with myocarditis, however, is high. Of those entered in a multicenter trial of immunosuppressive therapy for biopsy-proven myocarditis, the 5-year mortality was 50%.[74] In patients who present with syncope in the setting of acute or healing myocarditis, ventricular arrhythmias must be considered, particularly if LV function is significantly impaired. The Bethesda Conference recommends at least a 6-month convalescence period from exercise, although ventricular arrhythmias may persist beyond this period, even if biopsy-proven inflammation has resolved and LV function is normal.[75] Treatment options for ventricular arrhythmias in the acute or healing phase of myocarditis include drug therapy or the implantable defibrillator, but one should consider that the disease may be self-limited.

Valvular Heart Disease

Aortic stenosis and mitral valve prolapse (MVP) account for nearly all of the valvular lesions associated with sudden deaths in young individuals.[15,16,18,20,21,70–73] In one study, MVP was associated with exertional sudden cardiac death in 4 of 74 young individuals.[72] Chest pain, palpitations, presyncope, and syncope are commonly associated with MVP, although the true incidence is unknown since older studies use nonspecific echocardiographic criteria for diagnosing MVP. The incidence of ventricular or supraventricular arrhythmias is not significantly different in symptomatic MVP patients than in symptomatic patients referred for MVP who were later discovered not to have the mitral abnormality.[76,77] However, at least short runs of ventricular tachycardia may be seen in 35% of symptomatic patients with MVP and audible mitral regurgitation as compared with 5% of those without mitral regurgitation.[78] EPS are of limited value in assessing ventricular arrhythmias. Two of 20 patients with syncope and complex ventricular ectopy by ambulatory monitor had inducible sustained monomorphic ventricular tachycardia, and 3 had ventricular fibrillation. Eleven asymptomatic patients with complex ectopy had no inducible sustained arrhythmias. The prognostic value of EPS is therefore uncertain in this patient group. Sinus bradycardia or AV block are rarely seen in syncopal patients with MVP. Supraventricular arrhythmias are more common in MVP associated with mitral regurgitation, but they infrequently cause syncope. In athletes with syncope, MVP with mitral regurgitation, and ventricular arrhythmias, the causal relationship between ventricular tachycardia and symptoms should be determined before the initiation of treatment. The sudden death rate in athletes with MVP is low,[16] but the psychologic and monetary costs in treating ventricular arrhythmias with drug or device therapy are high. Loop monitoring and head-up tilt testing may be of additional diagnostic yield.

Exertional syncope is associated with sudden death in advanced aortic stenosis, although symptoms of exercise intolerance usually precede either syncope or sudden death,[79] since exercise is poorly tolerated. Multiple mechanisms of syncope are possible in advanced aortic stenosis. Such mechanisms include neurally mediated hypotension and bradycardia, ventricular arrhythmias, or supraventricular arrhythmias. The prognosis of exertional syncope associated with advanced aortic stenosis is poor and remains an indication for valve replacement surgery. Athletes with syncope and aortic stenosis should be advised not to exercise.

Drug Abuse

Cocaine has a well-known association with sudden death. Basketball enthusiasts remember Len Bias, the University of Maryland star who, soon after becoming the Boston Celtics number-one draft pick, had a cardiac arrest after snorting cocaine. Ventricular arrhythmias may be precipitated by cocaine's direct effects or may be mediated by coronary vasoconstriction and ischemia. Cocaine use may also lead to myocardial infarction or focal contraction band necrosis. Amphetamines and anabolic steroids are also associated with arrhythmias and myocardial ischemia. A careful drug history and screening in high-risk individuals should be a routine part of the evaluation in an athlete with syncope.

Wolff-Parkinson-White Syndrome

In patients with WPW, an AV accessory pathway is used during supraventricular tachycardia. AV reentrant tachycardia that uses the AV node in an anterograde direction and the accessory pathway in a retrograde direction is the most common form of narrow-complex tachycardia associated with WPW, the so-called orthodromic atrioventricular reciprocating tachycardia (AVRT). AVRT in the opposite direction produces a wide-complex tachycardia that may easily be mistaken for ventricular tachycardia, the so-called antidromic AVRT. Antidromic and orthodromic AVRT may produce significant symptoms, including syncope or presyncope. Accessory pathways in patients with WPW are able to conduct in the anterograde direction in sinus rhythm, and the resultant fusion complex between normal AV conduction and accessory AV conduction produces the characteristic electrocardiographic features of a short PR interval, widened QRS complex, and the delta wave. Rapid atrial arrhythmias such as atrial flutter or atrial fibrillation may conduct rapidly over an accessory pathway to the ventricles with rates in excess of 300 bpm. Syncope or sudden death may occur in athletes with rapidly conducting accessory pathways, although the reported incidence is low in most autopsy series.[14,16,21,70–73] In a study of 766 symptomatic athletes referred between 1974 and 1991, however, 16 had aborted sudden death. Five of these athletes were shown to have preexcited atrial fibrillation leading to ventricular fibrillation.[80]

In patients with syncope and WPW, an EPS should be performed to assess the refractory period and conduction characteristics of the accessory pathway. Additionally, ablation of an accessory pathway at the time of EPS can be performed safely with a high success rate. After a successful ablation the athlete may resume full activity.

Conduction Disease

First-degree AV block is seen in 10% to 33% of athletes,[81–83] and normalizes with exercise.[81,84–86] On ambulatory monitor, up to 40% of athletes demonstrate Mobitz type I block and up to 8% also demonstrate Mobitz type II block.[87] Acquired complete heart block is rare in athletes (approximately 0.02%),[88] but is 100-fold higher in athletes than in the healthy general population.[89] As with sinus bradycardia, AV block is overcome with exercise or atropine, suggesting that high vagal tone causes block at the level of the AV node in the vast majority of athletes.[90] Congenital complete heart block is also rare, but may cause significant exercise intolerance. Syncope would be an unusual manifestation of congenital complete heart block, since affected individuals usually have a stable junctional escape focus. There are case reports of sudden death associated with significant histopathologic evidence of conduction system fibrosis in young individuals with otherwise normal hearts. Rarely, conditioning can lead to symptomatic sinus bradycardia that usually resolves with deconditioning.

Miscellaneous

Rare causes of syncope in the athlete are pulmonary hypertension, left atrial myxoma, severe salt and water depletion, prescription drug therapy, and dysautonomias. These diagnoses should be evident after a careful history, physical examination, ECG, and echocardiogram.

Conclusions

Syncope may herald sudden death in the athlete, and if it occurs a careful evaluation including history, physical examination, ECG, and echocardiogram should be performed. Athletes greater than 35 years old or with exertional symptoms should undergo a treadmill exercise test. The presence of structural heart disease portends a relatively poor prognosis without specific therapy and, in some cases, restriction of physical activity should be prescribed. In these individuals cardiac catheterization and invasive electrophysiologic study may be useful for diagnosis and risk stratification. In athletes without evidence of structural heart disease, neurally mediated hypotension and bradycardia appears to be a frequent mechanism of syncope.

References

1. Savage D, Corwin L, McGee D, et al. Epidemiologic features of isolated syncope: The Framingham Study. *Stroke* 1985;16:626–629.
2. Dermkasian G, Lamb L. Syncope in a population of healthy young adults. *JAMA* 1958;168:1200.
3. Day SC, Cook EF, Funkenstein H, Goldman L. Evaluation and outcome of emergency room patients with transient loss of consciousness. *Am J Med* 1982;73:15–23.
4. Lin J, Ziegler D, Lai C, Mayer W. Convulsive syncope in blood donors. *Ann Neurol* 1982;11:525–528.

5. Burman W, McDermott M, Bornemann M. Familial hyperinsulinism presenting in adults. *Arch Intern Med* 1992;152:2125–2127.
6. Martin G, Adams S, Martin H, et al. Prospective evaluation of syncope. *Ann Emerg Med* 1984;13:499–504.
7. Pavlovic S, Kocovic D, Djordjevic M, et al. The etiology of syncope in pacemaker patients. *PACE* 1991;14:2086–2091.
8. McHenry L, Fazekas J, Sullivan J. Cerebral hemodynamics of syncope. *Am J Med Sci* 1961;214:173–178.
9. Kapoor W. Diagnostic evaluation of syncope. *Am J Med* 1991;90:91–106.
10. Kapoor W. Evaluation and management of the patient with syncope. *JAMA* 1992;268:2553–2560.
11. Kapoor WN. Workup and management of patients with syncope. *Med Clin North Am* 1995;79:1153–1170.
12. Manolis AS, Linzer M, Salem D, Estes NAM III. Syncope: Current diagnostic evaluation and management. *Ann Intern Med* 1990;112:850–863.
13. Corrado D, Basso C, Camerini F, et al. Is arrhythmogenic right ventricular dysplasia/cardiomyopathy a progressive heart muscle disease? A multicenter clinico-pathologic study. *Circulation* 1995;92:I–470.
14. Kramer MR, Drori Y, Lev B. Sudden death in young soldiers: High incidence of syncope prior to death. *Chest* 1988;93:345–347.
15. Maron B, Roberts W, McAllister H, et al. Sudden death in young athletes. *Circulation* 1980;62:218–229.
16. Maron BJ, Epstein SE, Roberts WC. Causes of sudden death in competitive athletes. *J Am Coll Cardiol* 1986;7:204–214.
17. Maron BJ, Fananapazir L. Sudden cardiac death in hypertrophic cardiomyopathy. *Circulation* 1992;85(suppl I):I-57–63.
18. Maron BJ. Sudden death in young athletes: Lessons from the Hank Gathers affair. *N Engl J Med* 1993;329:55–57.
19. Maron BJ, Isner JM, McKenna WJ. Task Force 3: Hypertrophic cardiomyopathy, myocarditis and other myopericardial diseases and mitral valve prolapse. *J Am Coll Cardiol* 1994;24:880–885.
20. Maron BJ, Shirani J, Poliac LC, et al. Sudden death in young competitive athletes: Clinical, demographic, and pathologic profiles. *JAMA* 1996;276:199–204.
21. Corrado D, Thiene G, Nava A, et al. Sudden death in young competitive athletes: Clinicopathologic correlations in 22 cases. *Am J Med* 1990;89:588–596.
22. Thiene G, Nava A, Corrado D, et al. Right ventricular cardiomyopathy and sudden death in young people. *N Engl J Med* 1988;318:129–133.
23. Burke AP, Farb A, Virmani R. Causes of sudden death in athletes. *Cardiol Clin* 1992;10:303–317.
24. Calkins H, Shyr Y, Frumin H, et al. The value of the clinical history in the differentiation of syncope due to ventricular tachycardia, atrioventricular block, and neurocardiogenic syncope. *Am J Med* 1995;98:365–373.
25. Kapoor WN. Evaluation and outcome of patients with syncope. *Medicine* 1990;69:160–175.
26. Grubb B, Temesy-Armos P, Samoil D, et al. Tilt table testing in the evaluation and management of athletes with recurrent exercise-induced syncope. *Med Sci Sports Exerc* 1992;25:24–28.
27. Horowitz L, Kay N, Kutalek S, et al. Risks and complications of electrophysiologic studies: A prospective analysis of 1000 consecutive patients. *J Am Coll Cardiol* 1987;9:1261–1268.
28. Schlesinger A. Life-threatening "vagal reaction" to physical fitness test. *JAMA* 1973;226:1119.

29. Fleg JL, Asante AVK. Asystole following treadmill exercise in a man without organic heart disease. *Arch Intern Med* 1983;143:1821–1822.

30. Hirata T, Yano K, Okui T, et al. Asystole with syncope following strenuous exercise in a man without organic heart disease. *J Electrocardiol* 1987;20:280–283.

31. Huycke E, Card H, Sobol S, et al. Post-exertional cardiac asystole in a young man without organic deart disease. *Ann Intern Med* 1987;106:844–845.

32. Pedersen W, Janosik D, Goldenberg I, et al. Post-exercise asystolic arrest in a young man without organic heart disease: Utility of head-up tilt testing in guiding therapy. *Am Heart J* 1989;118:410–413.

33. Tamura Y, Onodera O, Kodera K, et al. Atrial standstill after treadmill exercise test and unique response to isproternol infusion in recurrent post-exercise syncope. *Am J Cardiol* 1990;65:533–535.

34. Osswald S, Brooks R, O'Nunain S, et al. Asystole after exercise in healthy persons. *Ann Intern Med* 1994;120:1008–1011.

35. Buja G, Folino A, Bittante M, et al. Asystole with syncope secondary to hyperventilation in three young athletes. *PACE* 1989;12:406–412.

36. Sneddon JF, Scalia G, Ward DE, et al. Exercise induced vasodepressor syncope. *Br Heart J* 1994;71:554–557.

37. Sakaguchi S, Shultz JJ, Remole SC, et al. Syncope associated with exercise, a manifestation of neurally mediated syncope. *Am J Cardiol* 1995;75:476–481.

38. Calkins H, Siefert M, Morady F. Clinical presentation and long-term follow-up of athletes with exercise-induced vasodepressor syncope. *Am Heart J* 1995;129:1159–1164.

39. Kosinski D, Grubb BP, Kip K, Hahn H. Exercise-induced neurocardiogenic syncope. *Am Heart J* 1996;132:451–452.

40. Kapoor W. Syncope with abrupt termination of exercise. *Am J Med* 1989;87:597–599.

41. Lurie K, Benditt D. Syncope and the autonomic nervous system. *J Cardiovasc Electrophysiol* 1996;7:760–776.

42. Rasmussen V, Haunso S, Skagen K. Cerebral attacks due to excessive vagal tone in heavily trained persons. *Acta Med Scand* 1978;204:401–405.

43. Tse H-F, Lau C-P. Exercise-associated cardiac asystole in persons without structural heart disease. *Chest* 1995;107:572–576.

44. Rechavia E, Strasberg B, Agmon J. Head-up tilt table evaluation in a trained athlete with recurrent vaso-vagal syncope. *Chest* 1989;95:689–691.

45. Wigle E, Rakowski H, Kimball B, Williams H. Hypertrophic cardiomyopathy: Clinical spectrum and treatment. *Circulation* 1995;92:1680–1692.

46. Maron B, Roberts W, Epstein S. Sudden death in hypertrophic cardiomyopathy: A profile of 78 patients. *Circulation* 1982;65:1388–1394.

47. Spirito P, Seidman C, McKenna W, Maron B. The management of hypertrophic cardiomyopathy. *N Engl J Med* 1997;3336:775–785.

48. Gilligan D, Nihoyannopoulos P, Chan W, Oakley C. Investigation of a hemodynamic basis for syncope in hypertrophic cardiomyopathy: Use of a head-up tilt test. *Circulation* 1992;85(6):2140–2148.

49. Chmielewzki C, Riley R, Mahendran A, Most A. Complete heart block as a cause of syncope in asymmetric septal hypertrophy. *Am Heart J* 1977;93:91–93.

50. Joseph S, Balcon R, McDonald L. Syncope in hypertrophic obstructive cardiomyopathy due to asystole. *Br Heart J* 1972;34(9):974–976.

51. Fananpazir L, Chang A, Epstein S, McAreavey D. Prognostic determinants in hypertrophic cardiomyopathy: Prospective evaluation of a thera-

peutic strategy based on clinical, Holter, hemodynamic and electrophysiological findings. *Circulation* 1992;86:730–740.

52. Goodin J, Farb A, Smialek J. Right ventricular dysplasia associated with sudden death in young adults. *Mod Pathol* 1991;4:702–706.

53. Loire R, Tabib A. Mort subite cardiaque inattendue, bilan de 1000 autopsies. *Arch Mal Coeur* 1996;89:13–18.

54. Haisaguerre M, Le Metayer P, D'Ivernois C, et al. Distinctive response of right ventricular dysplasia to high dose isoproternol. *PACE* 1990;13: 2119–2126.

55. Wichter T, Haverkamp W, Martinez-Rubio A, Borggrefe M. Long-term prognosis and risk-stratification of arrhythmogenic right ventricular dysplasia/cardiomyopathy. Abstract. *Circulation* 1995;92:I-97.

56. Roden D, Lazzara R, Rosen M, et al. Multiple mechanisms in the long-QT syndrome. Current knowledge, gaps, and future directions. The SADS Foundation Task Force on LQTS. *Circulation* 1996;94:1996–2012.

57. Moss A, Schwarz P, Crampton R, et al. The long-QT syndrome: Prospective longitudinal study of 328 families. *Circulation* 1991;84:1136–1144.

58. Middlekauff HR, Stevenson WG, Stevenson LW, Saxon LA. Syncope in advanced heart failure: High risk of sudden death regardless of origin of syncope. *J Am Coll Cardiol* 1993;21:110–116.

59. Borggrefe M, Block M, Breithardt G. Identification and management of the high risk patient with dilated cardiomyopathy. *Br Heart J* 1994;72(suppl):S42–S45.

60. Milner PG, DiMarco JP, Lerman BB. Electrophysiological evaluation of sustained ventricular tachyarrhythmias in idiopathic dilated cardiomyopathy. *PACE* 1988;11:562–568.

61. Poll DS, Marchlinski FE, Buxton AE, Josephson ME. Usefulness of programmed stimulation in idiopathic dilated cardiomyopathy. *Am J Cardiol* 1986;58:992–997.

62. Turitto G, Ahuja RK, Caref EB, El-Sherif N. Risk stratification for arrhythmic events in patients with nonischemic dilated cardiomyopathy and nonsustained ventricular tachycardia: Role of programmed ventricular stimulation and the signal-averaged electrocardiogram. *J Am Coll Cardiol* 1994;24:1523–1528.

63. Anderson KP, Mason JW. Clinical value of cardiac electrophysiological studies. In Zipes DP, Jalife J (eds): *Cardiac Electrophysiology.* Philadelphia: W.B. Saunders Co.; 1995:1133–1150.

64. Luu M, Stevenson W, Stevenson L. Diverse mechanisms of unexpected cardiac arrest in advanced heart failure. *Circulation* 1989;80:1675–1680.

65. Coats A, Adamopolous S, Radaelli A. Controlled trial of physical training in heart failure. Exercise performance, hemodynamics, ventilation and autonomic function. *Circulation* 1992;85:2119–2131.

66. Kanter R, Garson AJ. Arrhythmia in congenital heart disease. In Podrid P, Kowey P (eds): *Cardiac Arrhythmia: Mechanisms, Diagnosis and Management, Volume 1.* Baltimore: Williams and Wilkins, 1995:1131–1160.

67. Garson A, Nihill M, McNamara D, Cooley D. Status of the adult and adolescent after repair of tetralogy of Fallot. *Circulation* 1979;59:1232–1240.

68. Garson AJ, Porter C, Gillette P, McNamara D. Induction of ventricular tachycardia during electrophysiolcgic study after repair of tetralogy of Fallot. *J Am Coll Cardiol* 1983;1:1493–1502.

69. Chandar J, Wolff G, Garson AJ, et al. Ventricular arrhythmias in postoperative tetralogy of Fallot. *Am J Cardiol* 1990;65(9):665–661.

70. Driscoll D, Edwards W. Sudden unexpected death in children and adolescents. *J Am Coll Cardiol* 1985;5:118B–121B.
71. Liberthson RR. Sudden death from cardiac causes in children and young adults. *N Engl J Med* 1996;334:1039–1044.
72. McCaffrey FM, Braden DS, Strong WB. Sudden cardiac death in young athletes. *Am J Dis Child* 1991;145:177–183.
73. Phillips M, Robinowits M, Higgins JR, et al. Sudden cardiac death in Air Force recruits: A 20-year review. *JAMA* 1986;256:2696–2699.
74. Mason J, O'Connell J, Herskowitz A. A clinical trial of immunosuppressive therapy for myocarditis. *N Engl J Med* 1995;333:269–275.
75. Friedman P, Kearney D, Moak J, et al. Persistence of ventricular arrhythmias after resolution of occult myocarditis in children and young adults. *J Am Coll Cardiol* 1994;24:780–783.
76. Kramer H, Kligfield P, Devereux R, et al. Arrhythmias in mitral valve prolapse: The effect of selection bias. *Arch Intern Med* 1984;144:2360–2364.
77. Savage D, Levy D, Garrison R, et al. Mitral valve prolapse in the general population. 3. Dysrhythmias: The Framingham study. *Am Heart J* 1983;106:582–586.
78. Kligfield P, Hochreiter C, Kramer H, et al. Complex arrhythmias in mitral regurgitation with and without mitral valve prolapse: Contrast to mitral valve prolapse without mitral regurgitation. *Am J Cardiol* 1985;55:1545–1549.
79. Selzer A. Changing aspects of the natural history of valvular aortic stenosis. *N Engl J Med* 1987;317:91–98.
80. Furlanello F, Bertoldi A, Bettini R, et al. Life threatening tachyarrhythmias in athletes. *PACE* 1992;15:1403–1411.
81. Nakamoto K. Electrocardiograms of 25 marathon runners before and after 100 meter dash. *Jpn Circ J* 1969;33:105–126.
82. Huston T, Puffer J, Rodney WM. The athletic heart syndrome. *N Engl J Med* 1985;313:24–32.
83. Venerando A, Rulli V. Frequency morphology and meaning of the electrocardiographic anomalies found in Olympic marathon runners and walkers. *J Sport Med Phys Fitness* 1964;4:135–141.
84. Bjornstad H, Storstein L, Dyre Meen H, Hals O. Electrocardiographic findings of heart rate and conduction times in athletic students and sedentary control subjects. *Cardiology* 1993;83:258–267.
85. Gibbons L, Cooper K, Martin R, Pollock M. Medical examination and electrocardiographic analysis of elite distance runners. *Ann N Y Acad Sci* 1977;301:283–296.
86. Van Ganse W, Versee L, Eylenbosch W, Vuylsteek K. The electrocardiogram of athletes: Comparison with untrained subjects. *Br Heart J* 1970;32:160–164.
87. Hanne-Paparo N, Kellerman J. Long-term Holter ECG monitoring of athletes. *Med Sci Sports Exerc* 1981;13:294–298.
88. Zehender M, Meinertz T, Keul J, Just H. ECG variants and cardiac arrhythmias in athletes: Clinical relevance and prognostic importance. *Am Heart J* 1990;119:1378–1391.
89. Hiss R, Lamb L. Electrocardiographic findings in 122,043 individuals. *Circulation* 1962;25:947–961.
90. Zeppilli P, Fenici R, Sassasra M, et al. Wenckebach second degree AV block in top-ranking athletes: An old problem revisited. *Am Heart J* 1980;100:281–294.

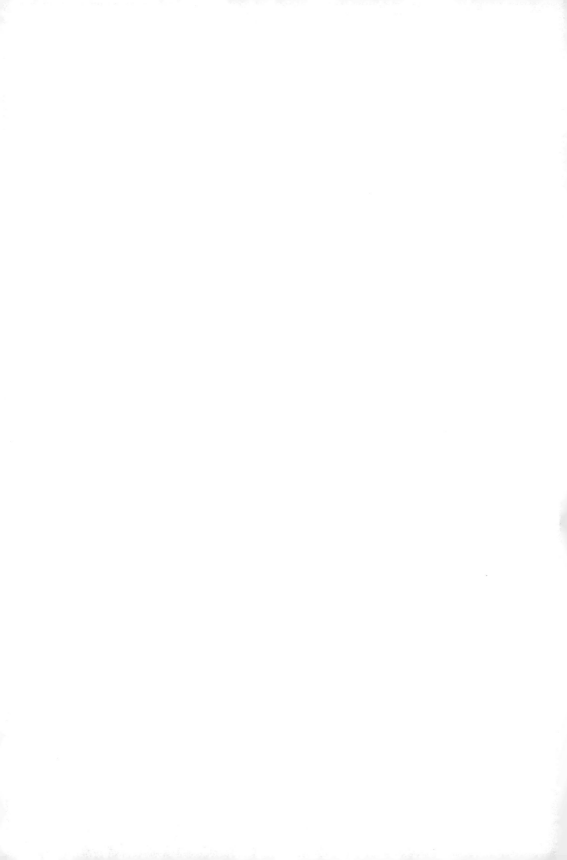

$$\boxed{25}$$

Illicit Drug Use in the Athlete as a Contributor to Cardiac Events

Robert A. Kloner, MD, PhD

Synopsis

There have been highly publicized cases of sudden cardiac deaths associated with use of illicit drugs in athletes. Sudden deaths after cocaine use followed by athletic activity have been reported. There are several mechanisms by which cocaine can precipitate sudden death in patients with otherwise normal hearts or in patients with underlying cardiac pathology. Cocaine has a local anesthetic property due to its ability to block sodium channels. This effect alters electrophysiologic parameters, increasing the PR, QT, and QTc intervals and precipitating arrhythmias. Cocaine also blocks the reuptake of neurotransmitters within the presynaptic membrane. As a result, norepinephrine and dopamine accumulate, leading to a sympathomimetic effect which can increase heart rate, blood pressure, and contractility—all of which can increase oxygen demand. In addition, sympathetic overload may predispose to arrhythmias. By stimulating α-receptors, cocaine causes an increase in coronary artery resistance and, perhaps in some patients, outright coronary vasospasm. Acute doses of cocaine appear to increase platelet aggregation in some patients. Thus, an acute dose of cocaine has the potential to trigger ischemia and arrhythmias even in

From Estes NAM, Salem DN, Wang PJ (eds). *Sudden Cardiac Death in the Athlete.* Armonk, NY: Futura Publishing Co., Inc.; ©1998.

a normal heart. In an athlete who is engaging in physical activity, the addition of cocaine to a cardiovascular system that is already stimulated by the sympathetic nervous system could mean disaster. In addition, the use of cocaine in an athlete with an element of underlying cardiac pathology (hypertrophic cardiomyopathy, coronary artery disease, etc.) might further precipitate arrhythmias or ischemia. There have been several case reports of ventricular fibrillation, with and without myocardial infarction, temporally associated with cocaine use. The cocaine needn't be taken intravenously or used in crack form; the most common use associated with cardiac events has been nasal insufflation (snorting). There have been no controlled clinical trials describing the best therapy for cocaine cardiotoxicity. Nitrates, calcium blockers, and α-blockers may play a role. If acute myocardial infarction occurs, thrombolytic therapy and aspirin can be considered if there are no contraindications. β-Blockers are controversial as they block the β-receptors, leaving the α-receptors unopposed (and hence there is an increased potential for coronary vasospasm). Antiarrhythmics such as quinidine have the potential to worsen arrhythmias precipitated by cocaine, as they further prolong the QT interval. Long-term cocaine use has been associated with acceleration of atherosclerosis, dilated cardiomyopathy, hypertrophic cardiomyopathy, and myocarditis.

Cardiac events, including myocardial infarction and sudden cardiac death, have been reported in athletes who use androgenic steroids to increase muscle mass. Amphetamines, which also are sympathomimetic, have been reported to precipitate cardiac events.

Cocaine and the Heart

In the mid-1980s there were a few highly publicized cases of prominent sports figures who died suddenly while engaged in physical activity following use of illicit drugs such as cocaine. These cases spurred interest in the effect of cocaine on the heart, and there now is a wide body of literature that has examined cocaine's deleterious effect on the cardiovascular system.[1] There also have been a growing number of case reports linking use of anabolic androgenic steroid use in athletes to cardiac events. This chapter summarizes how cocaine and anabolic steroids may adversely affect the heart.

Cocaine is an alkaloid that is derived from the erythroxylon coca. Cocaine has been used by humans for thousands of years.[2,3] The chewing of coca leaves remains common practice in parts of South America. Farmers and miners often chew the leaves to satisfy hunger and provide a sense of strength and stamina on the job; but use of coca leaves cuts across all social classes. It is likely that the amount of cocaine absorbed through the gastrointestinal tract is relatively small, and that the low pH of the stomach inactivates the substance.[4,5] In general, cardiac events reported with this form of cocaine use have either been rare or not reported.

In the United States the most common forms of cocaine use are intranasal insufflation (snorting) or smoking of crack cocaine. Intravenous injections of cocaine and smoking of "freebase" cocaine are less common. Since cocaine is rapidly absorbed through the respiratory tract, smoking of either crack or the freebase form results in rapid and high levels within the circulation within several seconds. Nasal insufflation of cocaine is associated with peak concentrations within 30 to 60 minutes of use.[5] The majority of cardiac events reported in the literature occurred after patients either used the intranasal route or smoked crack cocaine.

The effect of cocaine on the heart is complex. It has a local anesthetic property whereby it blocks sodium and potassium channels.[6] This local anesthetic effect blocks initiation and conduction of electrical impulses, prolongs the electrocardiogram (ECG) intervals, and may result in a proarrhythmic effect.[7] Cocaine also has a potent sympathomimetic effect that may contribute to arrhythmias or exacerbate ischemia.[6] It blocks the presynaptic uptake of neurotransmitters such as dopamine and norepinephrine. As a result, these neurotransmitters accumulate in the synaptic cleft, resulting in sympathomimetic responses including increases in heart rate, blood pressure, and contractility. In addition, stimulation of α-receptors in the vasculature causes vasoconstriction. Cocaine has a vagolytic effect, which can contribute to an increase in heart rate.[8] Some but not all studies report that cocaine can increase platelet aggregation.[9,10] It is not surprising that the sympathomimetic effect of cocaine can be exacerbated in athletes engaged in physical activity, in which the sympathetic nervous system is already stimulated.

Hale and colleagues[11] investigated the effect of an acute dose of cocaine (10 mg/kg intravenously) on cardiac dynamics, coronary diameter, and regional myocardial blood flow in an anesthetized canine model with an otherwise normal heart. Acute boluses or infusions of cocaine caused an acute depression of the change in left ventricular pressure over time (dp/dt), an increase in both end-systolic and end-diastolic ventricular areas assessed by echocardiography, a reduction in the diameter of epicardial coronary arteries, and a decrease in regional myocardial blood flow.[11-13] Since these dogs were anesthetized with sodium pentobarbital, it is likely that they already were under some degree of sympathomimetic stimulation and, hence, cocaine increased neither heart rate nor blood pressure in this preparation. However, in conscious animal preparations cocaine has been shown to increase heart rate, blood pressure, and contractility.[14,15] In rabbits that received acute doses of cocaine, regional wall motion abnormalities were observed on echocardiography, and some animals developed foci of contraction band necrosis.[16] Contraction band necrosis has been observed when animals were exposed to an excess of catecholamines or to calcium overload.

Experimental studies have shown that cocaine can alter cardiac rhythm. In anesthetized rats, an acute dose of cocaine consistently prolonged ECG intervals—RR, QRS, QT, and QTc. It also induced atrial and ventricular premature beats.[17] High doses induced asystole and conduction block in experimental models.[18,19] Cocaine has been shown to induce ventricular tachycardia and fibrillation during injections of catecholamines in anesthetized animals.[3] It induced ventricular fibrillation in conscious animals during exercise-induced ischemia.[3] There are at least six proposed mechanisms for cocaine's adverse effects on cardiac rhythms: (1) cocaine's local anesthetic effect (blocking sodium and potassium channels), which can inhibit the generation of action potentials and their conduction in nerve and heart tissue; (2) cocaine's sympathomimetic effect, which causes stimulation of both α- and β-receptors, which may increase ventricular excitability; (3) cocaine increases intracellular calcium (this may be linked to α-receptor stimulation), causing oscillatory afterdepolarizations which predispose to ventricular arrhythmias; (4) cocaine's vagolytic effect, which increases heart rate; (5) arrhythmias associated with cocaine-induced myocardial ischemia and/or reperfusion; and (6) arrhythmias associated with systemic effects such as hyperthermia, seizures, and acidosis.

When acute doses of cocaine are administered to awake human volunteers, the sympathomimetic effects predominate. Heart rate and blood pressure increase.[20] Low doses of intranasal cocaine administered in the cardiac catheterization laboratory have caused mild but diffuse reductions in coronary artery caliber, increases in coronary vascular resistance, and decreases in coronary sinus flow.[21–25] These changes appeared to be mediated by α-sympathomimetic stimulation and could have been blocked by α-blockers. Nitrates and calcium blockers have also reduced the degree of coronary artery vasoconstriction. The fact that cocaine increases oxygen demand (increasing heart rate and blood pressure) at the same time it reduces oxygen supply may help explain why it has been associated with myocardial infarction in humans. Cocaine use on top of exercise could further increase heart rate and blood pressure and hence, oxygen demand.

An acute dose of cocaine can induce arrhythmias in humans, as was observed when administration of cocaine as a local anesthetic agent for laryngoscopy increased ventricular premature beats.[26]

There are numerous clinical reports of cardiac events temporally associated with the use of cocaine.[1,2,27–33] These include chest pain typical of angina, myocardial infarction, and lethal ventricular arrhythmias. Again, there have been anecdotal reports of athletes who have died suddenly after using cocaine and then engaging in physical exertion. It is likely that cocaine induced ventricular arrhythmias in these patients with or without associated ischemia and with or without underlying cardiac pathology. The sympathomimetic effect of physical exertion, with increases in heart rate, blood pressure, and ventricular contractility, plus the sympathomimetic activity of cocaine, likely further worsens the potential for developing arrhythmias and ischemia.

At least 114 cases of acute myocardial infarction temporally related to the use of cocaine have been reported in the literature.[34,35] Infarction most commonly occurred within 3 hours of use of cocaine, with a range of a few minutes to 1 day. The quality of the chest pain of cocaine-related infarction is typical for infarction, and about half of patients have histories of previous episodes of angina. There does not appear to be a dose relationship between the amount of cocaine used and the development of infarction. The typical history is a young male in his late 20s or early 30s who develops an anterior myocardial infarction after cocaine use. The other most common risk factor for coronary artery disease is smoking. Patients need not be long-term users: first-time and occasional users have developed myocardial infarction. In one review of 91 cases of cocaine-induced myocardial infarction, there were several complications,[36] including 3 cases of ventricular fibrillation, 6 cases of ventricular tachycardia, 2 presentations as cardiac arrests, 3 deaths, 6 cases of congestive heart failure, and 3 cases of cardiogenic shock. Coronary angiographic and autopsy reports have revealed thrombus[36,37] with or without associated atherosclerotic narrowing. There are also a few documented cases of coronary spasm. Interestingly, plaque rupture, so common with most Q wave myocardial infarctions, was not a common finding.[37,38]

Not all chest pain following use of cocaine is due to either myocardial infarction or myocardial ischemia. In one series of 35 admissions for chest pain after cocaine use, 11 developed infarction.[35] Some episodes of chest pain have been associated with transient ST segment elevation, similar to that observed with Prinzmetal's vasospastic angina.[39] Some patients, however, describe a pleuritic type of chest pain that is most likely noncardiac in nature.

Most data regarding arrhythmias in humans are derived from uncontrolled case reports. Ventricular tachycardia and fibrillation have been described following cocaine use, with or without associated myocardial infarction.[1] A case of torsade de pointes[2] was described, in which the patient had prolongation of the QT interval, presumably related to cocaine.

Sloan and Mattioni[40] recently reported a case that typifies cocaine cardiotoxicity associated with physical exertion. *A 37-year-old man developed chest pain and ventricular tachycardia 30 minutes after intranasal cocaine hydrochloride use and jogging on a cold winter morning.* He developed a small myocardial infarction, atrial fibrillation, and a left-hemisphere cerebrovascular accident. The authors postulated that the stroke may have been related to an embolic source.

The most important long-term treatment is avoidance of cocaine. Short-term therapy for true myocardial infarctions associated with cocaine include thrombolytic therapy and aspirin if there are no contraindications (including intracerebral hemorrhage, seizure, and hypertension). Therapy for cocaine-related ischemic chest pain, which is anginal in nature, includes nitroglycerin, oxygen, aspirin, and benzodiazepines.[41–43] Calcium blockers and phentolamine have shown promise in investigational studies but there are limited clinical data available. β-Blockers are controversial because they leave α-receptors unopposed and this could potentially worsen coronary artery vasospasm.

There are little data available on the best approach to treating cocaine-induced arrhythmias.[2] In experimental studies sodium bicarbonate reversed QRS prolongation. Some studies suggested that lidocaine was safe if given several hours after cocaine use; however, lidocaine, as a sodium channel blocker and local anesthetic, theoretically could worsen the proarrhythmic effect of cocaine, especially if administered close to the time of cocaine intake. Verapamil was beneficial in experimental studies.

Long-term use of cocaine in humans has been associated with a number of other pathologies[2]: myocarditis, dilated cardiomyopathy, left ventricular hypertrophy (probably related to cocaine-induced hypertension), foci of myocardial contraction band necrosis, acceleration of atherosclerosis, and ruptured aortic aneurysms. It is likely that the abnormal cardiac substrate is then more susceptible to developing arrhythmias, either spontaneously or associated with the sympathomimetic effect of exercise, cocaine, or a combination of the two.

Anabolic Steroids

There have been several case reports of myocardial infarction and sudden cardiac death in weight lifters and other athletes who have used anabolic steroids in order to increase muscle mass.[44–52] Cases of myocardial infarction and sudden death have included thrombotic occlusion of the coronary artery.[46] Coronary arteries may appear normal.[46]

Some patients who have died suddenly have had very hypertro-

Table 1
Commonly Used Anabolic Steroids Associated
With Cardiovascular Events

1. Stanozolol
2. Oxandrolone
3. Testosterone
4. Methandrastenolone
5. Nandrolone
6. Oxymetholone
7. Oxymesterone

phied hearts, also without definite coronary artery disease. A report from Australia[52] describes the case of two football players, ages 18 and 24, who were using the anabolic steroid, oxymesterone, and had sudden cardiac arrests during training sessions. At autopsy, the 18-year-old had hypertrophic cardiomyopathy and the 24-year-old had myocarditis. Their coronary arteries were normal and without thrombi. These anabolic steroids may contribute to increase in heart mass in athletes. The inflammatory changes in the latter case may have contributed to development of an arrhythmic focus.

Other mechanisms by which anabolic steroids may adversely affect the cardiovascular system include worsening of atherogenic lipids,[53,54] hyperaggregation of platelets,[46,55] activation of the hemostatic system,[56] and hypertension. Commonly used anabolic steroids that have been associated with cardiovascular events are shown in Table 1.

Amphetamines

There have been several case reports of myocardial infarction and ventricular arrhythmias following amphetamine use in young persons.[57–61] In one case this was associated with angiographic normal coronary arteries. It has been suggested that amphetamines can induce coronary vasospasm. Amphetamine use has also been associated with cardiomyopathy.

Sudden Death and Dieting

There have been case reports of sudden cardiac death associated with starvation, semistarvation diets, and liquid protein diets.[63–65] The exact mechanisms for sudden cardiac death in these situations is not entirely clear. During severe weight loss both skeletal and heart muscle mass decrease. The decrease in cardiac muscle mass is associated with reduced myosin ATPase activity and development of insulin resistance.[63] The heart may also become more sensitive to adrenergic stimulation, which could increase its susceptibility to arrhythmias.[63,64] Deficiency of potassium, magnesium, and copper may occur with severe weight loss and could lead to electrical instability.[64] Obese patients with prolonged QT syndrome who are placed on severe diets may be especially prone to arrhythmias, although this concept remains controversial. In a recent study, Surawicz and Waller[65] examined the relationship between sudden cardiac death and dieting. An increase in sudden cardiac death and QT interval were associated with liquid protein diets but not other medically supervised weight loss programs.

Summary

As discussed by Wagner,[62] there are several reasons why athletes might use illicit drugs. These include therapeutic indications, recreational or social aids, as ergogenic aids, and to mask the presence of other drugs during drug testing. While this chapter has concentrated on cocaine, anabolic steroids, and amphetamines, there are several other drugs commonly used by athletes. Their possible effects related to exercise are shown in Table 2.

Table 2
Common Drugs that Athletes Use*

Amphetamines: stimulant; increase time to exhaustion masking physiologic response to fatigue.
Caffeine: stimulant; improves utilization of fatty acids sparing muscle glycogen.
Cocaine: stimulant; little or no effect on athletic performance. Recreational, social.
Clenbuterol: stimulant. β-agonist.
Anabolic steroids: increase lean muscle mass and strength under certain conditions.
Human growth hormone: possible anabolic effect.
Erythropoietin: increases red blood cell mass.
Narcotic analgesics: Mask discomfort and pain of injuries.
Alcohol: may reduce anxiety or tremor prior to competition.
Marijuana: social, recreational.
Tobacco: may control appetite.
β-blockers: control response to anxiety with competition.
Diuretics: weight control, mask drug contents to urine.
Probenecid: masks drug contents in urine.

*From Reference 62.

References

1. Isner JM, Estes M, Thompson PD, et al. Acute cardiac events temporaly related to cocaine abuse. *N Engl N Med* 1986;315:1438–1443.
2. Kloner RA, Hale S, Alker K, et al. The effects of acute and chronic cocaine use on the heart. *Circulation* 1992;85:407–419.
3. Billman GE. Cocaine: A review of its toxic actions on cardiac function. *Crit Rev Toxicol* 1995;25:113–132.
4. Warner EA. Cocaine abuse. *Ann Intern Med* 1993;119:226–235.
5. Warner EA. Is your patient using cocaine? Clinical signs that should raise suspicion. *Postgrad Med* 1995;98:173–180.
6. Das G. Cardiovascular effects of cocaine abuse. *Int J Clin Pharmacol Ther Toxicol* 1993;31:521–528.
7. Bauman JL, Grawe JJ, Winecoff AP, et al. Cocaine-related sudden cardiac death: A hypothesis correlating basic science and clinical observations. *J Clin Pharmacol* 1994;34:902–911.
8. Newlin DB. Effect of cocaine on vagal tone: A common factors approach. *Drug and Alcohol Dependence* 1995;37:211–216.
9. Togna G, Tempesta E, Togna AR, et al. Platelet responsiveness and biosynthesis of thromboxane and prostacyclin in response to in vitro cocaine treatment. *Haemostasis* 1985;15:100–107.
10. Rezkalla SH, Mazza JJ, Kloner RA, et al. Effects of cocaine on human platelets in healthy subjects. *Am J Cardiol* 1993;72:243–246.
11. Hale SL, Alker KJ, Rezkalla S, et al. Adverse effects of cocaine of cardiovascular dynamics, myocardial blood flow, and coronary artery diameter in an experimental model. *Am Heart J* 1989;118:927–933.
12. Hale SL, Alker KJ, Rezkalla SH, et al. Nifedipine protects the heart from the acute deleterious effects of cocaine if administered before but not after cocaine. *Circulation* 1991;83:1437–1443.
13. Abel FL, Wilson SP, Zhao RR, et al. Cocaine depresses the canine myocardium. *Circ Shock* 1989;28:309–319.
14. Stambler BS, Komamura K, Ihara T, et al. Acute intravenous cocaine causes transient depression followed by enhanced left ventricular function in conscious dogs. *Circulation* 1993;87:1687–1697.
15. Garfinkel A, Raetz SL, Harper RM. Heart rate dynamics after cocaine administration. *J Cardiovasc Pharmacol* 1992;19:453–459.
16. Gardin JM, Wong N, Alker K, et al. Acute cocaine administration induces ventricular regional wall motion and ultrastructural abnormalities in an anesthetized rabbit model. *Am Heart J* 1994;128:1117–1129.
17. Hale SL, Lehmann MH, Kloner RA. Electrocardiographic abnormalities after acute administration of cocaine in the rat. *Am J Cardiol* 1989;63: 1529–1530.
18. Nanji AA, Filipenko JD. Asystole and ventricular fibrillation associated with cocaine intoxication. *Chest* 1984,85:132–133.
19. Watt TB, Pruitt RD. Cocaine-induced incomplete bundle branch block in dogs. *Circ Res* 1964;15:234–239.
20. Fischman MW, Schuster CR, Resnekov L, et al. Cardiovascular and subjective effects of intravenous cocaine administration in humans. *Arch Gen Psychiatry* 1976;33:983–989.
21. Lange RA, Cigarroa RC, Yancy CW, et al. Cocaine-induced coronary-artery vasoconstriction. *N Engl J Med* 1989;321:1557–1562.
22. Lange RA, Ciagorroa RG, Flores ED, et al. Potentiation of cocaine-induced coronary vasoconstriction by beta adrenergic blockade. *Ann Intern Med* 1990;112:897–903.

23. Flores ED, Lange RA, Cigarro RG, et al. Effect of cocaine on coronary artery dimensions in atherosclerotic coronary artery disease: Enhanced vasoconstriction at sites of significant stenoses. *J Am Coll Cardiol* 1990; 16:74–79.

24. Brogan WC III, Lange RA, Kim AS, et al. Alleviation of cocaine-induced coronary vasoconstriction by nitroglycerin. *J Am Coll Cardiol* 1991;18: 581–586.

25. Brogan WC III, Lange RA, Glamann DB, et al. Recurrent coronary vasoconstriction caused by intranasal cocaine: Possible role for metabolites. *Ann Intern Med* 1992;116:556–561.

26. Orr D, Jones I. Anaesthesia for laryngoscopy. *Anaesthesia* 1968;23:194– 202.

27. Isner JM, Chokshi SK. Cardiac complications of cocaine abuse. *Annu Rev Med* 1991;42:133–138.

28. Lange RA, Willard JE. The cardiovascular effects of cocaine. *Heart Dis Stroke* 1993;2:136–141.

29. Om A. Cardiovascular complications of cocaine. *Am J Med Sci* 1992;303: 333–339.

30. Bunn WH, Giannini AJ. Cardiovascular complications of cocaine abuse. *Am Fam Physician* 1992;46:769–773.

31. Chakko S, Myerburg RJ. Cardiac complications of cocaine abuse. *Clin Cardiol* 1995;18:67–72.

32. Cregeler LL. Cocaine: The newest risk factor for cardiovascular disease. *Clin Cardiol* 1995;14:449–456.

33. Rezkalla SH, Hale S, Kloner RA. Cocaine-induced heart disease. *Am Heart J* 1990;120:1403–1408.

34. Minor RL, Brook BD, Brown DD, et al. Cocaine-induced myocardial infarction in patients with normal coronary arteries. *Ann Intern Med* 1991; 115:797–806.

35. Amin M, Gabelman G, Buttrick P. Cocaine-induced myocardial infarction. A growing threat to men in their 30s. *Postgrad Med* 1991;90:50–55.

36. Hollander JE, Hoffman RS. Cocaine-induced myocardial infarction: An analysis and review of the literature. *J Emerg Med* 1992;10:169–177.

37. Virmani R, Robinowitz M, Smialek JE, et al. Cardiovascular effects of cocaine: An autopsy study of 40 patients. *Am Heart J* 1988;115:1068–1075.

38. Dressler FA, Malekzadeh S, Roberts W. Quantitative analysis of amounts of coronary arterial narrowing in cocaine addicts. *Am J Cardiol* 1990; 65:303–308.

39. Nademanee K, Gorelick DA, Josephson MA, et al. Myocardial ischemia during cocaine withdrawal. *Ann Intern Med* 1989;111:876–880.

40. Sloan MA, Mattioni TA. Concurrent myocardial and cerebral infarctions after intranasal cocaine use. *Stroke* 1992;23:427–430.

41. Hollander JE. The management of cocaine-associated myocardial ischemia. *N Engl J Med* 1995;333:1267–1272.

42. Om A, Ellahham S, DiSciascio G. Management of cocaine-induced cardiovascular complications. *Am Heart J* 1993;125:469–475.

43. Olshaker JS. Cocaine chest pain. *Emerg Med Clin North Am* 1994;12: 391–396.

44. Welder AA, Melchert RB. Cardiotoxic effects of cocaine and anabolic-androgenic steroids in the athlete. *J Pharmacol Toxicol Methods* 1993;29: 61–68.

45. Kennedy C. Myocardial infarction in association with misuse of anabolic steroids. *Ulster Med J* 1993;63:174–176.

46. Ferenchick GS. Anabolic/androgenic steroid abuse and thrombosis: Is there a connection? *Med Hypotheses* 1991;35:27–31.
47. Appleby M, Fisher M, Martin M. Myocardial infarction, hyperkalaemia and ventricular tachycardia in a young male body-builder. *Int J Cardiol* 1994;44:171–174.
48. Huie MJ. An acute myocardial infarction occurring in an anabolic steroid user. *Med Sci Sports Exerc* 1994;26(4):408–413.
49. Kennedy MC, Corrigan AB, Pilbeam ST. Myocardial infarction and cerebral haemorrhage in a young body builder taking anabolic steroids. *Aust N Z J Med* 1993;23:713. Letter.
50. Dickerman RD, Schaller F, Prather I, et al. Sudden cardiac death in a 20-year old bodybuilder using anabolic steroids. *Cardiology* 1995;86:172–173.
51. Campbell SE, Farb A, Weber KT. Pathologic remodeling of the myocardium in a weightlifter taking anabolic steroids. *Blood Press* 1993;2: 213–216.
52. Kennedy MC, Lawrence C. Anabolic steroid abuse and cardiac death. *Med J Aust* 1993;158:346–348.
53. Glazer G. Atherogenic effects of anabolic steroids on serum lipid levels. A literature review. *Arch Intern Med* 1991;151:1925–1933.
54. Rockhold RW. Cardiovascular toxicity of anabolic steroids. *Annu Rev Pharmacol Toxicol* 1993;33:497–520.
55. Ferenchick G, Schwartz D, Ball M, et al. Androgenic-anabolic steroid abuse and platelet aggregation: A pilot study in weight lifters. *Am J Med Sci* 1992;303:78–82.
56. Ferenchick G, Hirokawa S, Mammen EF, et al. Anabolic-androgenic steroid abuse in weight lifters: Evidence for activation of the hemostatic system. *Am J Hematol* 1995;49:282–288.
57. Carson P, Oldroyd K, Phadke K. Myocardial infarction due to amphetamine. *Br Med J Clin Res Ed* 1987;294:1525–1526.
58. Dowling GP, McDonough ET III, Bost RO. "Eve" and "Ecstasy." A report of five deaths associated with the use of MDEA and MDMA. *JAMA* 1987; 257:1615–1617.
59. Suarez RV, Riemersma R. "Ecstasy" and sudden death. *Am J Forensic Med Pathol* 1988;9:339–341.
60. Packe GE, Garton MJ, Jennings K. Acute myocardial infarction, caused by intravenous amphetamine abuse. *Br Heart J* 1990;64:23–24.
61. Ragland AS, Isamil Y, Arsura EL. Myocardial infarction after amphetamine use. *Am Heart J* 1993;125:247–249.
62. Wagner C. Enhancement of athletic performance with drugs. An overview. *Sports Med* 1991;12:250–265.
63. Drott C, Lundholm K. Cardiac effects of caloric restriction-mechanisms and potential hazards. *Int J Obes Relat Metab Disord* 1992;16:481–486.
64. Fisler JS. Cardiac effects of starvation and semistarvation diets: Safety and mechanisms of action. *Lakartidningen* 1995;9:3411.
65. Surawics B, Waller BF. The enigma of sudden cardiac death related to dieting. *Can J Cardiol* 1995;11:228–231.

26

Care of the
High-Profile Athlete

David S. Cannom, MD

The care of the high-profile athlete becomes more difficult as sports dominate American nonworking life. At every level—from high school to college to the professional ranks—athletes seek to compete because of the enormous notoriety and even true wealth, for professionals, that come with success.

In an ideal world the various constituencies involved in determining whether an athlete can compete (including the athlete, physician, family members, and school or organization) would share the goal of putting the athlete's safety first. In fact, most such physician-athlete encounters are carried out in a professional manner and with good outcome. But in a world of nationally televised bowl games and multimillion dollar professional contracts, the seeds for strife can be quickly sown with the physician sometimes caught in the middle, both medically and legally. Schools can push doctors to play athletes, families and athletes can shop medical opinion until they hear what they want, and this unseemly behavior is often played out in the hot glare of national publicity.

The elements of the successful physician-patient relationship are basically the same for any physician-patient encounter. The relationship is based on competent clinical medicine, complete and unhurried communication, an atmosphere of mutual trust, and confidentiality.[1] The responsibilities of the physician differ somewhat, based on whether

From Estes NAM, Salem DN, Wang PJ (eds). *Sudden Cardiac Death in the Athlete.* Armonk, NY: Futura Publishing Co., Inc.; ©1998.

the physician is the designated team physician, a primary physician, or a consultant. Roles relate to issues of disclosure and care, which are discussed in this chapter.

Most of the high-profile athlete-physician encounters are resolved in the best interest of the patient with little or no publicity. Examples of this include Terry Cummings, Brian Williams, and recently, Hakeem Olajuwon. However, the early 1990s have seen at least three situations in which there has been a breakdown of the ideal model. These cases are briefly analyzed below, in order to see what lessons can be learned.

The Hank Gathers Case

Hank Gathers was a 23-year-old Loyola Marymount University basketball star who was expected to be an NBA first-round draft choice. His first symptom was a syncopal spell, which occurred on December 9, 1990 while he was shooting a foul shot during a game. He went on to have an inpatient work-up under the direction of a capable cardiologist and electrophysiologist. Electrocardiogram monitoring showed only ventricular premature contractions and an exercise test, three-beat runs of ventricular tachycardia (VT). A thallium scan showed only a small fixed apical defect, and left ventricular angiography confirmed an apical area of hypocontractility. The coronaries were normal. An echo showed wall thickness at the upper limit of normal. At electrophysiologic study, polymorphic VT was induced with triple extrastimuli.

A later Holter, acquired while he was playing very active basketball, disclosed repetitive polymorphic and monomorphic VT up to 21 beats in duration at 200 bpm. A divergence of opinion arose between the cardiologist and electrophysiologist as to whether the patient should play basketball. The patient and his family were involved with all of the doctors in one long discussion, during which the electrophysiologist said that Gathers should not play. The family was hurt and angered at this recommendation. Finally, all agreed that a trial of high-dosage propranolol (200 mg/day) should be tried. Surprisingly, on basketball Holters, this regimen suppressed the VT nearly completely. However, the patient was very sensitive to the drug and wanted to cut back the dosage. The patient and family broke off all association with the electrophysiologist, who said that Gathers could play only if all the VT was suppressed. A series of Holters was done as the dosage of propranolol was dropped eventually down to 80 mg/day. A Holter on this dosage showed three-beat runs. The patient dropped the dosage to 40 mg/day on his own and did not show up for his next basketball Holter. He died on that dosage of drug after a slam dunk on March 4, 1990, on national television (Figure 1).

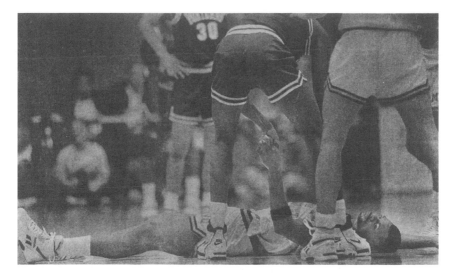

Figure 1. Photo taken just after Hank Gathers had a cardiac arrest following a successful slam dunk on March 4, 1991. Although there was a defibrillator at courtside, CPR was not begun for 3 minutes and there was no defibrillating shock given until the patient was outside the auditorium 7 minutes after his collapse. The resuscitation attempt was unsuccessful. Reprinted with permission.

The medical attention at the time of the cardiac arrest is also itself open to question. The school had bought an automatic defibrillator to be present at all of Gather's games, which itself suggests some uncertainty about the medical advice. The resuscitative effort was not begun for some 3 minutes, until the patient was taken out of the arena. There was uncertainty about how to work the defibrillator, so while cardiopulmonary resuscitation was done there was no defibrillation therapy until 7 minutes after the patient collapsed (a point later addressed in the lawsuit). At autopsy the heart weighed 480 grams and there were small patches of fibrosis.[2–4]

This was the first of the high-profile tragedies of the 1990s and a model of how things can go wrong. First, there was disagreement among the medical team about whether the patient should be playing at all and later on, about what dosage of β-blocker he should take. The cardiologist became very close to the patient and family but was less well equipped to make the difficult and controversial medical decisions. Many experts thought at the time that the patient should not be playing at all or possibly should receive an implantable cardioverter defibrillator (ICD). Communication about follow-up studies between the patient and cardiologist was poor and the patient did a lot on his own. Communication between the cardiologist, team physician, and electrophysiologist was nonexistent and the team physician ended up listening to the cardiologist for advice. Convincing outside second and third opinion was not requested. All of the seeds for catastrophe were present. The impending NCAA playoffs and the NBA draft and its riches both sped up the work-up and perhaps encouraged an atmosphere of risk minimization.

The Reggie Lewis Case

The Lewis and Gathers cases are very similar and are equally tragic. Lewis, a Boston Celtics superstar, suffered six dizzy spells in 4 months before collapsing during a playoff game on April 29, 1993 (Figure 2). He was subsequently hospitalized at Baptist Hospital in Boston and underwent a quick work-up including a thallium scan, magnetic resonance imaging, and cardiac catheterization showing a large apical defect with normal coronaries. Runs of nonsustained VT were noted on monitor. A panel of 14 electrophysiologists and cardiologists (later named the "Dream Team") was assembled and went over the data in a special 2-hour session at Baptist. It is important to note that they never saw or talked to the patient. They advised the team not to allow any further basketball for Lewis and to consider an ICD.

The family was very upset with this recommendation (which was conveyed by the team physician) and the patient was spirited off to the Peter Bent Brigham Hospital (PBBH) at midnight by van at the family's request. At the PBBH, data were reviewed and the anatomic abnormalities minimized. A tilt test was done and was positive. The diagnosis was changed from VT to vasodepressor syncope. The doctors developed an extremely close and positive relationship with the family. The patient was put on a β-blocker and told to do very little physically. The PBBH doctors stated publicly at press conferences that they thought Lewis could play basketball again. The patient had a cardiac arrest and died shooting baskets at Brandeis on July 27, 1993.[5,6]

There was a great deal of unpleasantness among the various parties. The Celtics' team physician initially called Lewis' condition life-threatening, but then did not speak out after the change in diagnosis at the PBBH. The team ownership took a neutral position after initially endorsing the PBBH diagnosis. The Lewis family felt abandoned by the team and by all doctors except the PBBH physicians; and the patient himself was very ambivalent about who was right. He sought a third opinion in California, but this also did not lead to clear resolution.

The tragedy of this case continues to haunt the city of Boston, the family (who just filed a lawsuit), the Celtics, and the physicians (one of whom has suffered death threats). As was clear from the outset, the diagnosis was serious and the preferred medical treatment, an ICD.

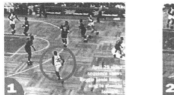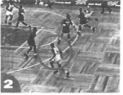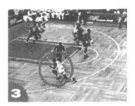

The death of Reggie Lewis:

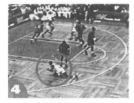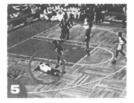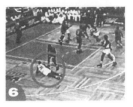

A search for

answers

Figure 2. Series of pictures taken during Reggie Lewis's cardiac arrest, which occurred during a playoff game on April 29, 1993. He subsequently had an extensive work-up but considerable disagreement ensued about which therapies to pursue (see text). He had a fatal cardiac arrest while shooting baskets at Brandeis on July 27, 1993. Reprinted with permission.

However, communication between the Dream Team and patient was nonexistent. A frightened patient and family clung to the alternative diagnosis of vasodepressor syncope. The extremely positive doctor-patient relationship at that center reinforced the second diagnosis. Tragically, a combination of good communication and bad science outdid that of good science and bad communication. It seems as if the Celtics organization was fragmented in its response, further alienating the patient and family.

The Case of Tony Penny

Tony Penny was a Central Connecticut State standout who suffered chest pain during a basketball game, was hospitalized, and even had a small infarction. Cardiac catheterization showed a cardiomyopathy and normal coronary arteries. He was told by Dr. Milton Sands, as well as by a group of cardiologists in Boston, to stop playing basketball (Figure 3). He was then cleared by other cardiologists and he sued Sands for $1 million. He went to England and died suddenly dur-

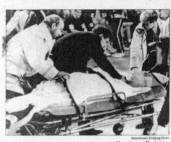

Figure 3. Newspaper article about Dr. Milton Sands, who saw Tony Penny after the athlete suffered chest pains during a basketball game and was diagnosed as having a cardiomyopathy. Dr. Sands told the patient to stop playing basketball, which the patient did not do. The patient went on to play Basketball in England and died during a professional basketball game. Reprinted with permission.

ing a professional game. This case emphasizes the need to stick to one's clinical guns, despite the frequent financial pressures.[7]

Milton Sands, the cardiologist involved, was under extreme pressure to allow Penny to play; plus there was the additional threat of a lawsuit if he did not. Sands never wavered from his initial clinical judgment, which was later proven to be entirely correct, he did not try the case in the press, and he never attempted to take advantage of the wisdom of his decisions. This is an example of the medical aspects of the cases having been dealt with adequately, but the outcome nonetheless tragic because of issues of inadequate communication with the athlete/patient, who never considered himself fallible.

The Role of The Media

The money and public fanfare that now define collegiate and professional athletics often inevitably make physician-athlete encounters objects of a media feeding frenzy. While the media has a right to know in many situations, in the cases of doctor-patient relationships the media has no rights and does have the potential to corrupt the relationship, inflicting great harm on patient and doctor alike. The Gathers case, and especially the Lewis case, point out the tragedies that can ensue if certain guidelines are not followed.

In the keynote address of the 1994 Bethesda Conferences,[8] Hutter addressed this issue and pointed out the essentials to remember when dealing with the press. He emphasized that the media should have access to protected information only if the patient and family give their permission; and even then, just as with any high-profile patient, there should be limits to the details offered to the public. If there are honest differences of opinion between treating physicians, these should not be played out in the public view. Of course, the Lewis case grotesquely violated this principle. Perhaps the best way to deal with the press is to have any and all statements made by a hospital or team spokesman. If an interview is granted, however, the details should not stray beyond those agreed upon with the patient.

Often physician experts are asked to comment on high-profile cases that they have not personally seen. In this situation there can be a temptation to second guess the treating physician; this is unfortunate for all. Such interviews can be used as an opportunity to educate the public about cardiac conditions, the need for careful work-up, and the general risks that some conditions impose. The names of appropriate not-for-profit institutions that have information to distribute (eg, the American Heart Association or Care Foundation) could be given out.

There is little doubt in this author's mind that the media goes overboard in these high-profile cases. They are incessant in their calls and requests for interviews. They want information, but also want to spark controversy. They are often not sophisticated medically and have inadequate regard for carefully checking quotes and facts. There are some extraordinarily gifted medical writers (Leonard Altman of the New York Times is one) who want information but only if it is accurate, and who seek to educate rather than to destroy. And, understandably, physicians are flattered to be called and often give statements on the spur of the moment that they later regret. A good rule to follow is to give interviews only with reporters who are known for accuracy and then to have everything you have said read back if it is to be used for the public record. Even with these rules, this author is usually disappointed when he reads a quote or sees an interview on television. We live in an era of sound bites and not context.

Conclusions

In caring for the high-profile athlete in 1998, we must engage a set of moral and legal issues that we have not resolved as a society, but which must be understood if both the athlete and the physician are to be protected. Given the incentives in today's sports world, the pressures on all concerned are intense.

The traditional components of the doctor-patient relationship are crucial to success in this often charged atmosphere. There are differences, of course, if the physician is the responsible team physician who has reporting obligations to the team. But even in this situation, his or her primary obligation is the well being of the athlete/patient.

The crucial components of the relationship include the following (see Table 1)

Table 1
Crucial Components of the Work-up of the High-Profile Athlete

- A thorough and unhurried medical work-up free of outside pressure
- A critical element of trust and communication between the physician and athlete-patient
- Follow appropriate guidelines such as the 1994 Bethesda Conference Eligibility for Competition Athletes with CV Disorders
- The patient-athlete and not the team organization or media should be the focus of attention
- Any decision regarding eligibility should be made by joint agreement of the physician, player, family, and team or sponsoring organization

CV = cardiovascular.

1. A thorough and unhurried medical work-up free of outside pressure or interference. This should differ from no other evaluation of a patient with a similar complaint whether he or she be a CEO, prince, cab driver, or capitated patient. Thorough and competent cardiology must be the only acceptable standard. It is this effort that assures that "good medical practice" is followed and, thus, removes the threat of litigation. Of course, appropriate subspecialists should be engaged when indicated.

2. There must be an element of trust and good communication between the physician and the athlete/patient. The patient must understand what his or her risks are if a certain course of action is pursued. While a close personal relationship with the family and patient is the ideal, the physician must maintain his objectivity. These relationships can be seductive and the physician can ignore or downplay important medical facts in an effort to please the patient and family and have the patient playing sports again. There was an element of this in both the Gathers and Lewis cases. Often a plainly written letter is a good way to communicate these risks.

3. Appropriate guidelines such as the 1994 Bethesda Conference on Eligibility for Competition in Athletes with Cardiovascular Disorders should be followed.[8]

4. The focus of attention is the athlete/patient and not the team, the organization, or the media. An occasional physician can become blinded to the facts of a case solely by the media attention. In the case of a consultant, communication with the school or organization should occur only with the permission of the athlete. The athlete must be responsible and finally decide what course of action to take.

5. The final decision regarding eligibility would best be made by joint agreement of the physician, player, family, and team or sponsoring organization. This outcome can be difficult to achieve, as seen in the Gathers and Lewis cases. Another idea that has been proposed is to set up an independent review board that has binding power in such disputes. This idea would likely be difficult to achieve and simply not trusted in a partisan world.

These guidelines are both simple and protective of all parties. The clinical work-up of the high-profile athlete with cardiological complaints is usually a very satisfying part of clinical practice and most cardiologists enjoy such encounters. It only becomes difficult when these standard models of good medical practice are not followed and the encounter quickly spirals out of control.

References

1. Cousins N. *The Healing Heart*. New York, London: WW Norton & Company; 1983:1–275.
2. Downey M. He didn't receive a fighting chance; and Drooz A. Loyola star, 23, taken off court during a game. *The Los Angeles Times* March 5, 1990;C1–C13.
3. Mayor BJ. Sounding board: Sudden death in young athletes. Lessons from the Hank Gathers affair. *N Engl J Med* 1993;329:55–57.
4. Wolf LJ, Brodsky MA. Arrhythmias and athletes. In Podrid PJ, Kowey PJ (eds): *Cardiac Arrhythmias: Mechanisms, Diagnosis and Management*. Philadelphia, PA: Williams and Wilkins; 1995:1175–1187.
5. Fainaru S, et al. The death of Reggie Lewis: A search for answers. *The Boston Sunday Globe* September 12,1993;69–74.
6. MacMullen J, et al. Reggie Lewis 11/21/65–7/27/93. *The Boston Globe* July 29,1993;62–68.
7. Altman LK. An athlete's health and a doctor's warning. *The New York Times* Medical Science, March 13,1990;B6.
8. The 26th Bethesda Conference Recommendations for Determining Eligibility for Competition Athletes with Cardiovascular Abnormalities. *J Am Coll Cardiol* 1994;24:845–899.

Part V

Pathologic Observations and Commotio Cordis

27

Molecular Biology and Genetics of Cardiac Disease Associated with Sudden Death:

Electrophysiologic Studies in Mouse Models of Inherited Human Diseases

Charles I. Berul, MD and
Michael E. Mendelsohn, MD

Background

Molecular biological and genetic approaches to the evaluation of sudden cardiac death have led to new insights regarding disease mechanisms and therapies. Genetic bases for electrophysiologic disorders are increasingly being recognized. Due to the advances in molecular biology and the exponential increase in transgenic strains, genetically engineered animals have become important models for human cardiovascular diseases.[1,2] Examples of murine models relevant to electrophysiology and cardiovascular disease include the mouse model of familial hypertrophic cardiomyopathy (FHC),[3] long QT syndrome (LQTS) models,[4–6] and myotonic dystrophy mice.[7] Murine models like these can now be

From Estes NAM, Salem DN, Wang PJ (eds). *Sudden Cardiac Death in the Athlete.* Armonk, NY: Futura Publishing Co., Inc.; ©1998.

used to study the effects of specific mutations on electrophysiologic phenotypes with a miniaturized electrophysiology study (EPS). Based on clinical protocols used to evaluate cardiac conduction in humans, this method allows assessment of the conduction characteristics of the murine heart in normal and transgenic animals, including evaluation of responses to programmed stimulation and pharmacological agents. This chapter reviews the mouse electrophysiology model and its application to several murine models of inherited human cardiovascular diseases associated with sudden cardiac death.

Murine Electrophysiology Studies

Berul and colleagues[8] recently reported the full details of an in vivo mouse EPS. In brief, mice are anesthetized, intubated, and mechanically ventilated, and a surface 12-lead electrocardiogram (ECG) is obtained. A midline sternotomy is performed under an operating microscope and epicardial pacing/recording wires are placed on the right ventricle, left ventricle, and right atrial surfaces.[8] Very recently, an endocardial approach to the murine EPS, which includes pacing, infusion of pharmacological agents, blood sampling, and pressure transduction,

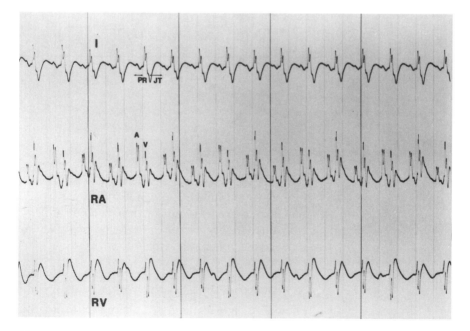

Figure 1. Three-channel recording (electrocardiogram lead, right atrial, and right ventricular intracardiac electrograms) obtained simultaneously via octapolar endocardial catheter in a normal mouse.

was developed and successfully implemented. Endocardial access is obtained via a right jugular vein cutdown approach. An octapolar electrode catheter was designed specially for simultaneous atrial and ventricular endocardial recording and pacing (see Figure 1). For both the epicardial and endocardial approaches, cardiac rhythm is monitored and recorded and all ECG frontal axes (P and QRS) and time intervals (PR, QRS, QT, JT, QTc, JTc, RR) are calculated.[9–12] For each approach, standard clinical electrophysiologic pacing protocols may be used to determine electrophysiologic parameters, and pharmacological manipulations are also feasible.[8,13–15]

Genetic Disorders Associated with Tachyarrhythmias

Cardiomyopathies

Familial Hypertrophic Cardiomyopathy

FHC is a relatively common genetic cardiac disease that is inherited in an autosomal dominant fashion and characterized by ventricular hypertrophy, arrhythmias, and sudden cardiac death. The cardiomyopathy results from a variety of mutations in cardiac myosin and other genes of the contractile apparatus.[16,17] Features of FHCs are ventricular hypertrophy, myocyte disarray and hypertrophy, interstitial fibrosis, and atrial and ventricular arrhythmias. The abnormal genes identified in FHC patients thus far encode for mutations in sarcomeric proteins including β-myosin heavy chain, α-tropomyosin, and cardiac troponin T.[17–19] The clinical course of FHC can range from the asymptomatic carrier state to premature sudden death in childhood. Risk factors for sudden death in FHC include young age at presentation, syncope, myocardial ischemia, inducible ventricular tachycardia during EPS, and a malignant family history.[20–23] In FHC patients who survive sudden death, electrophysiologic testing has often shown sinus node dysfunction, electrogram fractionation, and inducible ventricular arrhythmias.[24–26] Some FHC mutations are thought to be associated with a higher risk of ventricular hypertrophy and morphological abnormalities,[27] ventricular arrhythmias and other electrophysiologic abnormalities,[28,29] or sudden cardiac arrest.[30] However, echocardiography and cardiac catheterization are not accurate predictors of sudden death in FHC patients, and clinical electrophysiologic testing has had variable predictive value, possibly because it has not been feasible to perform EPS in large human cohorts with similar genotypes.[16,31]

One approach to examining directly the relationship between a specific genotype and its electrophysiologic phenotype is by designing a specific mutation in a mouse. The human FHC cardiac myosin heavy chain gene mutation Arg[403] Gln has been genetically engineered to create a murine model of FHC.[32] The homozygous mutation (α-MHC[403/403]) is uniformly fatal, while the heterozygous α-MHC[403/+] mice survive but with progressive development of the histologic and hemodynamic FHC phenotype.[32] Male mice and older mice develop a more severe pathology than their female and younger counterparts. The mutant FHC mice have sudden death during exercise testing, while wild-type littermate controls survive identical exercise testing.[32] The α-MHC[403/+] mutation studied in this group of mice is associated in humans with a relatively high risk of arrhythmia and mortality.[30]

Using the mouse electrophysiologic method, Berul and colleagues[33] found that these animals have distinct abnormalities in their ECGs (right axis deviation and prolonged repolarization times) and EPS (prolonged sinus node recovery times, heterogeneous ventricular conduction properties, and inducible ventricular ectopy). Figure 2 demonstrates an example of 12-lead ECGs and intracardiac electrograms from wild-type and mutant FHC mice. An example of inducible ventricular arrhythmia is shown in Figure 3. These data identify specific electrophysiologic abnormalities associated with the α-MHC[403/+] mutation and raise the possibility that prospective evaluation of ECG and EPS findings, as well as arrhythmia inducibility, may be of value in predicting which patients with α-MHC[403/+]-induced FHC are at risk for electrophysiologic sequelae and sudden death. There are at least 40 distinct mutations in cardiac myosin heavy chain gene, as well as other sarcomeric protein gene mutations, that lead to FHC. Determination of specific electrophysiologic abnormalities associated with other FHC-causing mutations may also be systematically assessed with use of these methods. Potential therapies for FHC may be evaluated during murine EPS as well, including assessment of drugs, pacing, and novel gene replacement approaches.

Dilated Cardiomyopathy

There are several examples of inherited dilated cardiomyopathy that are associated with varying degrees of risk for sudden cardiac death. The likelihood of sudden death in these cohorts is directly related to the likelihood of ventricular arrhythmia and cardiac dysfunction. *Familial dilated cardiomyopathy* (FDC) is a general term encompassing a spectrum of distinct genetic disorders with similar phenotypes. FDC is thought to account for approximately 20% to 30% of all "idiopathic" dilated cardiomyopathy cases.[34,35] The clinical presentation of inherited dilated cardiomyopathy usually begins with cardiomegaly and congestive cardiomyopathy, although the presenting symptom may be sudden

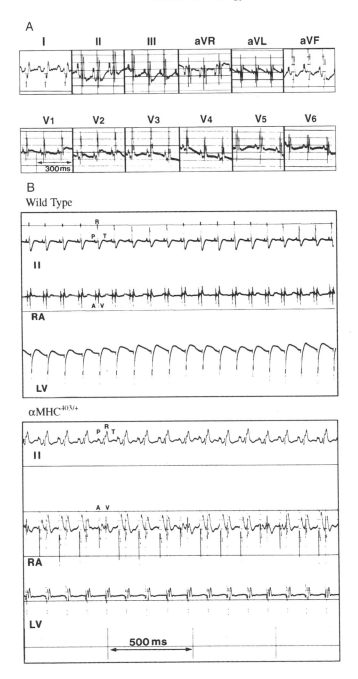

Figure 2. Twelve-lead electrocardiogram (**A**) and intracardiac electrograms (**B**) from heterozygous αMHC mutant male mouse.

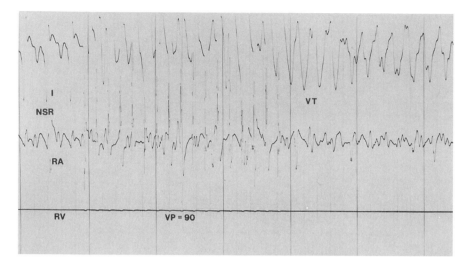

Figure 3. Ventricular tachycardia induced in a heterozygous αMHC mutant male mouse.

death due to arrhythmia. The majority of the FDC syndromes described have an autosomal dominant inheritance, with multiple genetic etiologies. One pedigree that has been evaluated has familial sinus node dysfunction, supraventricular tachycardias, cardiac conduction abnormalities, and dilated cardiomyopathy. Linkage analysis has mapped the gene responsible to the short arm of chromosome 3.[36] Additional mutations have been identified, including a large six-generation kindred mapped to the long arm of chromosome 9[37] and a separate kindred in which the locus is mapped to chromosome 1q32.[38] There are also some X-linked recessive forms of dilated cardiomyopathy presenting in males. These are often associated with abnormalities in the myocardial mitochondrial DNA.[39,40] At least one nonmitochondrial form of X-linked cardiomyopathy has been linked to deletions in the dystrophin gene, with a cardiac-specific myopathy that spares significant skeletal muscle involvement.[41] More severe X-linked FDC phenotypes present in infancy with congestive heart failure and unexplained sudden infant death; genetic linkage analysis has permitted mapping of several of these to distinct locations on chromosome X (Xp21, Xq28).[42] Mouse models of these disorders have recently been described using mice lacking the gene encoding for the muscle LIM protein (MLP). These MLP-deficient mice develop disrupted cytoskeletal architecture, leading to neonatal dilated cardiomyopathy.[43] As the genetic causes for these diseases are elucidated, murine models can be engineered and hemodynamic and electrophysiologic data can be systematically obtained. The identification and characterization of the electrophysiologic phenotypes may then allow for electrophysiologic abnormalities for these specific FDC gene defects to be identified, and potentially, for specific therapies to be designed for each disorder.

Storage Diseases

There are numerous disorders of glycogen metabolism that lead to childhood cardiomyopathy. The most severe type is Pompe's disease (glycogen storage disease type II), which has an autosomal recessive inheritance pattern, and has been mapped to human chromosome 17. This defect in the lysosomal enzyme α-glucosidase results in massive tissue accumulation of glycogen in the heart (as well as the rest of the body), which causes severe cardiomyopathy (Figure 4). In its most severe form, Pompe's disease leads to infantile sudden death, either from severe hypertrophic left ventricular outflow obstruction or from malignant ventricular arrhythmias in the first year of life. Thus far, there are no genetic animal models of Pompe's disease and no effective therapy or prevention of sudden cardiac death accompanying this disorder.

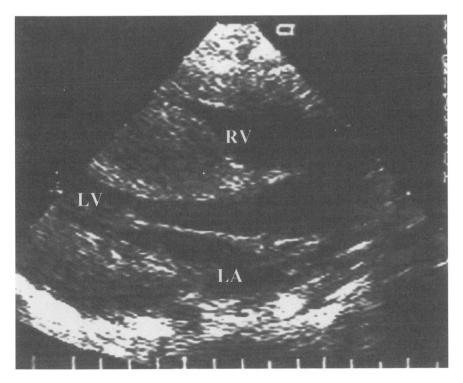

Figure 4. Echocardiogram of a baby with Pompe's disease.

Congenital Long QT Syndrome

As in the FHCs and FDCs, the congenital LQTSs are a collection of distinct genotypes that result in a similar phenotype.[44] The LQTS phenotype is characterized by the combination of several of the following clinical features: prolongation of the rate-corrected QT interval (or QTc) on the surface ECG, stress-induced syncope, polymorphic ventricular tachycardia (typically with a torsade de pointes pattern), and sudden cardiac death (Figure 5). These symptoms and ECG findings typically present during childhood, and sudden death is usually premature if the disease goes undiagnosed and untreated. Prior to the era of molecular genetics, congenital LQTS patients were subcategorized into three groups: autosomal dominant inheritance with variable penetrance (the Romano-Ward-type LQTS), autosomal recessive inheritance with associated congenital neural deafness (the Jervell-Lange-Nielson LQTS type), and sporadic mutations without clear inheritance

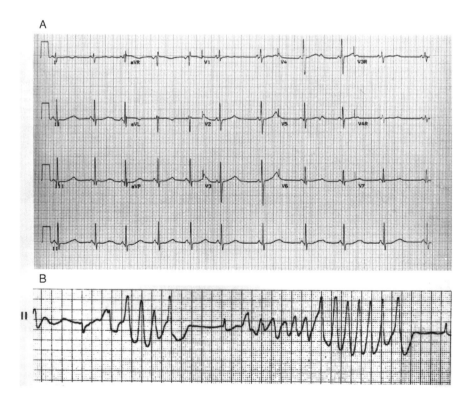

Figure 5. Twelve-lead electrocardiogram (**A**) and rhythm strip (**B**) of torsade de pointes in a child with congenital long QT syndrome.

patterns. The most common and best described group is the Romano-Ward type, which accounts for the majority of identified congenital LQTS cases. So far, at least 30 different mutations in at least four distinct sites responsible for Romano-Ward-type LQTS have been elucidated, and in each case distinct mutations in ion channel function underlie the phenotype.[45,46] These mutations have been aptly named LQT1, LQT2, LQT3, and LQT4. The two more common defects (LQT1 and LQT2) are due to potassium channel mutations leading to prolonged repolarization times, and the third (LQT3) is caused by a sodium channel defect. LQT4 has so far only been isolated in a single family pedigree, but appears to be due to a potassium channel defect as well. Like the FHC mutations, there are likely to be many more mutations leading to the LQTS clinical phenotype that have yet to be recognized. Murine models of LQTS have been developed by designing defects in several of the potassium channel subtypes that are associated with repolarization (I_{kr}, I_{ks}, I_{to}, I_{k1}). These mouse models of LQTS may prove useful for study with both in vivo whole animal EPS methods and for single-cell analysis (ie, dispersal of individual myocytes from these mice for single-cell patch-clamping studies).

Genetic Disorders with Cardiac Conduction Abnormalities

The Muscular Dystrophies

Duchenne's Muscular Dystrophy

Duchenne's muscular dystrophy (DMD) is a relatively common disorder (affecting 1 out of every 3500 live-born males) with an X-linked inheritance pattern. Approximately one third of cases are thought to be due to new sporadic mutations. The disease is characterized by focal but widespread muscle degeneration. Death is usually caused by malignant ventricular arrhythmias, cardiomyopathy, or respiratory failure/infection. The causative dystrophin gene has been localized to the short arm of the human X chromosome (Xp21), with successful isolation and cloning of the gene in multiple species. This gene is very large, which may account for the relatively high number of new clinical mutations. The dystrophin protein only accounts for roughly 0.002% of total myocyte protein in both skeletal and cardiac muscle. Whether the cardiomyopathy is a direct result of the abnormal protein content in the heart, preferential concentration or effect in the conduction system, or generalized muscle failure has not yet been fully defined.

Becker's Muscular Dystrophy

Becker's muscular dystrophy (BMD) is much less common (affecting 1 in 35,000 live-born males) than DMD, but has a similar autosomal recessive inheritance pattern and is due to defective dystrophin production. The clinical course is typically less severe, with less probability of sudden cardiac death from ventricular arrhythmias. However, some mutations, such as a dystrophin gene G-to-T transversion at the terminal end of exon13, can lead to cardiac involvement preceding skeletal myopathy.[47]

Myotonic Dystrophy

Myotonic muscular dystrophy is the most common adult-onset type of muscular dystrophy, with an incidence of more than 1 in 7500. The disease affects all muscle subtypes, including smooth, skeletal, and cardiac muscles, and leads to varying degrees of myotonia, skeletal wasting, and both cardiac muscle and conduction system disease. The cardiac symptoms relate to progressive atrioventricular (AV) block and bradycardia. Myotonic dystrophy is inherited in an autosomal dominant fashion with variable expression (again, similar to FHC, FDC, and Romano-Ward-type LQTS), and is thought to be due to repetitive expansion of a trinucleotide repeat sequence mutation in a protein kinase gene (DMPK), localized on chromosome 19.[48,49] A murine model of myotonic dystrophy has been designed recently by targeted disruption of the myotonic dystrophy protein kinase gene (DMPK$^{-/-}$ homozygous).[7] The DMPK-deficient mice display abnormalities in skeletal muscle with a progressive skeletal myopathy. However, their cardiac conduction characteristics have not yet been well defined. Berul and coworkers[50] therefore performed full in vivo EPS via epicardial and endocardial pacing/recording in 10 homozygous DMPK mutant mice and 10 age-matched wild-type controls. Complete 12-lead ECGs and electrophysiologic data were collected, including sinus node recovery times, AV and ventriculoatrial (VA) conduction properties, and atrial, AV, and ventricular effective refractory periods. On ECG, a prolonged PR interval was seen in all 10 mutants compared with wild-type mice (mean PR = 49.5±9 ms versus 33.2±5 ms, $P<0.001$), as exemplified in Figure 6. No wild-type mice had a PR greater than 35 milliseconds, while all homozygous DMPK mutant mice had a PR greater than or equal to 35 milliseconds, which may be analogous to first-degree AV block in humans. On electrophysiologic testing, 4 out of 9 of the mice with the targeted disruption in DMPK had second-degree AV block and 2 also developed third-degree AV block during atrial pacing (see Figure 7). None of the wild-type mice had any AV block. There were no examples of inducible

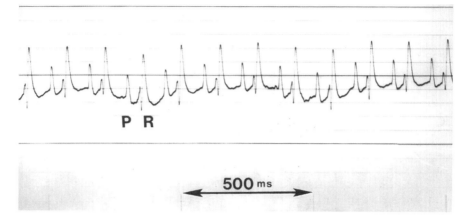

Figure 6. Electrocardiogram from a homozygous DMPK[-/-] mutant mouse, demonstrating first-degree atrioventricular block.

tachyarrhythmia or other electrophysiologic abnormalities with burst pacing or programmed atrial or ventricular stimulation. Thus, the homozygous DMPK-deficient mutant mice have distinct cardiac electrophysiologic abnormalities that specifically affect AV conduction. This mouse model of myotonic dystrophy may prove useful for the study of pharmacological and gene therapy approaches to cardiovascular complications seen in the inherited muscular dystrophies.

Emery-Dreifuss Muscular Dystrophy

This is a rare X-linked recessive disorder that is notable for its preferential cardiac conduction system abnormalities. The patients typically have severe cardiomyopathy and high-grade AV block. Survival requires permanent pacing in childhood for prevention of progressive (and sometimes sudden) AV block. No gene has been identified to date for Emery-Dreifuss muscular dystrophy and, therefore, there are no murine models of this rare disease and no effective therapy for the myopathy.

Connexin Defect Disorders

Gap junction proteins are critical to cardiac electrical signal conduction from cell to cell. There are multiple distinct protein members of the connexin family that are responsible for intermyocyte communication of electrical impulses.[51] In addition, different combinations of connexin subtypes are found in anatomically distinct regions of the heart (atrium versus ventricle versus specialized conduction tissue). Disorders of the cardiac gap junction channel proteins may lead to distinct

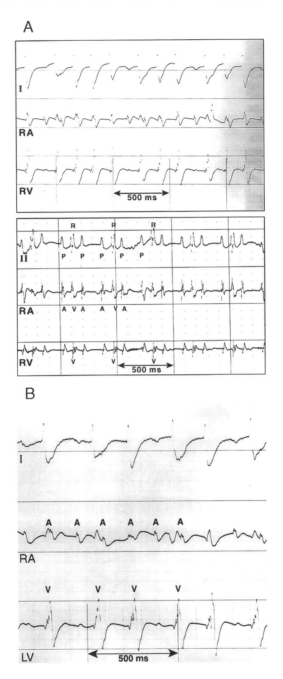

Figure 7. Electrocardiograms from homozygous DMPK[-/-] mutant mice, demonstrating second-degree (Mobitz type I and type II) (**A**) and third-degree (complete) (**B**) atrioventricular block.

forms of cardiac conduction abnormalities dependent on the spatial concentration of the individual connexin protein subtypes.[52] Developmental maturation of connexin spatiotemporal relationships occurs in human ventricular myocardium and may effect the alterations in functional requirements of the pediatric versus the adult heart.[53] Targeted mutagenesis of connexin43, one of the most prevalent gap junction proteins, has been performed, with homozygous mice surviving fetal life but dying at birth from congenital heart disease affecting the right ventricular outflow tract.[54] However, heterozygote mutant mice survive without obvious structural heart anomalies. Some studies have suggested that defects in connexin43 may be implicated in heterotaxy syndrome, a form of complex congenital heart and visceral abnormalities, while other authors have not found that association.[55,56] There has not been any systematic assessment of cardiac conduction thus far in connexin43 mutant mice, despite its biological role in intercellular electrophysiologic communication. Preliminary EPS of mice heterozygous for connexin43 mutations have been performed,[57] which demonstrated prolongation of the QRS complex duration on ECG in all mutant mice evaluated (see Figure 8). There were no other abnormalities on surface ECG

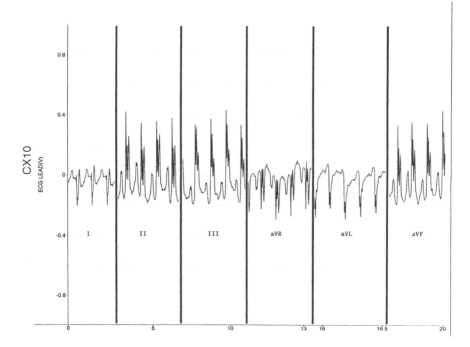

Figure 8. Electrocardiogram from a heterozygous connexin43 mutant mouse, demonstrating intraventricular conduction delay.

Table 1
Genetically Manipulated Mouse Models in the Study of Inherited Human Diseases

Disorder	Inheritance	Genes identified	Mouse Model	Mouse EP Data
Familial hypertrophic cardiomyopathy	Autosomal dominant, sporadic	sarcomeric proteins (myosin, tropomyosin, troponin)	Yes	Abnormal ECG & EPS Inducible VEA
Familial dilated cardiomyopathy	Autosomal dominant, sporadic, X-linked recessive, mitochondrial	dystrophin, MLP. chrom 3p, 9g, 1q, X	Yes	—
Storage diseases	Autosomal recessive	Chrom 17 - acid maltase	—	—
Congenital long QT syndrome	Autosomal dominant, autosomal recessive, sporadic	K⁺ - channel (KVLQT1, HERG, mink) Na⁺ - channel	Yes	—
Muscular dystrophies	Autosomal recessive, X-linked	DMPK, dystrophin	Yes	Prolonged PR; AV block
Connexin defects	?	connexin 43, connexin 40, connexin 45	Yes	Intraventricular conduction delay.

ECG = electrocardiogram; EPS = electrophysiologic study; VEA = ventricular ectopic activity.

or during electrophysiologic testing. There also were no differences in either mean PR interval, P wave duration, or atrial or AV conduction times. Thus, the only differences in mutant versus littermate controls noted were in the QRS duration, a correlate of prolonged intraventricular conduction times. These findings are consistent with an increased spatial density of connexin43 versus other connexin isoforms in ventricular muscle, compared with atrial muscle and specialized conduction tissue. The effects of connexin mutations on potential arrhythmias and sudden cardiac death remains to be determined.

Summary

Genetically manipulated animals are now becoming important models for the study of inherited human diseases associated with abnormal cardiac conduction and electrophysiology (see Table 1). The examples above highlight Berul and coworkers' initial studies of the in vivo murine electrophysiology of three genetic diseases: FHC due to the Arg[403]Gln mutation, myotonic muscular dystrophy due to disruption of the DMPK gene, and mice heterozygous for a disruption of the connexin43 gene. The mouse electrophysiologic model uses commercially available materials to measure the electrocardiographic and electrophysiologic data that are routinely collected in human clinical studies.

The development of a mouse model analogous to a human clinical cardiac EPS now allows for several types of electrophysiologic investigation in transgenic animals. First, specific disease models can be studied to better understand the relationship between single-gene defects and their electrophysiologic phenotype in whole animals. Second, transgenic animals harboring mutations in genes encoding proteins that are highly expressed in myocytes or that lead to cardiovascular abnormalities may prove to have interesting and informative electrophysiologic phenotypes.[1,2,6,58] Finally, mutations in or disruptions of individual ion channel genes in transgenic mice will allow the role of specific ion channels in in vivo cardiac conduction to be studied, which previously has not been possible.

References

1. Paigen K. A miracle enough: The power of mice. *Nat Med* 1995;1:215–220.
2. Lin MC, Rockman RA, Chien KR. Heart and lung disease in engineered mice. *Nat Med* 1995;1:749–751.
3. Geisterfer-Lowrance A, Christe M, Conner D, et al. A targeted missense mutation in α-myosin heavy chain gene leads to alterations in physiologic phenotype in the mouse. *Circulation* 1995;92:I233.
4. Wang Q, Shen J, Splawski I, et al. SCN5A mutation associated with an inherited cardiac arrhythmia-long QT syndome. *Cell* 1995;80:805–811.

5. Curran ME, Splawski I, Timothy KW, et al. A molecular basis of cardiac arrhythmias: HERG mutations cause long QT syndrome. *Cell* 1995;80: 795–803.
6. Grace AA, Chien KR. Congenital long QT syndromes: Toward molecular dissection of arrhythmia substrates. *Circulation* 1995;92:2786–2789.
7. Reddy S, Smith DBJ, Rich MM, et al. Mice lacking the myotonic dystrophy protein kinase develop a late-onset progressive myopathy. *Nat Genet* 1996;13:325–335.
8. Berul CI, Aronovitz M, Wang PJ, Mendelsohn ME. In vivo cardiac electrophysiology studies in the mouse. *Circulation* 1996;94:2641–2648.
9. Davignon A, Rautaharju P, Boisselle E, et al. Normal ECG standards for infants and children. *Pediatr Cardiol* 1980;2:123–131.
10. Berul CI, Sweeten TL, Dubin AM, et al. Use of the rate-corrected JT interval for prediction of repolarization abnormalities in children. *Am J Cardiol* 1994;74:1254–1257.
11. Zipes DP. Specific arrhythmias: Diagnosis and treatment. In Braunwald E (ed): *Heart Disease: A Textbook of Cardiovascular Medicine*. Philadelphia: WB Saunders Co.; 1992:667–725.
12. Hiss RG, Lamb LE. Electrocardiographic findings in 122,043 individuals. *Circulation* 1962;25:947.
13. Vetter VL. The pediatric electrophysiology study. In Liebman J, Plonsey R, Rudy Y (eds): *Pediatric and Fundamental Electrocardiography*. New York: Martinus Nijhoff; 1985:161–184.
14. Gillette PC, Buckles DS, Harold M, Garson A. Intracardiac electrophysiology studies. In Gillette PC, Garson A (eds): *Pediatric Arrhythmias: Electrophysiology and Pacing*. Philadelphia: WB Saunders Co.; 1990:216–248.
15. Kugler JD. Electrophysiology studies. In Emmanouilides GC, Reimenschneider TA, Allen HD, Gutgesell HP (eds): *Moss and Adams' Heart Disease in Infants, Children, and Adolescents, Including the Fetus and Young Adult*. Baltimore: Williams & Wilkins; 1995:347–366.
16. Seidman CE, Seidman JG. Gene mutations that cause familial hypertrophic cardiomyopathy. In Haber E (ed): *Molecular Cardiovascular Medicine*. New York: Scientific American Press; 1995:193–210.
17. Watkins H, McKenna W, Thierfelder L, et al. Mutations in the genes for cardiac troponin T and α-tropomyosin in hypertrophic cardiomyopathy. *N Engl J Med* 1995;332:1058–1064.
18. Thierfelder L, Watkins H, MacRae C, et al. Mutations in α-tropomyosin and in cardiac troponin T cause hypertrophic cardiomyopathy: A disease of the sarcomere. *Cell* 1994;77:701–712.
19. Watkins H, Anan R, Coviello DA, et al. A de novo mutation in α-tropomyosin that causes hypertrophic cardiomyopathy. *Circulation* 1995;91:2302–2305.
20. Fananapazir L, Chang AC, Epstein SE, McAreavy D. Prognostic determinants in hypertrophic cardiomyopathy: Prospective evaluation of a therapeutic strategy based on clinical, Holter, hemodynamic, and electrophysiological findings. *Circulation* 1992;86:730–740.
21. Epstein ND, Cohn GM, Cyran F, Fananapazir L. Differences in clinical expression of hypertrophic cardiomyopathy associated with two distinct mutations in β-myosin heavy chain gene. *Circulation* 1992;86:345–352.
22. Buja G, Miorelli M, Turrini P, et al. Comparison of QT dispersion in hypertrophic cardiomyopathy between patients with and without ventricular arrhythmias and sudden death. *Am J Cardiol* 1993;72:973–976.
23. Wigle ED, Rakowski H, Kimball BP, Williams WG. Hypertrophic cardiomyopathy: Clinical spectrum and treatment. *Circulation* 1995;92:1680–1692.

24. Fananapazir L, Epstein SE. Hemodynamic and electrophysiologic evaluation of patients with hypertrophic cardiomyopathy surviving cardiac arrest. *Am J Cardiol* 1991;67:280–287.
25. Maron BJ, Fananapazir L. Sudden cardiac death in hypertrophic cardiomyopathy. *Circulation* 1992;85:I57–I63.
26. Watson RM, Schwartz JL, Maron BJ, et al. Inducible polymorphic ventricular tachycardia and ventricular fibrillation in a subgroup of patients with hypertrophic cardiomyopathy at risk for sudden death. *J Am Coll Cardiol* 1987;10:761–774.
27. Solomon SD, Wolff S, Watkins H, et al. Left ventricular hypertrophy and morphology in familial hypertrophic cardiomyopathy associated with mutations of the beta-myosin heavy chain gene. *J Am Coll Cardiol* 1993;22:498–505.
28. Spirito P, Rapezzi C, Autore C, et al. Prognosis of asymptomatic patients with hypertrophic cardiomyopathy and nonsustained ventricular tachycardia. *Circulation* 1994;90:2743–2747.
29. McKenna WJ, Sadoul N, Slade AKB, Saumarez RC. The prognostic significance of nonsustained ventricular tachycardia in hypertrophic cardiomyopathy. *Circulation* 1994;90:3115–3117.
30. Watkins H, Rosenzweig A, Hwang D, et al. Characteristics and prognostic implications of myosin missense mutations in familial hypertrophic cardiomyopathy. *N Engl J Med* 1992;326:1108–1114.
31. Cannon CR, Reeder GS, Bailey KR, et al. Natural history of hypertrophic cardiomyopathy: A population-based study, 1976 though 1990. *Circulation* 1995;92:2488–2495.
32. Geisterfer-Lowrance A, Christe M, Conner D, et al. A mouse model of familial hypertrophic cardiomyopathy. *Science* 1996;272:731–734.
33. Berul CI, Christe ME, Aronovitz MJ, et al. Electrophysiological abnormalities and arrhythmias in αMHC mutant familial hypertrophic cardiomyopathy mice. *J Clin Invest* 1997;99:274–280.
34. Durand JB, Abchee AB, Roberts R. Molecular and clinical aspects of inherited cardiomyopathies. *Ann Med* 1995;27:311–317.
35. Michels VV, Moll PP, Miller FA, et al. The frequency of familial dilated cardiomyopathy in a series of patients with idiopathic dilated cardiomyopathy. *N Engl J Med* 1992;326:77–82.
36. Olson TM, Keating MT. Mapping a cardiomyopathy locus to chromosome 3p22–25. *J Clin Invest* 1996;97:528–532.
37. Norris JD, Fan DJ, Wagner BL, McDonnell DP. Identification of the sequences within the human complement 3 promoter required for estrogen responsiveness provides insight into the mechanism of tamoxifen mixed agonist activity. *Mol Endocrinol* 1996;10:1605–1616.
38. Durand JB, Bachinski LL, Beling LC, et al. Localization of a gene responsible for familial dilated cardiomyopathy to chromosome 1q32. *Circulation* 1995;92:3387–3389.
39. Ozawa T. Mitochondrial DNA mutations in myocardial disease. *Eur Heart J* 1995;16:10–14.
40. Remes AM, Hassinen IE, Ikaheimo MJ, et al. Mitochondrial DNA deletions in dilated cardiomyopathy: A clinical study employing endomyocardial sampling. *J Am Coll Cardiol* 1994;23:935–942.
41. Milasin J, Muntoni F, Severini GM, et al. A point mutation in the 5' splice site of the dystrophin gene first intron responsible for X-linked dilated cardiomyopathy. *Hum Mol Genet* 1996;5:73–79.
42. Gedeon AK, Wilson MJ, Colley AC, et al. X-linked fatal infantile

cardiomyopathy maps to Xq28 and is possibly allelic to Barth syndrome. *J Med Genet* 1995;32:383–388.

43. Arber S, Hunter JJ, Ross J Jr, et al. MPL-deficient mice exhibit a disruption of cardiac cytoarchitectural organization, dilated cardiomyopathy, and heart failure. *Cell* 1997;88:393–398.
44. Roden D, Lazzara MR, Rosen M, et al, and SADS Foundation Task Force on LQTS. Multiple mechanisms in the long-QT syndrome: Current knowledge, gaps, and future directions. *Circulation* 1996;94:1996–2012.
45. Towbin JA, Hua L, Taggart T, et al. Evidence of genetic heterogeneity in Romano-Ward long QT syndrome. *Circulation* 1994;90:2635–2644.
46. Tanaka T, Nagai R, Tomoike H, et al. Four novel *KVLQT1* and four novel *HERG* mutations in familial long-QT syndrome. *Circulation* 1997;95: 565–567.
47. Yu Y, Yamabe H, Fujita J, et al. Cardiac involvement in a family with Becker muscular dystrophy. *Intern Med* 1995;34:919–923.
48. Housman DE, Shaw DJ. Expansion of an unstable DNA region and phenotypic variation in myotonic dystrophy. *Nature* 1992;355:545–546.
49. Marian A J, Roberts R. Molecular basis of hypertrophic and dilated cardiomyopathy. *Texas Heart Inst J* 1994;21:6–15.
50. Berul CI, Reddy S, Aronovitz MJ, et al. Atrioventricular conduction abnormalities in a mouse model of myotonic dystrophy. *PACE* 1997;20:1101.
51. Saffitz JE, Davis LM, Darrow BJ, et al. The molecular basis of anisotrophy: Role of gap junctions. *J Cardiovasc Electrophysiol* 1995;6:498–510.
52. Davis LM, Kanter HL, Beyer EC, Saffitz JE. Distinct gap junction protein phenotypes in cardiac tissues with disparate conduction properties. *J Am Coll Cardiol* 1994;24:1124–1132.
53. Peters NS, Severs NJ, Rothery SM, et al. Spatiotemporal relation between gap junctions and fascia adherens junctions during postnatal development of human ventricular myocardium. *Circulation* 1994;90:713–725.
54. Reaume AG, deSousa PA, Kulkarni S, et al. Cardiac malformation in neonatal mice lacking connexin43. *Science* 1995;267:1831–1834.
55. Britz-Cunningham SH, Shah MM, Zuppan CW, Fletcher WH. Mutations of the connexin43 gap junction gene in patients with heart malformations and defects of laterality. *N Engl J Med* 1995;332:1323–1329.
56. Gebbia M, Towbin JA, Casey B. Failure to detect connexin43 mutations in 38 cases of sporadic and familial heterotaxy. *Circulation* 1996;94: 1909–1912.
57. Berul CI, Thomas SA, Aronovitz MJ, et al. Ventricular conduction abnormalities in heterozygous connexin 43 mutant mice. *Circulation* 1997;96: I673. Abstract.
58. Chien KR, Walter B. Cannon award lecture: Cardiac muscle diseases in genetically engineered mice—the evolution of molecular physiology. *Am J Physiol* 1995;269:H753–H766.

28

The Cardiac Conduction System in Sudden Death in Athletes

Saroja Bharati, MD

Although death may occur suddenly in the athlete, very little attention has been given to the study of the conduction system pathologically.[1] The study of the conduction system will be useful in the long run, especially in athletes who die suddenly with or without a previous history of arrhythmias. This chapter therefore deals with the pathologic findings in the conduction system in athletes who died suddenly. These findings are then compared with the findings in the conduction system in Alaskan sled dogs who died suddenly during the Iditarod race.

A study of the conduction system is mandatory in cases of sudden death in athletes, especially when death occurs during the sports activity or during training. It is presumed that the obvious cardiac and/or noncardiac causes of sudden death, as well as those found in the toxicological examination have been ruled out, and that despite a very thorough examination at postmortem including the microscopic findings at the light level, the cause of death could not be determined. It is then presumed that the death could be an arrhythmic event. Under these conditions, every attempt should be made to study the conduction system. It is also emphasized that a very careful gross anatomic examination may, in some cases, also give a clue as to the abnormalities that may be found

From Estes NAM, Salem DN, Wang PJ (eds). *Sudden Cardiac Death in the Athlete.* Armonk, NY: Futura Publishing Co., Inc.; ©1998.

in the conduction system. Thus, a detailed gross examination of the heart pertaining to the conduction system should be done first.[1,2]

Gross Examination of the Heart Relating to the Conduction System

The heart size, the chamber sizes, the wall thickness, the thickness of the ventricular septum, and the sizes of all of the four valves are taken and compared with those of a similar age group. In addition, special attention is given to: (1) The sinoatrial (SA) nodal area and its approaches, that is, at the junction of the superior vena cava as it enters the right atrial cavity. This includes the sulcus terminalis, the posterior crest, and the crista terminalis. (2) The atrial preferential pathways. This includes the atrial septum, the superior parietal wall, as well as the inferior wall close to the inferior vena cava. (3) The size and location of the coronary sinus and a left superior vena cava, if present, is noted. (4) The sizes and the location of the eustachian valve, thebesian valve, and other remnants of the sinus venarum valves in the atria. (5) The anatomy of the tricuspid, the aortic, and the mitral valves. (6) The membranous part of the atrioventricular (AV) septum. (7) The summit of the ventricular septum, including the right and the left sides.

What is the Conduction System?

The conduction system, although in a broad sense includes the entire heart, in a limited sense comprises the following: the SA node and its approaches, the atrial preferential pathways, the approaches to the AV node, the AV node, the AV bundle including the penetrating, branching, and the bifurcating portions, and the bundle branches up to the peripheral Purkinje network. In order to appreciate the pathologic and/or anatomic abnormalities in the conduction system, it is obvious that one should first understand the normal anatomy of the conduction system. This is dealt with briefly as follows.[3-7]

Normal Conduction System[3-13]

Sinoatrial Node and Its Approaches

The SA node is situated in the epicardial region of the sulcus terminalis, between the superior vena cava and the right atrial appendage. It is closely related to the Bachmann's bundle, the posterior crest including the crista terminalis, and the pectinate musculature of the right atrial appendage. At the light microscopic level, histologically (Figure 1), the node consists of small fusiform cells that are smaller than the remainder of the atrial cells and are arranged in a more or less serpiginous fashion with a tendency toward longitudinality along the course of the posterior crest and the crista terminalis. The cytoplasm stains lighter than the ordinary atrial cells. There is a large amount of elastic and collagenous tissue, distinctly more than the surrounding atrial myocardium in the node. The node more or less merges with the surrounding atrial myocardium by means of ordinary or working-type atrial cells. However, at the junctional areas there may be transitional cells. There is a distinct SA nodal artery within the substance of the node in almost all cases.

The Atrial Preferential Pathways

The entire atrial myocardium more or less forms a pathway for the conduction of impulses from the SA node to the AV node. Although it is believed that preferentially the conduction proceeds along the anterior, middle, and inferior pathways to the approaches to the AV nodal area, it is emphasized that the conduction also proceeds from the SA node anterosuperiorly via the pectinate muscles through the atrial appendage and reaches the anterior or superior pathway or may directly

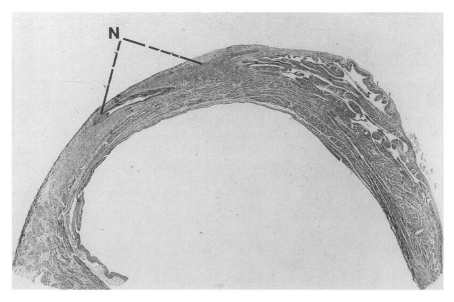

Figure 1. Normal sinoatrial node. Low-power photomicrograph showing the sinoatrial node and its approaches. Hematoxylin-eosin stain ×8. N = sinoatrial node. Reproduced from Reference 10, with permission.

reach the AV nodal area anterosuperiorly. It is likely that impulse transmission may occur faster through the pectinate muscles, since they are smaller (shorter) from the standpoint of size, and numerous from the standpoint of numbers.

The anterior pathway proceeds along the proximal or the upper part of the atrial septum and curves downward toward the AV nodal area. The middle pathway proceeds around the posterior part of the atrium and enters the atrial septum along the limbic margin. This then joins the anterior pathway to reach the superior or the anterior approaches to the AV node. The inferior or the posterior pathway proceeds along the crista terminalis and the inferior vena cava to the lower part of the atrial septum to the coronary sinus area and merges with the posterior approaches to the AV node. These three pathways consist of regular atrial myocardial cells at the light microscopic level. However, they vary in size, shape, and in the connective tissue component. These pathways are not specialized tracts separated by connective tissue from the remainder of the atria at the light microscopic level, but rather consist of wide areas of muscle making up more or less the entire atrial septum. These pathways may exhibit specific functional capabilities at the molecular level.

Approaches to the Atrioventricular Node

This is a wide area that varies considerably from heart to heart. The posterior approaches include the posterior or the inferior part of the right atrium, the posterior and part of the septal leaflet of the tricuspid valve, and the right ventricular aspect of the ventricular septum. The superior approaches include the myocardium from the right atrium, the left atrium, the atrial septum, the central fibrous body, and the mitral valve annulus. The atrial cells in the approaches become somewhat loosely arranged and become smaller than the surrounding atrial myocardial cells. It is again emphasized that the arrangement and the size and shape of the cells vary considerably from one approach to the other, with a distinct increase in elastic and collagen connective tissue, fat, and a fair amount of nerve fibers intermingling with the myocardial cells.

Atrioventricular Node

The AV node is situated in the distal part of the atrial septum between the mouth of the coronary sinus and the septal leaflet of the tricuspid valve. It is related to the right side of the central fibrous body and, in part, to the right side of the ventricular septum. The size and shape varies considerably from heart to heart. In the adult heart, it measures approximately 5 mm to 7 mm in length and 2 mm to 5 mm in width. At a light microscopic level (Figure 2), the cells are arranged in a plexiform

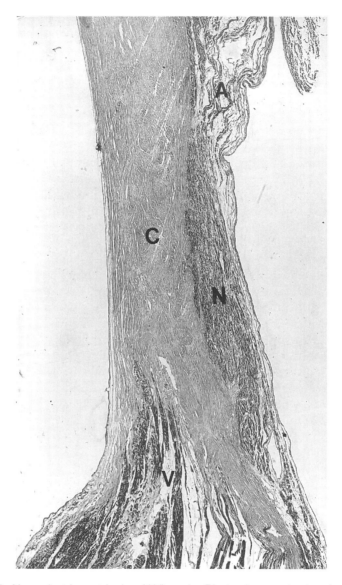

Figure 2. Normal atrioventricular (AV) node. Photomicrograph showing the AV node and its approaches and the summit of the ventricular septum. Hematoxylin-eosin stain ×10. N = AV node; C = central fibrous body; V = summit of the ventricular septum; A = approaches to the AV node. Reproduced from Reference 11, with permission.

manner and are larger than the SA nodal cells; the cytoplasm stains lightly with eosin or picric acid. The AV node also contains greater amounts of elastic and collagenous fibers compared with the atrial and the surrounding ventricular myocardium but lesser than the SA node.

Atrioventricular Bundle, the Penetrating, Branching, and Bifurcating Parts

As it penetrates the central fibrous body, the AV node becomes compact and forms the AV bundle. The AV bundle traverses through the central fibrous body as the penetrating part (Figure 3) and, at the lower margin of the membranous part of the ventricular septum, becomes the branching part. The branching part of the AV bundle is, in general, situated on top of the summit of the ventricular septum and gives off the posterior fibers of the left bundle branch. Thus, the branching part of the AV bundle gives off the posterior fibers of the left bundle branch in a wide fashion and it becomes the bifurcating bundle when it reaches the junction beneath the noncoronary and the right aortic cusp. At this area, the right bundle branch is given off with the remaining portion of the anterior fibers of the left bundle branch. Thus, the penetrating part of the AV bundle is related to the mitral annulus, the central fibrous body, and the AV part of the membranous septum, while the branching part of the AV bundle is related to the membranous part of the ventricular septum, the summit of the ventricular septum and, indirectly, to the base of the aortic valve. Histologically, the cells are arranged in a somewhat longitudinal fashion with some bridging fasciculi between the fibers. The diameter of these cells is the same as that of the cells of the ventricular myocardium, but they are lighter staining.

Left Bundle Branch

The main left bundle branch is given off in a fine, subendocardial fashion before the bifurcating bundle is reached. In general, therefore, the main left bundle branch gives off a larger posterior and a smaller anterior radiation. Both the radiations in general join together, forming a midseptal radiation and distally they end in a plexiform arrangement of Purkinje nets in the apical part of the ventricular myocardium. However, it is emphasized that no two left bundle branches look alike and they vary considerably from heart to heart. At a light microscopic level, as they become the Purkinje cells, the cells of the left bundle branch are larger, with pale, clear cytoplasm and a round or oval nuclei. They contain more elastic tissue than the surrounding ventricular myocardium.

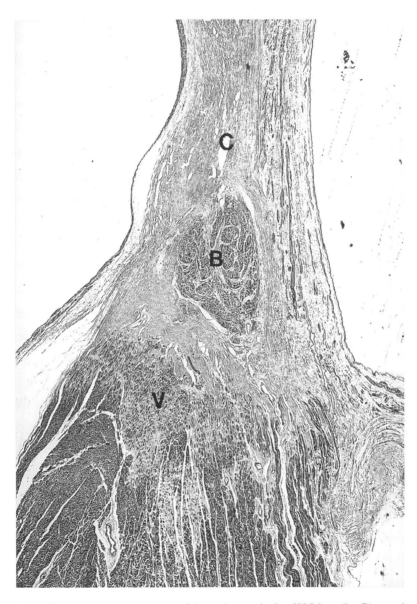

Figure 3. Normal penetrating part of the atrioventricular (AV) bundle. Photomicrograph showing the AV bundle within the central fibrous body. Hematoxylin-eosin stain ×20. B = penetrating AV bundle; C = central fibrous body; V = summit of the ventricular septum. Reproduced from Reference 12, with permission.

Right Bundle Branch

The right bundle branch proceeds from the bifurcating AV bundle along the lower septal band about 1 mm beneath the muscle of Lancisi (conal band) to the moderator band. The right bundle branch is divided into three components. The first and the third parts are subendocardial and, in general, the second part is intramyocardial. Histologically, the cells of the first part of the right bundle branch are the same size as the cells of the branching part of the AV bundle. In the second part, they are more or less the size of the surrounding ventricular myocardial cells, and in the third part they eventually become the Purkinje cells, which are larger than the surrounding ventricular myocardial cells. There is an increase in elastic fibers in the right bundle branch as compared with that of the ventricular myocardial fibers. In general, there is a large space surrounded by mesothelial cells surrounding the AV bundle, and the bundle branches up to the periphery.

The Usefulness of the Anatomy of the Normal Conduction System in Sudden Death

The above description of the normal conduction system is a summary, and readers who want more detailed information are encouraged to refer to our previous detailed studies of this vital system that includes the blood supply, the nerve supply, the other myocardial connections in and around the conduction system, as well as the variations.[1–13] We believe that a fair amount of knowledge of the normal conduction system is indeed essential while evaluating this vital system for congenital abnormalities and/or pathologic changes in sudden death in athletes.

Method of Study of the Conduction System

Blocks are taken from the SA node and its approaches, the atrial preferential pathways, the approaches to the AV node, the AV node, the AV bundle (including all parts), and the bundle branches up to the region of the moderator band and are serially sectioned. Every 20th or 30th section is retained and alternately stained with hematoxylin-eosin and Weigert-van Geison stain. In addition, several sections are taken from the atria and the ventricles from the remainder of the heart. The sections are then compared with those from an age-matched control conduction system.[8–13]

Why Should the Conduction System be Studied in the Above-Described Manner?

The reasons are: (1) the conduction system is in the form of a curve or an arc and is not in a straight line; (2) the conduction system is a relatively small structure and is situated in the strategic part of the heart; (3) various parts of the conduction system cannot be identified by random single sections; (4) it is important that this vital system is followed from the beginning to the end; and (5) the electrocardiogram represents the function of the conduction system and the entire heart. Therefore, it is obvious that a meaningful, semiquantitative analysis of the conduction system can only be accomplished by the above method of study.[8–13]

Conduction System in Sudden Death in Athletes

If the conduction system is examined in the above-described manner, one may find abnormal findings in the form of either congenital and/or acquired pathologic changes to a varying degree in the various parts of this system, such as: (1) the SA node and its approaches; (2) the atrial preferential pathways, the approaches to the AV node, and the AV node; (3) the AV bundle (the penetrating, the branching, and the bifurcating portions); (4) the bundle branches; and (5) the summit of the ventricular septum.[1] In this chapter, the emphasis is given *only* to the findings in the conduction system and the surrounding myocardium that are seen at the light microscopic level, which we believe may form an anatomic substrate for sudden death.

We examined the conduction system in 14 athletes who died suddenly. All were males, aged 14 to 47 years. The heart was hypertrophied and enlarged in all. An example of abnormal anatomic and/or pathologic findings related to the specific parts of the conduction system such as the SA node and its approaches, the AV node and its approaches, the AV bundle, the bundle branches, and the ventricular septum are discussed briefly. The interested reader may refer to the original work published previously.[1,14–17]

The Sinoatrial Node and Its Approaches

A 22-year-old black football player collapsed suddenly. He was found to have seizure, the carotid pulse was 56 bpm, and the initial monitor showed sinus bradycardia with wide QRS complexes. The heart weighed 380 grams. The conduction system revealed two SA nodes separated by ordinary atrial myocardium and fatty infiltration (Figure 4, panel A). One SA node was larger than the other and both were supplied by separate SA nodal arteries. The larger SA node had the smaller blood vessel and the smaller SA node had the larger blood supply. In addition to the above obvious congenital anomaly, there were chronic inflammatory cells in the approaches to the SA node (Figure 4, panel B). The AV node was situated close to the aorta, with marked fatty infil-

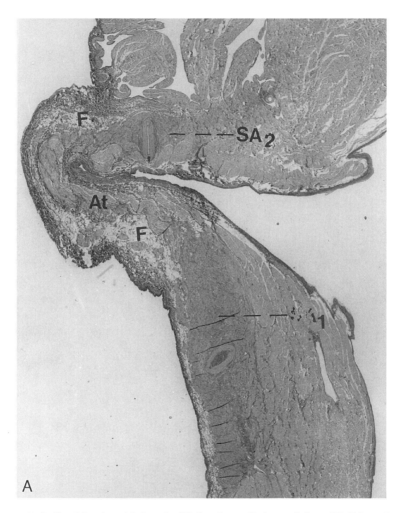

Figure 4. A. Double sinoatrial node. Weigert-van Geison stain ×12. SA_1 = larger sinoatrial node; SA_2 = smaller sinoatrial node; At = atrial muscle; F = fat. Reproduced from Reference 1, with permission. **B.** Accumulation of mononuclear cells in the approaches to the sinoatrial (SA) node. Hematoxylin-eosin stain ×25. A = approaches to the SA node. Arrows point to the accumulation of mononuclear cells. Reproduced from Reference 2, with permission.

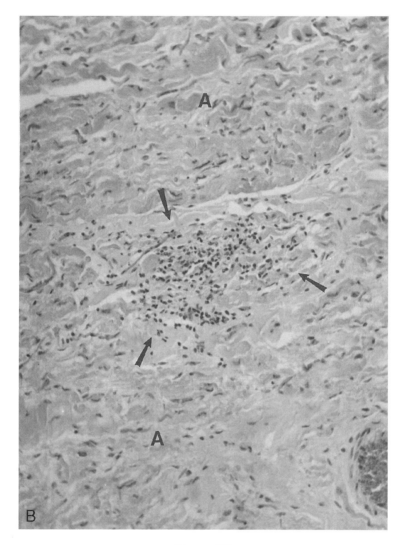

Figure 4B.

tration in and around the node with partial separation of the node from the surrounding atrial myocardium. Both the bundle branches revealed moderate to marked fibrosis.[1]

The function of the double SA node is unknown today. It is tempting, however, to hypothesize that both of the SA nodes may function alternately as the pacemaker and/or may inadvertently compete at times with each other; and during the latter, perhaps may create a reentry phenomenon or any other mechanism that may in turn produce varying types of arrhythmias, resulting in sudden death. The etiology of the chronic inflammatory cells in the approaches to the SA node and their functional significance is not known today.

The Atrioventricular Node and Its Approaches

A 34-year-old competitive bicyclist who, since the age of 12 and throughout his adulthood, had participated in bicycling competition, collapsed suddenly while cycling through a downtown area in preparation for a race.[1] He was found to be in coarse ventricular fibrillation and could not be resuscitated. The heart weighed 510 grams.

Histologically, the AV node was within the tricuspid valve annulus (Figure 5). The AV bundle was left sided and there was patchy fibrosis on the left side of the ventricular septum. Here again we are confronted with congenital and acquired pathologic changes in the conduction system. The congenital anomaly is the AV node situated in the tricuspid valve annulus with a left-sided AV bundle, and the acquired changes include the fibrotic, patchy areas in the ventricular septum. Thus, the AV node was practically isolated from the surrounding atrial myocardium—isolated from the superior and inferior approaches and obviously from the superior, mid, and inferior preferential pathways. We therefore hypothesize that the node situated within the tricuspid valve annulus may be subjected to the movement of the tricuspid valve, which may affect the function of the AV node. Further, the slowing of the conduction and organization of the impulses as they reach the AV node may be impeded to a varying degree that may promote a reentry type of an arrhythmic mechanism or some other type of a mechanism yet to be elucidated, resulting in premature ventricular contractions, which in turn may degenerate into ventricular tachycardia, fibrillation, and sudden death. The causes of the acquired fibrotic scars in the various parts of ventricular septum are unknown today. This may represent an end result of a previous myocarditis and/or an autoimmune reaction related to some foreign material during the athlete's life. On the other hand, could the fibrotic scars indeed represent the end result of athletic training?

Pathologic Findings in the Atrioventricular Bundle, Penetrating Portion, and Branching Portion

An athletic 14-year-old boy who practiced many sports complained of chest pains while playing soccer and collapsed and could not be resuscitated. The heart weighed 475 grams. The mitral valve was some-

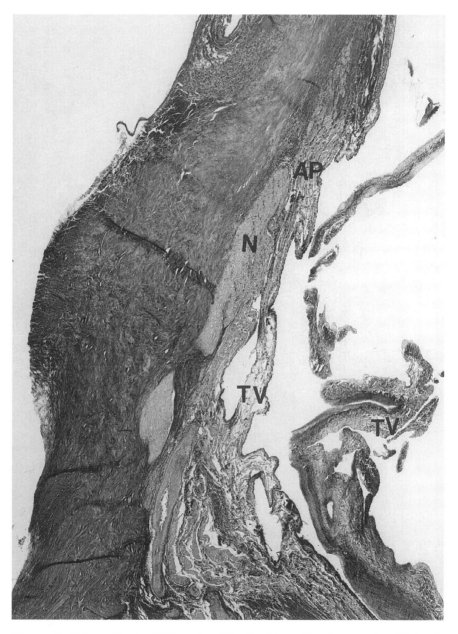

Figure 5. Atrioventricular (AV) node within the tricuspid valve annulus. Weigert-van Geison stain ×17. N = AV node; AP = approaches to the AV node; TV = tricuspid valve. Reproduced from Reference 1, with permission.

what floppy (moderate nature) with fibroelastic thickening beneath the aortic valve.[1]

Histologically, there was a left atrial His bundle connection, also called the atrio-Hisian connection (Figure 6, panel A). The bundle was

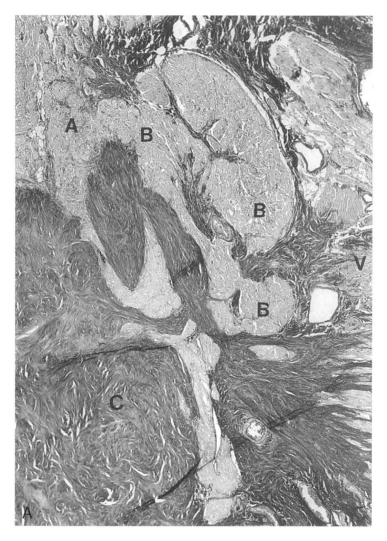

Figure 6. A. Atrio-Hisian connection with marked lobulation of the bundle of His. Weigert-van Geison stain ×45. A = atrial musculature; C = central fibrous body; V = ventricular septum; B = bundle. **B.** Left-sided branching bundle with minimal fibrosis and focal fibrotic scar areas in the left side of the ventricular septum. Weigert-van Geison stain ×22.5. B = branching bundle; V = ventricular septum; Fi = focal fibrotic scar areas. Figures **A** and **B** reproduced from Reference 1, with permission.

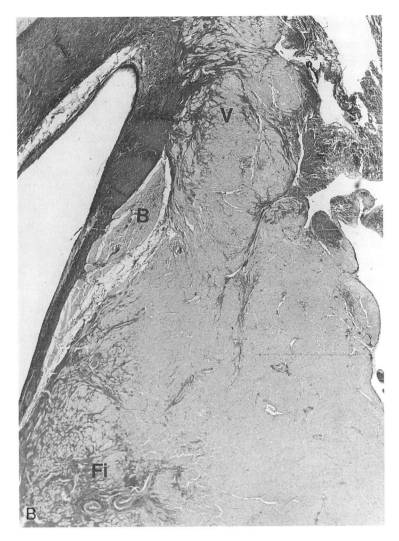

Figure 6B.

markedly septated and the branching bundle was distinctly situated on the left ventricular aspect a considerable distance away from the summit of the septum. In addition, there were focal fibrotic scar areas at the midpart of the septum on the left side (Figure 6, panel B). There was also epicarditis of the SA nodal area and the bundle branches revealed fibrosis.[1]

Similar to the previously described two cases, here we are confronted with both congenital and acquired pathologic changes in and around the conduction system. The congenital anomalies were the atrio-

Hisian connection, the septated AV bundle, and the left-sided branching bundle. The acquired changes were epicarditis in the SA node and its approaches, focal fibrotic scar areas in the ventricular septum, especially on the left side, with fibrosis of the bundle branches. An atrio-Hisian connection may promote a reentry or any other mechanism that may result in ventricular tachycardia and fibrillation. Likewise, the impulse conduction may be slowed at the junction of the fibrotic scar areas with the healthy myocardium, thereby forming a milieu for an arrhythmic event. The arrhythmic event may initially be in the form of a premature ventricular contraction that may proceed to ventricular tachycardia and fibrillation, especially during an altered physiologic state, and may result in sudden death. What are the causes for the epicarditis in the SA node and the fibrotic areas in the ventricular septum?

Pathologic Findings in the Atrioventricular Bundle and the Ventricular Septum on the Left Ventricular Aspect: Atypical Hypertrophic Cardiomyopathy?

A 25-year-old athlete collapsed suddenly while playing basketball, was found to be in ventricular fibrillation, and could not be resuscitated. The heart weighed 725 grams. The mitral valve was thickened and nodular. On the summit of the ventricular septum there was an irregular, thickened, fibroelastic ridge that extended from the anterior part of the ventricular septum to the aortic mitral annulus (Figure 7A). The fibroelastic plaque on the summit of the ventricular septum corresponded to the movement of the anterior leaflet of the mitral valve and also involved the region of the AV bundle and the left bundle branch fibers. In addition, there were several scars in the ventricular walls (Figure 7A).[1]

Histologically, there was a generalized epicarditis and neuritis of the SA node, with considerable amount of fibrosis and fat in an around it. The AV node was entrapped within the central fibrous body and most of it was situated within the atrial septum. There was marked fibrosis, lobulation and loop formation of AV bundle, and the bifurcating bundle revealed fibrosis, linear formation, and fatty infiltration affecting both the right and the left bundle branches. Further down, the left bundle branch fibers were replaced by space formation with distinct fibroelastosis in the endocardium. In addition, there were focal fibrotic scars in the ventricular septum (Figure 7B).[1]

Although the left ventricle was hypertrophied and enlarged, this is not a classic case of hypertrophic cardiomyopathy. On the other hand, there were distinct pathologic findings corresponding to the anterior movement of the mitral valve, thereby indicating that the movement of the mitral valve was probably abnormal, which suggests that

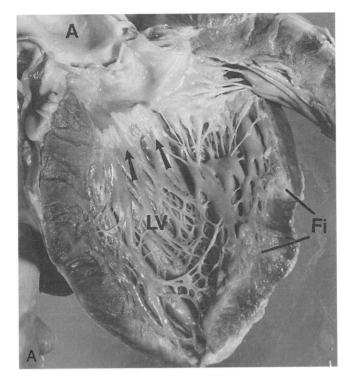

Figure 7A. Left ventricular outflow tract demonstrating the irregular fibroelastic ridge and thickening beneath the aortic valve corresponding to the movement of the anterior leaflet of the mitral valve and fibrotic scar areas in the left ventricular wall. LV = left ventricle; A = aorta; FI = fibrotic scar areas in the left ventricle. Arrows point to the irregular fibroelastic ridge in the summit of the ventricular septum beneath the aortic valve. Reproduced from Reference 2, with permission.

this may indeed be a variant form of hypertrophic cardiomyopathy. This was associated with marked focal fibrotic scars in the ventricular septum as well as the ventricular walls. It is well known that focal fibrotic scar areas at the junction with the healthy myocardium may give rise to delayed depolarization, thereby forming a milieu for a reentry phenomenon that may progress into ventricular tachycardia and further degenerate into ventricular fibrillation, resulting in sudden death. In addition to the above acquired changes, the AV node was situated within the central fibrous body. This is a congenital anomaly. Entrapment of the AV node within the atrial septum is frequently seen in cases of sudden death in the young and the healthy. It is also of interest that focal accumulation of mononuclear cells was again noted in the approaches to the SA node. However, it is not known why and when this occurred. What is its role in sudden death?

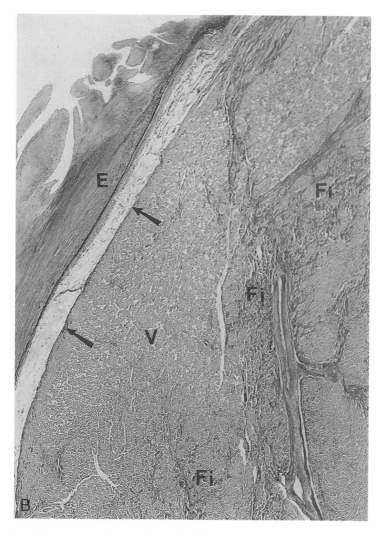

Figure 7B. Photomicrograph of the fibroelastic ridge shown in **A** pressing on the left bundle branch with almost total loss of left bundle branch fibers. Note the empty space and linear strands where the left bundle branch fibers should have been. Weigert-van Geison stain ×13. E = fibroelastic endocardial ridge corresponding to that shown in Figure 8; V = ventricular myocardium; Fi = scattered focal areas of fibrosis of the left ventricle. Arrows point to the empty space where the left bundle branch fibers should have been. Reproduced from Reference 1, with permission.

Conduction System in Athletically Trained Individuals with Familial Tendency to Sudden Death or Known Arrhythmias

Do the pathologic findings in the conduction system differ in athletically trained individuals or athletes with a familial tendency to sudden death and/or with known arrhythmias or diseases? In order to answer this question a few cases are illustrated here.

Familial Tendency to Sudden Death: Probable Hypertrophic Cardiomyopathy Affecting the Right Side of the Ventricular Septum

An apparently healthy, athletically trained 15-year-old boy died suddenly while swimming.[1,14] He had a family history of sudden death involving three consecutive generations, including a brother. The patient had a history of exercise-related syncope for which he was treated with nadolol. However, he was cleared to play sports. The heart weighed 333 grams with a right ventricular hypertrophy immediately beneath the septal leaflet of the tricuspid valve. The pulmonic valve was quadricuspid.

Histologically, the infundibular (the conal) muscle pressed on the penetrating part of the AV bundle, producing a distinct pressure hypertrophy. The right ventricular septal hypertrophy proceeded considerably up to the region where the AV bundle gave off the posterior radiation of the left bundle branch fibers (Figure 8). There was fibrosis and fatty infiltration of the penetrating and branching bundle, with distinct linear space formation and fatty metamorphosis within the left bundle branch fibers (Figure 8). The ventricular septum revealed arteriolosclerosis, fat, fibrosis, and linear formation. This extended up to the region of the bifurcating bundle involving the beginning of the right bundle branch and the anterior-most radiation of the left bundle branch fibers.

Because of the familial history of sudden death, one may hypothesize that there is a genetic tendency as such for sudden death. The genetic tendency may manifest in the abnormal formation and development of the conduction system including the summit of the ventricular septum. Thus, one may theorize that the infundibular myocardium of the right ventricle and/or the AV junctional area including the central fibrous body, the membranous septum, the main part of the ventricular septum, and the infundibular septum are predisposed to a genetic abnormality in the formation as well as the de-

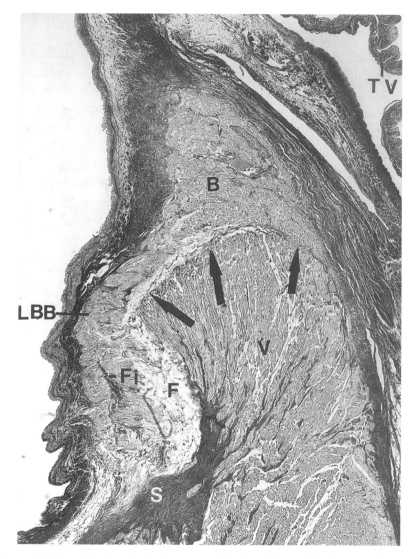

Figure 8. Branching bundle being pressed by the right ventricular septal muscle at the region of the posterior radiation of the left bundle branch. Weigert-van Geison stain ×22.5. B = branching bundle; LBB = posterior radiation of the left bundle branch; F = fat; FI = fibrous and linear change in the left bundle branch; V = summit of the ventricular septum, right side; S = increased sclerosis of the mid-septal region; TV = tricuspid valve. Arrows point to the pressure of the right ventricular septal muscle on the branching bundle at the level of the posterior radiation of the left bundle branch. Reproduced from Reference 14, with permission.

velopment. Since the AV bundle is intimately associated with all of the above structures, the bundle likewise may also be genetically predisposed to abnormal formation and development and/or affected by the surrounding abnormalities. Thus, all of the above abnormalities, or in any combination, may form a milieu for an arrhythmic event that may be precipitated during exercise. It is also conceivable that the right ventricular septal hypertrophy may indeed be genetically related to the classic hypertrophic cardiomyopathy seen predominantly on the left side.

History of Arrhythmias

Right Ventricular Premature Contractions

A 15-year-old boy was known to have had right ventricular premature contractions for a number of years but was totally asymptomatic. He suddenly collapsed while playing soccer.[1,15] The heart weighed 300 grams.

The SA node was markedly infiltrated with fat and was almost isolated from the surrounding atrial myocardium (Figure 9). There was moderate fibrosis of the right and left bundle branch fibers. In addition, the ventricular septum, especially on the right side, revealed focal fibrotic scar areas.

It is obvious that impulse conduction may be impeded at the junctional areas between the healthy myocardium and the fibrotic scar and may cause slowing of the conduction, promoting a reentry mechanism or any other mechanism for the development of an arrhythmic event and sudden death. Do the focal fibrotic scar areas represent an end result of a previous myocarditis? Or are they the end result of a myocardial reaction to repeated right ventricular premature contractions this young boy had? Or do they represent, at least to some extent, the end result of athletic training as such?

Sinus Bradycardia →First–Degree AV Block →Type I Second–Degree Block

A 47-year-old, extremely active, totally asymptomatic, trained jogger was found dead in bed.[1,16] He had a history of sinus bradycardia with first-degree AV block for 8 years and type I second-degree block for 5 years prior to death. A permanent pacemaker was implanted and he was apparently in good health and maintained his strenuous jogging program until he died suddenly. The sudden death occurred 3 months following the implantation of the pacemaker. The heart weighed 440 grams.

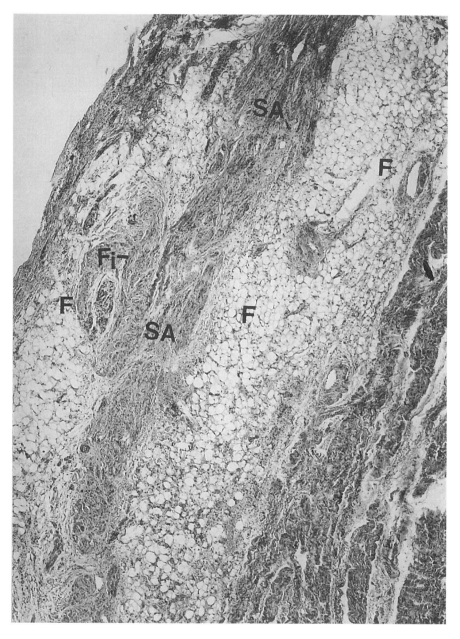

Figure 9. Approaches to the sinoatrial node and the sinoatrial node with marked fatty infiltration and mononuclear cells and fibrosis. Hematoxylin-eosin stain ×45. SA = sinoatrial node; F = fat; Fi = fibrosis of the SA node. Reproduced from Reference 2, with permission.

Histologically, the AV node was situated toward the left atrial aspect and was totally separated from the surrounding atrial myocardium by fat (Figure 10, panel A). There was marked fatty infiltration and moderate fibrosis in the approaches to the SA node, the atrial preferential pathways, and the AV node. The nodo bundle junction revealed mononuclear cell infiltration, fat, disarray, and areas of fibrosis. There was arteriolosclerosis of the ventricular septum with focal fibrotic scar areas. In addition, the left bundle branch revealed varying amounts of fibrosis (Figure 10, panel B).

Thus, pathologically, the AV node was not only situated on the left atrial aspect but practically had no continuity with the surrounding atrial myocardium. This is what we would call a lack of connection between the atria and the peripheral conduction system. This abnormality probably caused the first-degree AV block and eventually the type I second-degree block. Fundamentally, this was an abnormal location of the AV node and its discontinuity from the surrounding atrial myocardium with acquired changes in the nodo bundle junction as well as in the surrounding atrial myocardium. In addition, there was disarray of the AV bundle and fibrosis on the summit of the ventricular septum. The sudden death may be attributed to any one of the above findings or in any one of the above combinations.

In summary, it appears that athletically trained individuals with a familial tendency to sudden death or with a history of known arrhythmias do present significant pathologic findings in the conduction system and in the surrounding myocardium when compared with the findings in athletes without a history of arrhythmias or other known diseases.

The above data therefore suggest that when death occurs suddenly in athletes, there are significant congenital or acquired pathologic findings in the conduction system, the summit of the ventricular septum, and/or the surrounding myocardium to a varying degree, and these findings may form a milieu for an arrhythmic event that may promote a reentry mechanism or any other mechanism resulting in ventricular tachycardia, ventricular fibrillation, and sudden death.

The Athlete's Heart and the Acquired Changes

We are still perplexed with the question about the acquired pathologic findings such as mononuclear cells, fat, and fibrosis that are seen practically in all hearts in the conduction system and the myocardium to a varying degree. This raises the question as to whether these are indeed related, at least to some extent, to athletic training in some (genetically predisposed?).

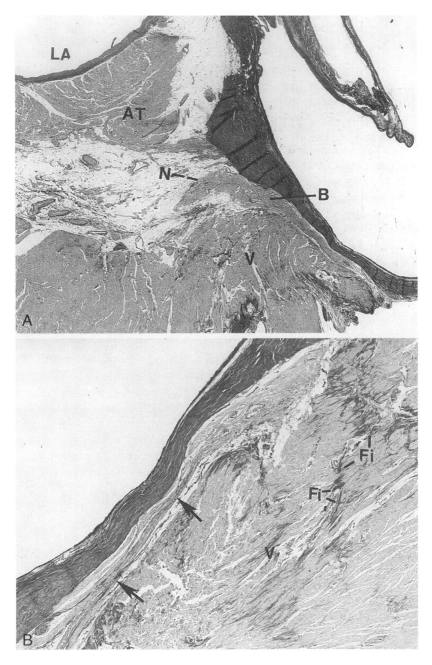

Figure 10. A. Oblique horizontal section through the atrioventricular (AV) node and the bundle of His. Weigert-van Geison stain ×9.7. AT = atrial septum; V = ventricular septum; N = AV node; B = bundle of His; LA = left atrial cavity. Reproduced from Reference 1, with permission. **B.** Photomicrograph showing the endocardial fibroelastosis, fibrosis of the midpart of the left bundle branch, and focal fibrotic scars in the ventricular myocardium. V = ventricular myocardium; FI = fibrosis. Arrows point to the fibrosis of the left bundle branch.

It is very likely that the focal fibrotic scars in the myocardium played a role in sudden death. It is, however, not clear what role the mononuclear cell infiltration, especially in the approaches to the SA node and the SA node, might have played in the sudden demise of these athletes. Is this a peculiar type of a focal myocarditis? Or, do they represent an allergic reaction to some foreign material the athlete might have encountered in the past? The findings are not sufficient enough to call it a myocarditis, but nevertheless they cannot be ignored and they require further research.

Conduction System Findings in Sudden Death: Human Athletes Versus Alaskan Sled Dogs

Are the acquired pathologic findings in the conduction system unique to human athletes? Do such changes occur in well-trained Alaskan sled dogs who might die suddenly during the Iditarod race or during training? In order to answer the above questions, we studied the conduction system of these well-trained and conditioned dogs to determine whether there are any pathologic findings in the conduction system and the surrounding myocardium and, if present, whether the findings are similar to the findings in the conduction system in sudden death in human athletes. The conduction systems of five Alaskan sled dogs who died suddenly, either during the Iditarod race or during training, were compared with the conduction systems of three sled dogs of similar age who died of other causes unrelated to the cardiovascular system.[17]

Findings in the Conduction System in Sudden Death in Alaskan Sled Dogs During the Iditarod Race or During Training Versus the Control Sled Dogs

The control group revealed mild fibro-fatty changes in the conduction system (Figure 11, panel A and Figure 12, panel A) *without fibrotic scar* in the ventricular myocardium.[17] In contrast to the control group, the conduction systems of sled dogs who died suddenly revealed marked fibrosis in the approaches and/or in the SA node with narrowing of the SA nodal artery in 3, fibrosis and fatty infiltration in the approaches and within the AV node in all, with almost total isolation of the AV node from its approaches by fat in 4 (Figure 11, panel B), fibrosis and fat to a varying degree in the AV bundle (Figure 12, panel B) and bundle branches in all, and focal fibrotic scars in the left ventricle with or without fat or disarray in 3 (Figure 13).[17]

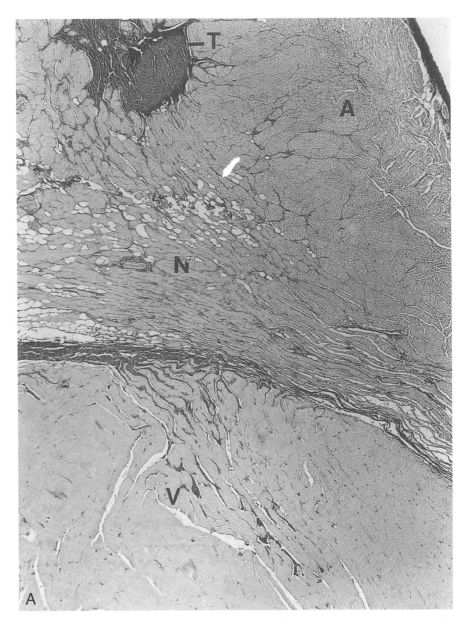

Figure 11. Comparison of the atrioventricular (AV) node and its approaches from **(A)** a normal control sled dog who died of natural causes with **(B)** an Alaskan sled dog who died suddenly during the race. Weigert-van Geison stain ×45 in control animal and ×24 in the sudden death dog. Note the marked fat in and around the AV node with thickening and narrowing of the small vessel in sudden death dog. N = AV node; T = tendon of Todaro; A = approaches to the node; V = summit of the ventricular septum; F = marked fat in and around the node. Arrows point to marked thickening of the small vessel. Reproduced from Reference 17, with permission.

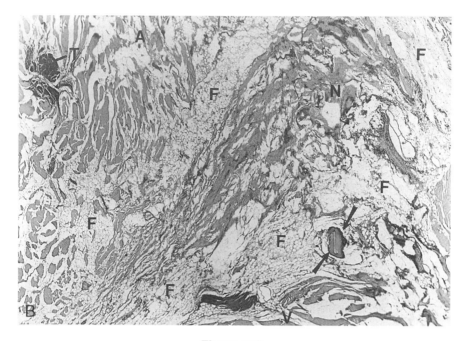

Figure 11B.

Are There Differences in the Conduction System in the Human and the Alaskan Sled Dog?

Similar to the human athletes, there is increase in fat in the vital parts of the conduction system in the Alaskan sled dogs. The marked fatty infiltration in and around the conduction system in the sled dogs may indeed be related at least to some extent to the increase in fat intake by the dogs as a part of preparation for the race. On the other hand, the focal fibrotic scar areas in the ventricular septum with or without fat and disarray of the myocardium may be related at least in part to the aging of the dog and/or to hypertrophy of the ventricular mass. Or, do these changes reflect the end result of chronic ischemic episodes of a hypertrophied heart? These findings likewise are similar to those seen in the human athletes. On the other hand, focal fibrotic scars in the left ventricle *were not present* in the control sled dogs.

Although at the light microscopic level the fat and fibrous tissue are the common denominators in both the human and the sled dog, *the findings are not identical* and the differences in these structures at the molecular level should be explored in the future.

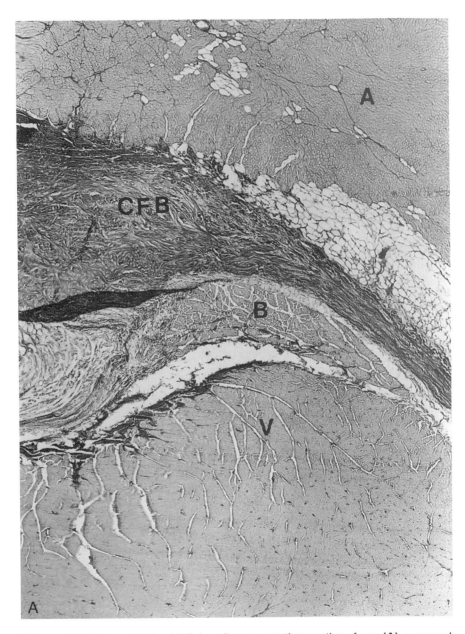

Figure 12. Atrioventricular (AV) bundle, penetrating portion, from **(A)** a normal control sled dog and **(B)** a sled dog who died during the Iditarod race. Weigert-van Geison stain ×45. CFB = central fibrous body; A = superior approaches to the node; F = fat; B = penetrating AV bundle; V = ventricular septum; CA = cartilage in the central fibrous body pressing the penetrating bundle. Reproduced from Reference 17, with permission.

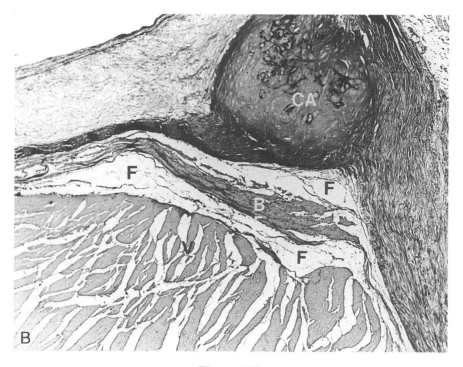

Figure 12B.

The above findings again emphasize the functional significance of fat and fibrosis in and around the conduction system that may be responsible for arrhythmogenesis and sudden death in athletes during an altered physiologic state. The altered physiologic state was exertional myopathy in one dog that demonstrated high levels of calcium and myoglobin; autopsy revealed acute severe myonecrosis in multiple skeletal muscle groups, pulmonary atelectasis, edema, and mesenteric fat necrosis. However, the early warning signals of exertional myopathy were not detected in this animal during the race. Nevertheless, this had resulted in acute skeletal muscle necrosis, hyperkalemia, ventricular fibrillation, and sudden death.[17] We[1] have previously demonstrated that ventricular tachycardia and fibrillation are the terminal events in almost all cases of sudden death in human athletes.

It is of interest that there *were no* congenital abnormalities of the conduction system in the Alaskan sled dogs, in both the control and the sudden death groups. Likewise, mononuclear cells in and around the SA node were only occasionally seen in the sudden death dogs.

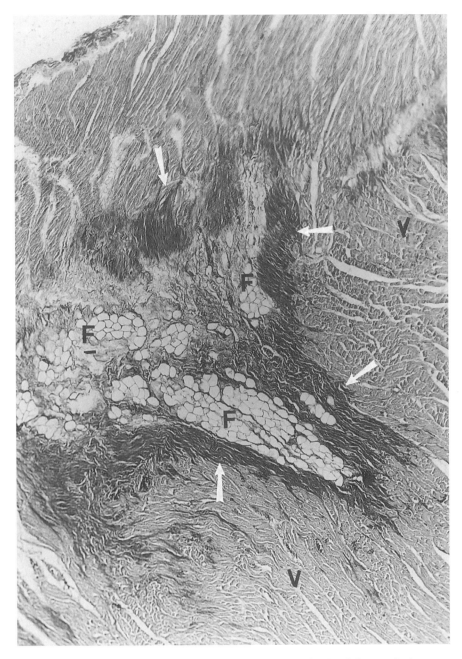

Figure 13. Focal fibrotic scars and fatty infiltration in the left ventricular myocardium in sudden death dog. Weigert-van Geison stain ×45. F = fat; V = ventricular myocardium. Arrows point to the irregular fibrotic scar area in the left ventricular myocardium with marked fatty infiltration. Reproduced from Reference 17, with permission.

Findings in the Conduction System and the Assumed Pathophysiology of Sudden Death in the Athlete

It is clear that the pathologic findings were present in the human athletes as well as in the sled dogs for a considerable period of time. The question, therefore, is why does death occur suddenly during participation in sports?

We hypothesize that the congenital and/or the acquired pathologic findings in the conduction system may indeed remain "silent" for a long time in one's life and may permit a normal life, especially in the athlete. However, during an altered physiologic or metabolic state, the acquired changes and/or the congenital abnormalities of the conduction system and/or the surrounding myocardium may become vulnerable or may promote a reentry mechanism or any other mechanism that may induce an arrhythmic event that may degenerate into ventricular tachycardia, fibrillation, and sudden death. It is also likely that there may be a tendency for sudden death in a genetically abnormally formed conduction system and/or the surrounding myocardium.

References

1. Bharati S, Lev M. *The Cardiac Conduction System in Unexplained Sudden Death.* Mt. Kisco, New York: Futura Publishing Co., Inc.; 1990:1–416.
2. Bharati S, Lev M. Sudden death in athletes—conduction system: Practical approach to dissection and pertinent pathology. *Cardiovasc Pathol* 1994;3:117–127.
3. Bharati S, Lev M. The anatomy of the normal conduction system: Disease-related changes and their relationship to arrhythmogenesis. In Podrid PJ, Kowey PR (eds): *Cardiac Arrhythmias: Mechanism, Diagnosis and Management.* Baltimore, MD: Williams and Wilkins; 1995:1–15.
4. Bharati S, Lev M. The anatomy and pathology of the conduction system. In Samet P, El-Sherif N (eds): *Cardiac Pacing, 2nd Edition.* New York: Grune & Stratton, Inc.; 1980:1–35.
5. Bharati S, Lev M. The anatomy and histology of the conduction system. In Chung EK (ed): *Artificial Cardiac Pacing: Practical Approach, 2nd Edition.* Baltimore, MD: Williams and Wilkins; 1984:12–27.
6. Lev M. The conduction system. In Gould SC (ed): *Pathology of the Heart and Blood Vessels, 3rd Edition.* Springfield, IL: Charles C. Thomas; 1968:180–220.
7. Lev M, Bharati S. Lesions of the conduction system and their functional significance. In Sommers SC (ed): *Pathology Annual, 1974.* New York: Appleton-Century Crofts; 1974;9:157–208.
8. Lev M, Bharati S. A method of study of the pathology of the conduction system for electrocardiographic and His bundle electrogram correlations. *Anat Rec* 1981;201:43–49.
9. Lev M, McMillan JB. A semiquantitative histopathologic method for the study of the entire heart for clinical and electrocardiographic correlations. *Am Heart J* 1959;58:140–158.
10. Lev M, Watne AL. Method for routine histopathologic study of the sinoatrial node. *Arch Pathol* 1954;57:168–177.

11. Lev M, Widran J, Erickson EE. A method for the histopathologic study of the AV node, bundle and branches. *AMA Arch Pathol* 1951;52:73–83.
12. Erickson EE, Lev M. Aging changes in the human atrioventricular node, bundle, and bundle branches. *J Gerontol* 1952;7:1–12.
13. Lev M. Aging changes in the human sinoatrial node. *J Gerontol* 1954;9:1–9.
14. Brookfield L, Bharati S, Denes P, et al. Familial sudden death: Report of a case and review of the literature. *Chest* 1988;94:989–993.
15. Bharati S, Bauernfeind R, Miller LB, et al. Sudden death in three teenagers: Conduction sytem studies. *J Am Coll Cardiol* 1983;1:879–886.
16. Bharati S, Dreifus LS, Chopskie E, Lev M. Conduction system in a trained jogger with sudden death. *Chest* 1988;93:348–351.
17. Bharati S, Cantor GH, Leach JB III, et al. The conduction system in sudden death in Alaskan sled dogs during the Iditarod race and/or during training. *PACE* 1997;20:654–663.

29

Commotio Cordis

Mark S. Link, MD, Barry J. Maron, MD, and N.A. Mark Estes III, MD

Introduction

Sudden death due to nonpenetrating chest wall impact in the absence of structural injury to the ribs, sternum, and heart is known as commotio cordis. This tragedy is a rare, albeit devastating, event. Commotio cordis usually occurs in young athletes when a baseball or other projectile strikes the victim in the precordium. Death is often instantaneous and unusually recalcitrant to standard resuscitative efforts. At autopsy, no cardiac pathology is found. The mechanism and pathophysiology of these rare but tragic events are not known. This chapter discusses possible mechanisms, risk factors, and preventive measures for commotio cordis. First, observations in commotio cordis victims are discussed, followed by an analysis of animal studies of chest wall trauma, and concluding with a discussion of possible mechanisms for commotio cordis, issues related to prevention, and what the future holds for commotio cordis research.

Human Observations (Tables 1, 2, and 3)

In a report from June of 1996, the US Consumer Product Safety Commission found that, between 1973 and 1995, there were 38 reported deaths from baseball blows to the chest.[1] This frequency is

From Estes NAM, Salem DN, Wang PJ (eds). *Sudden Cardiac Death in the Athlete.* Armonk, NY: Futura Publishing Co., Inc.; ©1998.

Table 1
Histogram of the Gender of all Commotio Cordis Cases
Reported in the Literature*

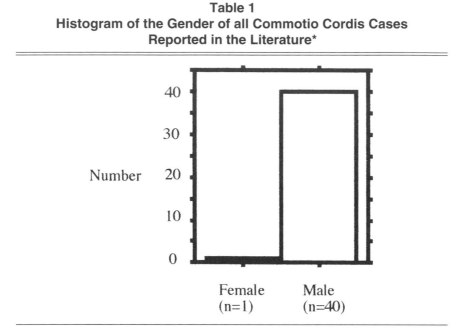

*References 2–9, 31. Note that the majority of the victims are male. Whether a gender pre-disposition exists is not clear from the current data on commotio cordis.

Table 2
Age at Occurrence of Commotio Cordis Cases
Reported in the Literature*

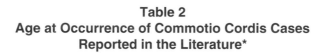

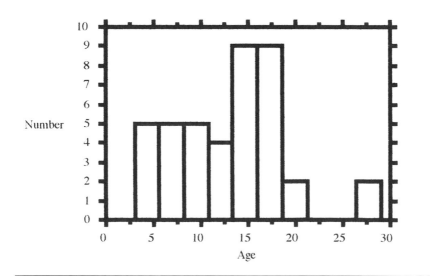

*References 2–9, 31. Note the majority of victims are between 4 and 18 years old.

Table 3
Sports Participated in by Victims of Commotio Cordis
Reported in the Literature.*

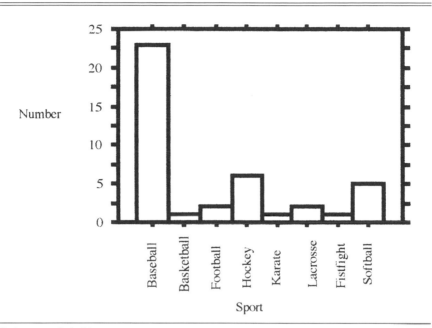

References 2–9, 31.

higher than the number of deaths due to baseball blows to the head during the same time period. It is quite possible that due to under-reporting of this unusual and little-known event, the number of deaths due to baseball impact to the chest is greater than the 2 to 3 reported cases per year.

The largest human series on commotio cordis was published in 1995 by Maron et al.[2] In this series, cases were gathered from the records of the US Consumer Product Safety Commission, the National Center for Catastrophic Sports Injury Research, Little League Baseball, and from newspaper reports. Of the 25 victims in the series by Maron et al, 24 were male. The ages ranged from 3 to 19 years, but most ages clustered from 7 to 16 years. A baseball blow to the chest caused the death in 16 victims; other causes of death were blows during football, softball, and hockey. Of the baseball injuries, 7 victims were struck by a batted ball, 6 were batters hit by a pitched ball, and 3 were players hit by a thrown ball. The force of the blow could be as light as a ball hit by a 6-year-old boy and as forceful as a body check during a hockey game. All impacts were to the anterior chest wall in the area overlying the heart. Instantaneous collapse occurred in 12 of the victims. The other 13 victims collapsed after a brief period of consciousness. Cardiopulmonary resuscitation (CPR) was begun within 3 minutes in 19 of the athletes. An initial rhythm following collapse was documented in 11 patients (B.J. Maron, personal communication, 1997). In seven of these, ventricular fibrillation (VF) was the initial rhythm. Two patients had initial ventricular tachycardia (VT), of which one degenerated into VF. One patient each had asystole and complete atrioventricular block. Only 2 of the 25 patients survived to the hospital and both of these died without regaining consciousness. Autopsies in 22 victims showed no evidence of acute (including myocardial hemorrhage, rupture, or infarction) or chronic cardiac abnormalities.

There have been very few reported cases of commotio cordis survivors. Doctors at the New England Medical Center have seen one patient who survived.[3] This 14-year-old patient was struck in the chest by a knee during a recreational game of football (Figure 1). He immediately complained of lightheadedness and then collapsed a few seconds later. CPR began within 1 minute; emergency medical technicians came within 6 minutes and found the patient in VF. He was cardioverted to sinus rhythm and brought to the emergency room. The

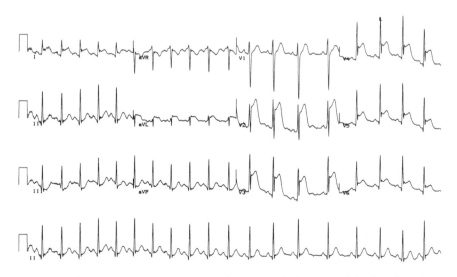

Figure 1 . Surface electrocardiogram of 14-year-old boy struck in the chest by a knee during a recreational game of football. Note the dramatic ST segment elevations in the anterior leads. These upsloping ST segment elevations are similar to those described in patients with coronary artery vasospasm. Cardiac catheterization performed 1 to 2 hours after the event revealed no hemodynamically significant coronary arterial narrowing or evidence of vasospasm. The ST segment elevations gradually normalized over 4 days.

initial 12-lead electrocardiogram (ECG) demonstrated marked ST elevations in the anterior chest leads (Figure 1). Because of the concern for acute ischemia, he was brought immediately to the cardiac catheterization laboratory. Coronary angiograms were remarkably normal, but a left ventriculogram showed anterior hypokinesis. Acute myocardial infarction was ruled out. Electrocardiographic abnormalities slowly resolved over 5 days and Q waves did not develop. His mental status slowly improved and he was discharged from the hospital.

There are only five other survivors reported in the literature. One of these was an 11-year-old boy who was struck in the chest by a baseball.[4] He fell forward and was unconscious for approximately 1 to 2 minutes. After 10 compressions of CPR he became responsive. The initial ECG showed minimal ST segment elevations that resolved after 24 hours. An echocardiogram was normal and a myocardial infarction was excluded. The patient was discharged 3 days later without any neurological sequelae. In a more recent case, a 17-year-old pitcher was hit in the chest by a batted ball.[5] He lost consciousness after a few seconds, but recovered within a few minutes. An initial ECG showed ST elevations in I, aVL, and in V_3 through V_6. Echocardiogram and technetium-pyrophosphate myocardial imaging were normal. Creatine kinase (CK) enzymes (495 units with normal <80 units) and myocardial band (MB) fraction (7.2%) were moderately elevated at admission. CK and MB enzymes decreased throughout admission. Cardiac catheterization 1 month later demonstrated normal coronary arteries but a small area of anterolateral hypokinesis.

Three survivors of commotio cordis were recently reported by Maron et al.[6] One was a 14-year-old boy who collided with a fellow baseball player. He collapsed and was found pulseless 10 seconds later. A chest "thump" was delivered 5 seconds later. Approximately 90 seconds after losing consciousness, the patient awoke without any neurological sequelae. The second commotio cordis survivor was a 12-year-old boy struck in the chest by a thrown ball. He collapsed five steps later and CPR was begun promptly. His pulse returned after 3 minutes. In the emergency room he was found in VT which degenerated into VF. The patient was successfully cardioverted. However, the patient suffered relatively severe neurological damage. The third patient is the oldest reported in the literature to date. This 29-year-old man was struck in the chest by a batted ball and collapsed seconds later. CPR was begun. When the paramedics arrived 8 minutes later, he was found to be in VF. After cardioversion to sinus rhythm he was in a coma for 5 days. An echocardiogram demonstrated mildly decreased global left ventricular dysfunction. His neurological function slowly improved, and 1 year later he showed mild neurological dysfunction.

Initial rhythms following collapse reported in victims who do not survive are predominantly VF,[4,7,8] but one case of complete heart block[7] and one case of idioventricular rhythm (after 10 minutes)[9] are also described.

Animal Experiments of Chest Wall Trauma

Efforts at experimentally producing commotio cordis in animals are limited by the severity of the cardiac damage resulting from the marked impact energies used. Consequently, these animal models are more representative of cardiac contusion than true commotio cordis. These animal models for chest wall trauma date to 1879.[10,11] In the early models, occasional sudden death was described and ascribed to heightened vagal stimulation. "Cardiac concussion," death due to chest wall trauma in the absence of morphological abnormalities, was first described in 1932 by Schlomka and Schmitz.[12] In their experiments, hammer blows to the chest of various animals caused frequent ECG changes (ST abnormalities) and occasional VF. The force of the blow was quantified only subjectively; most blows were of sufficient strength to cause readily evident cardiac damage. There was no gating to the cardiac cycle. Cutting or blocking the vagus nerve had no effect on ECG changes or death. Schlomka surmised that the short- and long-term changes were due to either coronary spasm (commotio cordis) or myocardial damage (contusio cordis).[13]

At the same time, Bright and Beck[14] were conducting their chest wall experiments in dogs. While they found a similar incidence of ECG abnormalities (25 of 25) and VF (2 of 25), all dogs had histologic evidence of myocardial hemorrhage. They reproduced the ECG changes by injecting blood into the myocardium. Thus, they ascribed the cardiac electrical abnormalities to myocardial contusion rather than to coronary spasm.

More sophisticated experiments with grading of force began in the mid 1960s. In Louhimo's series of 100 rabbits, weights were dropped equivalent to 1/3, 1/4, 1/6, and 1/8 of the animal weight.[15] All of the rabbits exposed to the impact of one third of their weight died. All of the group subject to the impact of only one eighth of their weight survived. Of the 47 animals that died, 43 had immediate VT, but this did not degenerate into VF in any animal. The only instance of VF was observed in an animal with respiratory arrest. A structural explanation for death was identified in each of those rabbits with VT. Transient ventricular asystole was seen in nine animals, but was not the cause of death. On autopsy, all of the 51 animals that died had injuries, including 48 with sternal fractures, 19 with ruptured aorta, and 23 with cardiac rupture or contusion.

In 1974, Liedtke et al[16] described a canine model of chest wall trauma. Dogs were subject to an impact of 650 joules, an energy level seen in motor vehicle accidents or in bombings. This energy of impact is equivalent to that of a baseball thrown at 228 mph. They pretreated some animals with vagotomy and β-blockers in an attempt to prevent death. Of the 9 animals not pretreated, 8 developed VT; 5 after varying periods of complete heart block. One of the eight animals with VT degenerated to VF, but the other animals reverted to sinus rhythm. Pretreatment with vagotomy did not appreciably alter the results, but pretreatment with a β-blocker caused death from complete heart block in four animals. Not surprisingly, almost all of these animals suffered cardiac contusions and other, more severe, cardiac injuries.

In the late 1970s, Vostal and Viano at General Motors worked with an animal model for chest wall trauma.[17] Dogs were administered direct cardiac trauma of an energy and velocity to simulate an auto accident. With an impact of 18 m/s, 68% of dogs died of fatal arrhythmias. With an impact of 12 m/s 40% of dogs died. Most commonly, VF developed instantly, but in some animals it was preceded by VT or complete heart block. Left ventricular pressures increased from 15 mm Hg to 520 mm Hg in the 12 m/s group, and to 750 mm Hg in the 18 m/s group. Cardiac contusions developed in all dogs.

At the same time, Cooper et al[18] developed a similar animal model. In their model the impact was gated to the cardiac cycle. VF was frequently seen in these experiments. They found that the T wave peak was the vulnerable segment of the cardiac cycle. These investigators also employed high-energy impact from 88 joules to 363 joules (mean of 188 joules), equivalent to being struck by a standard baseball at speeds of 83 mph to 171 mph (mean, 123 mph). All of their animals suffered relatively severe chest wall trauma, from sternal and rib fractures to joint displacement. In addition, most animals had cardiac injuries, from bruising to cardiac rupture, inconsistent with commotio cordis.

In the early 1990s Viano and colleagues[19] developed a baseball model of chest wall impact. The baseball was propelled at 95 mph to the chest wall of 16 swine. Two developed asystole, 2 had VT, 2 had VT that degenerated into VF, 4 had immediate VF, 4 had sinus rhythm or sinus tachycardia, and 1 had heart block. Given the energy involved in these experiments, it is not surprising that 14 of the 16 swine had histologic cardiac abnormalities, lesions not present in commotio cordis victims. Their impact was not gated to the cardiac or respiratory cycles, which may be important parameters in commotio cordis.

Data on coronary blood flow and coronary arteries in chest wall trauma are sparse. There are no chest wall trauma experiments that have used coronary angiography. Coronary blood flow measurements

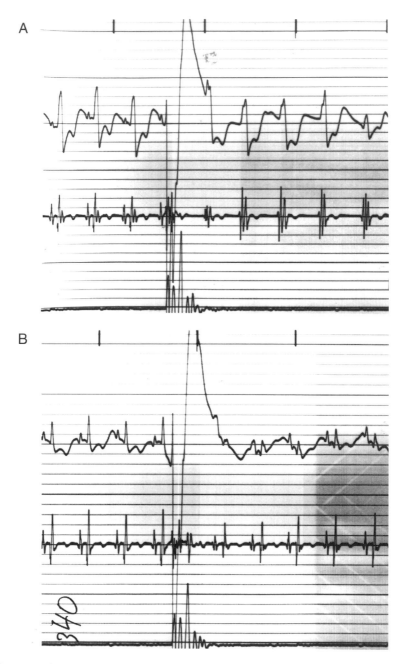

Figure 2. Surface electrocardiograms of a pig undergoing low-energy chest wall impact. These tracings are from our animal laboratory (Link and Estes). In **A,** a short run of an idioventricular rhythm is initiated by chest wall impact occurring during ventricular depolarization. In **B,** a premature ventricular beat is initiated by impact occurring during repolarization.

using radiolabeled microspheres have demonstrated increased blood flow to the area of cardiac injury,[20] and unchanged blood flow to contused areas.[21] Microscopy has generally shown no evidence of thrombosis, spasm, or luminal compromise,[20] although one group of investigators has demonstrated extrinsic compression of the coronary arteries following direct cardiac trauma.[22]

All of the models above have used very high energy projectiles, equivalent to motor vehicle accidents and bomb blast events. None of the series reported impacts that were less than 88 joules (83 mph baseball). With such force, most animals have evidence of severe cardiac and chest wall damage. Since commotio cordis deaths occur with low-velocity projectiles and cardiac or chest wall damage is absent, the aforementioned models do not necessarily reflect the true pathophysiology of commotio cordis.

Commotio Cordis: Possible Mechanisms

The absence of an appropriate animal model and the paucity of human data on commotio cordis have led to speculation regarding the etiology and pathophysiology of commotio cordis. The most widely held theory is that commotio cordis is primary VF occurring when chest wall impact occurs at a vulnerable time period of the cardiac cycle (generally thought to be the peak of the T wave).[2] This relatively minor impact causes a phenomenon similar to the R on T phenomenon, in which a ventricular premature contraction occurring at the peak of the T wave can cause VF.[23] Ventricular systoles can be induced in humans with thumping of the chest wall.[24] In this proposal, a precordial strike causes a premature ventricular contraction. The premature ventricular contraction happens to occur at the peak of the T wave, and VF ensues. In the human victims, the first documented rhythm after collapse was most frequently VF. The animal studies described above by Cooper et al and Viano et al, in which VF was produced by high-energy impact, also appear to substantiate this theory.[18,19] However, only one laboratory noted the importance of timing the impact to the cardiac cycle.[18] Other investigators have induced frequent VT,[15,16] but only rarely did this rhythm degenerate into VF. While primary VF may be a likely etiology, there are some features of commotio cordis that are not explained by primary VF. First, why is CPR so infrequently successful, given a structurally normal heart? One would expect that since VF is successfully resuscitated in up to 50% of patients with coronary disease,[25] the mortality in this young patient group without structural heart disease would be at least as favorable. Also, it is not clear that the electrical R on T phenomenon is replicated with chest wall trauma.

While VF is the most common initial rhythm documented following collapse, the number of observations is small. Furthermore, no victim has been electrocardiographically monitored at the time of chest impact, and VF may represent the terminal rather than the initial rhythm.

An alternate theory is that of blunt chest trauma-induced vasospasm. In fact, the first investigator to use the term *commotio cordis* was a proponent of this hypothesis.[13] According to this proposal, chest wall trauma causes coronary vasospasm, which produces myocardial ischemia, which in turn leads to VF. Most of the evidence for this theory comes from electrocardiographic monitoring of animals subjected to chest wall trauma. Ischemic ECG changes (most commonly ST segment elevation) are frequent.[13,26] However, coronary angiographic studies in chest wall trauma studies are rare. One such study examining the coronary vasculature after direct cardiac impact found no evidence of spasm, thrombosis, or hemorrhage.[20] Autopsies on commotio cordis victims are notable for the lack of coronary artery damage, thrombosis, or myocardial infarction, yet, case reports[3,5] of wall motion abnormalities consistent with coronary artery disease may provide some substantiation for the vasospasm hypothesis. Case reports showing ST segment elevation[3–5] are also consistent with coronary vasospasm. Immediate cardiac catheterization in a surviving commotio cordis victim has been reported only in the patient described above who had normal coronary arteries. This patient's presentation and clinical course are most consistent with coronary vasospasm.

A third major theory is the myocardial contusion theory, in which myocardial hemorrhage is thought to produce cardiac arrhythmias. Some support for this theory also comes from animal experiments showing a high frequency of ECG abnormalities and myocardial hemorrhages.[14,26] However, despite frequent ECG abnormalities in these experiments, VF was rare. Blood injected into the myocardium replicated the ECG changes but did not produce arrhythmias.[14] In human commotio cordis victims, myocardial hemorrhage is occasionally observed, but it is never extensive and is usually ascribed to the resuscitation efforts.[2] In one commotio cordis survivor described above,[5] the etiology of commotio cordis was thought to be a myocardial contusion based on an anterior left ventricular wall motion abnormality seen 1 month after injury.

Complete heart block and asystole have also been proposed mechanisms for commotio cordis.[27] However, these rhythms are only seen in 5% to 10% of animals subjected to chest wall trauma, and they are usually transient and do not lead to death.[15] Heightened vagal stimulation causing sudden death was an early hypothesis for sudden death in the chest wall trauma victim. However, in later animal experiments, vagotomy had little effect on ECG patterns or death.[13,16] Likewise, there are little animal or human data to support electromechanical dissociation or neurocardiogenic death.[27] While the long QT syndrome (and subsequent polymorphic VT) cannot be ruled out in victims of commotio cordis, there is no reason to suspect that a significant number of cases are explained by this syndrome.

Commotio cordis is seen almost exclusively in children and young adults. The reason for this predisposition is not entirely clear, but most authorities surmise that the pliability of the chest wall is a necessary condition. With this pliability of the chest wall, essentially the entire energy of a baseball or like object is absorbed by the chest and transmitted to the internal organs.[28] In animal experiments rib fractures are universal and, thus, the importance of chest wall pliability cannot be assessed. However, there may be other presently undefined factors for the predisposition of children and young adults to commotio cordis.

In conclusion, the most likely etiology for commotio cordis is VF. However, this etiology is far from confirmed and is based largely on circumstantial evidence in human commotio cordis victims and from animal models incorporating very high energy impacts. It is also possible that a single mechanism does not account for all commotio cordis deaths.

Preventive Measures

At present there are even less data on the prevention of commotio cordis than there are on the mechanism of this syndrome. In Maron's series of 25 victims of commotio cordis,[2] seven were wearing a commercially available chest wall protector (4 hockey players, 1 each of a football player, a baseball catcher, and a lacrosse goalie). Two other commotio cordis deaths in hockey have been reported despite chest protection.[7] Animal models have been used to evaluate chest wall protection in only one laboratory and this model used baseballs delivered at 95 mph.[29] In these experiments in six swine, there were minor reductions in fatalities when a softer-than-standard baseball was used in combination with commercially available chest wall protectors (ie, closed-cell foam and ABS plastic). However, chest wall protectors in combination with standard baseballs had little effect on the incidence of fatalities. This laboratory also used a human dummy model to evaluate chest wall protection in combination with standard baseballs and softer-than-standard baseballs.[29] In these studies, increased values for force and momentum were observed with chest protectors and standard baseballs. The values for force and momentum were even higher with the combination of softer-than-standard baseballs and chest wall protectors. A theoretical study using mathematical modeling found that the stiffness of a baseball is not as important as its mass chest wall injuries.[30]

Conclusions and Future Directions

Commotio cordis is a rare but devastating event. The exact incidence of this event is unknown. Self-limited cases due to nonsustained arrhythmias may be much more common than is realized. There are presently no indicators of which athletes are most susceptible to commotio cordis. Although the pathophysiology of this syndrome is most consistent with VF, there is little direct evidence to support this mechanism. Currently, preventive measures for commotio cordis do not exist.

Thus, more information is necessary concerning the mechanisms and prevention of the commotio cordis syndrome. A registry with systematic collection of all data has been established [Barry J. Maron, MD; US Commotio Cordis Registry, Minneapolis, MN; telephone: (612) 863–3984, Fax: (612) 863–3875]. This registry will be helpful in elucidating the clinical profile, prevalence, mechanism(s), and impact of any preventive measures. In addition, an appropriate animal model would be useful to more fully understand and prevent commotio cordis. With such an animal model of low-energy chest wall impact, better elucidation of the mechanisms of commotio cordis could result. These authors are currently developing a model using baseball impact at 20 to 40 mph (Figure 2). This model will incorporate timing of impact with the cardiac cycle. After the mechanisms of commotio cordis are better understood, they will proceed with evaluating measures for prevention of commotio cordis, including evaluating softer-than-standard baseballs and chest wall protection. It is their expectation that in the next few years, a fuller understanding of commotio cordis will be achieved.

References

1. Kyle SB. Study overview on baseball deaths, injuries, and protective equipment: US Consumer Product Safety Commission, 1996.
2. Maron BJ, Poliac LC, Kaplan JA, Mueller FO. Blunt impact to the chest leading to sudden death from cardiac arrest during sports activities. *N Engl J Med* 1995;3:337–342.
3. Link MS, Ginsburg SH, Wang PJ, et al. Commotio cordis: Cardiovascular manifestations of a rare survivor. *Chest* 1998; In press.
4. Abrunzo TJ. Cornmotio cordis, the single, most common cause of traumatic death in youth baseball. *Am J Dis Child* 1991;145:1279–1282.
5. Morikawa M, Hirose K, Mori T, et al. Myocardial contusion caused by a baseball. *Clin Cardiol* 1996;19:831–833.
6. Maron BJ, Strasburger JF, Kugler JD, et al. Survival following blunt chest impact induces cardiac arrest during sports activities in young athletes. *Am J Cardiol* 1997;79:840–841.
7. Kaplan JA, Karofsky PS, Volturo GA. Commotio cordis in two amateur ice hockey players despite the use of commercial chest protectors: Case reports. *J Trauma* 1993;34:151–153.

8. Dickman GL, Hassan A, Luckstead EF. Ventricular fibrillation following baseball injury. *Physician Sports Med* 1978;6:85–86.

9. Green ED, Simson LR, Kellerman HH, Horowitz RN. Cardiac concussion following softball blow to the chest. *Ann Emerg Med* 1980;9:155–157.

10. Meola F. La commozione toracica. *Gior Internaz Sci Med* 1879.

11. Riedinger F. *Die Verletzungen des Thoraz und Seines Inhaltes. Handbuch der Praktischen Chirurgie.* Stuttgart: Ferd. Enke; 1900.

12. Schlomka G, Schmitz M. Experimentelle untersuchungen uber den einfluss stumpfer brustkorbtraumen auf das electrokardiogramm. *S Ges Exp Med* 1932;85:171.

13. Schlomka G. Commotio cordis und ihre folgen, Vol. 47: *Med Kinderheilk,* 1934.

14. Bright EF, Beck CS. Nonpenetrating wounds of the heart. A clinical and experimental study. *Am Heart J* 1935;10:293–321.

15. Louhimo I. Heart injury after blunt thoracic trauma. An experimental study on rabbits. *Acta Chir Scand* 1967;380:7–60.

16. Liedtke AJ, Gault JH, Demuth WE. Electrographic and hemodynamic changes following nonpenetrating chest trauma in the experimental animal. *Am J Physiol* 1974;226:377–382.

17. Viano DC, Artinion CG. Myocardial conducting system dysfunctions from thoracic impact. *J Trauma* 1978;18:452–459.

18. Cooper GJ, Pearce BP, Stainer MC, Maynard RL. The biomechanical response of the thorax to nonpenetrating impact with particular reference to cardiac injuries. *J Trauma* 1982;22:994–1008.

19. Viano DC, Andrzejak DV, Potley TZ, King AI. Mechanism of fatal chest injury by baseball impact: Development of an experimental model. *Clin J Sport Med* 1992;2:166–171.

20. Liedtke AJ, Allen RP, Nellis SH. Effects of blunt cardiac trauma on coronary vasomotion, perfusion, myocardial mechanics, and metabolism. *J Trauma* 1980;20:777–785.

21. Utley JR, Doty DB, Collins JC, et al. Cardiac output coronary flow, ventricular fibrillation and survival following varying degrees of rnyocardial contusion. *J Surg Res* 1976;20:539–543.

22. Sabbah HN, Stein PD, Hawkins ET, et al. Extrinsic compression of the coronary arteries following cardiac trauma in dogs. *J Trauma* 1982;22:937–943.

23. Smirk FH, Palmer DG. A myocardial syndrome: With particular reference to the occurrence of sudden death and of premature systoles interrupting antecedent T waves. *Am J Cardiol* 1960;6:620–629.

24. Scherf D, Bornemann C. Thumping of the precordium in ventricular standstill. *Am J Cardiol* 1960:30–40.

25. Myerburg RJ, Kessler KM, Zaman L, et al. Survivors of prehospital cardiac arrest. *JAMA* 1982;247:1485–1490.

26. Scherf D, Terranova R. Estudio electrocardiografico de las desviaciones del segmento S-T e las contusiones toracicas experimentales. *Rev Argent Cardiol* 1942;9:157.

27. Estes NAM III. Sudden death in young athletes. *N Engl J Med* 1995;-333:380–381.

28. Viano DC, Andrzejak DV, King AI. Fatal injury by baseball impact in children: A brief review. *Clin J Sport Med* 1992;2:161–165.

29. Janda DH, Viano DC, Andrzejak DV, Hensinger RN. An analysis of preventive methods for baseball-induced chest impact injuries. *Clin J Sport Med* 1992;2:172–179.

30. Crisco JJ, Hendee P, Greenwald RM. The influence of baseball modulus and mass on head and chest impacts: A theoretical study. *Med Sci Sports Exerc* 1997;29:26–36.
31. Edlich RF, Mayer NE, Fariss BL, et al. Commotio cordis in a lacrosse goalie. *J Emerg Med* 1987;5:181–184.

30

Observations of the Consumer Product Safety Commission Staff

Susan B. Kyle, PhD

Background

The Consumer Product Safety Commission (CPSC) is an independent federal regulatory agency that was created in 1972 to protect the public from unreasonable risk of injury from consumer products. As an independent agency, CPSC is not under any executive-branch cabinet department. The agency has jurisdiction over approximately 15,000 types of consumer products found in and around the home, such as toys, children's nursery products, power tools and hand tools, furniture and appliances, and sporting equipment.

CPSC has the authority to ban or order the recall of hazardous products as well as to set mandatory safety regulations for products within its jurisdiction. The agency also works with manufacturers and other interested parties to develop voluntary standards for many of the

The opinions expressed in this chapter are those of the author and do not necessarily represent the views of the Commission. This material is in the public domain and may be freely copied or reprinted.

From Estes NAM, Salem DN, Wang PJ (eds). *Sudden Cardiac Death in the Athlete*. Armonk, NY: Futura Publishing Co., Inc.; ©1998.

products within its jurisdiction. In addition, CPSC develops and disseminates safety information.

To support these activities, the agency collects data on consumer product-related deaths and injuries. Some of these data may be useful to researchers interested in sudden cardiac death in athletes.

Data Collection Activities

CPSC collects information on deaths and injuries associated with consumer products in order to determine the extent and nature of the associated hazards. These data are used to determine which products are hazardous, what the magnitude of the hazard is, what the nature of the hazard is, and how the hazard should be addressed.

All CPSC raw data and completed data analyses are available to the public on request and can be obtained from the CPSC's National Injury Information Clearinghouse, Washington, DC 20207 or by calling (301) 504-0424.

CPSC has five major sources of data: the National Electronic Injury Surveillance System (NEISS), death certificates, Medical Examiners and Coroners Alert Project (MECAP), consumer complaints and news clips, and investigations.

The National Electronic Injury Surveillance System

NEISS is a network of 101 hospital emergency rooms across the country. These emergency departments report daily on injuries associated with some 800 consumer product categories. More than 300,000 cases are reported annually.

The emergency departments in the NEISS system are a stratified statistical sample, allowing national estimates to be made of the number of injuries associated with any one of the 800 product categories. The NEISS cases are also used for follow-up investigations to get more detail on particular types of injuries.

Information held in the NEISS system includes the following: the product involved in the injury, the age and sex of the injured person, the diagnosis (such as fracture, contusion, abrasion, etc), the body part injured (arm, leg, head), the disposition (whether the injured person was hospitalized or treated and released), the location at which the injury occurred (home, school, work, farm, etc), and up to two lines of text comment, which can provide useful insights into some of the circumstances of the injury.

Death Certificates

Deaths certificates are purchased from all 50 states and the District of Columbia. Only those E-codes that are generally associated with consumer products within CPSC's jurisdiction are purchased. For example, a motor-vehicle-related death certificate would not be purchased, but a bicycle-related death certificate would be purchased. About 8000 death certificates are purchased annually. Information includes age, sex, date of death, place of death, and cause of death. Death certificates are used to determine actual counts of deaths (rather than statistically derived estimates). They are also sources for potential follow-up investigations. It generally takes from 1 to 2 years from time of death until the death certificate is received by CPSC.

The Medical Examiners and Coroners Alert Program

MECAP is an informal, voluntary reporting system whereby some 2500 coroners and medical examiners across the country report product-related deaths to CPSC. This can be a source of extremely timely information, in contrast to the death certificates. CPSC receives approximately 2400 such reports annually. They are used to identify emerging hazards.

Consumer Complaints and News Clips

Consumers can report complaints or incidents involving consumer products directly to CPSC via the CPSC telephone hotline [(800) 638-CPSC] or by written complaint. Approximately 4000 hotline complaints were received in 1996. An additional 4000 written complaints are also received each year. CPSC's clipping services provide about 6000 newspaper articles annually about consumer product-related issues. All of these sources are used to identify emerging hazards and/or to follow-up cases that could provide more information on how injuries occur.

Investigations

In selected areas of interest, follow-up investigations are conducted, either by telephone or on site. These follow-up investigations are used to obtain more information about how the accident occurred, so that remedial strategies can be devised. Approximately 4000 follow-up investigations are conducted each year.

Example: Youth Baseball Protective Equipment

Introduction

In June, 1996, CPSC released the results of a project on Youth Baseball Protective Equipment.[1] The aim was to develop information for the general public about what types of available protective equipment could prevent or reduce the severity of baseball-, softball-, and tee–ball-related injuries and deaths to children ages 5 to 14.

Methods

Data on baseball-related (defined to include baseball, softball, and tee-ball) deaths and injuries to children ages 5 through 14 were collected and analyzed from all CPSC data bases. In addition, a special study was conducted to determine the specific ways in which children were injured while playing baseball. A random sample of injuries to this age group was chosen from the NEISS cases for a telephone follow-up survey to determine whether the injury occurred in circumstances where protective equipment might reasonably have been expected to prevent the injury. A review of the published scientific literature evaluating currently available protective equipment was conducted. Existing (voluntary) standards for protective equipment were evaluated. Types of protective equipment under consideration were softer-than-standard baseballs and softballs, face guards for batting helmets, modified "safety" bases, and chest protectors for batters.

Findings

In 1995 there were an estimated 162,100 baseball-related emergency-room-treated injuries to children ages 5 through 14. Results of a special study of baseball injuries to children[1] indicated that the most common cause of injury was ball impact, which accounted for 88,700 injuries, 55% of the total injuries. Eighty-eight baseball-related deaths to children ages 5 through 14 were identified between 1973 and 1995, an average of approximately 4 deaths per year. Sixty-eight of these deaths were due to ball impact. Of these 68, 38 were ball impact to the chest, 21 were ball impact to the head, and 9 were to other areas.[1]

Softer-than-standard baseballs and softballs are intended to reduce the risk of ball-impact injury, particularly ball-impact injury to the head. Ball impact to the head/neck region accounted for 54% of the emergency-room-treated ball-impact injuries in the CPSC special study, or

47,900 injuries. A CPSC-funded expert review of the applicable industry standard[3] concluded that softer-than-standard balls, which meet the standard, are generally safer than traditional balls in terms of risk of ball-impact head injury. Limited findings from the special study tended to support the effectiveness of softer balls in reducing the risk and severity of head-impact injury.

The available scientific literature on the ability of softer-than-standard balls to protect against chest-impact death has been controversial. The only published articles (a series of three articles[4-6]) concluded that softer balls (and chest protectors for batters) increased the risk of chest-impact death. CPSC funded an expert review of these articles[7] which concluded that the biological and biomechanical models used to mimic chest-impact death in children were not accurate. Therefore, CPSC staff concluded that the effect of chest protectors and softer balls on the risk of chest-impact death remains undetermined at this time.

Face guards for batting helmets are intended to protect the batter's face from being hit by the ball. In 1995 there were an estimated 59,400 emergency-room-treated facial injuries to children ages 5 through 14 associated with baseball. Facial injuries constituted 50% or more of total injuries for each year of age through age 9. Overall, approximately 74% of the facial injuries to children aged 5 through 14 were ball-impact injuries (44,000 injuries). Within this group, approximately 80% (35,200 injuries) occurred during organized play; 11% of these (or 3900) injuries occurred to batters. Although no published scientific studies were found evaluating face guards, staff review of the consensus voluntary standard for face guards[8] concluded that products meeting this standard would be effective in preventing facial injuries. Findings from the CPSC special study[1] supported this; none of the injured players who was wearing a face guard reported a facial injury.

Modified or "safety" bases are intended to reduce the risk of injury due to sliding into the base. Approximately 8% of the emergency-room-treated baseball injuries in 1995 were due to sliding (13,000 injuries). Of these, approximately 63% (8200 injuries) were due to contact with the base. Of these, approximately 80% (6600 injuries) occurred during organized games or practices. Approximately 53% of all base-contact sliding injuries occurred to girls, compared to 36% of overall baseball injuries. Two published scientific studies[9,10] found that the safety bases tested reduced the risk of injury. One of the safety bases tested and found effective is available in varying grades based on age, sex, and skill level. CPSC staff[1] concluded that safety release bases would be effective in reducing base contact sliding injuries in children. Because the proportion of girls injured sliding into base was higher than expected, staff concluded that an age- and sex-graded release base may provide the highest level of protection.[1]

Chest protectors for batters are intended to protect the heart (and, in some designs, the chest wall and other internal organs) from ball-impact injury. Ball impact to the chest was the most frequently reported cause of baseball-related death in children, accounting for 38 of the 88 reported deaths from 1973 through 1995. Expert review of the available scientific literature[7] indicated that the way in which baseball impact to the chest causes death is unknown at present. As mentioned above, CPSC staff concluded that the effect of any equipment on the risk of chest-impact death remains undetermined at this time.

Conclusions of the Protective Equipment Project

There were an estimated 162,100 baseball-related injuries to children ages 5 through 14 treated in hospital emergency rooms in 1995. Approximately one third of these injuries (more than 58,000 injuries) occurred in circumstances where available protective equipment could be expected to help reduce the severity of the injury or eliminate it altogether. The 47,900 injuries that involved ball impact to the head/neck area might have been lessened in severity or prevented by the use of softer balls. The 3900 facial injuries that occurred to batters in organized play could have been prevented by the use of face guards; and the 6600 base-contact sliding injuries that occurred in organized play might have been lessened in severity or prevented by the use of safety release bases.

Discussion and Conclusions

Youth Baseball Study

In considering how to address the estimated 162,100 annual injuries and 3 to 4 deaths per year in children ages 5 through 14 that are associated with playing baseball, softball, and tee-ball, the CPSC staff relied on its data collection and analysis capability to describe the nature and extent of the hazards associated with this sport in this age group.[1] Relevant product standards and published scientific literature on the available protective equipment were evaluated to determine whether currently available equipment would address the hazard patterns seen in the death and injury data.

Sudden Cardiac Death

CPSC data are available to any researchers interested in hazard analyses similar to that done in the youth baseball study.[1] All CPSC data bases are potential sources for identifying cases of sudden cardiac death in the athlete, since CPSC routinely collects information on deaths associated with sports. The amount and reliability of the information available on the cause of death vary depending on the source of the information in the data base. In addition, privacy considerations may limit the amount of identifying information available. However, careful analysis of the CPSC information could be helpful in estimating numbers of cardiac-related deaths in people participating in sports.

Perhaps the best use of CPSC data in establishing and maintaining a registry of sudden cardiac deaths is in partnership with interested cardiologists, as CPSC has no cardiologist on staff. CPSC staff are currently working with Dr. Barry Maron of the Minneapolis Heart Institute Foundation to evaluate the sports-related chest-impact deaths in CPSC data bases and to determine whether they are commotio cordis cases and, if so, to enter them into the registry he is maintaining. CPSC staff are interested in collaborating, when possible, to help in reducing deaths and injuries in sports.

References

1. Kyle SB. *Youth Baseball Protective Equipment Final Report.* Washington, DC, 20207: US Consumer Product Safety Commission; May, 1996.
2. Thibault LE, Goldsmith W. May 23, 1996. Letter to Susan B. Kyle. Re: *Evaluation of softer-than-standard baseballs and softballs.* TAB C. in Reference 1.
3. National Operating Committee on Standards for Athletic Equipment (NOCSAE). *Standard Method of Impact Test and Performance Requirements for Baseball/Softball Batter's Helmets, Baseballs and Softballs.* Overland Park, KS: NOCSAE; 1997.
4. Viano DC, Andrzejak DV, King AI. Fatal chest injury by baseball impact in children: A brief review. *Clin J Sport Med* 1992;2:161–165.
5. Viano DC, Andrzejak DV, Polley TZ, et al. Mechanism of fatal chest injury by baseball impact: development of an experimental model. *Clin J Sport Med* 1992;2:166–171.
6. Janda DH, Viano DC, Andrzejak DV, et al. An analysis of preventive methods for baseball-induced chest impact injuries. *Clin J Sport Med* 1992;2:172–179.
7. Kyle SB. March 18, 1996 memorandum to Robert E. Frye. *Summary of Expert Review of Baseball Protective Equipment Articles.* TAB D. in Reference 1.
8. ASTM. F910–86 *Standard Specification for Face Guards for Youth Baseball.* West Conshohocken, PA: ASTM; 1992.

9. Janda DH, Wojtys EM, Hankin FM, et al. Softball sliding injuries. A prospective study comparing standard and modified bases. *JAMA* 1988; 259:1848–1850.
10. Sendre RA, Keating TM, Hornak JE, et al. Use of the hollywood impact base and standard stationary base to reduce sliding and base-running injuries in baseball and softball. *Am J Sports Med* 1994;22:450–453.

Part VI

Legal, Medical, and Organizational Considerations

$$\boxed{31}$$

Legal Considerations in the Evaluation of the Athlete

Matthew J. Mitten, JD

Introduction

This chapter identifies important legal issues that arise in the diagnosis, evaluation, and treatment of athletes with heart disease or cardiovascular abnormalities and in the determination of their medical eligibility for athletic competition. There is currently very little case law or statutory authority that specifically establishes the legal duties of a physician providing cardiovascular care and treatment to athletes. Although there have been several recent lawsuits alleging physician malpractice in connection with medical treatment rendered to athletes, virtually all of them have been settled by the parties prior to judicial resolution of their merits. General legal principles regulating the physician-patient relationship and those authorities constituting the developing body of law governing the provision of cardiovascular care to athletes are analyzed and discussed herein.[1]

Nature of Physician–Athlete Relationship

The nature of the physician-athlete relationship differs in many respects from the ordinary physician-patient relationship. Athletes generally are highly motivated to participate in their chosen sports and

From Estes NAM, Salem DN, Wang PJ (eds). *Sudden Cardiac Death in the Athlete.* Armonk, NY: Futura Publishing Co., Inc.; ©1998.

are reluctant to spend time on the sideline because of an injury or illness. Both a typical patient and an athlete want a cure or treatment for a specific physical malady, but an athlete usually also seeks the quickest possible return to competition. Competitive athletes often feel invincible, have a strong desire to play a sport for psychological or economic reasons, and may be willing to sacrifice their bodies to accomplish an athletic objective. For these reasons, athletes may not readily accept physician medical recommendations that delay a return to play or advise against further participation in a desired activity.

Sports medicine physicians may encounter the sometimes conflicting objectives of protecting an athlete's health while minimizing the time spent away from athletic competition. Like many aspects of sports medicine, cardiovascular sports medicine is evolving and often lacks definitive scientific data on which a physician can rely when providing care and treatment to athletes. In addition to facing medical uncertainty, a physician may be subjected to extreme pressure from an athlete with a cardiovascular abnormality and/or team officials to provide medical clearance or treatment necessary for the athlete to play. This may create an environment that is not optimal for making well-considered and medically sound judgments that protect the athlete's health.

A physician has special knowledge, training, and skill (which a patient such as an athlete lacks) for diagnosing and treating diseases and injuries; this is the primary reason that patients seek medical services from physicians. Because an athlete entrusts his or her physical wellbeing to a physician and relies on the physician to protect his or her health by providing sports medicine care and treatment, the physician-athlete relationship is characterized as fiduciary in nature. This means that a physician has a legal obligation to act primarily for the athlete's benefit in connection with medical matters.

This fiduciary duty requires the physician to give advice consistent with an athlete's best health interests, even if a physician is selected and/or paid by an institution. It is important for a physician to be aware of the potential conflict of interest between the team's needs and the athlete's medical best interests and to recognize that although one of a sports medicine physician's objectives is to avoid the unnecessary restriction of athletic activity, his or her paramount responsibility is to protect the athlete's health, and his or her judgment should be governed only by medical considerations.

Physician's General Legal Duty of Care

While providing medical care to a patient, a physician has a legal obligation to have and use the knowledge, skill, and care ordinarily possessed and used by members of his or her specialty in good standing, considering the state of medical science at the time such care is rendered. The law generally permits the medical profession to establish the parameters of appropriate medical care as well as to designate any specific medical practices or treatment that a physician should follow within those boundaries. Thus, the medical standard of care, which must be established by physician expert testimony, becomes the legal standard of care for malpractice purposes. Malpractice liability for harm caused to an athlete may arise if a physician deviates from reasonable or accepted practices within his or her area of specialty in providing medical care; but he or she will not be liable for failing to use the *highest* degree of medical care, skill, and judgment exercised by physicians within his or her specialty.

In resolving malpractice claims involving medical specialists, the trend among courts is to apply a uniform national standard of care within a particular specialty, because national specialty certification boards, standardized training, and certification procedures now exist. In treating athletes with cardiovascular conditions, a cardiologist will be held to the standard of a reasonably competent cardiologist, and may be held to an even higher standard if he or she holds himself or herself out as having specialized expertise in cardiovascular sports medicine. A physician without specialized training in cardiovascular care may incur potential liability for not promptly referring a symptomatic athlete to a cardiologist for evaluation and treatment or for otherwise negligently providing cardiovascular care to an athlete. A physician also has a legal duty to inform an athlete of the medical risks of failing to see a cardiologist or other specialist for recommended evaluation and treatment of a cardiovascular condition.

During recent years, consensus guidelines concerning the cardiovascular care of athletes have been promulgated. In 1994 the 26th Bethesda Conference formulated guidelines for medically clearing or excluding competitive athletes with cardiovascular abnormalities from sports participation.[2] In 1996 the American Heart Association developed recommendations for cardiovascular preparticipation screening of competitive athletes.[3] These guidelines are intended to enhance the quality of cardiovascular care provided to athletes and improve self-regulation of the medical profession. Guidelines have the beneficial effect of pooling medical knowledge, distilling research and clinical experience, and enabling physicians to provide cardiovascular care to athletes on something other than their own background and experience.

Standing alone, consensus guidelines do not conclusively establish the legal standard of care that physicians must comply with. The legal standard of care is reasonable or accepted practice within a physician's specialty, but current medical guidelines are relevant in judicially resolving this issue. Under current law, consensus guidelines established by medical organizations and societies that are based on the present medical state of the art are admissible evidence of what constitutes good medical practice in malpractice litigation. For example, a monograph on preparticipation physical evaluations of young athletes developed by five organizations of family physicians, pediatricians, orthopedic surgeons, and sports medicine physicians recommends that medical clearance of athletes with cardiovascular abnormalities conform to the 26th Bethesda Conference guidelines.[4] The monograph's endorsement of these guidelines evidences that adherence to them constitutes reasonable or acceptable medical practice in providing cardiovascular medical clearance.

A physician's deviation from authoritative consensus guidelines regarding cardiovascular care of athletes may create malpractice liability. However, failing to follow such guidelines does not necessarily mean that a physician did not satisfy the proper medical and legal standard of care in treating an athlete. Deviations from guidelines are legally justifiable if they are medically acceptable and necessary in a specific situation. A physician should carefully document the medical basis for not following authoritative guidelines at the time cardiovascular care is provided to an athlete.

To summarize, in providing cardiovascular care to athletes, physicians must comply with the legal standard of care by following good medical practice within their respective specialties as determined by reasonable or accepted practices and state-of-the-art consensus guidelines. The most likely potential areas of malpractice liability are: failing to conduct appropriate screening or diagnostic tests, misinterpreting test results to determine cardiovascular fitness, providing improper treatment of a particular identified cardiovascular condition, improperly clearing an athlete to play with a known cardiovascular abnormality and/or inadequately disclosing the medical risks of doing so, or failing to follow generally accepted guidelines for sports medicine cardiovascular care of athletes. These specific topics are discussed in more detail in the following sections of this chapter.

Screening and Scope of Cardiovascular Examination

The law relies on the collective judgment of the medical profession to establish the appropriate nature and scope of a screening examination or preparticipation evaluation to discover cardiovascular abnormalities and potentially life-threatening conditions in athletes. This necessarily involves the development of reliable diagnostic procedures considering cost-benefit and feasibility factors as well as the current state of medical science. To further this objective, the American Heart Association recently developed consensus recommendations and guidelines for cardiovascular preparticipation screening of competitive athletes.[3] A consortium of five medical organizations whose members practice sports medicine also has developed a monograph which includes guidelines for the recommended scope of a preparticipation cardiovascular evaluation.[4] As more fully discussed in the preceding section of this chapter, such guidelines are some evidence of a physician's legal duty of care in screening athletes for cardiovascular conditions. The medical and legal acceptability or reasonableness of the comprehensiveness of a cardiovascular evaluation appears dependent on the individual athlete's level of competition, physical demands of the particular sport, and economic factors.

There is little judicial precedent regarding the legally required scope of a preparticipation physical examination. In *Ivey v Providence Hospital*,[5] the estate of a former Catholic University football player who died from respiratory distress during an asthma attack after football practice sued a physician for alleged negligence in conducting a preparticipation physical examination. The complaint asserted that the physician failed to conduct a proper and sufficient examination to determine whether the decedent could physically withstand the stress that intercollegiate football would place on his respiratory system. More specifically, the estate asserted that the physician did not obtain an adequate medical history of the player's respiratory condition and did not properly evaluate the effects that vigorous exercise placed on his condition. This case was settled by the parties prior to its judicial resolution. To establish the physician's legal liability for the player's death, the estate would have been required to prove by expert medical testimony and/or applicable guidelines that the physician did not follow reasonable or accepted medical practice in obtaining an athlete's full medical history or otherwise evaluating his fitness to play intercollegiate football.

A physician is not necessarily legally liable for failing to discover a latent cardiovascular condition during screening or evaluation of an athlete. Potential liability arises only if the examining physician deviates from accepted or reasonable medical practice, the use of which would have led to detection of the subject condition in the athlete. In *Rosensweig v State*,[6] the court ruled that a physician was not liable for failing to discover a boxer's preexisting brain injury from a previous fight. The court found that the physician had conducted a "standard examination" (without discussing its nature and scope) which did not reveal a prior brain injury. The court also observed that the boxer's medical history indicated no symptoms of concussions or brain injury and that the physician had relied on the opinions of other physicians who had examined the boxer after his prior fight without finding any indications of a brain injury. Similarly, in *Classen v State*,[7] the court found that a physician had conducted an extensive physical and neurological examination of a boxer in accordance with accepted medical practice and was not liable for malpractice in medically clearing the boxer to fight. It is important to recognize that a "standard examination" must conform to the medical state of the art and may not alone be sufficient for certain individual athletes.

An athlete's malpractice claim arising out of alleged negligence in connection with preparticipation screening or evaluation must be encompassed within the scope of the physician's understood duty to provide medical care or advice to the athlete. In *Murphy v Blum*,[8] the court held that a physician hired by the National Basketball Association (NBA) solely to advise it whether a referee would be physically capable of performing his duties did not have a physician-patient relationship with the referee that could form the basis of a malpractice claim. The NBA physician had informed an NBA official of the abnormal results of the referee's stress test. The NBA official then forwarded these results to the referee's personal physician. The NBA physician did not directly advise the referee of the abnormal test results and did not recommend or provide any treatment for his heart condition. After suffering a heart attack that prevented him from continuing to referee, the referee sued the NBA physician for malpractice in a suit that the court dismissed because of the lack of a physician-patient relationship between the parties.

The *Murphy* case suggests that a physician who conducts preparticipation examinations solely for the benefit of an athletic team is not legally required to directly inform an athlete of discovered cardiovascular abnormalities. Nevertheless, to minimize any potential legal liability, it is advisable for an examining physician to directly inform both the athlete and his or her personal physician of any such abnormalities in writing. Even if a physician who merely provides routine mass screening for certain medical conditions has no legal duty to provide follow-up cardiovascular care, it is strongly recommended that the physician inform all athletes of the limited nature of the medical services being provided when conducting preparticipation examinations, and promptly refer symptomatic athletes to cardiovascular specialists for fuller evaluation.

Testing and Diagnosis of Cardiovascular Condition

A physician may incur malpractice liability for not conducting appropriate diagnostic tests, which are required by the exercise of reasonable or accepted medical practice, in order to determine the nature of an athlete's cardiovascular condition. In *Goldman v St. Francis Hospital of Port Jervis*,[9] the court upheld a jury's finding that a thoracic surgeon deviated from good and accepted medical practice by not performing a stress test to determine the cardiovascular condition of a patient who had received a pacemaker and subsequently died while playing recreational basketball. Expert testimony indicated that performing a stress test would have disclosed that the patient had an arterial blockage and that strenuous exercise was contraindicated. It also was proven that the patient's death was related to the exercise he was doing at the time. The physician's failure to use proper diagnostic tests resulted in a misdiagnosis of the patient's condition and an erroneous failure to give cautionary instructions regarding appropriate exercise, culminating in the patient's death from ventricular fibrillation caused by circulatory failure. Based on this evidence, the jury found the physician liable for his patient's death.

In the well-publicized death of former Boston Celtics' basketball player Reggie Lewis, medical experts were sharply divided regarding their diagnosis of his cardiovascular condition and evaluation of the risks associated with continuing to play professional basketball. After collapsing during a Celtics game, Lewis was examined by numerous cardiologists. A team of 12 cardiologists assembled by the Celtics' team physician diagnosed Lewis as having cardiomyopathy, and concluded that this condition probably would prevent him from resuming his basketball career. A second medical opinion, rendered by other cardiologists at Lewis' request, concluded that Lewis had a relatively benign neurological condition that affected his heart beat, but that he had the normal heart of an athlete. A third medical opinion found evidence to support both opinions. Lewis died during a medically unsupervised workout, and autopsy results showed his heart to be abnormal, with ventricular cavity enlargement and extensive scarring, a finding consistent with healed myocarditis.

In April, 1996 Lewis' spouse filed a pending lawsuit against the physicians who concluded that Lewis did not have a potentially life-threatening heart condition.[10] Without asserting any specific acts of negligence, she broadly alleged that these physicians failed to care for and treat Lewis in accordance with the standard of care and skill ordinarily exercised by qualified cardiologists. This case probably will not be finally judicially resolved for several years but may establish important legal precedent regarding the cardiovascular care of athletes.

A physician generally does not guarantee the correctness of a diagnosis, and a doctor is not liable for a mere honest mistake of judgment if he or she has performed appropriate tests and the proper diagnosis or interpretation of test results is in reasonable doubt. However, a physician may be liable for malpractice for not using the requisite degree of care and skill ordinarily possessed by those within his or her specialty in interpreting test results and determining a patient's need for treatment. In *Gardner v Holifield,*[11] a basketball player's surviving mother alleged that a cardiologist misinterpreted two echocardiograms ordered to confirm an initial diagnosis during a routine physical examination that the player had Marfan syndrome. As a result, proper follow-up care, including the probable need for cardiovascular surgery, was not provided, and the athlete died 6 months after being initially evaluated by the cardiologist. Medical experts testified that a proper confirming diagnosis and treatment would have prevented the athlete's death and given him a normal life expectancy. This testimony created a factual issue regarding the physician's alleged malpractice for resolution by the jury.

Medical Treatment of Athlete's Known Cardiovascular Condition

A physician has a legal duty to either provide appropriate care or ensure that an athlete with a known cardiovascular condition receives medically necessary treatment in a timely manner. In *Dailey v Winston,*[12] expert medical testimony that a surgeon negligently failed to immediately hospitalize a basketball player for an arteriogram after he discovered that the athlete had an arterial blockage, and that he didn't inform him of the seriousness of his condition, created an issue of malpractice liability for resolution by a jury.

Two recent lawsuits alleged that the deaths of Hank Gathers and Earnest Killum were caused, at least in part, by the reduction of medication prescribed to treat the players' respective cardiovascular conditions below a therapeutic dosage to enable them to continue playing college basketball at a highly skilled level. In *Gathers v Loyola-Marymount University,*[13] the Gathers heirs asserted, along with claims of other negligent medical treatment, that Gathers was given a nontherapeutic dosage of heart medication to enable him to perform well in upcoming intercollegiate basketball tournament games. This action allegedly contributed to Gathers' collapse and death during a March, 1990 basketball game at Loyola-Marymount University.

In *Lillard v State of Oregon,*[14] Killum's mother alleged that his non-playing–field death was caused by physician malpractice. Killum had a history of two strokes and then experienced numbness and slurred speech during a recreational basketball game; tests determined that he had peripheral vascular disease. Physicians prescribed anticoagulant agents, and he was initially advised to withdraw from competitive basketball. Thereafter, his medications were reduced and he was cleared to resume playing college basketball despite recommendations to the contrary by a consultant. He died 1 month later, apparently of a massive cerebral infarction. A nontherapeutic dosage of medication to enable him to continue his intercollegiate career allegedly caused his death.

The *Gathers* and *Lillard* lawsuits raised important medical and legal issues concerning the appropriate care of an athlete with a known cardiovascular abnormality. Because both cases were settled out of court, these issues were not judicially resolved and no legal precedent was established. However, permitting nonmedical factors to interfere with the exercise of a physician's medical judgment breaches a physician's paramount responsibility to protect the athlete's health and would constitute malpractice. A court may allow a jury to award punitive damages against a physician to deter and punish this breach of the trust relationship between an athlete and the physician responsible for his or her medical care.

On the other hand, a physician is not legally liable merely because an athlete with an adverse cardiovascular condition who is under his or her care experiences a tragedy or undesirable result from treatment. Physicians generally do not guarantee that the effects of medical treatment will be favorable, and liability ordinarily does not result unless a particular result has been promised or the physician's care is outside medically acceptable norms. Physicians have a legal obligation to keep abreast of new developments and advances in cardiovascular treatment, and may be liable for using outdated treatment methods that no longer have a sound medical basis or do not currently constitute appropriate care.

The law permits the use of innovative cardiovascular care of athletes if it is within the bounds of reasonable or accepted medical practice under the circumstances. A physician may exercise judgment in choosing between medically recognized alternate methods of appropriate cardiovascular treatment. If competent and well-respected medical authority is divided over the appropriate method of cardiovascular treatment for an athlete, a physician will not be held legally responsible for adverse consequences that are caused by the exercise of his medical best judgment. Harm to an athlete that results from the physician's good-faith choice of one proper treatment method over another does not constitute malpractice.

Informed Consent Requirements and Medical Clearance Recommendations

A physician must have an athlete's informed consent before providing medical treatment. The informed consent doctrine is based on the principle of individual autonomy, namely that a competent adult has the legal right to determine what to do with his body. This autonomy includes the right to accept or refuse medical treatment. A competent adult athlete has the legal capacity to consent to medical care, but consent for treatment of athletes who are minors generally must be obtained from the athlete's parents or guardian.

For an athlete's consent to be legally valid, it must be the product of an informed decision regarding the proposed medical treatment. The average person has little understanding of medicine and relies on his physician to provide the information necessary to make a responsible decision regarding treatment. The extent of a physician's duty to disclose medical information to a patient traditionally has been determined by prevailing practices in the medical profession. Physician custom, or what a reasonable physician would disclose under the circumstances, has been the controlling legal standard. The recent judicial trend, however, is to focus on the patient and require physicians to disclose all material information to enable the patient to make an informed decision. A risk is material *when a reasonable person, in what the physician knows or should know to be the patient's position, would be likely to attach significance to the risk or cluster of risks in deciding whether or not to forego the proposed therapy.*[15] Thus, a physician should consider what information regarding his or her cardiovascular condition and treatment the athlete would want and need to know, and then disclose this medical information to the athlete in a timely manner.

A physician should fully disclose to an athlete the material medical risks of playing with the subject cardiovascular illness or abnormality and the potential health consequences of using or foregoing a given medication or treatment. The availability and pros and cons of accepted alternative methods of treatment must be considered and discussed with the athlete. All material short- and long-term medical risks of continued athletic participation and treatment, including any potentially life-threatening or permanently disabling health consequences, must be disclosed.

Treating physicians have a duty to disclose material medical risks to an athlete in plain and simple language. Information concerning the athlete's medical condition, proposed treatment and alternatives, probability of future injury and severity of harm from continued athletic participation, and potential long-term health effects should be preferably in writing or tape recorded when given verbally. It also is advisable to discuss any conflicting second opinions regarding appropriate cardiovascular care of the athlete, but not to downplay other physicians' conclusions about the athlete's medical condition and potential consequences of playing. A physician would be prudent to take affirmative steps to ensure that an athlete understands the available treatment options, side effects, and the potential consequences of engaging in athletics with a cardiovascular condition, which might include questioning or asking the athlete to write down his or her understanding of the medical information conveyed.

A failure to provide an athlete with full disclosure of material information about playing with a medical condition or the potential consequences of proposed treatment may create physician liability for negligence or fraud. In *Krueger v San Francisco Forty Niners,*[16] the court held that the conscious failure to inform a player that he risked a permanent knee injury by continuing to play was fraudulent concealment of a material fact in connection with his medical treatment. The court found that Charley Krueger was not informed by his physicians of the true nature and extent of his knee injuries, the consequences of steroid injection treatment, or the long-term dangers associated with playing professional football with his medical condition. The court also found that the purpose of this nondisclosure was to induce Krueger to continue playing football despite his injuries. The jury accepted Krueger's testimony that he would have rejected the proposed treatment and discontinued playing football, thereby preventing his subsequent permanent harm from occurring. The jury awarded Krueger $2.366 million in damages.

The *Krueger* case illustrates that a physician may incur legal liability for not fully disclosing material information about an athlete's cardiovascular condition that is necessary to enable the athlete to determine whether to accept proposed medical treatment or to continue playing a sport. To prevail in litigation against a physician for negligent or fraudulent nondisclosure of medical information, an athlete must prove that he or she would not have played or undergone the cardiovascular treatment causing harm if the material risks of doing so had been disclosed. Physicians who provide cardiovascular care to athletes can minimize potential liability and comply with the legal requirements of the informed consent doctrine by communicating openly and honestly with their patients.

Physicians should provide all material information about an athlete's cardiovascular condition directly to the athlete and obtain permission, preferably in writing, before communicating any medical information about the athlete to team officials. Ethically, a physician is prohibited from disclosing a patient's medical condition to others without patient consent or legal requirement. Unauthorized disclosure of information about an athlete's medical condition to third parties may create legal liability. In *Chuy v Philadelphia Eagles Football Club,*[17] a federal appellate court affirmed a jury finding that the Philadelphia Eagles' team physician intentionally inflicted emotional distress on a professional football player by falsely informing the press that the player suffered from a fatal blood disease. The physician's statement was found to be intolerable professional conduct because he knew that the player did not have the reported condition. Moreover, a physician's unauthorized disclosure of even accurate information about an athlete's medical condition creates potential legal liability for invasion of the athlete's privacy.

Even if an athlete's illness or condition has been properly diagnosed and the athlete has been warned of the potential health consequences of continued play, a physician may be liable for making a negligent medical clearance recommendation. In *Mikkelson v Haslam,*[18] a patient alleged that a physician negligently provided her with medical clearance to snow ski after she had undergone hip replacement surgery. The jury found the physician negligent based on undisputed testimony that advising a total hip replacement patient that skiing is permissible *is a departure from orthopedic medical profession standards.*[18]

The *Gathers*[13] and *Lillard*[14] litigations both involved unresolved allegations that physicians improperly cleared a college athlete to continue playing basketball with a serious cardiovascular abnormality. The Gathers lawsuit claimed that Hank Gathers was not fully informed of the seriousness of having ventricular tachycardia and should not have been medically cleared to play college basketball with this condition. This action, which was filed in 1990, asserted that physicians providing such clearance acted negligently because the 16th Bethesda Conference guidelines[19] (which were in effect at that time) recommended that persons with ventricular tachycardia should not participate in any competitive sports. The Gathers heirs contended that Gathers was *sacrificed on the altar of college basketball* in Loyola Marymount University's quest for basketball success, notoriety, and economic gain.

In the *Lillard* case, Earnest Killum's mother alleged that her son's physicians did not inform him of the material medical risks of playing college basketball with an impaired vascular condition caused by two prior strokes. She also claimed that these physicians negligently cleared her son to return to competition although doing so subjected him to an increased risk of death or serious injury. She further contended that the physicians breached their duty to: (1) refuse to provide medical clearance to avoid allowing an athlete to expose himself to an enhanced risk of death or serious harm; and (2) not compromise an athlete's medical care in order to advance a university's economic interests.

Both the *Gathers* and the *Lillard* lawsuits were settled before their judicial resolution established legal precedent regarding medical clearance recommendations. These cases, however, illustrate the need for physicians to consider carefully the parameters of the acceptable medical risks of athletic participation by athletes with known cardiovascular abnormalities and to always to adhere to their paramount obligation to protect an athlete's health. It is a serious violation of a physician's ethical and legal duties owed to an athlete to allow nonmedical factors to impair the exercise of medical best judgment in making clearance recommendations and/or to not fully inform an athlete of the health risks of athletic participation with his or her condition. A physician should refuse to clear an athlete to participate if there is a significant medical risk of harm from sports participation, irrespective of the team's need for the player or the player's strong psychological or economic motivation to play and willingness to take unreasonable health risks.

In formulating a participation recommendation, a physician should only consider the athlete's medical best interest. The following factors may be appropriately considered: the athlete's unique physiology; the intensity and physical demands of the subject sport; whether the athlete has previously participated in the sport with the subject physical condition; available clinical evidence; medical organization and society guidelines; the probability and severity of harm from athletic participation with the athlete's condition; and whether medication, monitoring, or protective devices will minimize potential health risks and enable safe athletic participation. In cases in which there is an uncertain potential for life-threatening or permanently disabling harm to an athlete with a cardiovascular condition, it appears advisable to err on the side of caution and recommend against athletic participation.

Consensus guidelines regarding participation recommendations for athletes with cardiovascular abnormalities, such as those established by the 26th Bethesda Conference,[2] provide a source of objective and collective guidance to physicians that may ultimately establish both the medical and the legal standard of care in making medical clearance recommendations. As the *Gathers*[13] case demonstrates, it is likely that, in litigation, noncompliance with such guidelines will be alleged to constitute malpractice.

There has been one case in which an athlete sued a physician for refusing to medically clear him to play a sport with a cardiovascular condition. In *Penny v Sands*,[20] Anthony Penny filed a malpractice suit against a cardiologist who diagnosed him as having cardiomyopathy and recommended against his continued participation in intercollegiate basketball. Two other cardiologists concurred with this opinion, and Central Connecticut State University refused to allow Penny to engage in its basketball program for 2 years. Penny ultimately obtained medical clearance from two other cardiologists to play competitive sports. He alleged that Dr. Sands' negligence caused economic harm to his anticipated professional basketball career because of his involuntary 2-year exclusion from college basketball. Penny voluntarily dismissed his malpractice suit before he collapsed and died while playing in a 1990 professional basketball game in England.

Although Penny's allegations were not judicially resolved, it is unlikely that a court would permit an athlete to recover any economic loss because team officials accept a physician's recommendation against permitting the athlete with a properly diagnosed cardiovascular abnormality to participate in a sport. Legal recognition of such claims would unduly impair a physician's medical judgment and may cause him to place greater weight on legal rather than medical considerations. This also would create the paradoxical and undesirable situation of imposing legal liability on a physician for complying with his or her primary obligation to protect an athlete's health.

Athlete's Responsibility to Protect Own Health

An athlete has a legal duty to reasonably protect his or her health. One court has defined a patient's duties regarding the receipt of medical care as follows:

A patient is required to cooperate in a reasonable manner with his treatment. This means that a patient has a duty to listen to his doctor, truthfully provide information to his doctor upon request, follow reasonable advice given by his doctor, and cooperate in a reasonable manner with his treatment. A patient also has a duty to disclose material and significant information about his condition or habits when requested to do so by his physician.[21]

An athlete must satisfy these obligations to satisfy the duty to reasonably protect one's health. Otherwise, the athlete may be contributorily negligent for exposing him- or herself to an unreasonable risk of harm.

Physicians and patients have corresponding legal obligations to facilitate the provision of quality medical care. A physician has a duty to obtain a complete and accurate medical history from an athlete. In turn, an athlete must exercise due care for one's health by truthfully relating his or her medical history to the physician. Although an athlete has no general duty to diagnose a medical condition or volunteer information, he or she should disclose known information about a cardiovascular condition that may create exposure to a risk of future harm if the physician has failed to ascertain these facts while taking his or her medical history. For example, an athlete would not be exercising reasonable care for his or her own safety by minimizing heart symptoms to avoid medical restriction of athletic activities.

An athlete generally may rely on the recommendations of treating physicians without seeking a second medical opinion. It ordinarily is reasonable for an athlete to rely on physicians' recommendations concerning cardiovascular care and treatment because of their superior knowledge and expertise. In *Mikkelson v Haslam*,[18] the court found that a patient was not contributorily negligent for following her physician's advice that she could snow ski after total hip replacement surgery without seeking a second opinion from other physicians. She did not assume the risk of her permanently disabling injury, which occurred while skiing, because her physician had not informed her of this potential risk and it was not an obvious risk to a lay person. Under *Mikkelson,* an athlete with a cardiovascular condition that does not expose him or her to an obvious risk of injury while engaging in athletics is not contributorily negligent for participating in an athletic activity with physician medical clearance, even if he or she does not consult with other physicians.

Courts have held that an athlete's failure to use reasonable care to protect his or her health may totally bar or reduce recoverable damages in a malpractice suit against his or her treating physicians. In *Gillespie v Southern Utah State College,*[22] a college basketball player was found to be solely responsible for aggravating an ankle injury by not following physician instructions. He iced his ankle for longer than the physician's prescribed period of time, causing thrombophlebitis and frostbite that required amputation of his toe and other foot tissue.

If an athlete fails to take prescribed medication in the required dosage to treat a heart condition or deliberately takes steps to reduce its therapeutic effectiveness, such conduct would be an unreasonable disregard for his or her own health. Similarly, disobeying physician restrictions on athletic activity by an athlete with a cardiovascular condition would constitute contributory negligence.

Legal Enforceability of Liability Waivers

Under certain circumstances, the law permits an adult to whom a legal duty of reasonable care is owed to waive, by contractual agreement among the parties, the right to recover damages in a negligence action for harm caused by another's breach of this duty. A waiver of legal rights signed by a minor usually is not enforceable even if it also is signed by his or her parents or guardian or entered into with their approval, because minors have only a limited legal capacity to enter into binding contracts. In general, an adult may prospectively agree to knowingly and voluntarily waive a legal right to recover for future harm attributable to another's wrongful conduct unless such an agreement violates public policy. In some instances, courts may uphold waivers of liability from future negligence but not more culpable conduct such as intentional, reckless, or grossly negligent torts.

As previously discussed, a physician providing cardiovascular care to an athlete has a legal duty to comply with reasonable or accepted medical practice and may be liable for malpractice for breach of this obligation. Courts generally will not enforce waivers purporting to release physicians from liability for negligent medical care of their patients. Such waivers have been held to violate public policy because medical services are essential public services; the patient places him- or herself under the physician's control but remains subject to the risks of negligence; and the physician may have the bargaining power to require a release from negligence liability as a condition of providing medical treatment.

Although a court may not enforce a waiver signed by an athlete agreeing not to hold a physician liable for providing negligent cardiovascular care that causes injury, a physician will incur malpractice liability only for deviation from the appropriate medical standard of care or failure to comply with the requirements of the informed consent doctrine. It is important to recognize that merely informing an athlete about the risks of participation with his or her condition does not discharge a physician's legal duty of care in providing cardiovascular care and providing medical clearance recommendations. For example, advising an athlete with a cardiovascular condition that he or she should not play a sport, but then providing medical clearance to play in exchange for a waiver of liability, probably will not protect a physician from malpractice liability if the physician acted negligently. Conforming to current standards of cardiovascular sports medicine practice and fully apprising the athlete of all material information about his or her condition are the best means by which a physician can avoid legal liability.

Immunity From Malpractice Liability

In some instances, physicians may be immune from legal liability for malpractice claims brought by athletes. Several states have enacted so-called "good Samaritan statutes," which protect licensed physicians from negligence liability for emergency medical care rendered to athletes in good faith and without compensation. These statutes apply when a physician provides emergency treatment to an athlete suffering from a cardiovascular problem. Immunity is generally not provided for emergency medical treatment found to be grossly negligent, reckless, or willful or wanton. Preparticipation physical exams, general nonemergency medical care rendered to athletes, and physician medical clearance recommendations are not normally subject to immunity.

In some jurisdictions state law immunizes physicians employed by public educational institutions from malpractice liability in suits brought by athletes. In *Gardner v Holifield*,[11] the court ruled that the alleged negligent medical care provided to a college basketball player by a physician was encompassed within the scope of tort immunity under Florida law if the physician was acting in his capacity as director of a public university's student health center when such treatment was rendered. Florida state employees, including physicians, are immune from liability for negligence committed within the scope and course of their employment.

Similarly, in *Sorey v Kellett*,[23] a federal court held that a public university's team physician was immune from a negligence suit by the mother of a deceased football player. The player collapsed during a football practice and was given medical treatment by the team physician, but died while being transported to the hospital. The court ruled that public employees have a qualified immunity from tort claims based on their discretionary acts. Finding that the physician was performing a discretionary function in administering emergency medical care to the decedent, the court dismissed the lawsuit.

A professional athlete's claim against a physician for negligent medical care may be barred by a state workmen's compensation statute prohibiting actions against co-employees for injuries caused to fellow employees when acting within the scope of their employment. If so, the athlete's legal remedy is limited to receipt of the statutorily determined workmen's compensation benefits under state law. In *Hendy v Losse*,[24] the court dismissed a professional football player's suit against a team physician for negligently diagnosing and treating his knee injury and medically clearing him to continue playing football. The court held that California's workmen's compensation law bars tort suits between co-employees for injuries caused within the scope of employment. The player's malpractice claim was dismissed because both he and the physician were employed by the San Diego Chargers team, and the physician acted within the scope of his employment in treating the player. However, the court stated that a physician who is an employee of a professional team is subject to malpractice liability for improper medical services provided to athletes that are outside of the scope of the services the physician agrees to provide to players pursuant to an employment agreement with the team.

In most instances in which cardiologists provide nonemergency medical care to athletes, there is no immunity for malpractice liability. There is no immunity for providing negligent cardiovascular care to an athlete unless a physician is both an employee of a public educational institution or professional team and is acting within the designated scope of his or her employment at the time treatment is rendered. Physicians serving as independent consultants rather than team employees do not satisfy these requirements.

Judicial Resolution of Athletic Participation Disputes

Ideally, the decision whether an athlete with a particular cardiovascular abnormality will participate in a sport should be the product of mutual agreement between the team physician and consulting cardiologists, team or school officials, and the athlete and family. It is not uncommon, however, for physicians to disagree in their medical clearance recommendations, or for highly motivated athletes at all levels of competition to be reluctant to accept a medical recommendation to not continue playing a sport. Disagreements regarding the propriety of participation in athletics by athletes with cardiovascular abnormalities is judicially resolved on an individual case-by-case basis under federal or state laws that prohibit discrimination against persons with physical impairments.

Both the Americans With Disabilities Act of 1990 (ADA)[25] and the Rehabilitation Act of 1973[26] prohibit unjustified discrimination against athletes with cardiovascular abnormalities or impairments. These federal laws apply to virtually all professional teams and intercollegiate or interscholastic sports programs, but do not appear to render a physician personally liable for determining that an athlete is medically ineligible to participate in a sport. State education, human rights, and/or employment laws also may prohibit medically unwarranted discrimination against athletes with physical impairments.

Federal law requires that an athlete with the physical capabilities and skills necessary to play a sport, despite a cardiovascular abnormality, is entitled to have his or her condition individually evaluated in light of current medical evidence. Exclusion from an athletic team or event must be based on reasonable medical judgments by physicians, given the state of medical knowledge. The ADA and Rehabilitation Act require a careful balancing of an impaired athlete's right to participate in athletic activities within his or her physical abilities, physician evaluation of the medical risks of athletic participation, and the team's interests in conducting a safe athletics program.[27]

Exclusion of an athlete because a cardiovascular condition increases the risk of personal injury to others or to him- or herself while engaging in athletic activity must be based on *reasonable medical judgments given the state of medical knowledge*.[28] Relevant medical factors include the nature, duration, probability, and severity of harm from athletic participation as well as whether the risk of injury can be effectively reduced by medication, monitoring or protective devices, or other reasonable accommodations to enable athletic participation.

An athlete may be legally excluded from an athletic event or competition if his or her participation exposes others to significant health and safety risks. In *Myers v Hose*,[29] a federal court held that a county transit authority's determination that a person with chronic heart disease, hypertension, and uncontrolled diabetes was not qualified for employment as a bus driver did not violate the ADA. He failed to pass a medical examination establishing certain minimum health requirements to operate county vehicles. The court found that his poor cardiovascular condition prevented him from operating a bus in a responsible fashion *that does not threaten the safety of his passengers or of other motorists.*[29] Under *Myers,* a team or entity sponsoring an athletic competition may exclude an athlete with a cardiovascular abnormality from participation in a sport (*eg,* auto racing) if doing so is medically necessary to prevent a significant risk of harm to others.

Even if such participation does not expose others to significant harm, developing judicial precedent holds that a college or high school athlete with a cardiovascular condition may be excluded from a sport to prevent exposing the athlete to a significant risk of injury. To date, there have not been any cases in which a professional athlete with a cardiovascular abnormality has asserted a legal right to play a sport. Although the medical issues may be the same, courts may develop a different legal framework for resolving participation disputes involving professional athletes, because sports is their livelihood rather than an extracurricular activity that is merely a component of a high school or college education.

In *Larkin v Archdiocese of Cincinnati,*[30] a federal court held that a high school could exclude Stephen Larkin from its football team because he was diagnosed with structural heart disease. Larkin and his family were informed of the medical risks of future athletic competition and were willing to waive any future legal claims against the school if he was permitted to play football. Because examining cardiologists unanimously recommended against Larkin's continued participation in competitive interscholastic sports and Larkin was unable to satisfy an Ohio high school athletic association bylaw requiring physician medical clearance, the court held that the school's decision did not violate the Rehabilitation Act.

In *Knapp v Northwestern University,*[31] a federal appellate court held that Northwestern University did not violate the Rehabilitation Act in following its team physician's recommendation that an athlete with idiopathic ventricular fibrillation not play intercollegiate basketball. As a high school senior, Nicholas Knapp suffered sudden cardiac arrest while playing recreational basketball, which required cardiopulmonary resuscitation and defibrillation to restart his heart. Thereafter, he had an internal cardioverter defibrillator implanted in his abdomen. He subsequently has played competitive recreational basketball without any incidents of cardiac arrest and received medical clearance to play college basketball from three cardiologists who examined him.

Northwestern agreed to honor its commitment to provide Knapp with an athletic scholarship, although it adhered to its team physician's medical disqualification from intercollegiate basketball. This recommendation was based on Knapp's medical records and history, the 26th Bethesda Conference[2] guidelines for athletic participation with cardiovascular abnormalities, and opinions of two consulting cardiologists who concluded that Knapp would expose himself to a significant risk of ventricular fibrillation or cardiac arrest during competitive athletics.

All medical experts agreed that Knapp had suffered sudden cardiac death due to ventricular fibrillation. Even with the internal defibrillator, playing college basketball places Knapp at a higher risk for suffering another event of sudden cardiac death compared to other male college basketball players; the internal defibrillator has never been tested under the conditions of intercollegiate basketball; and no person currently plays or has ever played college or professional basketball after suffering sudden cardiac death and having a defibrillator implanted.

The court held that a university may legally establish legitimate physical qualifications that an individual must satisfy to participate in its athletic program. An athlete can be disqualified from athletics if necessary to avoid a significant risk of personal physical injury that cannot be eliminated through the use of reasonable medical accommodations. The court explained that Knapp's exclusion from Northwestern's basketball team was legally justified:

We disagree with the district court's legal determination that such decisions are to be made by the courts and believe instead that medical determinations of this sort are best left to team doctors and universities as long as they are made with reason and rationality and with full regard to possible and reasonable accommodations. In cases such as ours, where Northwestern has examined both Knapp and his medical records, has considered his medical history and the relation between his prior sudden cardiac death and the possibility of future occurrences, has considered the severity of the potential injury, and has rationally and reasonably reviewed consensus medical opinions or recommendations in the pertinent field—regardless whether conflicting medical opinions exist—the university has the right to determine that an individual is not otherwise medically qualified to play without violating the Rehabilitation Act. The place of the court in such cases is to make sure that the decision-maker has reasonably considered and relied upon sufficient evidence specific to the individual and the potential injury, not to determine on its own which evidence it believes is more persuasive.

We do not believe that, in cases where medical experts disagree in their assessment of the extent of a real risk of serious harm or death, Congress intended that the courts—neutral arbiters but generally less skilled in medicine than the experts involved—should make the final medical decision. Instead, in the midst of conflicting expert testimony regarding the degree of serious risk of harm or death, the court's place is to ensure that the exclusion or disqualification of an individual was individualized, reasonably made, and based upon competent medical evidence. So long as these factors exist, it will be the rare case regarding participation in athletics where a court may substitute its judgment for that of the school's team physicians.

In closing, we wish to make clear that we are not saying Northwestern's decision necessarily is the right decision. We say only that it is not an illegal one under the Rehabilitation Act. On the same facts, another team physician at another university, reviewing the same medical history, physical evaluation, and medical recommendations, might reasonably decide that Knapp met the physical qualifications for playing on an intercollegiate basketball team. Simply put, all universities need not evaluate risk the same way. What we say in this case is that if substantial evidence supports the decision-maker—here Northwestern—that decision must be respected.

It is important to note that the *Knapp* case holds that it is legally appropriate for physicians to follow consensus medical opinions such as those established by the 26th Bethesda Conference[2] when making participation recommendations for athletes with cardiovascular abnormalities. This view is consistent with the essential requirement of both the ADA and Rehabilitation Act that there be a reasonable medical basis for excluding an athlete from a sport. Thus, consensus guidelines and recommendations probably will play an important role in future participation disputes involving athletes with cardiovascular conditions, both in preventing and resolving litigation.

References

1. Mitten MJ. Team physicians and competitive athletes: Allocating legal responsibility for athletic injuries. *U Pitt L Rev* 1993;55(1):129–169.
2. 26th Bethesda Conference. Recommendations for determining eligibility for competition in athletes with cardiovascular abnormalities. *J Am Coll Cardiol* 1994;24(4):845–899.
3. Mason BJ, Thompson PD, Puffer JC, et al. Cardiovascular preparticipation screening of competitive athletes. *Circulation* 1996;94:850–856.
4. American Academy of Family Physicians, American Academy of Pediatrics, American Medical Society for Sports Medicine, American Orthopaedic Society for Sports Medicine, American Osteopathic Academy of Sports Medicine. *Preparticipation Physical Examination, Second Ed.* 1997;34–45.
5. Civil Action No. 93-010-330 (Dist. Col. Super Ct, filed Sept 10, 1993).
6. 171 NYS 2d 912 (NY App 3d Dept), *aff'd,* 185 NYS 2d 521 (NY 1958).
7. 500 NYS 2d 460 (NY Ct Cl 1985).
8. 554 NYS 2d 640 (NY App 2d Dept 1990).
9. No. 80 Civ 1729 (CBM) (WDNY Aug. 31, 1981) (slip opinion available on LEXIS).
10. *Lewis v Mudge,* No. 96-2349-F (Mass Super Ct., filed on April 30, 1996).
11. 639 So2d 656 (Fla.App 1994).
12. 1986 WL 12063 (Tenn. App 1986) (slip opinion available on LEXIS).
13. No. C 795027 (Los Angeles, CA Super Ct, filed April 20, 1990).
14. No. BC 2941 (Los Angeles, CA Super Ct, filed Jan. 19, 1993).

15. Canterbury v Spence, 464 F2d 772, 787 (DC), *cert denied,* 409 US 1064 (1972).
16. 234 Cal Rptr 579 (Cal Ct App 1987).
17. 595 F2d 1265 (3d Cir 1979).
18. 764 P2d 1384 (Utah Ct App 1988).
19. Mitchell JH, Maron BJ, Epstein SJ. 16th Bethesda Conference: Cardiovascular abnormalities in the athlete: Recommendations regarding eligibility for competition. *J Am Coll Cardiol* 1985;6:1186–1232.
20. No. H89–280 (D. Conn., filed May 3, 1989).
21. Benedict v St. Luke's Hospital, 365 NW 2d 499, 505 (ND 1985).
22. 669 P2d 861 (Utah 1983).
23. 849 F2d 960 (5th Cir 1988).
24. 819 P2d 1 (Cal. 1991).
25. 42 USCA §§ 12101-12213 (West 1995 and 1996 Supp.).
26. 29 USCA §§ 701–796 (West 1995).
27. Mitten MJ. Amateur athletes with handicaps or physical abnormalities: Who makes the participation decision? *Neb L Rev* 1992;71:987–1032.
28. School Board of Nassau County, Florida v Arline, 480 US 273 (1987).
29. 50 F3d 278 (4th Cir 1995).
30. No. C-90–619 (SD Ohio, Aug 31, 1990) (oral findings of fact and conclusions of law supporting denial of injunctive relief and dismissal of complaint) (Partial Transcript of Proceedings).
31. Knapp v Northwestern University, 101 F3d 473 (7th Cir 1996).

32

The Role of the Team Physician in the Prevention of Sudden Cardiac Death:

The Orthopedist's Perspective

John C. Richmond, MD

The main function of all team physicians is basically the same: to assure, as fully as possible, the health and safety of the athletes. The orthopedic surgeon as a team physician is likely to have a perspective on the issue of sudden cardiac death in the athlete that is significantly different from that of other physicians functioning in that capacity. Due to background and training, the orthopedist is likely to be less familiar with the potential cardiac problems of the athlete than the primary care physicians or medical specialists who care for athletes. This lack of familiarity should not translate into reduced care, but should channel the orthopedic surgeon team physician into developing a system of team care and referral patterns that assure the utmost in safety for the athlete.

The orthopedic surgeon as a team physician is often well known to the players, coaches, and trainers, due to presence on the sideline and in the training room. He or she will often have treated a significant percentage of the team for many different musculoskeletal injuries. The orthopedic surgeon may therefore be the physician that the players,

From Estes NAM, Salem DN, Wang PJ (eds). *Sudden Cardiac Death in the Athlete.* Armonk, NY: Futura Publishing Co., Inc.; ©1998.

coaches, and trainers are most comfortable with. It is this comfort level and accessibility that results in team members approaching the orthopedist with any medical problem. It is as important to encourage the athletes and coaching staff to come to the team physician for any health concern, as it is crucial that the orthopedic surgeon rapidly recognize and triage all potentially serious medical problems to the appropriately qualified physician. If he or she maintains high visibility and accessability for all players, coaches, and trainers, the players will come early to the physician if problems are developing. Being a member of the social structure of the team and athletic department will facilitate this. This is best accomplished for the team physician by taking extra time to participate in team social events such as awards banquets. The rapport built with the team at these events increases the chance that an athlete will seek the physician out, as opposed to hiding a potential problem.

At all levels of play, a large percentage (nearly 20% in one recent survey) of head team physicians are orthopedic surgeons.[1] This introduces the issues of setting up and following protocols for screening, prevention, and emergent treatment in disciplines of medicine with which the orthopedist may be unfamiliar. The orthopedic team physician must be a true sports medicine practitioner, must make him- or herself well versed in the skills necessary to administrate this program, and must enlist the assistance of appropriate medical physicians with the appropriate knowledge base. By accepting the position as team physician, the orthopedic surgeon makes the commitment to oversee the entire program and ensure not just the musculoskeletal health and well-being of the athletes but also their medical and cardiovascular health.[2]

There are various age and performance levels that may be encountered by the team physician. These include high school, college, professional, and organized amateur teams. At the high school level, most participants still have their pediatrician as their primary care physician. For any medical problem that is identified in the athlete, through screening or other means, it is most important that the lines of communication from primary practitioner to team physician be kept open. At the college level and beyond, it is unusual for the athlete to have a primary care doctor beyond the school or team unless there is an ongoing medical problem. It is obviously of benefit for the team physician to gain any pertinent information from the athlete's physician. Proper respect of patient confidentially issues require a release to obtain information.

For each level—high school, college, professional, or organized amateur—it is incumbent on the team physician to be sure that there are protocols in place for preparticipation screening, return to play, and emergent treatment. Each level may have its own requirements determined by its governing body, and the team physician should be familiar with and adhere to these. At the high school level, the National Federation of State High School Associations publishes guidelines, which each state's interscholastic athletic association may adopt with or without modification. The preparticipation evaluation guidelines endorsed by the National Federation of State High School Associations are those which have been recommended by multiple medical societies including the American Academy of Family Physicians, the American Academy of Pediatrics, the American Heart Association, the American Medical Society for Sports Medicine, the American Orthopaedic Society for Sports Medicine, and the American Osteopathic Academy of Sports Medicine. These evaluations include a history and physical examination form that can be obtained from any of these organizations. At the collegiate level, the National Collegiate Athletic Association (NCAA) regularly publishes and distributes a *Sports Medicine Handbook,* which covers these topics.[3] This handbook does cover in generalities these preparticipation requirements, but the details of implementation are up to each institution. At the professional level in the United States and Canada, the major professional leagues recommend or require yearly cardiovascular screening to include not only history and physical examination, but electrocardiograms. The individual teams are responsible for implementing this, and they have often worked out detailed evaluation criteria.[4]

Due to the broad application of the NCAA guidelines to all intercollegiate sports, and the fact that they act as a model for many states, it makes sense to review the NCAA guidelines as they apply to cardiovascular issues.[3]

Preparticipation Medical Evaluation

This is required at the student/athlete's entry into a given institution's intercollegiate athletic program. It should include a comprehensive health history and relevant physical examination.[5] The cardiovascular history should include: recent conditioning status, syncope or near syncope with exercise, cardiac symptoms or history of cardiac disease, and family history to include sudden death of a family member under the age of 50 from nontraumatic cause or a family history of Marfan syndrome.

Clearly, the health care professional charged with performing the physical examination should have appropriate skill for that portion of the examination for which he or she is responsible. There are few orthopedic team physicians who maintain the skill to do a thorough and adequate cardiac examination.

Annual Updates

While the NCAA does not believe that further routine physical examinations are necessary, an updated history should be performed annually. It is key that trained medical personnel review the annual history and require appropriate examinations where indicated by the history.

Follow-Up Examinations

The student/athlete with a significant illness during an athletic season should be given a follow-up examination to reestablish fitness for participation. Clearance for an athlete to return to activity *is solely the responsibility of the team physician or that physician's designated representative.*[3]

Withholding a Student/Athlete from Activity

It is the team physician that has the final responsibility to determine if the student-athlete is allowed to participate in light of an illness.

Throughout these guidelines it is clear that the team physician has the ultimate responsibility to decide the athlete's fitness to participate.[6] When the team physician is an orthopedic surgeon and the medical issue is cardiac in nature, it is mandatory that the team physician access the best medical advice available. To simply rely on "clearance" from an unknown practitioner is inappropriate. The orthopedic surgeon team physician must be familiar with the cardiac issues that are involved and must have full faith in the medical practitioner to adequately assess the problem and reach an appropriate conclusion as to that athlete's fitness to participate safely. Publication of readily accessed, up-to-date guidelines for athletic participation in those patients with cardiovascular abnormalities, such as was done at the 26th Bethesda Conference, can be extremely helpful to the team physician.[7]

Another significant issue is that of the athlete with a cardiac abnormality who desires to play in spite of an increased risk of sudden death. This has come into sharp focus over the past few years with the tragic deaths of Hank Gathers and Reggie Lewis. While the orthopedic surgeon as the team physician may have the final say whether an athlete can play with such a potentially catastrophic condition, no orthopedic surgeon is qualified to make that decision. The final determination should be made by an appropriately qualified cardiologist. Potential legal ramifications arise when the athlete wishes to play in spite of medically determined major risk. While this is unlikely to occur at the lower levels of competition such as NCAA Division III, it may cause problems at higher levels. The team physician can help to deter the athlete from playing by bringing together all involved parties. This may simply involve a meeting with the athlete, his or her family, coaches and trainers, the consultant specialist, and the team physician. Often this meeting will focus the athlete and family to the undue risks involved with continued participation, and a consensus for the athlete to stop may be reached. If the athlete and his or her family insist that the athlete continue, the team physician should be ready to seek legal counsel from the team involved, be it school district or university. If the team physician believes that excessive risk is involved with the continued participation of that athlete, the institution must be fully aware of that fact and appropriate legal steps must be taken. This author believes that it is imperative that the institution fully support the team physician in his or her decision to exclude an athlete from play. If the institution fails to support the decisions of the team physician, then "doctor shopping" by athletes looking for easy clearance may ensue, undermining the entire structure of the sports medicine team.

While it is clear cut that the team physician must make the school administration or team aware of those conditions in which he or she feels it is medically unsafe for the athlete to play, in all other conditions patient confidentiality remains paramount. If the athlete's condition does not preclude him or her from participation, then any wishes of the athlete for confidentiality must be honored. While it may be assumed that the athlete would allow the physician to discuss the time frame for return to participation from any minor condition, the physician must be sensitive to the issues of the athlete's confidentiality in virtually all other matters. The physician must seek a release from the athlete prior to discussing these issues with team or school officials. At the professional level, state laws pertaining to the release of information to the employer may come into play as well. In many states, laws mandate that the employer is entitled to a full and timely report for any treatment for a condition for which the athlete is claiming workman's compensation.

While the orthopedic surgeon is well versed in the on-the-field treatment of traumatic injuries, he or she is less likely to be skilled in the management of cardiac arrest or arrhythmias. There should be a system for the emergent treatment of the athlete at all games and practices. In the most basic form, this should be the means of communication with emergency support personnel via phone or radio. Optimally, this would include trainers and/or coaches that are trained in CPR to provide support until emergency personnel arrive. If a defibrillator is to be supplied on the field or in the field house, it is useless without the proper training of the athletic staff.

Based on a knowledge of the musculoskeletal system and the ability to diagnose and treat injuries to the musculoskeletal system, the orthopedic surgeon has unique qualifications to be a team physician. In order to truly function as a team physician, the orthopedist must be prepared to deal with many other issues for the athlete. Among these is the potential of a catastrophic cardiac event. To be the team physician, the orthopedist must have a working knowledge of the potential cardiac problems of the athlete and must establish a working relationship with physicians appropriately skilled in the diagnosis and treatment of the athlete's heart. The orthopedic surgeon/team physician should invest the time and energy necessary to understand the cardiac and other medical conditions that might seriously impact on the athlete. The ability to recognize Marfan syndrome or other life-threatening conditions in the athlete may prevent a sudden catastrophe. Time spent by the orthopedist reading about or at courses involving the medical aspect of sports is invaluable. The team physician ultimately has responsibility for all aspects of the athlete's health and well-being and he or she must assert this responsibility.

References

1. Gallup EM. *Law and the Team Physician.* Champaign, IL: Human Kinetics; 1995:1–87.
2. Herbert DL. *Legal Aspects of Sports Medicine, 2nd Edition.* Canton, OH: PRC Publishing, Inc.; 1995:1–66.
3. Benson M (ed): *1995–1996 NCAA Sports Medicine Handbook.* Overland Park, KS: NCAA; 1995:1–14, 46–47.
4. Scheller A, Rask B. A protocol for the health and fitness assessment of NBA players. *Clin Sports Med* 1993;12:193–205.
5. Lombardo JA. Preparticipation examination. In Cantu RC, Micheli LJ (eds): *ACSM's Guidelines for the Team Physician.* Malvern, PA: Lea and Febiger; 1991:71–94.
6. Puffer JC. Organizational aspects. In Cantu RC, Micheli LJ (eds): *ACSM's Guidelines for the Team Physician.* Malvern, PA: Lea and Febiger; 1991: 95–100.
7. Maron BJ, Mitchell JH, Hutter AM, et al. Revised eligibility recommendations for competitive athletes with cardiovascular abnormalities. *Med Sci Sports Exerc* 1994;26:S223–S283.

33

The Role of Athletic Organizations

Christopher A. McGrew, MD

There are a multitude of athletic organizations in the United States and worldwide that oversee and regulate competitive sports, ranging from "pee wee" leagues involving young children up to the most elite level of professional sport. These organizations vary tremendously in the range of their resources and their governing structure, but they all have interests in sports safety and injury prevention. These interests are represented in a variety of programs, publications, and special committees, as well as in the activities of the individual members. In this country, some of the most wide-ranging groups that oversee nonprofessional sports include the National Collegiate Athletic Association (NCAA), the National Association for Intercollegiate Athletics (NAIA), and the National Federation of State High School Associations (NFSHSA). Included in the guiding principles of these and most other athletic organizations is the concept of the "health and welfare" of the athlete. In fact, some groups owe their origins to this concept; for example, the NCAA was formed in 1906 as a response to threats from then US President Theodore Roosevelt to abolish the game of football because of a rash of fatalities that had become prevalent.[1] This chapter reviews the areas of the prevention of injury/mortality in which athletic organizations have traditionally been involved, and explores the role of athletic organizations in the prevention of sudden cardiac death.

From Estes NAM, Salem DN, Wang PJ (eds). *Sudden Cardiac Death in the Athlete.* Armonk, NY: Futura Publishing Co., Inc.; ©1998.

The key areas that have been addressed by athletic organizations for the purpose of prevention of illness and injury from athletic participation have included: (1) epidemiologic research and record keeping; (2) modifications of rules that regulate participation and competition; (3) emergency planning; (4) development and promulgation of guidelines concerning preparticipation screening and athletic health care; and (5) drug education and testing. In the NCAA, the NAIA, and most professional teams, the traditional conduit for the inflow and outflow of information concerning these areas has been the athletic trainer. The majority of high schools do not have athletic trainers and information primarily flows through the athletic director or principal of the school. The NCAA, the NAIA, and most professional leagues have some sort of "sports medicine/athletic health care" committees that coordinate the review of this information at a central level. The NFSHSA is currently organizing such a group. Also, ongoing dialogue among some athletic organizations and sports medicine groups takes place through annual meetings of the Joint Commission of Sports Medicine and Science [7611 Elmwood Ave, Suite 203, Middleton, WI 53562; (608) 836–4792]. Although primarily a sports medicine group, the Joint Commission actively works with athletic organizations.

Epidemiologic information concerning sudden cardiac death comes from a variety of sources. Athletic organizations have played a role in the collection of much of these data and some individual organizations such as the NCAA have their own injury surveillance systems. In the area of sudden cardiac death, one valuable resource is the National Center for Catastrophic Sports Injury Research (NCCSIR),[2] which collects data on sudden cardiac death. The NCCSIR has been supported by combined efforts of the NCAA, the American Football Coaches Association, and the NFSHSA. Support comes from these groups in the form of financial grants, administrative support, information concerning specific sudden cardiac deaths, and participation numbers from which exposure rates can be developed.[2] Data from such epidemiologic resources should be used to monitor trends in injury/mortality. This information should also be used as a balance against the dramatic effect of intense news media coverage of isolated events that makes sudden cardiac death in athletes seem more prevalent than it actually is. Athletic organizations should continue to play a supportive role in cooperative efforts to track catastrophic injuries including sudden cardiac death. At the very least, athletic organizations should encourage their members to cooperate fully in the timely and accurate reporting of such events to a central organization such as the NCCSIR.

Another primary role of athletic organizations is the modification of rules that exist to make the specific sport being monitored potentially safer for the participant. In general, the role of rules has been seen to: (1) permit congruent transitions within contests; (2) maintain consistency in the mechanics of games and contests; and (3) promote the safety of participants.[3] In particular, rules that affect safety can involve changes in equipment, playing techniques, conduct of the game, and on-the-field behavior and practice parameters. Within a given athletic organization, input for rules changes may come from coaches, athletic trainers and their families, injury surveillance groups, medical personnel, and administrators.

Examples of how rules changes have affected mortality include the following: (1) direct fatalities caused by catastrophic head and neck injuries have been reduced by changes in the equipment (ie, the helmet) and coaching techniques (changing the method for tackling or blocking, known as spearing)[2] as well as in specific on-the-field conduct (penalties against spearing); (2) indirect fatalities caused by heat illness[3] have been reduced by changes mandated in preseason and out-of-season practices. These changes include allowing adequate time for acclimatization and access to fluids. In the area of sudden death, however, it is not clear whether rules changes would specifically have any impact. Certainly, allowing for an appropriate amount of preseason conditioning might seem intuitively helpful but because a large majority of sudden cardiac deaths are caused by structural heart disease, it is unlikely that a few days of preseason conditioning will have much of an effect.

One topic that should be specially mentioned is commotio cordis, as discussed in chapter 29. Some sports organizations, especially at the level of the younger athlete (such as Little League and youth hockey), look at information concerning the development of equipment for protection of the chest.[4] There is no clear indication from research available to date that gives a definitive direction in this area. If and when a definitive answer is available concerning such equipment change, then sports organizations could mandate their use.

Another role that sports organizations can play is that of encouraging institutions to have formal emergency plans in the case of the sudden collapse of an athlete. Sports organizations play an important role in developing and promulgating guidelines for their membership that concern appropriate standards for an emergency response plan tailored to community resources. This can be on a very basic level and does not necessarily require having a physician or other health care personnel on site (for many institutions, especially at the high school level, this is likely to be the case). The most important part of an emergency plan involves a responsible person (eg, coach, athletic director, EMT, physician, athletic trainer, official) who attends the contest or practice and has the ability to perform initial life support maneuvers such as basic first aid, cardiopulmonary resuscitation, and accessing the local emergency medical services system (automatic external defibrillators are currently under discussion for use in athletic settings, but no definitive answer is available at this time). Athletic organizations should make strong recommendations and/or requirements that all coaches and officials be proficient in these basic skills. On a local level, sports organizations such as coaches associations, state athletic associations, and community sports leagues could offer group training at reduced cost for coaches and officials. Additionally, an appropriate route of evacuation along with ready access to working communications devices is also essential.[5]

Athletic organizations also play an important role in the promulgation of standards concerning preparticipation screening as well as guidelines for participation by athletes with known cardiovascular abnormalities. One example of the way in which these organizations can cooperate is the recent summit, held in Dallas, Texas in 1996, concerning sudden death in the athlete. The key purpose of this summit was to decide how to efficiently disseminate recently revised information concerning cardiovascular preparticipation screening of competitive athletes.[6] The organizations at this summit included traditional athletic organizations along with sports medicine groups and representatives from the American Heart Association. Other examples of promulgation of such standards include publications and other educational materials put out by the organizations themselves, such as the *NCAA Sports Medicine Handbook*.[5] Monitoring the adoption of such guidelines can be done through surveys by the organizations of their members. It is important for the athletic organizations to be invited to play a role in the developments of such guidelines. For example, the NCAA was invited to have a representative at the 26th Bethesda Conference on Recommendations for Determining Eligibility for Competition of Athletes with Cardiovascular Abnormalities[7] as well as the American Heart Association Writing Group, which developed the guidelines concerning cardiovascular preparticipation screening of competitive athletes.[6] Such a close working relationship is more conducive to producing guidelines which will be practical and more readily accepted by the membership of such groups. In turn, athletic organizations could consider sponsoring workshops at medical meetings where health care providers could receive training in performing appropriate history and physical examinations.

The more difficult role for athletic organizations is in the area of setting standards for participation by the athlete who has known cardiac conditions. The recent Bethesda Conference provides useful guidelines and there are references in the publications of some athletic organizations (eg, *NCAA Sports Medicine Handbook*.) Athletic organizations have not seen it as their role to mandate a standard procedure

seen to: (1) permit congruent transitions \
consistency in the mechanics of games and
the safety of participants.[3] In particular, rules
volve changes in equipment, playing technique,
and on-the-field behavior and practice parameter,
letic organization, input for rules changes may com
letic trainers and their families, injury surveillance
personnel, and administrators.

Examples of how rules changes have affected mortal
following: (1) direct fatalities caused by catastrophic head
juries have been reduced by changes in the equipment (ie, t.
and coaching techniques (changing the method for tackling
ing, known as spearing)[2] as well as in specific on-the-field c
(penalties against spearing); (2) indirect fatalities caused by he
ness[3] have been reduced by changes mandated in preseason and o
of-season practices. These changes include allowing adequate time fo
acclimatization and access to fluids. In the area of sudden death, however, it is not clear whether rules changes would specifically have any
impact. Certainly, allowing for an appropriate amount of preseason
conditioning might seem intuitively helpful but because a large majority of sudden cardiac deaths are caused by structural heart disease, it
is unlikely that a few days of preseason conditioning will have much of
an effect.

One topic that should be specially mentioned is commotio cordis,
as discussed in chapter 29. Some sports organizations, especially at the
level of the younger athlete (such as Little League and youth hockey),
look at information concerning the development of equipment for protection of the chest.[4] There is no clear indication from research available to date that gives a definitive direction in this area. If and when a
definitive answer is available concerning such equipment change, then
sports organizations could mandate their use.

Another role that sports organizations can play is that of encouraging institutions to have formal emergency plans in the case of the
sudden collapse of an athlete. Sports organizations play an important
role in developing and promulgating guidelines for their membership
that concern appropriate standards for an emergency response plan
tailored to community resources. This can be on a very basic level and
does not necessarily require having a physician or other health care
personnel on site (for many institutions, especially at the high school
level, this is likely to be the case). The most important part of an emergency plan involves a responsible person (eg, coach, athletic director,
EMT, physician, athletic trainer, official) who attends the contest or
practice and has the ability to perform initial life support maneuvers
such as basic first aid, cardiopulmonary resuscitation, and accessing

for implementing such guidelines and have preferred that such issues be resolved on a local basis. However, there are well-publicized cases in which local decision making seems to have gone astray. Some have suggested a national oversight group to which such situations could be referred to for nonbiased binding arbitration and decision making.[8] Ideally, such an "umbrella" group could also serve as a steering organization which could coordinate issues of safety and health among athletic organizations. Practical concerns such as how such a group would operate as well as be supported financially and administratively have not yet been answered.

One role for athletic organizations, which might not be commonly thought of as concerning the prevention of sudden cardiac death, is that of drug education and testing. There are several high-profile cases of drug-related sudden death in athletes. Dissemination of information concerning the adverse effects on the cardiovascular system form the use of illicit and/or so-called ergogenic drugs (eg, cocaine, amphetamines, and anabolic steroids) is well within the realm of athletic organizations. Although the number of sudden cardiac deaths is very small from drug use (as best as can be determined from the literature), it is still an important area that should be addressed. Because of legal and economic restraints, drug testing will probably remain limited in scope, to the upper levels of sports competition such as collegiate, Olympic, and professional levels.

Finally, although not a strategy for preventing sudden cardiac death in sports, athletic organizations can play a role in educating the public about the reality of the very low risk of sudden cardiac death during competitive sports. There is no indication that this risk is higher in organized athletic competition that these groups regulate as compared to general athletic activity in the nonorganized or recreational setting. On the other hand, most sudden deaths in young athletes occur during sports-related activity compared to non-sports–related activity. From the standpoint of public health and quality of life, it is desirable that children, teenagers, and adults of all ages be encouraged to exercise and participate in sports, and not be discouraged by dramatic media coverage of relatively rare events. Additionally, coaches, athletes, families, and the general public all need to be educated that the preparticipation screening exam is limited in its ability to predict those who might be at risk for sudden death and offers no guarantees. Athletic organizations should further realize that "high-tech and expensive" (such as echocardiograms for routine screening) is not necessarily better, and they should promote adherence to a sensible and cost-effective protocol as outlined in the most recent consensus guidelines. These recommendations should be within the means of all members, not just an elite few. Additionally, athletic organizations must be responsible in pointing out that just because a few of their members may decide to do things outside of recognized guidelines (eg, routine screening electrocardiograms or echocardiograms), such behavior does not represent a standard that other members should be held to.

In summary, athletic organizations have a role in the ongoing effort to prevent sudden cardiac death in athletes. Despite wide variations in the resources and administrative structure of these groups and their respective members, there are several areas that can be addressed by all. At a most basic level these include active participation in sudden death case surveillance, dissemination of the most recent information concerning preparticipation screening and participation guidelines, promotion of adequate emergency preparedness, and drug education.

References

1. Metzler B. *A Century of Rules Changes in Sidelines.* Boulder, CO: College Football Association; 1996;9:8–11.
2. Mueller F, Cantu R, VanCamp S. Catastrophic injuries in high school and college sports. *HK Sports Monograph Series* 1996;8:1–39.
3. Nelson DM. The role of sports rules and safety. In Mueller F, Ryan AJ (eds): *Prevention of Athletic Injuries. The Role of Sports Medicine Team.* Philadelphia: F.A. Davis Co; 1991:64–70.
4. Maron B, Poliac L, Kaplan J, et al. Blunt impact to chest leading to sudden death from cardiac arrest during sports activities. *N Engl J Med* 1995;333:337–342.
5. Benson M. *1996–1997 NCAA Sports Medicine Handbook.* Overland Park, KS: The National Collegiate Athletic Association.
6. Maron BJ, Thompson PD, Puffer JC, et al. Cardiovascular pre-participation screening of competitive athletes: A statement for health professionals. *Circulation* 1996;94:850–856.
7. Recommendations for determining eligibility for competition in athletics with cardiovascular abnormalities. 26th Bethesda Conference. *Med Sci Sports Exerc* 1994;26(10 suppl):S223–S283.
8. Maron B, Brown R, McGrew C, et al. Ethical legal and practical considerations affecting medical decision making in competitive athletics. *J Am Coll Cardiol* 1994;24:854–860.

34

Research Imperatives and Future Directions

Sanjeev Saksena, MD, FACC and Irakli Giorgberidze, MD

Introduction

The syndrome of sudden cardiac death in the athlete has undergone profound changes in its perception and understanding in the medical community. It is now a subject of public discussion and concern. However, the development of a concerted plan to investigate and evaluate this medical dilemma has been difficult and in need of clearer definition. It is relatively clear that this uncommon syndrome is a multifaceted disorder and, as such, requires study at multiple levels. Basic research at molecular, genetic, cellular, and electrophysiologic levels, and in in vivo animal models is sorely needed. Clinical investigation needs range from the whole gamut of epidemiologic data to laboratory studies of anatomic and electrophysiologic markers. Finally, further attention is needed for the selection of interventional therapy as well as for the public health issues that arise for patients, high-risk individuals, and sports organizations. It is the purpose of this chapter to highlight major areas suitable for investigation and to suggest directions for research initiatives in the near future.

From Estes NAM, Salem DN, Wang PJ (eds). *Sudden Cardiac Death in the Athlete.* Armonk, NY: Futura Publishing Co., Inc.; ©1998.

Potential Role for Basic Research

The ability to delve into the basic structural and physiologic mechanisms of sudden death in the athlete is confounded by the multiple disease states that are associated with this clinical syndrome. Table 1 is a partial list of cardiac and other disorders that manifest in this presentation. Many of these disorders are myocardial disease states characterized by tissue hypertrophy, infiltration, and hemodynamic embarrassment. Myerburg et al[1] have highlighted the complex interaction between structural and functional abnormalities in the genesis of sudden cardiac death. While patients with coronary disease have some similarities in structural abnormalities to patients with primary myocardial disease (including presence of fibrosis, hypertrophy, and ventricular dilatation), the electrophysiologic mechanisms for initiation of ventricular tachyarrhythmias may be similar or quite different based on the

Table 1
Potential Etiologies of Sudden Death
in Adolescent and Adult Athletes

Primary myocardial disease
 Hypertrophic cardiomyopathy: obstructive and nonobstructive
 Idiopathic dilated cardiomyopathy
 Arrhythmogenic right ventricular dysplasia
 Myocarditis
 Infiltrative cardiomyopathy eg, sarcoidosis

Specific arrhythmic disorders
 Long QT syndrome
 Right ventricular outflow tract ventricular tachycardia
 Idiopathic left ventricular tachycardia
 Brugada syndrome
 Atrioventricular conduction system disease

Primary electrical disease
 Idiopathic ventricular fibrillation

Hemodynamic/vascular disorders
 Atherosclerotic coronary artery disease
 Valvular heart disease eg, aortic stenosis
 Anomalous origin of a coronary artery
 Marfan syndrome with arteriopathy
 Kawasaki's disease
 Thromboembolic events eg, cerebral, pulmonary

Toxic conditions
 Drug abuse eg, cocaine

Miscellaneous disorders
 Sickle cell disease
 Mitral valve prolapse

myocardial disease. For example, recurrent sustained ventricular tachycardia as characterized in healed myocardial infarction may also be elicited in arrhythmogenic right ventricular dysplasia. In both instances, the site of ventricular disease (infarct scar or dysplastic fibrolipomatous changes) provides the substrate for intramyocardial reentry. Similarly, in certain phases of acute ischemia, release of lipid metabolites can result in sudden changes in electrophysiologic properties of the myocardial membrane.[2] This results in reduction in membrane potential and conditions suitable for reentrant excitation. While this cascade of events is characteristic of acute coronary artery obstruction, ischemic mechanisms potentially exist in hypertrophied hearts due to vascular mismatch and hemodynamic derangements that can elicit ischemia. Zee Cheng et al[3] described initiation of supraventricular tachycardia in a patient with hypertrophic cardiomyopathy resulting in presumably hypotension and ischemia, triggering ventricular tachycardia and fibrillation. Figure 1 shows an example of sinoatrial reentrant tachycardia in a symptomatic patient with familial long QT syndrome, syncope, and palpitations. The probability of initiating a triggered or reentrant ventricular tachyarrhythmia by the rapid ventricular rate or long-short sequences at tachycardia onset or termination is uncertain as a mechanism for serious symptomatic arrhythmias.

Dissimilar mechanisms for arrhythmogenesis can, however, exist in cardiomyopathy. Abnormalities in cellular calcium currents with alteration in diastolic relaxation have been described in hypertrophic cardiomyopathy. These ionic currents can possibly also mediate the development of afterdepolarizations and triggered electrical activity.[4,5] In patients with dilated cardiomyopathy, macroreentrant circuits involving the bundle branches as well as intramyocardial reentry have been described, but the relative contribution of each mechanism is unclear.[6] Animal models for some of these disease states exist but are rather sparsely used. They clearly must be standardized and analyzed for concordance with the clinical disorder.

Primary arrhythmia syndromes can be involved in this syndrome. In a study of Italian athletes, Furlanello[7] reported the initial presentation of symptomatic Wolff-Parkinson-White syndrome as sudden cardiac death. In patients with the long QT syndrome, genetically mediated abnormalities in specific ionic currents can result in triggered arrhythmias that may become sustained by use of automatic or reentrant excitation.[8,9] Even more recently, a specific syndrome of "primary ventricular fibrillation" in young adults, associated with electrocardiographic abnormalities (right bundle branch block and ST segment elevation in right precordial leads—the Brugada syndrome) has been described in sporadic and familial form.[10] Abnormalities in repolarization currents have been postulated but remain to be conclusively established. Figure 2 is an

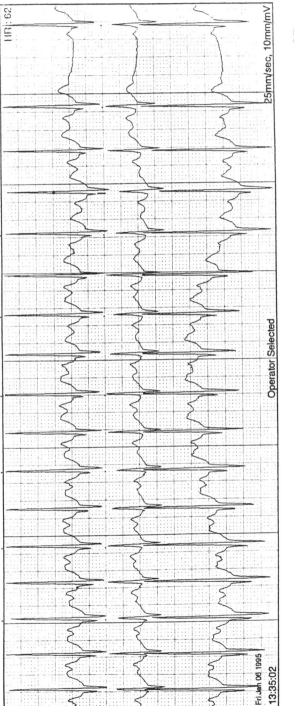
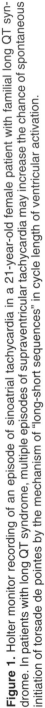

Figure 1. Holter monitor recording of an episode of sinoatrial tachycardia in a 21-year-old female patient with familial long QT syndrome. In patients with long QT syndrome, multiple episodes of supraventricular tachycardia may increase the chance of spontaneous initiation of torsade de pointes by the mechanism of "long-short sequences" in cycle length of ventricular activation.

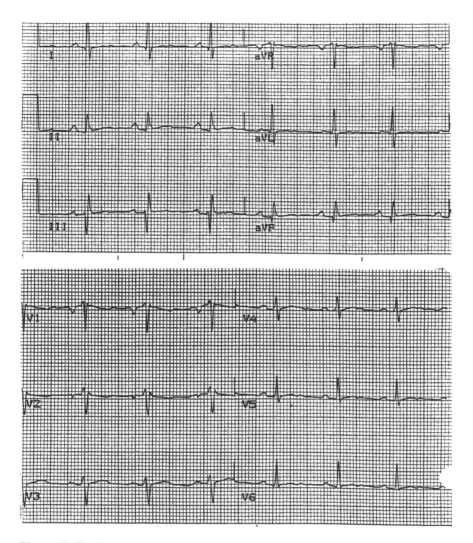

Figure 2. Twelve-lead electrocardiogram of a 23-year-old male athlete with exercise-related aborted sudden cardiac death. Electrocardiogram showed incomplete right bundle branch block, isoelectric or biphasic T waves in precordial leads, and slight ST segment elevation and small Q waves in inferior leads. Echocardiography and cardiac catheterization showed normal appearance of cardiac chambers, valvular apparatus, and coronary arteries, as well as normal left and right ventricular function. Myocardial biopsy samples were consistent with chronic focal myocarditis. Patient subsequently underwent electrophysiologic study and had easily inducible ventricular tachycardia in drug-free state. Patient refused antiarrhythmic drug trial and received an implantable cardioverter defibrillator.

electrocardiogram in a young male who experienced a cardiac arrest during sports activity. He was noted to have ventricular fibrillation and was resuscitated. The electrocardiogram shows incomplete right bundle branch block and minimal ST elevation. Myocardial biopsy showed focal myocarditis without coronary disease. It is relatively clear that each individual disease state requires specific studies directed at its particular mechanism for sudden cardiac death.

More recently, basic research at another level has extended our understanding of the basis of many of these disorders. Genetic and molecular studies have identified the β-myosin heavy chain gene on chromosome 14q11-q12 in some hypertrophic cardiomyopathy families. Specific amino acid mutations (leucine-valine and arginine-glutamine) were noted with varying degrees of disease expression, with the latter being invariably associated with left ventricular hypertrophy.[11] Subsequently, additional mutations have been identified, often being observed in patients of specific ethnic origin.[12,13] Finally, new morbid gene loci are also being reported, pointing out the genetic heterogeneity of this condition.[14] Mutations in genes for α-tropomyosin and troponin T have been documented in hypertrophic cardiomyopathy.[15] Yet, the complexity of the findings is obvious, and it is more than likely that individual disease states will manifest similar heterogeneity in genetic studies. Explanations for sporadic and familial disorders may be forthcoming from such investigations.

Basic research imperatives in these conditions should focus on each individual disease state, ranging from applicable animal models to tissue and molecular biological studies of affected individuals. These latter studies may indeed present us with a large and heterogenous group of biochemical disorders. Cell culture models can define pathways for cellular hypertrophy and signals for this process.[16] Electrophysiologic studies in excised tissues, as well as genetic and molecular studies of these tissues, must be prosecuted. Efforts to develop relevant animal models should be fostered.[17] Genetically engineered animal models may be necessary in order to study the diversity of disorders involved. In vivo animal studies would be particularly valuable in defining the role of the autonomic nervous system and cardiac electrophysiology in these conditions.

Clinical Research Needs in Athletes

Epidemiologic Data

In the clinical arena patient investigations remain sparse. It would be accurate to state that this field remains, despite its recent visibility, a fertile area for future study. While pathologic data have been the main source for the anatomic basis of the constellation of conditions leading to sudden death in this patient population, premorbid clinical studies are still rare.[18–20] Epidemiologic assessment of the disorder in this population is warranted. While the prevalence of this syndrome has been variously estimated at 1 in 100,00 to 1 in 300,000 in high school athletes to 1 in 15,000 to 1 in 50,000 in older athletes, individual disorders such as hypertrophic cardiomyopathy are often quite prevalent in the general population.[21] Particular ethnic predispositions must be identified. Pathologic studies suggest a predominance of hypertrophic cardiomyopathy in black athletes who experience sudden death.[19] In one study of patients with hypertrophic cardiomyopathy at two referral centers, patterns of left ventricular hypertrophy also differed in young and older patients.[18] Epidemiologic studies can help define disease patterns in the different subgroups; for example adolescents, young adults, or even particular athletes.

Clinical Laboratory Models

A particular need is for clinically relevant laboratory models for study of symptomatic patients and asymptomatic high-risk individuals. While the electrophysiology laboratory has served as an indispensable tool for initiation and study of ventricular tachyarrhythmias associated with coronary artery disease, arrhythmogenic right ventricular dysplasia, and right ventricular outflow tract or left ventricular septal tachycardia,[22–24] similar reproducible results are less likely in dilated or hypertrophic cardiomyopathy.[25,26] Significant debate exists regarding the value of noninducible tachycardia in dilated cardiomyopathy, and inducible tachycardia in hypertrophic cardiomyopathy. In the Brugada syndrome, ventricular tachycardia or fibrillation can be provided by programmed stimulation. Interestingly, the patient illustrated in Figure 2 had easily provokable ventricular fibrillation which was suppressed by phenytoin at electrophysiologic study. Newer protocols for study in the electrophysiology laboratory that can be applied to this population may include different pacing protocols, autonomic stress, and volume loading conditions.[27] Long-short pacing sequences often elicit bundle branch reentrant tachycardia in dilated cardiomyopathy. Saumarez et al[27] reported increased fragmentation and latency in right ventricular electrograms during pacing. Newer stimulation protocols for eliciting atrial arrhythmias such as atrial fibrillation have been investigated in the laboratory at the Eastern Heart Institute. Sensitivity and specificity of such protocols is now comparable to ventricular stimulation protocols.[28] Mapping and regional electrophysiologic study of sites of atrial disease is thus becoming feasible.[29,30] Autonomic system activity has been evaluated in hypertrophic cardiomyopathy by use of heart rate variability.[31] Atrial distension has enhanced atrial vulnerability and atrial fibrillation induction.[32]

Management Dilemmas

The limited understanding of the pathogenetic mechanisms for sudden death in this population reflects directly on the therapeutic alternatives offered to symptomatic patients. Only a few well-targeted clinical therapies are widely accepted, such as permanent pacemaker insertion in conduction disorders, or catheter ablation of supraventricular tachycardias, right ventricular outflow tract tachycardia, and left ventricular septal tachycardias. Occasionally drug therapy and its rationale have been defined, although outcome data are uncommon. β-Blockers and sodium channel blockers are available for different variants of the long QT syndrome.[8] For the vast majority of patients, such as the patient illustrated in Figure 1, the clinician faces the dilemma of offering generic therapy such as an implantable defibrillator for a suspected ventricular tachyarrhythmia, or drug therapy with an unknown outcome.[33] In patients with hypertrophic cardiomyopathy for example, amiodarone therapy has been reported to have variable outcome.[34,35] The use of implantable defibrillators and their long-term performance is unclear in this condition. In contrast, data on patients with long QT syndrome, dilated cardiomyopathy, and pediatric sudden death victims are now forthcoming (Figure 3).[36,37] It is important to note the marked differences in outcome based on the underlying myocardial disease.

The need for targeted therapy in the form of drugs, pacing, ablation, or defibrillation is obvious. However, an equally important area for expert consensus is the defininition of the principles that should underlie the investigation and selection of treatment in these patients. It is important to highlight and discuss unusual disorders currently being studied, such as the Brugada syndrome, and the use of newer, less utilized diagnostic aids, such as magnetic resonance imaging or myocardial biopsies, in order to define myocardial diseases. The proper work-up of these patients, and the cost-effectiveness of each approach will need vigorous analysis.

Psychologic and Socioeconomic Issues

Critical to the discussion of future directions is the psychologic and socioeconomic impact of this condition and its therapy on the individual. The younger the victim, the greater the need for long-term psychological support. Rehabilitation of the victim into the workforce and familial involvement in the long-term course of the condition is necessary. Quality-of-life assessments, in the opinion of these authors, are important in

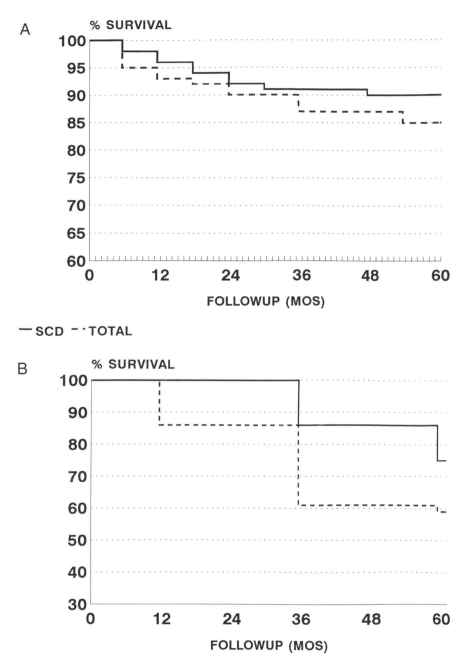

Figure 3. Total and sudden death survival in pediatric patients with various cardiac diseases (**A**) and adult patients with dilated cardiomyopathy (**B**) receiving treatment with implantable cardioverter defibrillator. From References 34 and 35.

the selection of different therapeutic options. In stark contrast to patients with epilepsy, these patients may face greater limitations in work and physical activity. The correct balance between the normalization of the patient's lifestyle and workforce safety must be struck with a better data base on patient outcomes. For example, combined drug and defibrillator therapy may both provide the mortality benefits of device therapy and reduce recurrences to limit symptoms during follow-up.[38]

Identification of the Asymptomatic and High-Risk Individual and Public Education

The recently published medical scientific statement from the American Heart Association paid early attention to this issue.[39] Due to recognition of the infrequent nature of this condition in the general population, the use of general screening investigations has been examined. Electrocardiography may be the most cost-effective method at present. However, in individuals manifesting symptoms such as chest pain, palpitations, or presyncope, further investigations for structural and electrical disorders are necessary. Echocardiography, ambulatory monitoring, and exercise testing are important in this regard. Heart rate variability may have a role in specific subgroups such as hypertrophic cardiomyopathy.[26] Invasive studies must be considered on an individual patient basis. Certainly, in familial high-risk individuals more detailed evaluation is needed prior to athletic competition.

An important aspect, which is often neglected, is the need for a clear set of informational messages for public education. The warning symptoms and signs in an athlete must be widely appreciated. The ability to diagnose and manage a large proportion of those at risk and to improve outcome by careful medical management should be communicated by all involved in this field. National medical and philanthropic groups should join forces in such an effort. There is a pressing need to bring together the many national athletic, medical, and scientific groups involved. This will allow us to approach the research challenges in a concerted and coordinated manner. Such an initiative will bear important fruits for the younger population and lead to safer practices in the athletic arena.

References

1. Myerburg RJ, Kessler KM, Bassett AL, et al. A biological approach to sudden cardiac death. *Am J Cardiol* 1989;63:1512–1516.
2. Creer MH, Dobmeyer DJ, Corr PB. Amphipathic lipid metabolites and arrhythmias during myocardial ischemia. In Zipes DP, Jalife J (eds): *Cardiac Electrophysiology From Cell to Bedside.* Philadelphia, PA: WB Saunders Co.; 1990:417–433.

3. Zee Cheng C-S, Quattromani A, Barbey JT, et al. Aborted sudden death in a young adult with hypertrophic cardiomyopathy and atrioventricular nodal tachycardia. *J Electrophysiol* 1988;2:251–254.

4. Gwathmey JK, Warren SE, Briggs GM, et al. Diastolic dysfunction in hypertrophic cardiomyopathy: Effect on active force generation during systole. *J Clin Invest* 1991;87:1023–1031.

5. Marban E, Robinson SW, Wier WG. Mechanisms of arrhythmogenic layed and early afterdepolarizations in ferret ventricular muscle. *J Clin Invest* 1986;78:1185–1192.

6. Tchou P, Jazayeri M, Denker S, et al. Transcatheter electrical ablation of right bundle branch: A method of treating macro-reentrant ventricular tachycardia due to bundle branch reentry. *Circulation* 1988;78:246–257.

7. Furlanello F, Bettini R, Bertoldi A, et al. Competitive sports and cardiac arrhythmias. In Luderitz B, Saksena S (eds): *Interventional Electrophysiology*. Mount Kisco, NY: Futura Publishing Co., Inc.; 1991:41–47.

8. Schwartz PJ, Priori SG, Locati EH, et al. Long QT syndrome patients with mutations of the SCN5A and HERG genes have differential responses to Na^+ channel blockade and to increases in heart rate. Implications of gene-specific therapy. *Circulation* 1995;92:3381–3386.

9. Roden DM, Lazzara R, Rosen M, et al. Multiple mechanisms in the long QT syndrome. *Circulation* 1996;94:1996–2012.

10. Brugada P, Brugada J. Right bundle branch block, persistent ST segment elevation and sudden cardiac death: A distinct clinical and electrocardiographic syndrome. A multicenter report. *J Am Coll Cardiol* 1992;20:1391–1396.

11. Epstein ND, Cohn GM, Cyran F, et al. Differences in clinical expression of hypertrophic cardiomyopathy associated with two distinct mutations in the beta-myosin heavy chain gene. A 908[Leu—Val] mutation and 403[Arg—Gln] mutation. *Circulation* 1992;86:345–352.

12. Fananapazir LM, Epstein ND. Genotype-phenotype correlations in hypertrophic cardiomyopathy of kindreds with distinct and identical beta-myosin heavy chain gene mutations. *Circulation* 1994;89:22–32.

13. Ko YL, Chen JJ, Tang TK, et al. Malignant familial hypertrophic cardiomyopathy in a family with a 453 Arg—Cys mutation in the beta myosin heavy chain gene: Coexistence of sudden death and end-stage heart failure. *Hum Genet* 1996;97:585–590.

14. Hengstenberg C, Carrier L, Schwartz K, et al. Clinical and genetical heterogeneity of familial cardiomyopathy. *Herz* 1994;19:84–90.

15. Watkins H, McKenna WJ, Thierfelder L, et al. Mutations in the genes for cardiac troponin T and alpha tropomyosin in hypertrophic cardiomyopathy. *N Engl J Med* 995;332:1058–1064.

16. Morkin E, Bahl JJ, Flink IL, et al. Molecular analysis of human and rate alpha-myosin heavy chain genes. In Chien S (ed): *Molecular Biology of the Cardiovascular System*. Philadelphia, PA: Lea & Febiger; 1990:45–51.

17. Berul CI, Aronovitz MJ, Wang PJ, et al. In vivo cardiac electrophysiologic studies in the mouse. *Circulation* 1996;94:2641–2648.

18. Corrado D, Thiene G, Nava A, et al. Sudden death in young competitive atheletes: Clinicopathologic correlations in 22 cases. *Am J Med* 1990;89:588–596.

19. Klues HG, Schiffers A, Maron BJ. Phenotypic spectrum and patterns of left ventricular hypertrophy in hypertrophic cardiomyopathy: Morphologic observations and significance as assessed by two dimensional echocardiography in 600 patients. *J Am Coll Cardiol* 1995;26:1699–1708.

20. Maron BJ, Shirani J, Poliac LC, et al. Sudden death in young competitive athletes. Clinical, demographic and pathological profiles. *JAMA* 1996;276: 199–204.

21. Maron BJ, Gardin JM, Flack JM, et al. Prevalence of hypertrophic cardiomyopathy in a general population of young adults: Echocardiographic analysis of 4111 subjects in the CARDIA Study-Coronary Artery Risk Development in (Young) Adults. *Circulation* 1995;92:785–789.

22. Waldo AL, Akhtar M, Brugada P, et al. The minimally appropriate electrophysiologic study for the initial assessment of patients with documented sustained monomorphic ventricular tachycardia. *J Am Coll Cardiol* 1985;6:1174–1177.

23. Nakagawa H, Beckman KJ, McClelland JH, et al. Radiofrequency catheter ablation of idiopathic left ventricular tachycardia guided by a Purkinje potential. *Circulation* 1993;88:2607. 24. Klein LS, Shih HT, Hackett FK, et al. Radiofrequency catheter ablation of ventricular tachycardia in patients without structural heart disease. *Circulation* 1992;85:1666.

25. Poll DS, Marchlinski FE, Buxton AE, et al. Usefulness of programmed stimulation in idiopathic dilated cardiomyopathy. *Am J Cardiol* 1986;58: 992.

26. Naccarelli GV, Prystowsky EN, Jackman WM, et al. Role of electrophysiologic testing in managing patients who have ventricular tachycardia unrelated to coronary artery disease. *Am J Cardiol* 1982;50:165.

27. Saumarez RC, Camm AJ, Panagos A, et al. Ventricular fibrillation in hypertrophic cardiomyopathy is associated with increased fractionation of paced right ventricular electrograms. *Circulation* 1992;86:467–474.

28. Krol RB, Saksena S, Giorgberidze I, et al. Prospective evaluation of a minimally appropriate programmed electrical stimulation protocol for induction of atrial fibrillation. (Abstract) *Circulation* 1995;92(I):I-404.

29. Saksena S, Giorgberidze I, Prakash A, et al. Endocardial mapping during induced atrial fibrillation. *Circulation* 1996;94(I):I-555.

30. Prakash A, Hill M, Giorgberidze I, et al. Propagation of atrial premature beats during atrial pacing: Insights from regional atrial mapping. *PACE* 1996;19(II):642.

31. Counihan PJ, Fei L, Bashir Y, et al. Assessment of heart rate variability in hypertrophic cardiomyopathy. Association with clinical and prognostic features. *Circulation* 1993;88:1682–1690.

32. Vester EG, Klein MR, Schultheiss HP, et al. Effect of an immunosuppressive therapy on cellular structure, hemodynamics and ventricular vulnerability in patients with malignant arrhythmia and chronic myocarditis. *Circulation* 1996;94:I-626. Abstract.

33. Jackman WM, Friday KJ, Anderson JL, et al. The long QT syndromes: a critical review, new clinical observations and unifying hypothesis. *Prog Cardiovasc Dis* 1988;31:115.

34. Fananapazir L, Leon MB, Bonow RO, et al. Sudden death during empiric amiodarone therapy in symptomatic hypertrophic cardiomyopathy. *Am J Cardiol* 1991;67:169–174.

35. McKenna WJ, Oakley CM, Krikler DM, et al. Improved survival with amiodarone in patients with hypertrophic cardiomyopathy and ventricular tachycardia. *Br Heart J* 1985;53:412.

36. Fazio G, Veltri EP, Tomaselli G, et al. Long-term follow-up of patients with nonischemic dilated cardiomyopathy and ventricular tachyarrhythmias treated with implantable cardioverter defibrillators. *PACE* 1991;14: 1905–1910.

37. Silka MJ, Kron J, Dunnigan A, et al. Sudden cardiac death and the use of implantable cardioverter-defibrillators in pediatric patients. *Circulation* 1993;87:800–807.
38. Bocker D, Haverkamp W, Bock M, et al. Comparison of d,l-sotalol and implantable defibrillators for treatment of sustained ventricular tachycardia for fibrillation in patients with coronary artery disease. *Circulation* 1996; 94:151–157.
39. Maron BJ, Thompson PD, Puffer JC, et al. Cardiovascular preparticipation screening of competitive athletes. A statement for health professionals from the Sudden Death Committee (Clinical Cardiology) and Congenital Defects Committee (Cardiovascular Disease in the Young), American Heart Association. *Circulation* 1996;94:850–856.

Index